Brain Imaging in Behavioral Medicine and Clinical Neuroscience

Ronald A. Cohen • Lawrence H. Sweet
Editors

Brain Imaging in Behavioral Medicine and Clinical Neuroscience

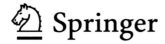

Editors
Ronald A. Cohen
Department of Psychiatry and Human Behavior and the Institute for Brain Science
Warren Alpert Medical School of Brown University
Providence, RI 02912, USA
RCohen@lifespan.org

Lawrence H. Sweet
Department of Psychiatry and Human Behavior
Warren Alpert Medical School of Brown University
Providence, RI 02912, USA
lawrence_sweet@brown.edu

ISBN 978-1-4419-6371-0   e-ISBN 978-1-4419-6373-4
DOI 10.1007/978-1-4419-6373-4
Springer New York Dordrecht Heidelberg London

Library of Congress Control Number: 2010937678

© Springer Science+Business Media, LLC 2011
All rights reserved. This work may not be translated or copied in whole or in part without the written
permission of the publisher (Humana Press, c/o Springer Science+Business Media, LLC, 233 Spring Street,
New York, NY 10013, USA), except for brief excerpts in connection with reviews or scholarly analysis. Use
in connection with any form of information storage and retrieval, electronic adaptation, computer software,
or by similar or dissimilar methodology now known or hereafter developed is forbidden.
The use in this publication of trade names, trademarks, service marks, and similar terms, even if they are
not identified as such, is not to be taken as an expression of opinion as to whether or not they are subject
to proprietary rights.
While the advice and information in this book are believed to be true and accurate at the date of going
to press, neither the authors nor the editors nor the publisher can accept any legal responsibility for any
errors or omissions that may be made. The publisher makes no warranty, express or implied, with respect
to the material contained herein.

Printed on acid-free paper

Springer is part of Springer Science+Business Media (www.springer.com)

Foreword

The past two decades have witnessed an explosion of imaging research focused on the human brain. In large part, this growth has been fueled by the emergence of non-invasive, widely available, and relatively low-cost imaging tools that provide precise measurements of brain anatomy and function. The beginning of this era can be tied to the development of functional magnetic resonance imaging (fMRI) in the early 1990s. Prior to this, knowledge of human brain function was derived primarily from the careful study of patients with focal brain lesions. In the decade following its development, fMRI provided the neuropsychologist and cognitive neuroscientist with an implement to validate lesion models by examining brain function in healthy individuals. This trend lead to the development and validation of a wide range of task activation paradigms for probing higher-order cognitive processes, such as language, memory, and attention. As novel and refined models of cognitive systems emerged from fMRI studies of intact individuals, neuroscientists began to apply fMRI to understanding brain disorders. The volume edited by Cohen and Sweet is both unique and timely, since it distills the most important scientific discoveries derived from imaging investigations conducted on clinical populations.

The book begins with clear and concise descriptions of the technical and physiological underpinnings of imaging tools that play key roles in investigating clinical disorders. Although fMRI is highlighted, a series of chapters also describe perfusion and diffusion MRI, MR spectroscopy, and optical imaging. The chapter provides critical background information that is comprehensible to the reader without formal training in MR physics. Most contemporary imaging studies take the advantage of multiple imaging strategies for interrogating brain function in clinical populations. As an example, it is no longer unusual for such a study to examine the integrity of white matter fiber tracks, using diffusion tensor imaging (DTI), that interconnect gray matter regions activated by fMRI. The reader will not only understand the strengths and weaknesses of each imaging method, but also acquire an appreciation for how these techniques complement each other.

Imaging studies of clinical populations present unique challenges for imaging studies. Relative to healthy participants, patients exhibit higher rates of claustrophobia, head movement, brain structure abnormalities (e.g., atrophy), impaired cognitive task performance, mood disturbances, and decreased motivation, to name a few. The reader is provided with a thorough understanding of how such factors can influence imaging results along with methods for addressing such problems.

A quite unique feature of this volume is its emphasis on exploring brain imaging in conditions commonly addressed in the field of behavioral medicine. The middle and largest section of the book contains chapters devoted to the effects of eating disorders, drug abuse, cardiovascular disease, and chronic pain on brain structure and function. A chapter also examines the role of exercise as an important factor influencing cognitive brain function. Imaging results hold the potential for better understanding the early brain changes resulting from these lifestyle factors. Eventually, one could foresee imaging data being used to examine the success of intervention programs designed to influence the course of such conditions.

The remaining third nicely summarizes the results of imaging studies conducted in neurological disorders related to Alzheimer's disease (AD), HIV, multiple sclerosis, stroke, and fatigue. One goal of such research is to develop valid imaging biomarkers that can be used to accurately identify early brain changes, even before cognitive symptoms emerge. Another is to determine the most sensitive imaging biomarkers to assess the efficacy of interventions designed to prevent or to treat these brain disorders. This volume provides a "fact check" on the status of the imaging field in addressing these lofty goals that have tangible societal consequences.

To summarize, the volume by Cohen and Sweet provides a compact and comprehensive summary of the state-of-the-art in advanced imaging research applied to clinical populations. Findings from such research may eventually lead to the widespread expansion of imaging tools in clinical practice. In the USA, fMRI is currently a reimbursable procedure for presurgical mapping in patients with epilepsy and brain tumors. With additional validation studies, one could foresee the clinical application of advanced imaging tools, like fMRI and DTI, in the diagnosis and management of a wide range of conditions and diseases in neurology and behavioral medicine. Sensitive imaging tools also hold the promise of reducing the time and expense associated with screening potentially efficacious drug, surgical, and lifestyle interventions. This scholarly volume provides the reader with a sense for how close we are to achieving these objectives.

Stephen M. Rao Ph.D.
Ralph and Luci Schey
Director, Schey Center for Cognitive Neuroimaging,
Professor, Cleveland Clinic Lerner College of Medicine at
Case Western Reserve University
Neurological Institute, Cleveland Clinic,
Cleveland, OH, 44195, USA

Preface

Rapid developments in brain imaging have occurred over the past decade. These advances have revolutionized cognitive and behavioral neuroscience, and are likely to have major influence on clinical psychological, psychiatric, and neurological practice over the coming years. News stories now appear on almost a daily basis in the national and international media describing findings from neuroimaging studies that have application to health and behavior. Interest in these neuroimaging efforts stems from the innate human curiosity to better understand how one's mind works, and the nature of brain dysfunction. There has been a greater realization by the layperson, scientist, and health care practitioner over the past decade that the mind and behavioral processes play an essential role in preventive health, response to illness, and the basic underlying mechanisms of many diseases. Brain imaging seems to be inherently interesting, and has increasingly drawn the efforts of large numbers of talented young behavioral scientists who strive to integrate these approaches with their research and clinical work.

The number of published empirical research studies incorporating neuroimaging methods to explore clinical and more basic neuroscience questions has increased exponentially over the past two decades. Structural neuroimaging data is now routinely included in neurological, neuropsychiatric, and neuropsychological studies, often as a way of verifying the brain disturbance that is the focus of investigation. In fact, failure to include neuroanatomic evidence of the location of brain lesions in neuropsychological studies of disorders in which there is localized damage (e.g., stroke) is often grounds for manuscripts being rejected for publication. Many excellent scientific journals now exist that provide a vehicle for disseminating neuroimaging research findings. Some focus specifically on brain imaging methods, such as Neuroimage and Human Brain Mapping, while others come from specific fields, including neuropsychology. Most of these journals are oriented toward cognitive and clinical neuroscience or applied medicine, including a large number of journals from the fields of neurology, neuropsychiatry, and radiology. With the exception of the recently launched journal, Brain Imaging and Behavior, few journals are oriented toward neuroimaging in the context of the clinical behavioral sciences. However, increasingly niche journals focusing on particular behavioral topics are publishing neuroimaging studies as well. For example, the American Journal of Clinical Nutrition has published recent studies on brain imaging findings in obesity, while journals like Nicotine and Tobacco Research publish studies on brain mechanisms underlying nicotine dependence and smoking behavior. In sum, neuroimaging has proliferated into the research literature on many topics in behavioral science, although to date this research is quite scattered across disciplines and journals, and not well integrated.

Books provide a vehicle for integrating information from emerging fields, such as neuroimaging. The majority of neuroimaging books have focused on the use of particular imaging methods in clinical medicine, with neuroradiology and neurology being primary sources. A number of books dealing with the more technical aspects of magnetic resonance and radiological physics and engineering also exist. Cognitive psychology and neuropsychology books now often include chapters addressing neuroimaging applications related to the study of brain and cognition. Furthermore, cognitive neuroscience texts have increasingly incorporated functional neuroimaging as a major topic. There are excellent books that address basic functional neuroimaging methods and concepts, such as the "Functional MRI: an introduction to methods."[1]

Yet, there are few books to date that consider and review emerging research in the application of brain neuroimaging methods for the study and assessment of behavioral and cognitive disorders. The "Handbook of Functional Neuroimaging of Cognition" is an example of a book that does an excellent job with respect to integrating knowledge on functional imaging in the cognitive sciences.[2] Frank Hillary and John Deluca, contributors to the current text, recently published a book "Functional Neuroimaging in Clinical Populations," that addresses the use of functional imaging for the study and assessment of clinical brain disorders.[3] It is one of the only books on the topic with a neuropsychological orientation to date.

It is quite remarkable that virtually no book currently exists that addresses the application of brain imaging to behavioral medicine, especially in light of the large number of research projects that have been initiated over the past several years, and the interest of the National Institutes of Health in this area of investigation. Most of the books previously mentioned were either written from a cognitive neuroscience perspective, from the standpoint of clinical medicine and standard clinical practice, or they are heavily focused on basic imaging physics and methods. Books that do focus to a greater extent on neuropsychological and behavioral topics have tended to primarily cover functional brain imaging, with little emphasis on related types of neuroimaging, such as diffusion-weighted, perfusion-weighted, and metabolic imaging methods, such as magnetic resonance spectroscopy. Furthermore, they have addressed topics of relevance to behavioral medicine and neuropsychology to only a very limited degree. Accordingly, there seemed to be a compelling need for a book to introduce clinical and behavioral scientists to a broader range of neuroimaging methods and their application to behavioral medicine and clinical neuroscience questions.

These considerations motivated the writing of this book. Our goal was to provide relatively broad coverage of current research trends in the clinical application of brain neuroimaging methods in the context of behavioral medicine, neuropsychology, and related areas of medical psychology, as well as to introduce readers to the spectrum of neuroimaging methods that are currently available.

Objectives. This book is a response to a need within behavioral medicine, neuropsychology, and more broadly the clinical and behavioral neurosciences for an integrated review of current neuroimaging methods and their clinical and research applications. The book canvases a relatively broad range of topics, covering not only functional neuroimaging, but also structural imaging, as well as neuroimaging methods that provide information underlying pathophysiology. The goal is to provide an introduction to these neuroimaging approaches, and their potential value in the assessment and treatment of medical and behavioral disorders. In this regard, we believe this book may be valuable not only for specialists in behavioral medicine and neuropsychology, but also for clinical psychologists, psychiatrists, neurologists, and physicians and clinical health providers who are interested in the neurobiological and brain-behavior contributions to health and medical disorders, and seek to understand how neuroimaging may be useful in their clinical practice. The topics covered in this book may also help to stimulate new ideas among researchers using neuroimaging methods to study the brain and behavior. The broad objectives of the book are outlined below.

Provide an introduction to a variety of neuroimaging methods for clinicians working in the field of behavioral medicine, as well as neuropsychologists, neuroscientists, and clinicians of psychology, psychiatry and neurology.

Consider the strengths and limitations of specific methods, including constraints that may impact their future use in clinical situations.

Provide an integration and synthesis of current research and thinking on neuroimaging in behavioral medicine and clinical neuroscience.

Review current clinical and research evidence regarding the use of these methods for the assessment of specific brain and behavioral disorders.

Consider how these methods can be used in combination to understand the relationships among brain structure, pathophysiology, and function.

Consider current research questions being examined through neuroimaging within behavioral medicine and clinical neuroscience, and provide insights into future directions of research.

Organization. The book is organized into three sections. Part One introduces neuroimaging, including basic concepts, theoretical considerations, and methods. It consists of chapters that address theoretical and methodological considerations and constraints on the clinical application of neuroimaging. This is followed by chapters providing overviews of specific imaging approaches, along with some technical information about each approach, methodological constraints, and a discussion of what type of information each method provides.

Part Two consists of chapters that discuss the use of neuroimaging methods in behavioral medicine. Specific areas of focus will include obesity and eating disorders, physical activity and exercise, nicotine and amphetamine effects, pain, fatigue, and emotional experience in the context of medical disorders.

Part Three considers neuroimaging in clinical neuroscience for the study and assessment of brain disorders affecting behavior and cognition. This chapter emphasizes brain disorders that have major medical implications, including Stroke, cardiovascular disease, HIV, Alzheimer's disease, and Multiple Sclerosis. This section of the book emphasizes how multimodal imaging can help to disentangle neuropathological mechanisms underlying these conditions and brain-behavioral relationships.

Ronald A. Cohen
Lawrence H. Sweet

References

1. Jezzard P, Matthews PM, Smith SM, eds. *Functional MRI: an Introduction to Methods.* New York, NY: Oxford University Press; 2001.
2. Cabeza R, Kingstone A, ed. *Handbook of Functional Neuroimaging of Cognition,* 2nd ed. Cambridge, MA: MIT Press; 2006.
3. Hillary F, DeLuca J, *Functional Neuroimaging in Clinical Populations* New York: Guilford Press; 2007.

Contents

1 Brain Imaging in Behavioral Medicine and Clinical Neuroscience: An Introduction 1
Ronald A. Cohen and Lawrence H. Sweet

2 Basic MR Physics: Considerations for Behavioral Medicine and Neuropsychology 11
Edward G. Walsh

3 Functional Magnetic Resonance Imaging 37
Lawrence H. Sweet

4 Diffusion-Tensor Imaging and Behavioral Medicine 49
Stephen Correia and Assawin Gongvatana

5 Perfusion MRI 67
Richard Hoge

6 Proton Magnetic Resonance Spectroscopy (^{1}H MRS): A Practical Guide for the Clinical Neuroscientist 83
Andreana P. Haley and Jack Knight-Scott

7 Functional Near-Infrared Spectroscopy 93
Farzin Irani

8 Methodological Considerations for Using Bold fMRI in the Clinical Neurosciences 103
Kathy S. Chiou and Frank G. Hillary

9 Application of Functional Neuroimaging to Examination of Nicotine Dependence 117
Sean P. David, Lawrence H. Sweet, Ronald A. Cohen, James MacKillop, Richard C. Mulligan, and Raymond Niaura

10 The Relationship Between Mood, Stress, and Tobacco Smoking 147
Espen Walderhaug, Kelly P. Cosgrove, Zubin Bhagwagar, and Alexander Neumeister

11 Imaging Substance Use and Misuse: Psychostimulants 163
Tara L. White

12 Eating Disorders 179
Angelo Del Parigi and Ellen Schur

13 Structural and Functional Neuroimaging in Obesity 193
Kelly Stanek, Joseph Smith, and John Gunstad

14 Neuropsychology and Neuroimaging in Metabolic Dysfunction 201
Jason J. Hassenstab

15 Neuroimaging of Cardiovascular Disease 215
Ronald A. Cohen

16 Exercise and the Brain 257
Uraina S. Clark and David Williams

17 Neuroimaging of Pain: A Psychosocial Perspective 275
Tamara J. Somers, G. Lorimer Moseley, Francis J. Keefe,
and Sejal M. Kothadia

18 Neuroimaging in Acute Ischemic Stroke 293
Shashidhara Nanjundaswamy, Ronald A. Cohen, and Marc Fisher

**19 Neuroimaging of Alzheimer's Disease, Mild Cognitive
Impairment, and Other Dementias** 309
Shannon L. Risacher and Andrew J. Saykin

**20 Application of Neuroimaging Methods to Define Cognitive
and Brain Abnormalities Associated with HIV** 341
Jodi Heaps, Jennifer Niehoff, Elizabeth Lane, Kuryn Kroutil, Joseph Boggiano,
and Robert Paul

21 Neuroimaging and Cognitive Function in Multiple Sclerosis 355
Lawrence H. Sweet and Susan D. Vandermorris

22 Neuroimaging of Fatigue 369
Helen M. Genova, Glenn R. Wylie, and John DeLuca

**23 Brain Imaging in Behavioral Medicine and Clinical
Neuroscience: Synthesis** 383
Ronald A. Cohen and Lawrence H. Sweet

Index 395

Contributors

Zubin Bhagwagar, MD
MRCPsych Assistant Professor Department of Psychiatry, Yale School of Medicine, 300 George St., Suite 901, New Haven, CT 06511, USA

Joseph Boggiano
Division of Behavioral Neuroscience, Department of Psychology, University of Missouri, St. Louis, St. Louis, MO, USA

Kathy S. Chiou, MS
Doctoral Candidate Department of Psychology, Pennsylvania State University, University Park, PA, USA

Uraina S. Clark, PhD
Department of Neuropsychology, The Warren Alpert Medical School of Brown University, The Miriam Hospital, Providence, RI, USA

Ronald A. Cohen, PhD
Department of Psychiatry and Human Behavior, Brown University, Providence, RI 02912, USA

Stephen Correia, PhD
Department of Psychiatry and Human Behavior, Brown University, Providence, RI, USA

Kelly P. Cosgrove, PhD
Department of Psychiatry, Yale School of Medicine, 300 George St., Suite 901, New Haven, CT 06511, USA

Sean P. David, MD, SM, DPhil
Division of Family & Community Medicine, Department of Medicine, Stanford University School of Medicine, Stanford , CA, USA
and
Policy, SRI International, Menlo Park, CA, USA
and
Family Medicine, Alpert Medical School of Brown University, Providence, RI, USA

Angelo Del Parigi, MD
Clinical Development Endocrime, Pfizer Inc., 235 East 42nd Street, Mailstop
219/8/2, New York, NY 10017, USA

John DeLuca, PhD, ABPP
Kessler Foundation Research Center, 1199 Pleasant Valley Way, West Orange, NJ
07052, USA
and
Department of Physical Medicine and Rehabilitation, University of Medicine and
Dentistry of New Jersey – New Jersey Medical School, Newark, NJ, USA

Marc Fisher, MD
UMASS-Memorial Medical Center, Belmont St., Worcester, MA 01506, USA

Helen M. Genova, PhD
Research Associate Kessler Research Center, West Orange, NJ, USA

Assawin Gongvatana, PhD
Department of Psychiatry and Human Behavior, Brown University, Providence,
RI, USA

John Gunstad, PhD
Summa Health System, Kent State University, 221 Kent Hall Addition, Kent, OH,
USA

Andreana P. Haley, PhD
Assistant Professor, Department of Psychology, The University of Texas at
Austin, Austin, TX, USA

Jason J. Hassenstab
Departments of Neurology and Psychology, Washington University Medical School
in St. Louis, St. Louis, MO 63108, USA

Jodi Heaps
Division of Behavioral Neuroscience, Department of Psychology, University
of Missouri, St. Louis, St. Louis, MO, USA

Frank G. Hillary, PhD
Department of Psychology, Pennsylvania State University, 223 Moore Building,
University Park, PA 16802, USA

Richard Hoge, PhD
Department of Physiology and Institute of Biomedical Engineering, Université de
Montréal, Centre de recherche de l'institut universitaire de gériatrie de Montréal,
Montréal, QC, Canada

Farzin Irani, PhD
Department of Psychiatry, Neuropsychiatry Division, University of Pennsylvania,
3400 Spruce Street, Gates Builing–10th Floor, Philadelphia, PA 19104, USA

Francis J. Keefe
Duke University Medical Center, Durham, NC, USA

Jack Knight-Scott, PhD
Department of Radiology, Children's Healthcare of Atlanta, Atlanta, GA, USA

Kuryn Kroutil
Division of Behavioral Neuroscience, Department of Psychology, University of Missouri, St. Louis, St. Louis, MO, USA

Sejal M. Kothadia
Duke University Medical Center, Durham, NC, USA

James MacKillop, PhD
Division of Behavioral Neuroscience, Department of Psychology, Elizabeth Lane, University of Missouri, St. Louis, St. Louis, MO, USA

G. Lorimer Moseley
Prince of Wales Medical Research Institute, Australia

Richard C. Mulligan, PhD
Department of Community Health, Center for Alcohol and Addiction Studies, Brown University, Providence, RI, USA

Shashidhara Nanjundaswamy, MD
Department of Neurology, University of Massachusetts Medical Center, Worcester, MA, USA

Alexander Neumeister, MD
Molecular Imaging Program of the National Center for PTSD, Clinical Neuroscience Division, VA Connecticut Healthcare System, (116-A) 950 Campbell Avenue, Bldg. 1, Room 9-174 (MSC 151E), West Haven, CT, 06516, USA
Mount Sinai School of Medicine, New York, NY, 10029, USA

Raymond Niaura, PhD
Associate Director for Science, Professor of Psychiatry and Human Behavior at the Alpert Medical School of Brown University Schroeder Institute for Tobacco Policy and Research Studies at the Legacy Foundation, Providence, RI, USA

Robert Paul
Department of Psychology, Division of Behavioral Neuroscience, University of Missouri, One University Blvd., Stadler, 412, St. Louis, MO 63121, USA

Shannon L. Risacher
Department of Radiology and Imaging Sciences, IU Center for Neuroimaging, Medical Neuroscience Program, Indiana University School of Medicine, Stark Neurosciences Research Institute, Indianapolis, IN, USA

Andrew J. Saykin
Center for Neuroimaging, Department of Radiology and Imaging Sciences, Indiana
Alzheimer Disease Center, Medical Neuroscience Program, Stark Neurosciences
Research Institute, Indiana University School of Medicine, Indianapolis, IN, USA

Ellen Schur, MD, MS
Assistant Professor Division of General Internal Medicine, Department of
Medicine, Harborview Medical Center, Seattle, WA, USA

Joseph Smith, BA
Kent State University, Kent, OH, USA

Tamara J. Somers
Duke University Medical Center, Durham, NC, USA

Kelly Stanek, MA
Kent State University, Kent, OH, USA

Lawrence H. Sweet, PhD
Department of Psychiatry and Human Behavior, Alpert Medical School
of Brown University, Providence, RI, USA

Susan D. Vandermorris, PhD
Post-Doctoral Fellow Rotman Research Institute, Baycrest, Toronto, ON, Canada

Espen Walderhaug, PhD
Department of Psychiatry, Yale University School of Medicine, West Haven,
CT, USA
Center for the Study of Human Cognition, Department of Psychology, University of
Oslo, Oslo, Norway

Edward G. Walsh, PhD
Brown University, Departments of Neuroscience and Diagnostic Imaging, Institute
for Brain Science, Providence, RI, USA

Tara L. White, PhD
Center for Alcohol and Addiction Studies, Department of Community Health,
Brown University, Box G-S121-4, Providence, RI 02912, USA

David Williams, PhD
Program in Public Health, Institute for Community Health Promotion, Brown
University, Providence, RI, USA

Glenn R. Wylie, DPhil
Research Scientist, Assistant Professor of Physical Medicine and Rehabilitation
Kessler Research Center, West Orange, NJ, USA
University of Medicine and Dentistry of New Jersey – New Jersey Medical School,
New York, NJ, USA

Chapter 1
Brain Imaging in Behavioral Medicine and Clinical Neuroscience: An Introduction

Ronald A. Cohen and Lawrence H. Sweet

We are living in a remarkable time in the history of neuroscience. A little over a century ago, neuropsychology had not yet emerged as a formal area of scientific inquiry, and knowledge regarding brain function was largely limited to pioneering studies of the effects of brain damage on cognitive functions. Demonstration by Broca and Wernicke of expressive and receptive aphasia associated with focal brain lesions resulted in an initial understanding of the functional neuroanatomy of language,[1,2] while observation of effects of frontal lobe damage in the famous case of Phineus Gage spurred initial speculation about the role of the frontal lobes in behavior and emotional control.[3] This led to a steady increase in scientific research in the clinic and laboratory over the first half of the twentieth century to understand brain function, providing a foundation of knowledge for the field of Neuropsychology.

Early efforts to localize brain functions largely involved analyzing the effects of naturally occurring focal lesions among patients with neurological disorders, most commonly stroke. This work was extremely important, as clinical observation provided the foundations for many brain science methods and theories. The fields of behavioral neurology, neuropsychology, and cognitive neuroscience evolved directly from these efforts. Yet, the information that can be derived from the assessment of patients with brain lesions is limited by certain conceptual and methodological factors intrinsic to such neurological cases. For example, naturally occurring lesions vary in volume and location, so that it is difficult to achieve precise localization in the context of single studies. Knowledge about specific brain regions usually has to be extracted from meta-analysis of a large set of studies showing converging functional neuroanatomic findings regarding particular areas of the brain. Occasionally, a unique patient is discovered with a lesion that is so well localized as to provide conclusive information about the role of a particular brain structure in cognitive function, such as the famous case of H.M., which enabled localization of declarative memory processing to the anterior temporal lobe.[4] While such cases have been essential to current memory theories, it is difficult to develop an entire field of cognitive neuroscientific inquiry based on such individual cases, as they are very rare.

Parallel research involving ablation of focal brain areas in laboratory animals provided a partial remedy to this limitation, as this approach enabled greater experimental control of the areas of the brain to be removed and individual differences in functional neuroanatomy, although not all findings from studies of laboratory animals can be extrapolated to conclusions about higher cognitive functions and subjective experience in humans. Therefore, there continues to be a strong need for human-based research aimed at understanding brain–behavior relationships.

Another now well-recognized limitation of the lesion analysis approach stems from the fact one could usually not be certain that conclusions about the role of particular brain areas in cognitive function would hold true for people without brain lesions. In other words, were lesion effects truly indicative of the role of damaged brain areas in cognition, or simply reflecting how the rest of the brain behaves in the presence of focal damage? Two other limitations associated with traditional lesion analysis methods are more difficult to circumvent: (1) Brain lesions inform about the effects of complete structural damage involving

R.A. Cohen (✉)
Department of Psychiatry and Human Behavior
and the Institute for Brain Science
Warren Alpert Medical School of Brown University,
Providence, RI 02912, USA
e-mail: RCohen@lifespan.org

R.A. Cohen and L.H. Sweet (eds.), *Brain Imaging in Behavioral Medicine and Clinical Neuroscience*,
DOI 10.1007/978-1-4419-6373-4_1, © Springer Science+Business Media, LLC 2011

specific brain areas but are less useful in helping to understand the physiological substrates underlying these effects. (2) Lesion analysis lends itself well to a modular view of the brain function but is more difficult to integrate into brain theories that consider cognition to be a function of distributed brain systems. With respect to the first point, there is now an abundance of clinical evidence for both neurological and psychiatric disorders that involve either neurophysiological disturbances in which structural damage to the brain is not apparent, or microstructural abnormalities that lead to gross neuroanatomic change only as the disease progresses. Major depression exemplifies the first scenario, and Alzheimer's disease the second. Clearly, lesion analysis methods have only limited value for understanding such disorders. For many years, inferences about the brain systems thought to be involved in neuropsychiatric disorders were based largely from patterns of deficits on neurocognitive assessment and from psychopharmacological studies of the effects of particular drugs on the brain using humans and laboratory animals. Many of the clinical brain imaging applications that will be explored in this book are for disorders of this type; that is, cognitive, emotional, and behavioral disturbances not resulting from localized lesion.

The "modular" view of brain function, which is a natural outgrowth of the lesion analytic method, continues to have strong support. Indeed there is considerable evidence that the brain is modular, at least to a point. For example, the pre-central frontal region is universally accepted as a primary motor area, while the occipital lobe clearly is involved in primary visual processing. Furthermore, there is compelling evidence that certain cognitive processes, such as attention, can be explained by the interaction of specific brain areas acting as a functional system.[5] Neuropsychological models that have been developed to account for the interaction of "modules" across multiple brain areas typically evolved based on cumulative evidence arising from a large number of separate studies showing the effects of damage to separate brain areas on the processes thought to be necessary for the cognitive function of interest. Fortunately, many of the functional neuroanatomic systems delineated through such meta-analyses have been validated in recent years by other methodological approaches. Yet, from a neuroscientific perspective, it is ultimately difficult to draw definitive conclusions about how the brain is functioning as a whole in a particular person based on analysis of cognitive dysfunction from a large set of patients with discrete brain lesions. Furthermore, cognitive functions that are thought to be broadly distributed across particular cortical areas are less easily studied by this method. In sum, the lesion analytic approach works best for cognitive functions that are clearly a byproduct of interacting modular processes. It works less well for understanding associative phenomena and other cognitive processes that are less modular in nature.

Psychophysiological Perspective

The limitations associated with the lesion localization approach provided a clear catalyst for the development of other methods that could provide complementary data to validate brain localization findings. Psychophysiology emerged in response to this need, as well as the broader goal of linking cognitive and behavioral processes to underlying physiological processes. Psychophysiology provided a means of measuring physiological response associated with behavioral, cognitive, and emotional processes. Methods were developed to measure both systemic autonomic reactivity (e.g., heart rate, muscle activity, pupil dilation, etc.),[6-8] as well as central nervous system activity.[9] By recording physiological responses occurring in conjunction with cognitive and behavioral responding, there was hope that researchers might obtain objective measures separate from, but functional related to, the behavior of interest. While the physiological metrics derived from early psychophysiological investigations were typically distal to the phenomena of interest, these methods enabled investigators to begin with the "mind and body."

Electroencephalographic (EEG) methods to record and stimulate activity in specific brain areas represented major advances in this regard. By recording changes in the electrical activity in particular brain regions during cognitive processing, researchers hoped to show that the brain–behavior relationships revealed by lesion analyses had physiological underpinning.[10,11] Correlating physiological responses from particular brain areas with cognitive processes could provide independent functional neuroanatomic validation apart from the results of lesion analysis.

Electrophysiological methods proved to be a powerful neuroscientific tool, particularly when used in the context of direct recording from the surface of the brain and single unit studies of laboratory animals.[12-16] These methods enabled measurement of changes in the response of individual neurons to different sensory and cognitive conditions. The power of these methods stems from the tight temporal coupling between the stimulation provided to the animal and the physiological response. Recording the electrical activity in small regions of the brain provided a window into how physiological response was changing on a moment by moment basis. The temporal resolution of electrophysiology was one of its strongest features, along with the fact that the electrical activity that was being recorded was presumably directly related to the electric signaling upon which communication in the brain was based.

In humans efforts to derive similar types of electrophysiological data are constrained by major logistical issues, most notably the fact that for health and ethical reasons electrodes cannot be placed into brain of healthy study participants. While intriguing data has come from electrophysiological studies of patients undergoing neurosurgery for epilepsy, tumor, and other neurological disorders, there are limitations to the types of experiments that can be conducted during these medical procedures. Consequently, the bulk of human electrophysiological brain research has come from the record of surface EEG from the scalp. There is now a large research literature of human EEG with studies that have employed innovative experimental paradigms, such as the measurement of evoked potentials record event-related brain activity (ERPs) associated with specific cognitive, emotional, and behavioral tasks.[9,11,17]

This line of research has provided considerable insight about key information processing events occurring during cognition, with greatest power derived from the ability of these techniques to detect processes occurring within the first 1 s after a stimulus has been presented. For example, the N100, a component of the ERP that involves a negative electrical potential occurring at around 100 ms post-stimulus presentation has been associated with initial attentional response to visual and auditory stimuli, and reliably differs from the P300 response, which occurs when novel stimuli occur that standout from the background of typical stimuli in a particular context.[17-20] This level of tempo-

ral precision in the measurement of brain activity remains superior to other brain imaging methods even today. Historically, the primary limitation associated with these methods arose from the fact that scalp recordings did not allow for high spatial resolution. It was difficult to know the exact anatomic sources of specific ERP components, even when a large number of electrodes were used, in part because of constraints associated with spread off electrical activity across the scalp. This limitation is associated with the inverse problem derived from Helmholtz's principle[21] and the first law of thermodynamics. The inverse problem dictates that there is not one unique solution when trying to work backwards from the recording site to determine the electrical source. Over the last 20 years, computational approaches have been developed that partially overcome this problem,[22,23] and magnetic encephalography (MEG) offers considerable promise for imaging short-duration processes with high temporal resolution,[24,25] though the spatial resolution of EEG including MEG continues to be weaker compared to that which is possible with functional magnetic resonance imaging (fMRI).

Besides enabling the measurement of neural activity associated with brain processes, electrophysiology provided means of validating the localization of brain functions by actively altering specific responses. For example, by stimulating a specific brain region electrically, it was possible to elicit a physiological and functional change that enabled a direct functional neuroanatomic manipulation. Penfield's ability to elicit specific behavioral responses or subjective experiences by stimulating focal brain regions provided compelling evidence for the role of these brain areas in particular cognitive functions.

In sum, electrophysiology continues to provide extremely valuable neuroscientific methods, particularly for characterizing brain function during cognitive processes with excellent temporal resolution. However, logistic and interpretive complexities associated with these methods have limited their clinical application. EEG remains a primary neurodiagnostic tool for assessing seizure activity and basic sensory and motor disorders, but it has been overtaken by other functional imaging methods for neuropsychological and cognitive neuroscientific inquiry. Many books have been published over the past 30 years that address research and clinical findings derived from EEG. Accordingly, EEG methods will not be a focus of this book. Instead we will focus on radiological and magnetic resonance (MR)-based functional brain imaging methods that provide excellent spatial resolution for characterizing neuroanatomy, along with different levels of temporal resolution.

Vascular Psychophysiology

Beyond EEG, the field of psychophysiology was strongly influenced by efforts to better understand the relationship between systemic physiological activity and psychological experience. Vascular physiology was of particular interest given the emerging view that stress and other emotional and behavioral factors could lead to alterations in the vascular health, including the development of disorders such as hypertension. Furthermore, efforts were directed at using behavioral methods together with physiological measurement to train people to modify their vascular response (i.e., biofeedback). This work had a dominant influence in the emerging field of behavioral medicine. One of the outcomes of this line of work was the observation by a number of researchers that systemic physiological response was coupled with cognitive processing, and that different vascular responses accompanied specific cognitive processes. For example, heart rate acceleration was shown to occur during tasks involving focused attention and working memory, whereas heart rate deceleration occurred during states of vigilant, but passive attention to stimuli in the environment, when strong demands to respond are not present. From a clinical neuroscience perspective, measures of vascular and other psychophysiological responses were seen as having potential value in that they provided a physiological biomarker of cognitive processes, such as orienting and habituation in the context of attention.

While most of the early neuropsychological research on psychophysiology focused on using systemic vascular response as a correlate of cognitive processes, neuroscientists have long recognized a strong link between vascular and brain functions. In the late nineteenth century, Roy and Sherrington in their seminal neurophysiological studies of laboratory animals observed a link between the cerebral circulation of blood and brain metabolism.[26] Subsequently, isolated experiments were conducted

in the context of individual clinical cases that demonstrated that cerebral vascular response varied as a function of the demands placed on the patient. For example, Fulton demonstrated that the intensity of a bruit that was heard from the scalp of a patient with an occipital arterial–venous malformation increased when the patient read vs. when they sat passively with eyes open, suggesting that cerebral blood flow was changing in response to the complexity of visual processing demand. Yet, the link between cerebral vascular response and neuronal activity was not the subject of much research until well into the twentieth century. This was partly due to early findings which suggested that the relationship between cerebral circulation and neuronal function was not very strong, and perhaps even more importantly because of the lack of technological capability to adequately address this question.

Radiological Imaging

A major breakthrough in both structural imaging occurred with the development of X-ray computed tomography (CT) methods in the mid-1970s that led directly to functional imaging methods as well. Until that time, radiological imaging was limited by the two-dimensional nature of standard X-ray procedures, which were capable of primarily detecting skull abnormalities, with minimal detail of brain structure. While the principles underlying CT imaging seem almost intuitive today, the conceptual innovation of placing X-ray devices in a circle around the cranium, enabling a three-dimensional brain image to be constructed was a major innovation.[27] In fact, cognitive psychology courses during the 1970s used CT as an illustration of how problem solving often involves a quantum leap in the approach taken to reach a solution.[28]

From a neuroscience perspective, the development of CT imaging was extremely important, as it provided the first good noninvasive "in vivo" method for imaging brain neuroanatomy. Compared to all methods that preceded it, CT had incredible spatial resolution and could be obtained relatively quickly, making it a vital and relatively routine part of clinical practice by the 1980s. CT imaging continues to be widely used today, as it offers certain advantages over MRI, is less expensive for clinical settings to implement, and is useful for detecting many disorders, such as tumors. However, from the standpoint of our current focus, CT has been largely overshadowed by MRI, which provides much higher spatial resolution and the ability to image different types of brain tissue without the use of X-rays or radioactive ligands.

Very soon after the introduction of CT methods for structural brain imaging, radiological researchers realized that this general approach of using detectors placed around the cranium could be combined with "autoradiography" to measure blood flow, glucose metabolism, and oxygen consumption.[29-31] These autoradiographic methods had been employed in laboratory animals using invasive procedures previously. The application of the principles associated with CT to measure brain physiology represented a logical extension of these ideas, although one that was highly innovative in its own right. Two major techniques, positron emission tomography (PET) and single photon emission computed tomography (SPECT) evolved from this work. A key element of both methods is the introduction of a radioactive agent into the blood stream, which is metabolized at differing rates by the brain, as a function of the blood flow and glucose metabolism characteristics of different types of brain tissue. Furthermore, it soon became evident that besides showing differential activity across brain areas at rest, these methods were able to detect subtle differences in the response of particular brain structures to cognitive and behavioral challenges.

While the majority of chapters in this book focus on MR-based methods, functional radiological imaging remains very important, particularly because it can be used to image specific neurotransmitter, peptides, and metabolic byproducts during functional imaging, which remains a major challenge for MR-based methods. This is particularly important when studying psychiatric disorders and substance abuse. Chapter 10 discusses the application of neuroradiological methods for the study of nicotine dependence, stress response, and mood. Overview of functional radiological methods. Magnetic resonance spectroscopy (MRS) offer a potential alternative for measuring brain metabolites, although for purposes of imaging brain neurotransmitter systems PET remains a better alternative to MRI methods.

Functional Magnetic Resonance Imaging

Approximately, a decade after the emergence of CT imaging as a clinical radiological tool, magnetic resonance imaging (MRI) evolved to the point that it could be employed clinically as an alternative for anatomic imaging. As its name suggests, MRI was possible because strong magnetic fields cause the alignment of nuclei of hydrogen atoms in the water content of the different tissues of the body. Radiofrequency fields are used to alter the magnetic fields created by a large magnet. This causes the hydrogen nuclei to spin with a particular resonance. When the radiofrequency is turned off or the magnetic field is altered by some other manipulation, there is a relaxation of the spin of the hydrogen nuclei and recovery back to its original state. This recovery occurs along different spatial dimensions. Along the longitudinal axis the magnetic response is referred to as T_1 relaxation, as it occurs exponentially with a time constant T_1. In contrast, the loss of phase coherence of the spin in the transverse plane is called T_2 relaxation. T_1 is associated with the enthalpy of the spin, whereas T_2 and $T_2{}^*$ are associated with its entropy. In the soft tissues of the body, T_1 is around 1 s while T_2 and $T_2{}^*$ are much shorter, typically under 100 ms. However, the exact value for T_1, T_2, and $T_2{}^*$ vary dramatically depending on external magnetic fields and the type of tissue being imaged. This fact provides MRI with very high soft tissue contrast. From a practical standpoint, T_1, T_2, and $T_2{}^*$ differ in their sensitivity and resolution of particular types of tissue. The biophysics of MRI is discussed in greater detail in Chap. 2, and is covered in greater detail in recent books on MRI methods (e.g., Jezzard and Mathews[32]). The important consideration for the moment is that MRI provides extremely strong spatial resolution to different types of brain tissue under varying physiological conditions.

As originally conceived for purposes of clinical brain imaging, structural imaging makes use of redundant scanning sweeps which are summed. This has the effect of reducing variance in the signal that is obtained on a single image. For purposes of structural imaging, this variance is a source of noise that diminishes the resolution of the anatomy of interest. Yet, in reality the variation in the MRI response that occurs across successive magnetic pulses is actually a function of many biologically important factors and contains much potential information. Pauling and Coryell observed that by changing the amount of oxygen carried in the blood, it was possible to cause perturbations in magnetic fields.[33] Accordingly, if instead of summing across all of the trials involved in a typical structural imaging session, MRI acquisition trials are grouped based on some factor that changes systematically over time, it is possible to extract information that may have physiological value.

In the early 1990s, based on Pauling and Coryell's earlier observation, Kwong and colleagues and Ogawa and colleagues separately demonstrated that in vivo changes in blood oxygenation could be obtained using MRI, with these changes detected across acquisition trials.[34-37] This phenomenon was described as blood oxygen level dependent (BOLD) signal and became the basis for fMRI. Not long after this initial experiment, a series of studies were published that employed this method in conjunction with simple functional tasks, with the results demonstrating that changes in the BOLD response occur in association according to these functional demands.[38-40] This led to a virtual explosion of research employing MRI to study brain function in relationship to neuroanatomy and physiology.

The early work on FMRI attributed observed effects to BOLD. However, it has become apparent in subsequent years that other factors also affect the brain activation detected during imaging. For example, BOLD is influenced by the amount of cerebral blood flow that is occurring from moment to moment. Furthermore, the glucose utilization that occurs in association with the BOLD response is greater than the amount of oxygen actually being consumed. This energy differential is not fully understood. Studies have focused metabolic activity associated with the excitatory neurotransmitters, in particular glutamate,[41] although ultimately knowledge of how neuronal activity is translated into changes in the BOLD response and functional brain response is still in its infancy. Fortunately, from a clinical neuroscience perspective it has been possible to obtain reliable brain responses to specific cognitive and behavioral challenges, suggesting that the general method has strong validity, even though it is not completely understood.

Evolution of Functional Brain Imaging as Tool for Neuroscientific Research

Rapid developments in structural and functional neuroimaging methods have occurred over the past two decades. These advances have revolutionized cognitive and behavioral neuroscience, and are likely to have major influence on clinical psychological, psychiatric, and neurological practice over the coming years.

The evolution of brain imaging methods and research has consisted of several important phases. During the first phase of research in the early 1990s, studies were directed at demonstrating that reliable BOLD signals could be obtained and analyzed in response to changes in well-controlled physiological conditions. This was followed by studies focusing on basic sensory and motor functions, again demonstrating consistency of activation across brain regions known to be involved in particular processes. For example, activation of the occipital region was reliably shown to occur when healthy participants were presented to with alternating visual stimuli (e.g., checkerboard pattern). Similarly, activation of the motor strip could be reliably elicited when participants tapped with their finger. Work in this basic area of functional imaging investigation has continued, with effort directed at examining functional brain response relative to concurrent physiological or anatomic data. For example, while the BOLD signal reflects oxygen utilization, it is strongly coupled with cerebral blood flow. There is still much be learned about how hemodynamic function as measured by perfusion imaging and BOLD response relate to one another. Similarly, the metabolic activity that presumably underlies FMRI is ultimately linked to the electric activity of the brain. Changes in electrical activity at the level of individual neuronal units are considered to be the basis for communication throughout the brain. Accordingly, studies that integrate MRI and EEG methods continue to be at the cutting edge of the field. These are two of the many areas of development that continue at a rapid pace.

The next developmental phase began soon after the first and was characterized by cognitive studies aimed at showing activation of brain regions of interest in response to specific cognitive processes involving language, visual–spatial processing, memory, and higher order functions such as problem solving. Studies were also aimed at characterizing the response of limbic and other cortical brain regions to emotional stimuli. To a large extent, the primary focus of these efforts was to validate the role of particular brain areas in these cognitive processes, and to show that brain activation was sensitive to changes in task parameters. For most of these investigations individual differences were a source of noise, and a factor that was controlled for experimentally to the extent possible. These studies tended not to focus on establishing normative data on for the various imaging metrics of interest, but rather aimed at showing dissociations in cognitive processes. This line of research continues to be a major thrust of ongoing brain imaging research and has made a great contribution to the development of cognitive and affective neuroscience.

There are now several excellent books that focus on specific neuroimaging methods, such as FMRI, and also the application of these methods to cognitive psychology and cognitive neuroscientific inquiry. While this research will be addressed to some extent in this text, it is not our primary focus.

The third phase of brain imaging application has been a natural outgrowth of the first two phases: the application of imaging methods and experimental paradigms to the study of brain disorders. Research in this area has grown exponentially over the past decade and is beginning to have a significant impact in neurology and other clinical neurosciences. For example, functional and structural imaging methods are now an important part of the clinical assessment of Alzheimer's disease and related dementias. PET and SPECT imaging have been approved by insurance providers for use in determining whether patients are exhibiting decreased brain activation in brain regions, such as the temporal and parietal lobes, thought to be affected early in the disease course. Increasingly, FMRI is being used along with radiological imaging to examine early markers of Alzheimer's disease. In Chap. 19, Dr. Saykin addresses the use of functional and related brain imaging methods for the study and assessment of dementia. Other imaging methods have made an impact in the neurodiagnostic assessment of other neurological disorders. For example, diffusion and perfusion weighted imaging methods are now considered to be important tools for assessing the evolution of cerebral infarctions by neurologists working in the field of stroke (see Chap. 18). Major efforts are also underway to employ multiple imaging modalities, including MRS, diffusion tensor imaging, and advanced mor-

phometric analyses of structural images for the study of brain abnormalities that occur secondary to HIV. These areas of investigation are still early in their development, and will likely be important parts of clinical neuroscience for years to come. There is a strong need for normative data for the various brain imaging modalities that are currently being employed, as well as studies aimed at establishing the reliability and comparability of findings across scanners and laboratories.

The fourth and most recent area of brain imaging study has focused on the application of brain imaging methods in the context of behavioral medicine. Increasingly, grant submissions to the National Institutes of Health have proposed to employ functional and other imaging methods to study human behavior, risk factors, and brain functions associated with the development of systemic diseases, such as cancer and heart disease. Much of our current research at Brown University has been directed at such applications. For example, we have ongoing studies employing FMRI, perfusion-, and diffusion imaging to characterize early brain changes associated with cardiovascular disease. Other lines of work of relevance to the field of behavioral medicine include the use of functional imaging to study chronic pain, chemotherapy response, predisposition and response to exercise, obesity, and eating behaviors. Another important direction of work includes studies aimed at understanding the basis for nicotine dependence and other forms of substance abuse. Of course, this work dovetails into now more established lines of research aimed at understanding the brain disturbances underlying major affective disorders, schizophrenia, post-traumatic stress syndrome, and a various other psychiatric conditions.

Conceptual and Methodological Considerations

Before we become fully immersed into the contents of this book, there are several conceptual, philosophical, and methodological issues that warrant consideration. These include the following: (1) The spatial and temporal resolution of the different imaging methods. (2) What types of information can be derived from each method. (3) The extent to which particular methods are useful for identifying underlying neuronal mechanisms. (4) The experimental task requirements to obtain meaningful data. (5) How the data obtained from imaging will be used to answer an experimental or clinical question. (6) The philosophical and ethical implications of findings obtained from brain imaging studies.

Brain Imaging in Behavioral Medicine and Clinical Neuroscience

In summary, this text is aimed at introducing readers to research now underway in the third and fourth areas of brain imaging inquiry as described above. While there are books directed at the basic theories and techniques underlying functional and structural brain imaging, and increasingly books directed at the imaging in the context of cognitive neuroscience, there has been few efforts to date to present the broader scope of work that is now beginning to emerge in the application of brain imaging methods in clinical neuroscience and behavioral medicine.

References

1. Broca PM. The discovery of cerebral localization. *Rev Prat.* 1999;49(16):1725–1727.
2. Geschwind N. *Wernicke's Contribution to the Study of Aphasia.* New York: Butterworth-Heinemann; 1997.
3. Harlow JM. Passage of an iron rod through the head. *J Neuropsychiatry Clin Neurosci.* 1999;11(2):281–283.
4. Milner B. The medial temporal-lobe amnesic syndrome. *Psychiatr Clin North Am.* 2005;28(3):599–611. 609.
5. Heilman KM, Valenstein E. Mechanisms underlying hemispatial neglect. *Ann Neurol.* 1979;5(2):166–170.
6. Bradshaw FL. Pupil size and problem solving. *Q J Exp Psychol.* 1968;20:116–122.
7. Cohen RA, Waters W. Psychophysiological correlates of levels and states of cognitive processing. *Neuropsychologia.* 1985;23(2):243–256.
8. Jennings J, Hall SW. Recall, recognition, and rate: memory and the heart. *Psychophysiology.* 1980;17:37–46.
9. Wilkinson RT, Seales DM. EEG event-related potentials and signal detection. *Biol Psychol.* 1978;7(1–2):13–28.
10. Ciganek L. A comparative study of visual and auditory EEG responses in man. *Electroencephalogr Clin Neurophysiol.* 1965;18:625–629.
11. Mirsky AF, Tecce JJ. The analysis of visual evoked potentials during spike and wave EEG activity. *Epilepsia.* 1968;9(3):211–220.

12. Humphrey NK. Responses to visual stimuli of units in the superior colliculus of rats and monkeys. *Exp Neurol.* 1968;20(3):312–340.
13. Penfield W, Perot P. The brain's record of auditory and visual experience. A final summary and discussion. *Brain.* 1963;86:595–696.
14. Mishkin M, Ungerleider LG. Contribution of striate inputs to the visuospatial functions of parieto-preoccipital cortex in monkeys. *Behav Brain Res.* 1982;6(1):57–77.
15. Jagadeesh B, Chelazzi L, Mishkin M, Desimone R. Learning increases stimulus salience in anterior inferior temporal cortex of the macaque. *J Neurophysiol.* 2001;86(1):290–303.
16. Morrell F, Engel JP Jr, Bouris W. The effect of experience on the firing pattern of visual cortical neurons. *Electroencephalogr Clin Neurophysiol.* 1967;23(1):89.
17. Picton TW. The P300 wave of the human event-related potential. *J Clin Neurophysiol.* 1992;9(4):456–479.
18. Hillyard SA, Hink RF, Schwent VL, Picton TW. Electrical signs of selective attention in the human brain. *Science.* 1973;182(108):177–180.
19. McEvoy LK, Pellouchoud E, Smith ME, Gevins A. Neurophysiological signals of working memory in normal aging. *Brain Res Cogn Brain Res.* 2001;11(3):363–376.
20. Squires KC, Squires NK, Hillyard SA. Decision-related cortical potentials during an auditory signal detection task with cued observation intervals. *J Exp Psychol Hum Percept Perform.* 1975;1(3):268–279.
21. Desolneux A, Lionel Moisan L, Morel JM. *The Helmholtz Principle from Gestalt Theory to Image Analysis: A Probabilistic Approach.* New York: Springer; 2008:31–45.
22. Hjorth B, Rodin E. Extraction of "deep" components from scalp EEG. *Brain Topogr.* 1988;1(1):65–69.
23. O'Donnell BF, Cohen RA, Hokama H, et al. Electrical source analysis of auditory ERPs in medial temporal lobe amnestic syndrome. *Electroencephalogr Clin Neurophysiol.* 1993;87(6):394–402.
24. Halgren E, Raij T, Marinkovic K, Jousmaki V, Hari R. Cognitive response profile of the human fusiform face area as determined by MEG. *Cereb Cortex.* 2000;10(1):69–81.
25. Vieth J. Magnetoencephalography, a new function diagnostic method. *EEG EMG Z Elektroenzephalogr Elektromyogr Verwandte Geb.* 1984;15(2):111–118.
26. Roy C, Sherrington CS. On the regulation of the blood-supply of the brain. *Physiology.* 1890;11(1–2):85–108.
27. Findlay GF. Computer-assisted (axial) tomography in the management of subarachnoid haemorrhage. *Surg Neurol.* 1980;13(2):125–128.
28. Dunker K. *On Problem Solving.* Washington, DC: American Psychological Association; 1945.
29. Ackerman RH, Subramanyam R, Correia JA, Alpert NM, Taveras JM. Positron imaging of cerebral blood flow during continuous inhalation of C15O2. *Stroke.* 1980;11(1):45–49.
30. Yamamoto YL, Thompson CJ, Meyer E, Robertson JS, Feindel W. Dynamic positron emission tomography for study of cerebral hemodynamics in a cross section of the head using positron-emitting ^{68}Ga-EDTA and ^{77}Kr. *J Comput Assist Tomogr.* 1977;1(1):43–56.
31. Hill TC. Single-photon emission computed tomography to study cerebral function in man. *J Nucl Med.* 1980;21(12):1197–1199.

32. Jezzard P, Matthews PM, Smith SM, eds. *Functional MRI: An Introduction to Methods.* New York, NY: Oxford University Press; 2001.
33. Pauling L, Coryell CD. The magnetic properties and structure of the hemochromogens and related substances. *Proc Natl Acad Sci U S A.* 1936;22:159–163.
34. Kwong KK, McKinstry RC, Chien D, Crawley AP, Pearlman JD, Rosen BR. CSF-suppressed quantitative single-shot diffusion imaging. *Magn Reson Med.* 1991;21(1):157–163.
35. Rosen BR, Belliveau JW, Buchbinder BR, et al. Contrast agents and cerebral hemodynamics. *Magn Reson Med.* 1991;19(2):285–292.
36. Ogawa S, Lee TM, Kay AR, Tank DW. Brain magnetic resonance imaging with contrast dependent on blood oxygenation. *Proc Natl Acad Sci U S A.* 1990;87(24):9868–9872.
37. Ogawa S, Lee TM, Nayak AS, Glynn P. Oxygenation-sensitive contrast in magnetic resonance image of rodent brain at high magnetic fields. *Magn Reson Med.* 1990;14(1): 68–78.
38. Crosson B, Rao SM, Woodley SJ, et al. Mapping of semantic, phonological, and orthographic verbal working memory in normal adults with functional magnetic resonance imaging. *Neuropsychology.* 1999;13(2):171–187.
39. Rao SM, Harrington DL, Haaland KY, Bobholz JA, Cox RW, Binder JR. Distributed neural systems underlying the timing of movements. *J Neurosci.* 1997;17(14):5528–5535.
40. Binder JR, Frost JA, Hammeke TA, Cox RW, Rao SM, Prieto T. Human brain language areas identified by functional magnetic resonance imaging. *J Neurosci.* 1997;17(1):353–362.
41. Gsell W, Burke M, Wiedermann D, et al. Differential effects of NMDA and AMPA glutamate receptors on functional magnetic resonance imaging signals and evoked neuronal activity during forepaw stimulation of the rat. *J Neurosci.* 2006;26(33):8409–8416.

Chapter 2
Basic MR Physics: Considerations for Behavioral Medicine and Neuropsychology

Edward G. Walsh

Origin of the Nuclear Induction Signal

From its beginnings as a medical imaging modality in the mid-1980s, magnetic resonance imaging (MRI) has become a dominant modality, combining the ability to provide both structural and physiologic information. The physical principles relating to the production of the nuclear signal were described in the mid-twentieth century, with the publication of the first demonstration of nuclear induction taking place in 1946.[1-3]

Nuclear induction is understood using a quantum mechanical approach. Fortunately, the magnetic resonance phenomenon also lends itself to a classical formalism when dealing with a large number of nuclei, which is always the case when discussing magnetic resonance as an imaging modality. Protons possess properties of mass and momentum, and a quantized property known as spin angular momentum. Spin is a property of both individual particles, and of nuclei. Not all nuclei possess spin. The basic conditions for the existence of spin:

- Nuclei with even mass and charge numbers have zero spin (e.g., ^{12}C).
- Nuclei with odd mass numbers have half integral spin (e.g., ^{13}C).
- Nuclei with odd mass and even charge numbers have integral spin (e.g., ^{14}N).

^{13}C and ^{31}P, for example, have been used for in vivo magnetic resonance spectroscopic studies. For MRI, the ^{1}H nucleus is used due to its abundance and favorable molecular dynamics of water molecules. As a quantized property, nuclear spin can take on only specific values, related to the composition of the nucleus. In the case of ^{1}H, the nuclear spin is 1/2, because the nucleus consists of a single proton, which is a spin 1/2 particle. A consequence of the spin is the generation of a magnetic moment. The spin number of a nucleus dictates the number of orientations that the moment axis can take. For a spin 1/2 particle, there are two possible orientations of the spin axis. In the absence of an external magnetic field, the energy states associated with the two orientations are identical (said to be degenerate). No difference in energy exists between the orientations. This degeneracy is lifted when a nucleus is placed in an external magnetic field.

Prior to placement of a sample (or patient) in a magnetic field (designated $\mathbf{B}_0$), the orientation of the spin axes is random, and the nuclear magnetic dipoles essentially sum to zero, so no net magnetization is developed. When the sample (or patient) is placed in the static field of an MRI scanner, the degeneracy is lifted and the hydrogen nuclei (protons) assume one of the two states describing the alignment of their magnetic moments: either aligned with or against the static field of the scanner (Fig. 2.1). Owing to the fact that the thermal energy of the system is larger than the energy difference between the two alignment states, the population of spins aligned against the static field is nearly identical to the population aligned with the field. Since alignment in the direction of $\mathbf{B}_0$ represents the lower energy state, there is a slight surplus (a few ppm) of spins aligned in the direction of $\mathbf{B}_0$, and a net magnetization in the direction of $\mathbf{B}_0$ is developed within the sample. This is referred to as polarization. Establishment of this distribution

---

E.G. Walsh (✉)
Brown University, Departments of Neuroscience and Diagnostic Imaging, Institute for Brain Science, Providence, RI, USA
e-mail: Edward_Walsh@brown.edu

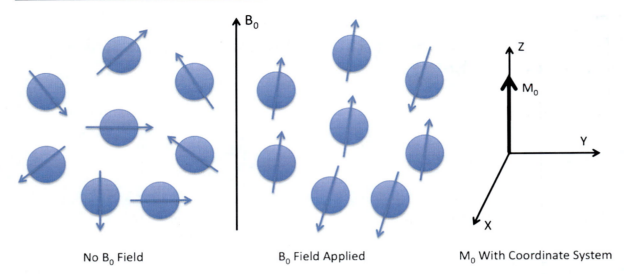

Fig. 2.1 *Left*: In the absence of an applied magnetic field, nuclear magnetic moments are randomly oriented and sum to zero. *Middle*: Application of magnetic field (B_0) causes polarization and resultant sample magnetization. *Right*: Coordinate system used to describe magnetic resonance experiments. Magnetization developed from polarization is defined as being in the z-direction

requires some time, and when the process is complete, the system is said to be in its equilibrium state. Static field strength is expressed in units of Tesla (T). 1 T=10,000 Gauss (G). By way of comparison, the Earth's magnetic field strength is about 0.5 G. Increasing the strength of B_0 from 1.5 to 3 T, for example, increases the difference in the size of the two spin populations, and therefore the magnitude of the sample magnetization (designated M_0). The maximum size of the MR signal is proportional to M_0, so increasing field strength (B_0) increases M_0 and therefore the maximum size of the MR signal. For clinical scanners, field strength ranges from 0.35 (for some open permanent magnet designs) to 3 T. Scanners used in research applications can have higher field strengths. As of this publication, the Food and Drug Administration (FDA) has defined field strengths greater than 8 T as representing a significant risk for humans over 1 month in age.

There is a second aspect to the behavior of the spins in an external magnetic field. The alignment of the spins with and against B_0 is not complete, in that an angle exists between the nuclear magnetic moments and B_0. This results in a precession of the moment about B_0. The frequency of this precession is known as the Larmor frequency and is given by:

$$\omega_L = \gamma B_0 \qquad (2.1)$$

where the constant of proportionality γ is known as the gyromagnetic ratio and is unique for each isotope. For ^1H, $\gamma = 42.58$ MHz/T, so at clinical field strengths, the range of precession frequencies falls within the range of frequencies used for radio communications. It is important to note that the splitting of the spin population into the two states, and resulting precession, does not result in a detectable MR signal. At this point, the phases of the individual spins in precession are random, so the component of the sample magnetization perpendicular to B_0 is zero.

The MRI process involves the manipulation of the magnetization vector **M** in order to produce a detectable signal. This process can be described using a classical formalism. To begin with, once a sample has been placed in the scanner, the net sample magnetization M_0 is developed over a few seconds. M_0 is aligned with B_0 as shown in Fig. 2.1. In the Cartesian reference frame, B_0 is defined as being in the z-direction. In conventional scanners, the z-direction is along the bore, with the x-direction being left-right and the y-direction being up-down. A rotating reference frame (x,y-axes rotate about the z-axis at the Larmor frequency) greatly simplifies the description of the imaging process and is normally used in analyzing MRI acquisition sequences. A radiofrequency magnetic field (designated $\mathbf{B}_1$) applied perpendicular to $\mathbf{B}_0$ *with a frequency equal to the Larmor frequency* will cause some spins in the low-energy state to move to the high-energy state, at the same time placing the precession of the spins in phase. The result is that the vector $\mathbf{M}$ is seen to rotate into the *x–y* plane in the rotating reference frame (Fig. 2.2). In a stationary reference frame $\mathbf{M}$ would be seen to be precessing at the Larmor frequency as it tips down toward the *x–y* axis plane (typically referred to as the transverse plane since it is perpendicular to $\mathbf{B}_0$). This is described as being a *resonance* phenomenon since the application of a $\mathbf{B}_1$ field at a frequency away from the Larmor frequency will not have an effect on the spin population and therefore no action on $\mathbf{M}$.

A radiofrequency resonator, or coil, is configured and oriented to produce a $\mathbf{B}_1$ field perpendicular to $\mathbf{B}_0$. This coil can also detect the precessing magnetization $\mathbf{M}$. The precessing $\mathbf{M}$ will induce a voltage in the coil at the precession (Larmor) frequency that can be amplified and processed. The resonator itself is a resonant circuit at the Larmor frequency. This tuning provides for improved response (stronger signal) at the Larmor frequency and for attenuation of noise away from the Larmor frequency.

The angle (θ) through which $\mathbf{M}$ rotates away from the *z*-axis while under the influence of $\mathbf{B}_1$ is known as the flip angle and is given by:

$$\theta = \gamma B_1 t \quad (2.2)$$

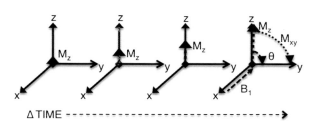

Fig. 2.2 Development of longitudinal magnetization over time following placement of a sample in a static magnetic field ($\mathbf{B}_0$). *Right*: Delivery of an RF pulse ($\mathbf{B}_1$) rotates magnetization into the transverse plane by an angle θ. If the *x,y*-axes rotate about the *z*-axis at the Larmor frequency, precession of the $\mathbf{M}$ vector is removed simplifying visualization of relaxation and the effects of RF pulses. This also reflects the recovery of magnetization following a 90° pulse. Delivering another pulse during the recovery will produce a signal with intensity proportional to the degree of recovery

where B_1 is the strength of the radiofrequency field and t is its duration. Flip angle is an important adjustable contrast parameter for some imaging sequences as will be seen later. Note that like $\mathbf{B}_0$, $\mathbf{B}_1$ is a vector quantity and has both magnitude and direction.

Relaxation

When the spin population has been perturbed by the application of a $\mathbf{B}_1$ field, this new distribution does not remain indefinitely following the termination of $\mathbf{B}_1$. Instead, the equilibrium distribution will re-establish itself over time. The rate at which the equilibrium is restored is given by the longitudinal relaxation time constant, designated T_1. In the rotating reference frame, termination of $\mathbf{B}_1$ stops the rotation of $\mathbf{M}$. In the absence of $\mathbf{B}_1$, the $\mathbf{M}$ vector will be seen to begin moving back toward its equilibrium position on the *z*-axis (aligned with $\mathbf{B}_0$). This recovery (often referred to as relaxation) is described by the longitudinal Bloch equation[1]:

$$\frac{dM_z}{dt} = \frac{M_0 - M_z}{T_1} \quad (2.3)$$

where M_z is the longitudinal (*z*) component of the magnetization ($\mathbf{M}$), M_0 is the equilibrium magnetization (prior to any excitation), and T_1 is the longitudinal relaxation time constant, which is a material-dependent property. Since molecules tumble and translate, a given spin is subjected to a fluctuating magnetic field owing to the motion of nearby nuclear magnetic moments. If the frequency of fluctuation approaches the Larmor frequency, for example, relaxation becomes very efficient and T_1 will be very short. This is the effect exploited by contrast agents such as Gd-DTPA that act to reduce the T_1 of tissues in which they accumulate.

There is a second relaxation process at work simultaneously with the one just described. This process relates to the individual spin precession frequencies. Recall that ω_L varies with the external field strength. A given nucleus is also in the presence of other nuclei, and electrons, and is therefore subject to tiny fluctuations in the field that it experiences (due to the magnetic moments of nearby particles). These in turn produce tiny fluctuations in ω_L. Since these interactions are essentially random, the effect is that the spins gradually go out of phase, and therefore the transverse summation of the magnetic moments decays over time, resulting in a reduction in the transverse component of $\mathbf{M}$ (commonly known as $\mathbf{M}_{xy}$). This is seen as a loss in the amplitude of the observed signal coming from the resonator. Such signals are referred to as free induction decays (FID). The decay rate constant for this process is known as T_2, the spin–spin relaxation rate constant. The transverse magnetization decay is given by the transverse Bloch equation[1]:

$$\frac{dM_{xy}}{dt} = \frac{-M_{xy}}{T_2} \qquad (2.4)$$

The preceding describes the process based on the true T_2 of the sample, the decay rate characteristic to the material. There is another process to consider, and it relates to the fact that the static field produced by the scanner magnet is not perfectly uniform (homogeneous). The actual strength of $\mathbf{B}_0$ can vary by a few ppm over the imaging volume. This field imperfection produces a corresponding distribution in ω_L across the sample, and this distribution also contributes to signal dephasing. Field variations also result from the presence of materials with differing magnetic susceptibility (differing tendency to generate magnetization). The observed decay rate of the signal in the presence of field inhomogeneity is given by the rate constant T_2^*. These two transverse relaxation rates are related as:

$$\frac{1}{T_2^*} = \frac{1}{T_2} + \frac{1}{T'_2} \qquad (2.5)$$

where T_2' is the contribution resulting from field imperfections. It will be seen that T_2^* relaxation processes play a major role in functional MRI of the brain. The decay of the transverse signal is given by the same expression (2.4) used for transverse decay, substituting T_2^* for T_2. It will be shown later that it is possible to separate T_2 and T_2^* using appropriate pulse sequences. Scanners also provide a mechanism for improving the uniformity of the field. The process typically referred to as shimming involves the use of field gradient coils to modify $\mathbf{B}_0$ in order to maximize homogeneity over the volume to be scanned.

Values for T_1 and T_2 depend on field strength and material properties (e.g., molecular correlation times).

Of benefit for MR imaging is that different tissues often have different relaxation time constants. These differences can be exploited for the purpose of generating soft tissue contrast. For example, at 3 T the T_1 of grey matter is about 1,400 ms, while for white matter T_1 is about 800 ms. This difference allows for the generation of excellent contrast between grey and white matter without the use of any exogenous contrast agent.

Now it is appropriate to introduce the concept of flip angle (θ) in the context of signal strength and relaxation. Of particular interest in structural brain imaging is the generation of contrast among grey matter, white matter, and cerebrospinal fluid (CSF). Turning first to longitudinal magnetization, there are two flip angle examples that are relevant for generating contrast. Recall that flip angle is the extent to which the sample magnetization vector $\mathbf{M}$ is rotated by an RF excitation ($\mathbf{B}_1$). If $\mathbf{M}$ is rotated onto the transverse (x–y) plane, a 90° excitation (pulse) has been delivered. In this case, the longitudinal magnetization M_z is zero, and the system is said to be saturated (the populations of spins in the high- and low-energy states are equal). It is possible to continue rotating $\mathbf{M}$ past this point, continuing the excitation until $\mathbf{M}$ lies on the negative z-axis. In this case, a 180° excitation (pulse) has been delivered, and the system is said to be inverted. The inversion excitation is so named since the populations of spins in the two energy states have been exchanged (inverted), with the (same equilibrium) majority of spins now aligned against the field. Based on these excitations, the longitudinal magnetization as a function of time is given as:

$$M_z(t) = M_0(1 - e^{-t/T_1}), \quad \theta = 90° \qquad (2.6)$$

$$M_z(t) = M_0(1 - 2e^{-t/T_1}), \quad \theta = 180° \qquad (2.7)$$

where t is the elapsed time following the termination of the RF excitation. For the transverse magnetization following a 90° pulse:

$$M_{xy}(t) = M_0 e^{-t/T_2^*} \qquad (2.8)$$

where t again represents the elapsed time following the termination of the RF excitation. These expressions (which are solutions to the Bloch equations) assume that the RF pulse is delivered with the spin system at equilibrium (full longitudinal recovery). In imaging studies, it is generally not practical to deliver all excitations with the spin system at equilibrium, as the scans would become prohibitively long.

We now have the information available to measure the T_1 of a sample. Returning to Fig. 2.2, a 90 or 180° can be delivered, followed by a gradient pulse to destroy (spoil) any transverse signal. Gradients will be discussed later, but suffice it to say at this point that turning on a field gradient produces a huge field inhomogeneity that results in very rapid signal dephasing (loss of the transverse component of **M**). Following this, a delay (t) is allowed, during which some longitudinal relaxation takes place. If another 90° pulse is delivered (readout pulse), and the signal received, it is seen that the transverse magnetization intensity is proportional to that of the longitudinal magnetization at the time of the delivery of the readout pulse. If signals are obtained for a range of values of t, the T_1 of the sample (or tissue) can be determined by a curve fit (signal intensity vs. t) to (2.6) (Fig. 2.3). This is T_1 measurement by saturation recovery. It is also possible to use a 180° (inversion) pulse prior to the readout pulse, in which case (2.7) is used. This inversion recovery method has the advantage of doubling the dynamic range of longitudinal magnetization and produces more accurate T_1 estimation (or more contrast in images). It will be seen that these methods can also produce soft tissue contrast, for example, between grey and white matter since they possess different T_1 values. For imaging, the initial 90 or 180° pulse is known as a contrast pulse, or contrast preparation pulse, and will be followed by a pulse sequence (readout sequence) for reading spatially encoded image information.

Turning now to T_2 and T_2^*, it was noted that the first value is a property of the material under consideration, and the second adds the effects of static field inhomogeneity. To separate these two effects, a pulse sequence is needed that can "undo" the effect of the static (time invariant) inhomogeneities. Such a sequence can be formed using two RF pulses, a 90° pulse followed by a 180° degree pulse. This is shown in Fig. 2.4. Note that there are no spoiler gradients. The transverse magnetization is preserved throughout the sequence. As shown

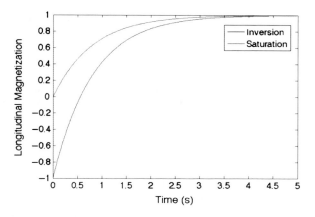

Fig. 2.3 Magnetization vs. postsaturation or inversion time of a material with a T_1 of 1 s. Use of inversion doubles the dynamic range in the longitudinal magnetization

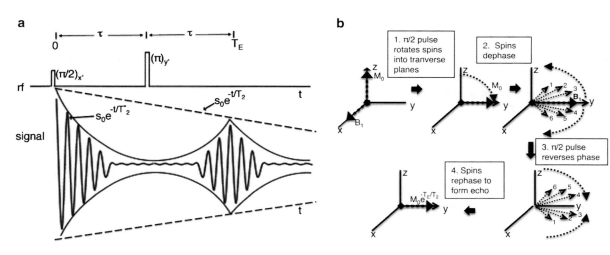

Fig. 2.4 *Left*: Spin echo pulse and signal diagram. The 90° ($\pi/2$) pulse produces a free induction decay (FID) that decays according to T_2^*. The 180° (π) pulse refocuses an echo at the echo time with amplitude reflecting the true T_2. *Right*: Effect of the refocusing pulse on the temporal evolution of magnetization in different parts of an inhomogeneous field

in Fig. 2.4, a 90° pulse (**B**₁) delivered on the *x*-axis rotates **M** onto the *y*-axis. The transverse magnetization (M_{xy}) now begins to dephase in the presence of static field inhomogeneity. In regions of lower field, precession takes place more slowly, and vice versa. After a delay (designated TE/2), a 180° pulse (**B**₁) is delivered on the *y*-axis. This rotates the vectors such that those that had fallen behind in phase (lower field strength) have been placed ahead in phase, and those that had been precessing faster (higher field strength) have been placed behind in phase. Note, however, that the static field has not changed its configuration (pattern of inhomogeneity). Those spins in higher field strength regions still process faster than those in lower field strength regions. As seen in the rotating (at the Larmor frequency) reference frame, the spin vectors converge on the *y*-axis, and full "refocusing" takes place after another interval TE/2. At this point, the signal intensity reaches a maximum. This is known as a spin echo,[4] and at its peak intensity, the signal loss against M_0 is the only result of random dephasing effects from spin interaction, which cannot be recovered. The effect of the static field inhomogeneity was removed by the 180° pulse. Thus, the spin echo allows signal strength measurement (and image contrast) based on the true T_2 of the sample. The elapsed time from the center of the 90° pulse to the peak of the spin echo is known as the echo time, designated TE. Measurement of T_2 can be carried out by acquiring a number of signals corresponding to different values of TE. A curve fit (signal intensity vs. TE) to (2.8) can be performed to determine T_2.

We can now modify these expressions to take into account excitation repetition times (designated TR) in order to compute signal strengths for cases where repetition times are much shorter than the time required for full recovery of longitudinal magnetization (typically defined as $5T_1$). Figure 2.5 shows the longitudinal magnetization starting at equilibrium (M_0) when subjected to a string of 90° pulses when TR is too short to permit full recovery to M_0. In this situation, M_z does not recover to M_0, but rather, arrives at some intermediate value at the moment that the next excitation is delivered. That value is given by:

$$M_z(\text{TR}) = M_0(1 - e^{-\text{TR}/T_1}) \quad (2.9)$$

In the case of inversion recovery:

$$M_z(\text{TR,TI}) = M_0(1 - 2e^{-\text{TI}/T_1} + e^{-\text{TR}/T_1}) \quad (2.10)$$

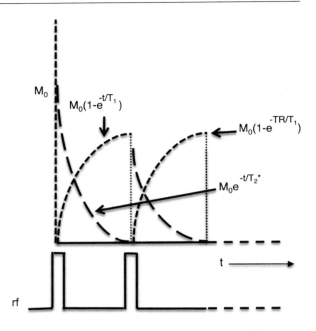

Fig. 2.5 Longitudinal magnetization over a string of 90° pulses. Reducing TR reduces available time for the recovery of longitudinal magnetization and therefore less signal results

where TI (the inversion time) is the interval between the 180° preparation pulse and the 90° readout pulse. As in the case of the fully relaxed initial condition, it is possible to use these expressions to determine T_1 using a curve fit. Imaging of patients is almost always done using sequences with repetition times much shorter than $5T_1$. In general, total scan session times of less than 1 hour are desired from the standpoint of patient tolerance. Patient tolerance can vary considerably depending on patient condition, and imaging protocols are designed with physiological and behavioral characteristics taken into account to the extent possible.

Spatial Encoding

MRI is a tomographic technique, in that it produces image information representing cross-sections through the patient. A significant advantage for MRI is that tomographic planes can be arbitrarily selected. In addition to the standard (orthogonal) transverse, sagittal, and coronal views, it is possible to angle tomographic planes according to the individual anatomy to be examined. Clinical scanners facilitate this process by allowing graphic prescription of image planes based on a fast scout scan. The operator simply moves an outline overlay over the displayed scout images to define the tomographic slices to be obtained in the subsequent scan. The scanner software takes care of the mathematics relating the selected image planes to the standard orthogonal views.

In the previous discussions, the processes of signal formation and decay were discussed. These signals did not contain any spatial information, and arose from the entire sample (or patient) in the scanner. In order to produce tomographic images, it is necessary to have three dimensions of spatial encoding imposed on the MR signals. This is accomplished using linear field gradients,[5–8] which can be switched on and off very rapidly. Every patient scanner is equipped with a set of field windings that can generate a linear field gradient on each (x,y,z) axis. The individual gradient channels (one for each direction) can be independently switched. These gradient systems are manufactured to high tolerances such that a field linearity specification of at least 95% can be achieved, typically over a diameter spherical volume (DSV) of 45–50 cm. The purpose of the field gradients is to cause the static field (B_0) to vary in a linear fashion with distance on each axis from the central point of the scanner's defined imaging volume. The consequence of turning on a gradient is that the Larmor frequency (ω_0) will also vary in a linear fashion with position along the gradient direction. The gradient systems are designed such that there is a point where the field does not vary when a gradient is turned on. This point is common for all three gradient axes, and is known as the isocenter. The isocenter represents the center of the DSV mentioned above. Figure 2.6 shows what happens when a gradient is turned on. On one side of isocenter, the field decreases, and on the other, it increases, and at isocenter, it does not change. The B_0 field strength and Larmor frequency now become:

$$B(x) = B_0 + Gx \quad (2.11)$$

$$\omega(x) = \gamma(B_0 + Gx) \quad (2.12)$$

where x is the distance from isocenter (and can be positive or negative depending on direction), and G is the gradient strength, typically expressed in units of G/cm or mT/m. Current clinical scanners can generate maximum field strengths ranging up to 4.5 G/cm (implications for rapid imaging performance). As opposed to the main field windings of superconducting magnets, the resistive gradient field windings are designed to be switched on and off very rapidly. Switching times are typically on the order of a few hundred microseconds. Gradient switching rate is also an important specification with respect to rapid imaging performance.

At this point it is necessary to introduce the Fourier transform. The Fourier transform is an operation that relates a time domain signal (the FID or spin echo) to its frequency spectrum. As noted above, delivering a 90° excitation to a water sample produces a monoexponential decay at the Larmor frequency. The Fourier transform of that signal will be a single peak at the Larmor frequency. If this simple spectrum is shifted to the rotating reference frame, the peak moves to a frequency of zero relative to the Larmor frequency.

It was previously mentioned that a gradient is a form of B_0 inhomogeneity that results in very rapid decay of signals. For the time being, dephasing will be ignored in this discussion of spatial encoding. Dephasing, and the means of undoing it, will be discussed in the section on image acquisition pulse sequences. Delivering a 90° excitation produces a signal (FID) at the Larmor frequency that decays over time in a monoexponential fashion. Now consider the case of an object in the scanner, at some distance from isocenter in the x-direction (horizontal displacement). This object is a cube filled with water and is 1 cm on each side, and the center of the cube is 2 cm from the isocenter. After delivering the 90° excitation, a gradient in the x-direction is turned on with strength equal to 1 G/cm. The first observation is that the signal has a complex appearance (Fig. 2.7). Recall that the Larmor frequency now varies as a function of position in the x-direction. Since the object is of finite extent, it is producing a signal whose frequency

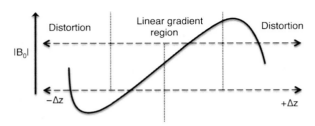

Fig. 2.6 Effect of linear gradient application. B_0 and therefore the Larmor frequency vary linearly with distance from the isocenter (the point where B_0 does not change when the gradient is switched on). Beyond the designed linear region of the field gradient coils, linearity is lost and geometric distortion results

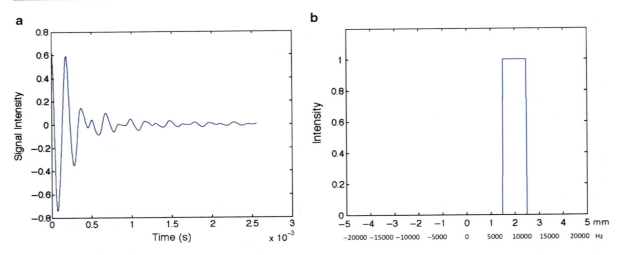

Fig. 2.7 *Top*: Signal produced by a 1 cm cube centered 2 cm from the isocenter. *Bottom*: Fourier transform of the signal showing frequency offset and extent

content is determined by its spatial distribution. The 1 cm cube is centered 2 cm from isocenter in the *x*-direction, therefore its spatial extent covers from 1.5 to 2.5 cm away from the isocenter. Using (2.12), this means that its extent in frequency space is 6,387–10,645 Hz. The Fourier transform shows the presence of signal covering that frequency range (Fig. 2.7). Signal intensity in the transform is uniform across that frequency range indicating that there is the same amount of material at all frequency components. There is no signal at any other frequency component since there was only a single object present. Thus, by turning on the gradient during signal collection, it was possible to determine the location and spatial extent of the object in the gradient direction by examining the frequency content of the signal (as well as estimating the shape of the object). This method is known as frequency encoding, and is used to spatially encode one of the in-plane dimensions of MR images.

MR imaging is a tomographic method, and in order to form tomographic images, it is necessary to possess the capability of exciting a thin slab of spins in the patient, while leaving everything else unaffected. We only want signal to arise from the slice of interest. How is this accomplished? Two components are needed: a gradient and a frequency selective RF excitation. Recall from the section "Origin of the Nuclear Induction Signal" that an RF excitation was delivered at the Larmor frequency to the entire sample to produce a FID. Now, a frequency selective pulse and a gradient will be used to limit the excitation to a defined range of frequencies, corresponding to a specific spatial extent within the scanned object. With respect to the cube example, suppose we want to excite a slab of that cube, 5 mm wide, and centered within the cube. This would place the center of the excited slab 2 cm from isocenter in the *x*-direction. If we turn on the 1 G/cm gradient, a distance of 2 cm corresponds to a frequency offset of 8,516 Hz. We have also specified a slab thickness of 5 mm. A spatial extent of 5 mm centered at $x=2$ cm implies a frequency range of 7,452–9,581 Hz according to (2.12). This frequency range is contained completely within the frequency range for the entire cube. If we offset the frequency of the pulse by +8,516 Hz, its frequency will now correspond to the Larmor frequency at the center of the cube when the gradient is turned on. We need, however, to excite material over the range of frequencies just mentioned while excluding the rest. Therefore, we need an excitation that has a matching frequency content. Ideally, this excitation should have a frequency content of uniform intensity, beginning at +7,452 Hz and ending at +9,581 Hz, and having no other frequency components. This corresponds to a spectral width of 2,129 Hz. Taking the Fourier transform of such a rectangular function in frequency space results in a function in the time domain of the form:

$$B_1(t) = \frac{\sin(t)}{t} \quad (2.13)$$

This waveform is shown in Fig. 2.8, and it often referred to as a sinc pulse. The frequency content of

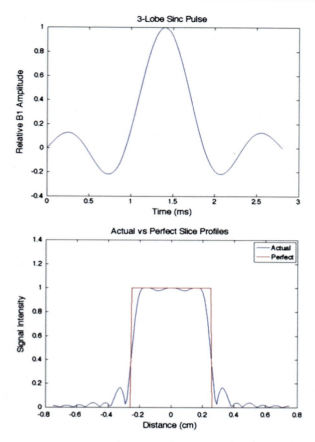

Fig. 2.8 *Top*: Typical three-cycle sinc pulse suitable for use in imaging sequences. *Bottom*: Corresponding slice profile showing the effects of truncation to limit pulse duration to an acceptable value

this pulse is determined by the interval between the zero-crossings of the waveform, with the bandwidth given by:

$$\Delta t = \frac{2}{\Delta f} \quad (2.14)$$

where Δt is the interval between zero-crossings and Δf is the bandwidth of the excitation. For the situation that we are currently considering, a bandwidth of 2,129 Hz is needed, and this corresponds to a zero-crossing interval of 0.939 ms. It should be noted at this point that the Fourier transform of a perfectly rectangular frequency function is a sinc function of infinite extent. RF excitations of infinite extent are not compatible with minimizing the duration of imaging studies for patient tolerance. Therefore, the sinc pulse is truncated. A three-lobed waveform can be used as shown in Fig. 2.8. The duration of this pulse will be $3\Delta t$ or 2.82 ms. This pulse duration is compatible with MR imaging requirements. The consequence of truncating the sinc waveform is some degree of compromise in the excitation profile as shown in Fig. 2.8, where it is seen that there is some out-of-slice excitation accompanied by some "ripple" across the excited slab. This plot was generated using a numerical solution of the Bloch equation describing the motion of **M** during the application of $\mathbf{B}_1$ (the RF excitation). For typical diagnostic imaging applications, these compromises have negligible effect on the images. Other waveforms are available for use when tailoring some aspect of the slice profile (e.g., out-of-slice excitation) to reduce interaction between neighboring slices.

From the foregoing, the procedure for slice positioning is clear. The plane of the slice is determined by the gradient that is turned on during delivery of the RF excitation: z-gradient gives a transverse slice, x-gradient gives a sagittal slice, and y-gradient gives a coronal slice. Gradient channels can be combined to give angulated slices. For example, if both the z- and y-gradients are turned on at the same time, and with the same strength during excitation, the resulting slice will be angulated 45° off the transverse orientation toward the coronal plane. Fortunately, the scanner operator does not have to perform any computations to obtain such angulations. Scanner software takes care of all calculations relating to gradient assignment in a user-transparent fashion. The operator simply selects the desired plane (and other relevant imaging parameters) and initiates the scan. Slice offset (from isocenter) and slice thickness are determined by the frequency offset and bandwidth of the RF excitation, and by the gradient strength. The dependencies are:

- For fixed gradient strength:
  - Increasing frequency offset increases slice offset
  - Increasing excitation bandwidth increases slice thickness
- For fixed frequency offset:
  - Increasing gradient strength reduces slice offset
  - Changing gradient polarity moves slice to opposite side of isocenter with the same offset distance

- For fixed excitation bandwidth:
  - Increasing gradient strength reduces slice thickness

The opposites apply for the above, so for example, decreasing gradient strength for fixed frequency offset increases the slice offset. As with gradient assignments for selection of image planes, these parameters are all set in a user-transparent fashion.

We now have two dimensions of spatial encoding and it remains to describe the process for generating the remaining in-plane spatial encoding, but first it will be helpful to introduce the concept of k-space.[9] As seen in the discussion on frequency encoding, the profile of the object was revealed by taking the Fourier transform of the MR signal. For images, the Fourier transform relates the spatial representation of an object to its spatial frequency representation. In MR imaging, the signals that are being produced by the pulse sequences are pieces of the spatial frequency representation of the object. When the signals are assembled into a matrix, this matrix will be the frequency space representation of the viewable image. The Fourier transform is then applied to produce the viewable image

The remaining spatial encoding process is known as phase encoding, and is a bit more complicated in its description than the processes for the other two dimensions in that it "builds up" information using a succession of gradient pulses. As shown in Fig. 2.9, the application of the short duration pulse changes the start location in the other in-plane direction for the k-line to be sampled. This phase shift is proportional to the shape, strength, and duration of the gradient pulse, and also on the distance of the object from the isocenter:

$$\Delta \varphi = \gamma x \int_0^T G(t) \, dt \qquad (2.15)$$

where $\Delta \phi$ is the phase shift, x is the distance from the isocenter, $G(t)$ is the gradient waveform shape function, and T is the duration of the gradient waveform. As seen in Fig. 2.9, if this process is repeated for a number of times, then it is possible to build up the same sort of information that was obtained using the frequency encode gradient applied in the other direction. The reason for using such a method to build information for one of the spatial dimensions will become clear in the discussion on image acquisition pulse sequences. With slice selection, frequency encoding, and phase encoding, we now have three orthogonal dimensions of spatial encoding that permit magnetic resonance to be used as a tomographic imaging modality. Two of the gradient assignments will always be used for in-plane spatial encoding and the third will be used for slice selection.

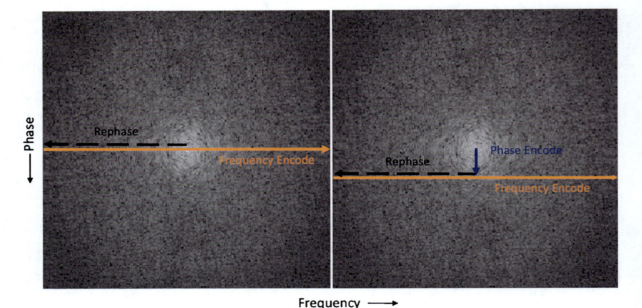

Fig. 2.9 Assembly of raw frequency space image data from MR signals acquired using multiple phase encode steps. The phase encode gradient pulse determines the starting position for the line to be read out using the frequency encoding gradient pulse

For the basic orthogonal planes (transverse, sagittal, and coronal), example gradient assignments would be:

- Axial (transverse)
  - Slice select $= z$
  - Frequency encode $= y$
  - Phase encode $= x$

- Sagittal
  - Slice select $= x$
  - Frequency encode $= z$
  - Phase encode $= y$

- Coronal
  - Slice select $= y$
  - Frequency encode $= z$
  - Phase encode $= x$

Note that for the two in-plane dimensions, the gradient assignments can be exchanged. In some applications, however, the patient geometry with respect to the desired field of view (FOV) dictates a specific assignment. The reason for this is that in the phase encode direction, any material outside of the specified FOV will be aliased back into the image (known as a fold-over artifact), a consequence of the Nyquist sampling condition.

Field of view in the frequency encode direction is determined by the range of frequencies that the scanner is instructed to receive. Recall from the preceding discussion that in the presence of a gradient, a range of Larmor frequency exists across an object. By restricting the range of frequencies that the scanner processes, the FOV can be limited. Specifically:

$$FOV_{Freq} = \frac{SW}{G_{Freq}} \qquad (2.16)$$

where the FOV_{Freq} is in units of cm, SW is the spectral width (receive bandwidth) in units of Hz, and G_{Freq} is the frequency encode gradient strength in units of Hz/cm (for example, a 1 G/cm gradient corresponds to 4,258 Hz/cm). In the phase encode direction, the FOV is determined by the amount by which the area under the gradient waveform is incremented, which is also equal to the smallest gradient pulse to be applied:

$$FOV_{Phase} = \frac{1}{\gamma \int_0^T G_{min}(t)\,dt} \qquad (2.17)$$

This increment insures that the Nyquist sampling theorem is observed in order to prevent aliasing. As with other parameters mentioned, the operator simply specifies the FOV, and the calculations for establishing encoding gradient strengths, durations, and the phase encode increment are performed in the background.

Although one cannot make a diagnosis from the frequency space representation of a brain image, there are certain characteristics to the k-space formalism that are helpful to know when selecting or designing acquisition sequences. Figure 2.10 shows how information is distributed in k-space. From the brain image example, it is seen that most of the signal energy is contained near the center of the k-space representation. The center of k-space ($k=0$) is the zero spatial frequency point. Spatial frequency, expressed in units of inverse distance (e.g., cm^{-1}) increases with increasing distance from $k=0$. Low spatial frequency information (near the center) deals primarily with contrast and representation of large areas. High spatial frequency information (away from $k=0$) deals with edges and fine details. How far out into k-space one samples determines the spatial resolution of the images. Figure 2.11 shows the effect of altering information content in k-space. In the low-pass filter example, it is seen that by removing high spatial frequency information, that contrast is preserved, but the image is blurred (edges and fine detail are lost) and has a lower effective spatial resolution. In the opposite case, removing the low spatial frequency information removes most of the contrast, but edge and fine detail information are preserved. The image acquisition pulse sequences are designed to fill k-space to a degree adequate for various applications within the limits of scanner performance and scan time tolerance.

Image Acquisition Pulse Sequences

Having discussed the three dimensions of spatial encoding, it is now appropriate to assemble the encoding tasks into a single sequence of events that will yield data that can be reconstructed into viewable images. For the purpose of simplification, the discussion of spatial encoding did not take into account the dephasing effect of gradient application. This dephasing will now be dealt with, and the solution to gradient dephasing involves, not surprisingly, additional gradients. To begin with, we will construct a gradient echo sequence. This is the

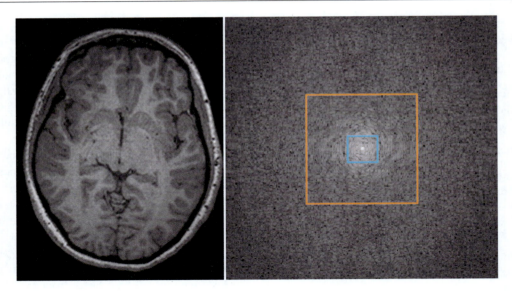

Fig. 2.10 Distribution of signal energy in *k*-space. *Left*: Brain image and *Right*: Fourier transform of the brain image. Most signal energy is near the center (*blue box*) corresponding to low spatial frequencies (large features and contrast). Higher spatial frequency information (*orange box*) defines edges and fine detail

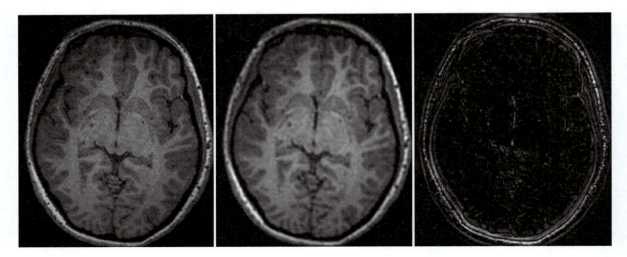

Fig. 2.11 Effect of altering *k*-space content. *Left*: Acquired full *k*-space brain image. *Center*: Blurring effect of removing outer 60% of *k*-space data. *Right*: Effect of removing inner 12% of *k*-space data (essentially a high pass filter leaving mostly edge information)

simplest sequence and it is used to generate images with T_1 and/or T_2^* contrast. Beginning with slice selection (Fig. 2.12), it was shown that the delivery of a frequency selective excitation in the presence of a gradient allows for excitation of a designated slab. It is now necessary to take into account the fact that the slice selection gradient also dephases the transverse magnetization. The solution to this problem is the application of a second gradient pulse, opposite in polarity to, and half the duration of the slice select pulse (assuming the same amplitude but opposite polarity). The effect of this pulse is to undo the dephasing that took place during the slice select excitation. Note that the duration of the slice rephasing gradient can be reduced by increasing its amplitude. The important condition is that the area under the gradient waveform (its integral) be half that of the slice select gradient.

Next we will add the phase encode gradient. In Fig. 2.12, the phase encode gradient is shown as occurring in the same time interval as the slice rephase gradient.

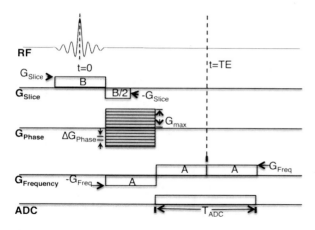

Fig. 2.12 Gradient echo pulse sequence. Following slice selection, the slice rephase, phase encode, and read rephase gradients occur in the same time interval since these activities are mutually orthogonal. The phase encode increment (ΔG_p) is given by (2.17)

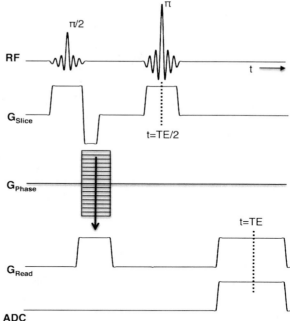

Fig. 2.13 Spin echo sequence. The 180° refocusing pulse reverses the temporal arrangement of the individual spin vectors as shown in Fig. 2.4, resulting in the formation of an echo whose peak intensity arrives at $t=TE$, which is twice the interval between the 90 and 180° pulses. The frequency encode gradient rephasing pulse is of the same polarity as the frequency encode gradient itself due to the presence of the 180° RF pulse

This is valid because the two gradients are orthogonal. They do not have any mutual effect. In the diagram, the horizontal bars indicate that the phase encode gradient amplitude is incremented on successive repetitions of the sequence by an amount given by (2.17). For example, if a 256^2 image is being acquired, there will be 256 repetitions of the sequence, each with a different value of the phase encode gradient (other pulses remain unchanged). There is no rephase gradient associated with the phase encode gradient in the basic gradient echo sequence.

The remaining function is frequency encoding. This gradient also requires a rephase gradient, and it is placed before the encoding gradient, in the same time interval containing the slice rephase and phase encode gradients. As with the slice select rephase, the frequency encode rephase gradient is opposite in polarity to the frequency encode gradient, and the integral under the waveform is 1/2 that of the frequency encode gradient. Again, this placement is valid since the gradients are orthogonal and there is no mutual interaction. The benefit to placing these three functions into the same time interval is that the minimum achievable echo time (TE) is reduced over the case where the gradient pulses occur consecutively. This reduction in sequence execution time also allows for a reduction in the minimum achievable repetition time (TR) and for improved immunity to motion artifacts. Finally, the read gradient is turned on, along with the receiver in order to capture the signal. The sequence is referred to as a gradient echo (or gradient refocused echo) since the frequency encode rephase gradient is used to prepare the transverse magnetization to be refocused by the frequency encode gradient. This differs from the spin echo sequence that uses a 180° RF pulse to refocus spins to produce an echo. A significant difference between the two is that the spin echo sequence removes the effect of static field inhomogeneity, and this produces images that are contrast weighted according to T_2. The gradient echo sequence does not eliminate the effects of static field inhomogeneity (the echo is produced by gradient polarity switching) and produces images that are contrast weighted according to T_2^*. These contrast weightings assume that $TR \gg T_1$ so that there is no T_1 contribution to the result. By reducing TR, some T_1 character can be imparted to the contrast.

The spin echo sequence adds a 180° pulse for echo formation. In Fig. 2.13, it is seen that this pulse is also slice selective in order to excite the same material as excited by the 90° pulse. Note that there is no rephase gradient. Since a 180° excitation undoes the dephasing effect of static field inhomogeneities, it also undoes the dephasing effect of its own slice select gradient. Optionally, the slice selective 180° excitation can be centered between two gradient pulses of equal amplitude and same polarity. These gradients (sometimes called "primer-crusher" gradients) spoil undesired transverse magnetization produced as a result of the imperfect slice profile (discussed previously) as well as that resulting from slight variations in the actual flip angle of the 180° excitation across the FOV. Both the spin echo and the gradient echo sequences can be preceded by a saturation or inversion pulse for the production of contrast weighted by T_1.

A third pulse sequence is a variation on the gradient echo and is designed for rapid image acquisition. It is known as the echo-planar method and it is the most common technique used for image acquisition in brain fMRI studies. The echo-planar imaging (EPI) method can acquire all the information needed for image formation using a single RF excitation. For a given level of gradient performance, the matrix size limit (number of phase encode lines) is limited by the T_2^* of the tissue (since this is a variation on the gradient echo acquisition). The basic idea is to take advantage of the ability to refocus echoes by reversing frequency encode gradient polarity (as seen in the gradient echo). Figure 2.14 shows a pulse sequence diagram for a basic EPI acquisition. Slice selection takes place with the sequences mentioned previously. The frequency encode gradient starts with the rephase pulse as seen with the gradient and spin echo sequences. In EPI, the frequency encode gradient is then repeatedly switched in polarity to produce a string of echoes. The receiver is turned on for the entire readout duration. On the phase encode channel, a gradient pulse positions the acquisition at the end line of k-space. As the frequency encode gradient is switched, the phase encode gradient is pulsed very briefly to advance the phase to the next line to be acquired. The frequency encode and phase encode processes continue until the specified number of lines have been acquired. Since the frequency encode gradient is switching polarity on each line of data acquired, it is necessary to "reverse" one half of the lines prior to the Fourier transform when reconstructing EPI images. A limiting factor in the achievable spatial resolution of EPI is the T_2^* of the sample. As the string of echoes is being generated, transverse magnetization is decaying

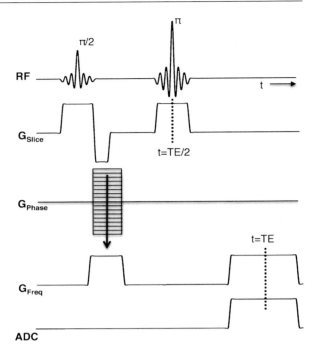

Fig. 2.14 Echo-planar sequence. Following a single RF pulse, reversals of the read gradient polarity refocus echoes. Short phase encode pulses are used to advance lines through k-space as shown in Fig. 2.9

according to the T_2^* of the tissue. If the sequence execution time is, for example, longer than $2T_2^*$, the echoes acquired at the end of the sequence will have very little amplitude compared with the echoes taken near the start of the sequence and will not contribute anything of significance to the image information. In other words, that part of k-space will have very little amplitude, and it will be as if a filter were applied to the data. For this reason, single-shot EPI acquisitions typically use matrix sizes of 64^2–128^2. Of particular concern for brain fMRI imaging is a requirement that the effective echo time of the acquisition (the point where the $k=0$ and nearby lines are acquired) be approximately equal to the T_2^* of grey matter, which is approximately 30 ms at 3 T. Use of this echo time maximizes the contrast effect produced by blood flow and deoxyhemoglobin changes associated with (and occurring subsequent to) cerebral activation. Single-shot EPI resolution is significantly less than that is obtained using conventional gradient echo or spin echo structural imaging where matrix sizes of 256^2–512^2 are common. Multiple-shot EPI acquisitions are possible, where a different segment of k-space is sampled on each acquisition in order to increase the matrix size (and spatial resolution) but motion effects produce artifacts when the individual groups of lines are combined for reconstruction (correction methods are available for reducing such artifacts). Multiple-shot acquisitions also reduce the temporal resolution for fMRI time series imaging protocols since multiple repetition time intervals are needed to form one image frame.

For the imaging sequences just described, it is not unusual to have TR much longer than the time required to execute the sequence. This allows for interleaved slice acquisition. Rather than acquire all the image information for one slice before moving on to the next, a number of sequence executions can take place in the TR interval in which each individual sequence execution uses a different slice selection frequency offset to excite individual slices. For example, if 12 ms are required to execute a gradient echo sequence, and the TR is 1,000 ms, it is possible to execute the sequence 83 times, with each execution exciting and retrieving information from a different slice (by changing the RF pulse frequency offset). By this means, one can acquire image data for 83 slices in the same amount of time required for the acquisition of a single slice. To minimize any "crosstalk" effects resulting from imperfect slice profiles, the slices can be acquired in such a manner that the odd numbered slices (1,3,5,...) are acquired in the first half of the TR interval, then the even numbered slices (2,4,6...) in the second half.

It is also possible to use phase encoding in the slice direction. This is done with so-called 3D acquisitions. Slice phase encoding is done by using a non-selective RF excitation (or excitation of a wide slab corresponding to the entire stack of slices desired). The RF excitation is then followed by a phase encode gradient in the slice direction. For a gradient echo sequence, this slice phase encoding takes place in the same time interval as the in-plane phase encoding and frequency encode rephase gradients. A significant advantage to these acquisitions is the ability to generate very thin slices, typically thinner than possible using conventional slice selection methods due to gradient strength limits. With 3D acquisitions, it is possible to generate image datasets with isotropic resolution (slice thickness equal to the in-plane resolution) of better than 1 mm for whole-head scans. A caveat is that since the slice direction is phase encoded, there must not be any tissue outside of the volume to be imaged in the slice direction or else aliasing will result. Another caveat is that these acquisitions can be lengthy if TR is not very short. Contrast preparations can be used with 3D sequences by segmenting the acquisition of k-space data. An advantage for isotropic resolution datasets is that a single acquisition can be reformatted for viewing in different orientations. For example, a dataset acquired in the transverse orientation can be easily reformatted for viewing as sagittal or coronal images.

Contrast

MRI has the ability to generate contrast between many types of soft tissue without the need for contrast agents. Generally, this is done by exploiting differing T_1, T_2, and $T_2{}^*$ values between tissue types. For anatomic (structural) imaging of the brain, the materials of interest are grey matter, white matter, and CSF. Table 2.1 shows the approximate relaxation time constants for brain[10–18]:

At 3 T, it is seen that the percent difference in T_1 for grey and white matter is greater than that for T_2. For generating contrast between grey and white matter, it is preferable to generate contrast by using sequences with T_1 contrast weighting. This approach also allows the use of minimum echo times to reduce motion sensitivity.

One mechanism for generating T_1 contrast is known as partial saturation. As mentioned in "Relaxation" section, by delivering excitation with a repetition rate $TR < 5T_1$, that longitudinal recovery will not be complete when successive excitations take place. Materials with different T_1 will recover to different degrees, and therefore the signals produced will differ in amplitude. Figure 2.15 shows a plot of signal intensity vs. TR for grey and white matter at 3 T. Taking the difference between the two curves shows the TR at which the signal difference (contrast) is maximized. By acquiring a gradient echo image at that value of TR, a T_1 weighted image will be produced. In this case, the echo time (TE) is set to the shortest possible value in order to

Table 2.1 Approximate Relaxation Time Constants for Brain at 1.5 T and 3 T

Tissue	T_1 1.5 T	T_2 1.5 T	T_1 3 T	T_2 3 T
Grey	1,090	100	1,400	80
White	630	70	805	50
CSF	3,840	2,600	4,200	3,000

minimize T_2^* contribution to the contrast. As seen in the left image of Fig. 2.16, there is contrast between the grey and white matter.

It is possible, however, to improve the level of contrast over that available using partial saturation. As discussed in "Relaxation" section, the T_1 of a sample can be measured using inversion recovery. This involved placing a 180° (inversion) excitation and delay in front of a signal readout pulse. Such a process can also be used for imaging. In this case, the 180° excitation and delay can be placed in front of a gradient echo sequence. One can even set the inversion recovery delay (TI) to null either grey or white matter, which can be considered the ultimate in contrast. As shown in (2.10), the value of TI required to null signal from a tissue is also influenced by the selection of TR. Inversion recovery is the preferred method for generating grey–white contrast in structural brain imaging. It is also possible to generate T_1 contrast using a 90° excitation in front of the image readout. This is known as saturation recovery. Inversion recovery, however, doubles the dynamic range $(-M_0 \to M_0)$ of the longitudinal magnetization over saturation recovery $(0 \to M_0)$ and therefore produces more contrast (Fig. 2.16), and allows for the nulling of one component based on its T_1 if desired.

T_2 contrast weighting is also of use in brain imaging. Note that from Table 2.1 it is seen that there is a very substantial difference between the T_2 of CSF and those of grey and white matter. This is a consequence of CSF consisting largely of free water. The small mobile water molecules experience considerable motion, such that the interactions between neighboring magnetic dipoles are more completely randomized and cancel to a greater degree than for less mobile molecules, resulting in a very long T_2 compared with tissue water, which is much less mobile and therefore subject to greater dephasing effects. T_2 contrast is generated using the spin echo sequence, which has the ability to cancel effects due to $\mathbf{B}_0$ inhomogeneity, leaving only the true T_2 decay of the signal. In this case, one sets the TE based on the maximum difference between the signal curves (signal vs. TE) based on the T_2 values to be distinguished. In the case of CSF, a long echo time, typically 100–200 ms, will be used such that some tissue

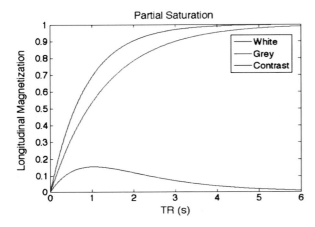

Fig. 2.15 Partial saturation signal intensity vs. TR for grey and white matter at 3 T. Also shown is the difference signal, which reaches its maximum at TR ≈ 1,000 ms. This TR value will produce the maximum grey–white contrast for a partial saturation acquisition

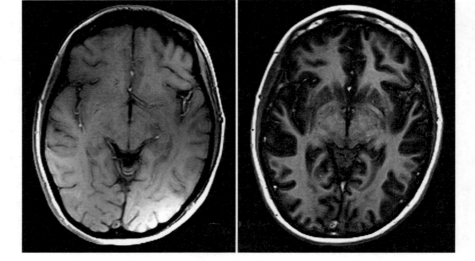

Fig. 2.16 Contrast examples at 3 T: partial saturation with TR = 1,000 ms gives grey–white contrast. *Right*: Inversion recovery produces substantially more contrast between grey and white matter

signal remains for reference purposes, and the CSF compartments return high signal intensity. This sensitivity to free water makes T_2 contrast a preferred method for imaging following stroke, where regions of edema (accumulation of extracellular water) will return higher signal intensity than normal tissue (Fig. 2.17).

It is also possible to generate contrast based on T_2^*. This is done using a gradient echo or echo-planar sequence with a suitable TE. As indicated in "Relaxation" section, the gradient echo does not compensate for the effects of static field ($\mathbf{B}_0$) inhomogeneity. T_2^* weighted sequences are therefore useful for examining tissues where susceptibility gradients on a small scale can exist, for example, from iron deposition in tissue. Brain fMRI scanning is done using T_2^* weighted sequences since the objective is to be sensitive to blood oxygenation changes, and the magnetic susceptibility of oxyhemoglobin is less than that of deoxyhemoglobin. A caveat regarding T_2^* weighting relates to the range of echo times that are feasible. Increasing TE increases the sensitivity of the sequence to $\mathbf{B}_0$ inhomogeneity – any inhomogeneity, whether it arises from tissue structure on a small scale, or from large susceptibility gradients that result from air–tissue interfaces as seen with the orbitofrontal cortex (which borders the sinuses), or from inhomogeneity resulting from field shim errors. Long echo times in the presence of such inhomogeneities results in geometric distortion or even signal loss as shown in Fig. 2.18.

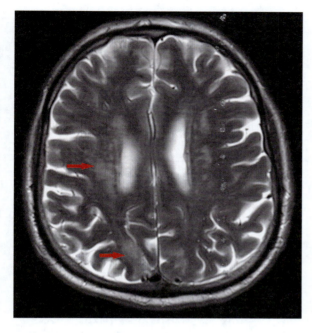

Fig. 2.17 T_2 contrast weighting. Example of poststroke acquisition showing regions of edema (arrows) as increased signal intensity resulting from increased extracellular water

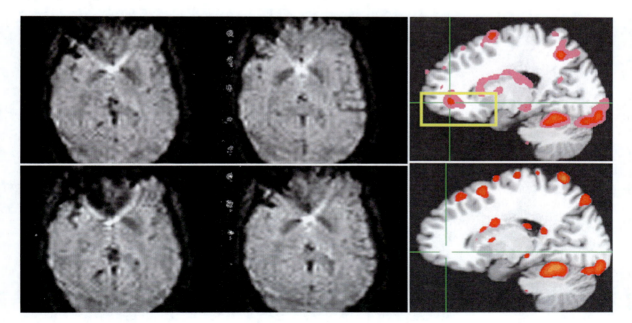

Fig. 2.18 Echo-planar image examples from the orbitofrontal cortex showing the effect of the air–tissue susceptibility difference. *Top*: Images acquired using a localized shim on the orbitofrontal cortex. *Bottom*: Same data acquired using the default shim condition. In the default shim case, there is substantial signal loss in the orbitofrontal cortex. Localized shimming restores intensity. F-statistic maps on the *right* show activation data that was not seen with the default shim

MRI is also capable of generating images with contrast weighting based on some aspects of physiologic function. For example, maps of flow velocity can be generated using a sequence in which gradient pulses will produce phase shifts in flowing spins, as compared to stationary spins.[19, 20] Using expressions relating flow velocity to phase shift, it is possible to build maps of flow velocity in arteries and veins, which is helpful in assessing vessel patency and determining total blood flow to specific regions. Of particular relevance to neuroimaging studies are the fMRI techniques for detecting hemodynamic events relating to cerebral activation (Chap. 4), diffusion weighted and diffusion tensor imaging (Chap. 5), and quantitative perfusion imaging (Chap. 6). Magnetic resonance can also be used for producing information related to the presence of specific metabolites, using spectroscopic techniques. In fact, for most of the history of use of the magnetic resonance phenomenon, analytic spectroscopy has been the primary application.

Signal-to-Noise Ratio

In order to distinguish structures, it is necessary to have contrast. It is also necessary that the contrast be distinguishable in the presence of noise. Noise will be a factor in any measurement and is a form of uncertainty in the measured parameter. Noise arises from random electron motion in the receiver electronics, RF coils, and the subject. This noise is characterized by having equal power at all frequencies within the receiver bandwidth, and is sometimes referred to as white noise. White noise appears in images as a uniform speckling with no distinguishable texture (Fig. 2.19). The effect of improving signal-to-noise ratio (SNR) is to reduce the magnitude of speckling and improve the ability to distinguish small differences in signal intensity between different structures or to visualize fine detail. The variance of noise is proportional to temperature, the resistance of the loaded RF

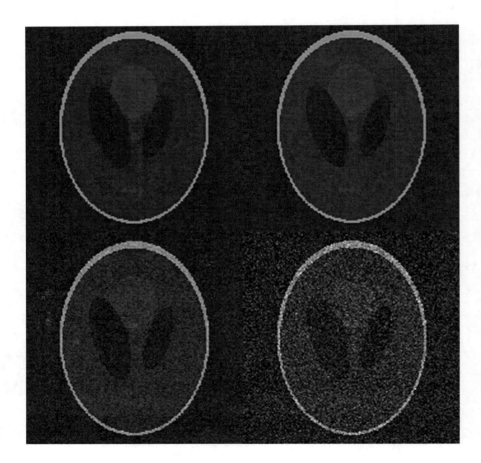

Fig. 2.19 Simulated head phantom images with varying degrees of noise: Noise-free (*upper left*), SNR=50 (*upper right*), SNR=10 (*lower left*), and SNR=4 (*lower right*). Ability to observe small contrast variations is compromised in the image center at SNR=10 and the small features located at the lower center of the image are essentially lost at SNR=4. SNR values are referenced to the bright border of the "head"

coil, and the receiver bandwidth. The receiver bandwidth is the one factor in this relationship over which the scanner operator (or sequence programmer) can exercise some control.

As seen in Fig. 2.19, noise can overwhelm small contrast variations, compromising the ability to make a diagnosis or to extract a quantitative parameter from images. There are a number of relationships that exist between scan parameters and SNR that can be varied in order to generate images with adequate SNR for a particular purpose. SNR varies with these parameters:

1. Voxel size (linear dependence)
2. Repetition time (monoexponential dependence according to T_1)
3. Echo time (monoexponential dependence according to T_2 or T_2^*)
4. Flip angle (interactive dependence with repetition time and T_1)
5. Receiver bandwidth (square root dependence)
6. Choice of resonator (linear dependence with fill factor which is the ratio of the volume of excited tissue to the volume of the resonator)

Voxel size is determined by the slice thickness and the in-plane resolution. Higher-resolution images not only require more time for acquisition, but for all other parameters fixed, they will also have reduced SNR. Voxel size is the product of the two in-plane pixel dimensions and the slice thickness. For example, doubling the slice thickness will double the SNR, but this change must be weighed against the effect of additional partial volume effects due to the additional anatomy contained in the larger slice.

As shown in the example in Fig. 2.15, increasing TR increases the available signal in a partial saturation acquisition. This change must be weighed against the effect on contrast. For grey and white matter, optimum contrast was achieved with a TR of about 1 s. The critical factor for distinguishing two structures from each other is the contrast-to-noise ratio (CNR), which is the ratio of the signal difference between two structures and the noise. For most situations, these tradeoffs have been determined by the scanner manufacturer, and optimized protocols are included in the scanner software package.

A reduction in echo time will result in greater SNR. In general, for acquisitions other than T_2 or T_2^* weighted imaging, the echo time will be set to the minimum possible value in order to maximize SNR and to minimize motion sensitivity and T_2 or T_2^* contributions

to the contrast. For most T_2 weighted imaging, the echo time will be set to retain some tissue detail while providing for a high signal from free water (CSF). For BOLD fMRI scans, the echo time will be set to the T_2^* of grey matter in order to maximize the BOLD susceptibility contrast.

Flip angle is also a contrast parameter, and its relationship to signal intensity is more complex than that for TR and TE. When TR is set to allow for complete recovery of longitudinal magnetization (TR > $5T_1$), a flip angle of 90° will produce the largest possible signal. When operating at shorter TR values, the signal that will be obtained is a function of the flip angle, the TR, and the T_1 of the tissue in question. For a basic gradient echo acquisition, the signal dependence is given by:

$$M_{xy}(\theta,\text{TR},\text{TE},T_1,T_2) = \frac{M_0 \sin\theta (1-e^{-\text{TR}/T_1})e^{-\text{TE}/T_2}}{(1-\cos\theta)e^{-\text{TR}/T_1}} \quad (2.18)$$

For T_1 weighted imaging, the TE will be set to the shortest possible value, and the last term in the numerator becomes negligible. For maximizing SNR for a structure of known T_1, it is necessary, for a given TR, to determine the flip angle giving the largest signal. This flip angle is known as the Ernst angle, and is given by:

$$\theta_E = \arccos(e^{-\text{TR}/T_1}) \quad (2.19)$$

For rapid gradient echo imaging, where TR values can be on the order of 7 ms, the Ernst angle for grey matter at 3 T will be approximately 6°. Using (2.19), the signal intensity for TR = 7 ms and $\theta = 6°$ from grey matter will be $0.096M_0$. While this represents the largest signal that can be obtained from grey matter for a TR of 7 ms, it is clear that the contrast available will be meager, and the SNR will likely be poor. The preferred approach for generating rapid T_1 weighted images, therefore, is to use contrast preparation, typically inversion recovery, and then use a segmented rapid gradient echo readout to obtain the spatially encoded data.

Receiver bandwidth affects SNR with a square root dependence. Doubling the receiver bandwidth results in a factor of $\sqrt{2}$ reduction in SNR. Receiver bandwidth setting is generally transparent to the user, although it is generally possible to drop into a lower-level menu for setting such system parameters. Receiver bandwidth (BW) is a function of the signal sampling time per point (Δt), and the faster the data is sampled, the wider the receiver bandwidth will be:

$$BW = \frac{2}{\Delta t} \qquad (2.20)$$

The tradeoff here is sampling rate vs. time required to read a line of data. Longer sampling time results in smaller bandwidth and improved SNR. However, longer sampling time per point results in a longer frequency encode interval, which increases the minimum echo time. For rapid gradient echo imaging, this also implies a longer minimum TR and longer scan time. Longer echo time also translates into increased motion sensitivity and increased susceptibility artifact. Generally, these tradeoffs have been taken into account in the design of the default protocols provided as part of the scanner's software package. Specific circumstances might dictate deviation from default bandwidth settings when the shortest echo time possible is needed (e.g., presence of strong susceptibility gradients) or if getting all the possible SNR available becomes critical (e.g., arterial spin labeled perfusion imaging).

For resonators, the general practice is to use the one that provides the best fill factor for the anatomy to be scanned. For heads, array receive resonators are now commonly used. In some cases, when a specific grey matter region is to be scanned (e.g., occipital cortex for visual studies involving V_1 and V_2), an array surface resonator may be used. As the name implies, this resonator is placed directly on the surface of the head, and will return a large signal from the tissue directly underneath. For scans not requiring whole-brain data, surface resonators provide a means of gaining a substantial improvement in the effective fill factor over a whole-head volume resonator for cortical imaging.

A common method for improving SNR is signal averaging. This is the acquisition of the same image data two or more times, with the data summed (or averaged, the difference is only a scaling factor). Since the signal adds linearly, and the noise adds with a square root dependence, the SNR improves by a factor equal to the square root of the number of acquisitions. Acquiring the same image data four times and summing results in a doubling of the SNR. Since the scan time increases linearly with the number of averages, scan time and patient tolerance must be taken into consideration when using averaging. For example, to double the SNR of a 4 min acquisition using averaging, four acquisitions will be necessary, totaling 16 min. Motion correction may be necessary if the data were acquired as successive complete scans.

MRI Hardware

The Magnet

With an understanding of the imaging process, it is useful to examine the machinery that brings it all about. The most obvious component of an MRI scanner is the magnet that produces the static field ($\mathbf{B}_0$). In most cases, this is a superconducting solenoidal design in which the main field is produced within a cylindrical bore. The superconducting design possesses some important advantages. A very uniform field can be produced over a DSV on the order of 50 cm, allowing for coverage of a large FOV in a single acquisition. The magnet does not require a constant input of electric current, as would be required with a conventional resistive electromagnet. Superconductivity implies that there is no heat generated as a result of resistive losses in the field windings. Once a superconducting magnet has been energized, the current in the field windings circulates indefinitely (for all practical purposes) with no further input of energy. There is a loss of current over a very long time scale due to electron–electron interactions, but these do not influence the routine operation of the system. The disadvantage of superconducting systems relates to the cost of cryogens required to maintain the superconductivity of the field windings. The niobium-titanium alloy typically used in this application has a critical temperature of about 11.7 K, below which the alloy is superconducting. In order to maintain the field windings below the critical temperature, they are immersed in liquid helium, which has a boiling point of 4.2 K. Older magnets enclosed the liquid He vessel inside another filled with liquid nitrogen (boiling point 77 K) to limit heat transfer from the environment to the He vessel. The housing containing the cryogen vessels is pumped down to a vacuum to eliminate air as a heat transfer medium. Newer magnet designs eliminate the nitrogen vessel, and have reduced the He fill interval compared with the original generation of clinical scanners. The development of an alloy that would be reliably superconducting at liquid nitrogen temperature would be very welcome, in that liquid nitrogen is inexpensive and is also much easier to handle. The field winding set consists of multiple elements. These are designed to increase the size of the most uniform part of the field (variation of a few ppm) to permit imaging at a FOV as large as 50 cm (centered on isocenter) in all possible tomographic planes. When a new scanner is delivered, it is first cooled by repeated fillings with liquid He. Once the magnet temperature is stabilized, it is brought up to field using a power supply connected to the main field windings through a superconducting switch. In a manner resembling the charging of a battery, current is added to the system over a period of a few hours until the main field winding is carrying the current required to generate the specified B_0. At this point, the superconducting switch is closed, and the current in the field windings continues to circulate. There will be a slight reduction in the field winding current over the next 24 h or so after which it stabilizes, at which point the field strength is measured by measuring the resonant frequency (2.1). Once the field strength and stability are confirmed, a shimming process takes place to further improve the uniformity of the field over the imaging volume. This is done following placement of the gradient set and whole-body RF coil. This process takes into account imperfections in the field windings as well as interactions from nearby metal structures. On some magnet designs, this involves adjusting the current in a set of superconducting shim windings. Other designs use a passive method in which metal plates of various size are placed in holders that line the bore of the magnet. A field map sequence is executed with results fed to a program that instructs the service engineer regarding the placement of plates with respect to quantity and location.

Permanent magnet-based "open" designs are also available. These tend to be of lower field strength (typically 0.35 T) and the less uniform static field limits the usable FOV. The SNR and susceptibility contrast implications of the lower field strength and the gradient performance available do not render permanent magnet systems as the first choice for functional neuroimaging applications. Permanent magnet systems do possess two advantages over superconducting systems: no cryogens are used and the open design is more easily tolerated by claustrophobic patients.

The Gradient System

Spatial encoding of the MR signals is accomplished through the use of linear magnetic field gradients. These linear gradient fields are superimposed on the static magnetic field and are switched on and off as necessary to accomplish image acquisition as described in the section on image acquisition pulse sequences. The gradient system consists of two major components: the gradient field windings and the gradient amplifiers.

To provide for three-dimensional spatial encoding, it is necessary to produce linear field gradients in three directions corresponding to the orthogonal axes of the spatial reference frame. For MR imaging, these are defined as the z-direction (along the bore of the magnet) and the x,y-directions (horizontal and vertical). For each of these directions, a set of field coils are provided that will produce a linear field gradient when current is passed through the coil. These coils are resistive (not superconducting) and only produce gradient fields when current is sent through them. Resistive coils are necessary since imaging sequences require that the gradients fluctuate quickly.

Gradient amplifiers are used to produce the large current pulses that are required to drive the gradient coils. These currents will be in the range of hundreds of amperes. Typical maximum gradient strengths now exceed 40 mT/m in clinical systems, with gradient slew rates as high as 200 T/m/s. For a given gradient coil, the strength of the gradient field is linearly proportional to the current flowing through the coil. Gradient strength has implications with respect to the speed of imaging. Strength also influences minimum echo times and time required, for example, for diffusion encoding. Another important factor, especially for echo-planar fMRI is the slew rate (or ramp time) that is achievable in a given gradient system. The greater the maximum slew rate, the less time is required for the gradient field to reach its assigned strength (and to be changed or switched off). Maximum slew rate is a function of the characteristics of both the gradient coils and of the amplifiers. Any conductor has an associated inductance (L) and since $V = L(dI/dt)$ where V is the amplifier output voltage and dI/dT is the rate of current change (slew rate), it is seen that the greater the maximum output voltage of the amplifier, the greater the slew rate will be. Alternatively, reducing the inductance of the gradient coil will also increase the slew rate for a given applied voltage.

Increasing gradient slew rates allows reduction in the echo time (TE) of both gradient echo and spin echo acquisitions (not to mention echo-planar and spiral scan techniques[21, 22]). Unless the objective is a deliberately long echo time for T_2 or T_2^* contrast weighting, reducing the minimum TE brings some important benefits:

1. Greater immunity to motion artifacts relating to blood and CSF pulsatility.
2. Reduced artifacts arising from susceptibility gradients, very important in the orbitofrontal cortex.
3. Reduced signal acquisition time in EPI allowing for more slices per TR period in fMRI studies.
4. Ability to reduce repetition time (TR) in rapid gradient echo imaging for reduced imaging time in T_1 weighted anatomic structure imaging (e.g., T_1 MP-RAGE[23]).

For whole-body gradients with slew rates on the order of 150–200 T/m/s concerns exist regarding peripheral neurostimulation that can result from currents induced in the body from the rapidly switching gradient field (a time varying magnetic field will induce a current in a conductor). However, for the gradient switching rates available in clinical scanners (adhering to FDA guidelines), neurostimulation is not a significant issue, and generally will not be a factor at all if the patient is advised prior to scanning.

The rapidly switching gradient fields can also induce currents in other components of the magnet. These induced currents, in turn, will generate their own gradient fields that act to degrade image quality. As with the static magnetic field, these effects can be reduced through the use of active shielding in which additional coils are used to cancel the gradient field outside of the gradient coil set. Such gradient sets involve greater purchase cost than unshielded gradient sets and require greater currents and drive voltages (owing to increased inductance). However, such gradient systems are essential for functional neuroimaging (and diffusion tensor) applications. The lifetime of induced currents in the magnet structure from unshielded gradients is typically longer than the desirable echo time desirable (TE < 2.5 ms) for T_1 weighted (e.g., T_1 MP-RAGE) gradient echo structural imaging.

Another specification to consider for gradient systems is the linearity. A gradient coil set is intended to produce linear gradient fields on the three spatial axes. However, this linear portion of the gradient field does not cover the full extent of the magnet bore. As mentioned previously, the isocenter of the magnet is defined as the point where the magnetic field strength does not change when a gradient is turned on. Slice offsets are defined with the isocenter as a reference (i.e., slice offset = 0 mm). For images to appear without geometric distortion, the gradient fields must be linear throughout the region defined for the tomographic plane to be acquired. If this is not done, any anatomy outside of the linear region of the gradient set will be rendered with geometric distortion. For clinical scanners, a typical linearity specification would permit the use of FOV settings as large as 50 cm. Over this volume, the gradient linearity is at least 95% (typical specification). For imaging heads, this volume is more than adequate.

During operation, the gradient coil set can produce a considerable sound pressure level. When a current is passed through a conductor that is in a magnetic field, the conductor will experience a force. This principle is exploited in the design of electric motors. In a clinical scanner, the large static magnetic field, combined with the high currents and rapid switching used for the gradient pulses, results in large forces generated in the gradient conductors, with resulting sound. The characteristic sounds produced are a function of the type of imaging sequence, the repetition and echo times, number of slices, etc. Higher slew rates generally correspond to greater loudness. Patients are provided with hearing protection during studies, typically in the form of disposable ear plugs.

RF Coils

The RF coil, also referred to as a resonator, acts as the antenna for transmission of the RF excitation ($\mathbf{B}_1$) and for reception of the resulting MR signals. Although an antenna is typically thought of as a device intended to transmit a radiofrequency field away from the transmitter site, an RF coil for MR imaging is designed to confine the RF magnetic field to the imaged volume. At the same time, this RF field is intended to be as uniform in intensity as possible over the imaging volume. Coils fall into two classes: volume coils and surface coils (with a further subdivision known as array coils for both classes). In all cases, the RF coils are resonant circuits, intended for operation at a specific (Larmor) frequency (although some coils permit operation at two frequencies for spectroscopy). A resonant coil develops stronger transmit fields (for a given transmit power) and is capable of receiving weaker signal strengths than a non-resonant device. In addition, the frequency selectivity (bandwidth) of the coil improves receive SNR by imposing an additional degree of selectivity to the receive system. For imaging, coils are resonant at the proton (^{1}H) frequency of the scanner. On a 1.5 T system, this is approximately 63 MHz, for 3 T, approximately 128 MHz. Most scanners are equipped with a large volume coil (generally referred to as the body coil) that actually forms the innermost "layer" of the scanner bore (it is located inside the gradient set). This coil has an inner lining and is not visible to the patient. A common configuration for volume coils is the "birdcage" configuration (Fig. 2.20). In this design, one or two legs are driven, with the remainder acting as passive radiators such that a uniform radiofrequency field is produced within most of the volume of the coil. The inner diameter of the body coil actually defines the usable diameter of the scanner bore. Although a magnet may have a 90–100 cm bore, once the gradient and shim coil sets, and the body RF coil are inserted, the remaining diameter available to accommodate the patient will be on the order of 55–70 cm. The body coil is intended to produce an adequately uniform RF field over a volume corresponding approximately to the linear region of the gradient set. The most basic mode of operation for the body coil is the one in which it is used for both transmit and receive. This is a convenient mode of operation, especially for scout imaging in which a large volume is to be imaged quickly for purposes of identifying the regions of interest and establishing tomographic planes for detailed study. In general, the larger the coil, the greater the transmit power required to produce a given flip angle in the region of interest. Thus, the body coil requires more transmit power than the other coils used on a clinical scanner. For the 180° pulses required for spin echo imaging, several kilowatts peak power can be needed in order to permit the use of adequately short RF pulses.

The SNR of an image depends (among other factors) on the fill factor. The fill factor is defined as the ratio of the volume of tissue excited to the sensitive volume of the coil. Typically, the ratio of the volume of a tomographic slice to the sensitive volume of the body coil is very small. In order to improve the SNR for specific studies and to permit the use of smaller FOV settings, smaller volume coils and surface coils are employed. For brain imaging, a head coil is routinely used. As the name suggests, head coils are designed to accommodate a head only. The advantage is that the improved fill factor results in improved SNR over what would be achieved using the body coil for transmit and receive. Traditionally, the head coil was a transmit/receive device producing an adequately uniform B_1 field over a head. More recent scanner designs take advantage of multielement receive coils as will be discussed below.

A surface coil is placed on the body, as close as possible to the structure to be imaged. Surface coils may be used as transmit/receive antennas, or they may be used in a mode in which the body coil transmits the RF field, and the surface coil is used as the receive antenna. The latter approach has the advantage of providing a uniform transmit field, effectively improving the intensity profile of the image. The reason for this is that a surface coil produces a non-uniform field when used as a transmit coil. The field intensity falls off with distance from the plane of the surface coil. This same dependence applies to sensitivity for receiving the signal. Use of the body coil as the transmit antenna removes the spatial dependency of the transmitted RF field. The spatial dependence in the receive profile can be exploited to improve the spatial resolution of images. If the FOV of the scanner in the phase encode direction is set smaller than the size of the subject, signal from outside the

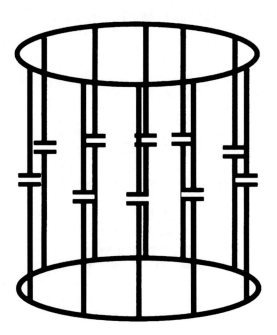

Fig. 2.20 A birdcage volume resonator consists of multiple radiating elements intended to produce a uniform **B**$_1$ distribution and receive sensitivity profile across a specified volume. Capacitors along with the inductance of the elements along with a matching network determine the resonant frequency

FOV will alias ("fold-over") into the image. Since the surface coil will pick up signal only from its vicinity, the FOV can be set to smaller values, corresponding to the size of the surface coil without the possibility of fold-over since there is no signal arising from outside the region of interest. Since the FOV can be set smaller, for a given matrix size (e.g., 256×256), the pixel size will be smaller, and finer detail can be resolved. Surface coils contain a decoupling circuit that shifts the resonant frequency of the coil when the volume coil is transmitting in order to prevent retransmission resulting in artifacts or even RF burns.

A class of RF coils that are increasingly used in neuroimaging studies is the array coils. As the name indicates, such coils consist of multiple elements that are arranged in a housing and connected in such a manner that they can be as simple to use as a conventional coil. With some coil designs, the housing can be flexible such that the coil array can conform to the geometry of the patient. For imaging heads, volume array coils (Fig. 2.21) are available that resemble the conventional transmit/receive head coils traditionally used on clinical scanners. The purpose of array coils is to attempt to combine the best aspects of surface coils and volume coils. Surface coils are intended to produce images of improved SNR over a specific region (when compared with the same images acquired with a body coil). Volume coils provide a more uniform RF field homogeneity to provide consistent intensity and contrast across the entire FOV. A phased-array receive coil can provide receive sensitivity over a larger area (since it consists of multiple coil elements) and can rely on the body coil for a uniform transmit field. Use of array coils requires the ability to receive the individual element signals and combine them in the proper manner to produce the composite receive signal. This generally requires the use of multiple receiver channels on the scanner, with appropriate signal processing capability. Although these capabilities add to the cost of the scanner, the results justify the costs with SNR improvements of more than a factor of 2 available. Array coil capabilities have therefore become standard on scanners intended for neuroimaging applications. While some variation of signal intensity characteristic of surface coils is seen in the array coil image, the difference in SNR is readily apparent.

Array surface coils with multiple receivers permit the use of techniques to increase the speed of image acquisition. This class of parallel imaging acquisitions

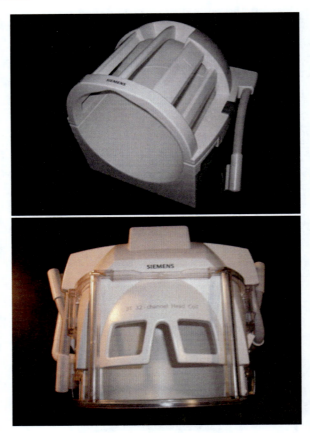

Fig. 2.21 Two examples of volume array head coils. On the *top* is a 12-channel unit with a 32-channel unit on the *below*. Preamplifers for each channel are located at the back of the housing for improved receive signal-to-noise performance (Siemens AG Medical Solutions)

such as SMASH (Simultaneous Acquisition of Spatial Harmonics),[24] SENSE (Sensitivity Encoding),[25] UNFOLD (Unaliasing by Fourier-Encoding the Overlaps Using the Temporal Dimension, itself not a parallel method but can be combined with a parallel method),[26] and GRAPPA(Generalized Autocalibrating Partially Parallel Acquisition)[27] make use of the known sensitivity profiles of array coil elements to simultaneously acquire information corresponding to more than one k-space line at a time. With the use of appropriate postprocessing to resolve the spatial harmonics in order to produce the complete k-space representations of the images, scan time reductions on the order of two- to fourfold can be achieved, with a factor of 2 producing acceptable results for a 12-channel head coil and a factor of 4 practical for use with a 32-channel head coil. Such parallel methods can be applied to most fast imaging methods, further multiplying the speed of these techniques without incurring an unacceptable signal-to-noise penalty. These parallel imaging methods also go by several trade names as used by the various scanner manufacturers.

Safety

Safety in MRI centers on three considerations: the static magnetic field ($\mathbf{B}_0$), the radiofrequency field ($\mathbf{B}_1$), and the gradient fields. Of these three considerations, the static field is the one typically associated with contraindications to MR scanning.

The static field of clinical scanners ranges from 0.35 (for some open permanent magnet systems) to 3 T (for cylindrical bore superconducting systems) and higher for some research scanners. The primary concern relates to biomedical implant devices. These consist of a wide range of geometries and materials, and include both passive and active devices (such as pacemakers and cardioverter/defibrillators). Devices are classified as MR-Safe (no danger in any MRI environment), MR-Conditional (safe at some field strengths), or MR-Unsafe (dangerous at any clinical field strengths). Standard testing procedures have been published for assessing ferromagnetic force and torque that include criteria for a Safe designation. The general criteria for the Safe designation being that a device experience no more force or torque from the magnetic field than it does from gravity. Given the extent of tissue damage that can result from implant device migration due to ferromagnetic force or torque, it is essential that the manufacturer and specific model of implant device in a patient be unambiguously determined. This information should be available in the medical records, and publications exist that allow an MRI technician to confirm the MR safety status of a given implant device. If any doubt exists regarding the identity of an implanted device, the patient enclosing the device should not be scanned. A technician will typically go over a screening form listing contraindications to imaging with each patient to be scanned to insure that the questions are clearly understood, especially with regard to implanted devices or residual metal fragments from a previous injury.

Safety concerns extend to any equipment to be brought into the scanner room. MRI compatible medical equipment (e.g., monitoring devices, IV poles, oxygen tanks, etc.) is available and should be clearly marked regarding their safety status. If there are any doubts, a handheld magnet can be kept at the scanner facility for testing questionable items for ferromagnetic force development.

There are safety issues relating to the $\mathbf{B}_1$ field as well. These all relate to radiofrequency energy absorption by tissue, over a large volume, or on a very localized basis. Radiofrequency energy absorption by tissue results in an increase in temperature, so the FDA has issued guidelines regarding the rate at which RF energy can be applied. The specific absorption rate (SAR) is expressed in units of W/kg and for the whole body averaged over 15 min, the maximum SAR is 4 W/kg. For heads, the limit over 10 min is 3 W/kg. When scan parameters are being set, an estimation of the SAR is provided to the operator. Excessive SAR values will require modification of one or more scan parameters. For example, increase in TR (to reduce deposition rate) or reduction in flip angle (to reduce RF transmit power). Rapid spin echo sequences are of particular concern due to the extensive use of 180° pulses over short time intervals. Higher flip angles correspond to stronger $\mathbf{B}_1$ fields, which in turn correspond to higher RF transmit powers. RF absorption increases with frequency, so the SAR issue becomes more prominent as main field strength (B_0) increases.

SAR is influenced by scan type and parameters, and affects all the tissue within the usable volume of the transmit coil. There exist RF safety issues of a more focal nature. One relates to the use of surface coils. During volume coil transmit, the surface coil is deliberately detuned (a user-transparent process) to move its resonant frequency away from the Larmor frequency. If this were not done, a very strong RF current would be induced in the surface coil, with resultant retransmission of an intense RF field by the surface coil. This retransmitted field can be strong enough to produce RF burns on the skin underneath the coil. If surface coils are being used, they should be checked periodically using a phantom for proper detuning. If the detuning mechanism is losing effectiveness, artifacts will be seen in the test images owing to the retransmitted field producing its own excitation in the phantom near the coil. If a patient or subject reports a warm sensation under a surface coil during scanning, the scan should be stopped immediately. A similar concern exists for monitoring leads. The leads used for electrocardiogram monitoring and other purposes can act as antennas to retransmit the RF field if they are allowed to form loops within the volume of the transmit coil. This can result in RF burns. It is very important that all monitoring leads be as straight as possible, and out of contact with bare skin as practical.

References

1. Bloch F. Nuclear induction. *Phys Rev*. 1946;70:460-474.
2. Bloch F et al. The nuclear induction experiment. *Phys Rev*. 1946;70:474-485.
3. Purcell EM, Torrey HC, Pound RV. Resonance absorption by nuclear magnetic moments in a solid. *Phys Rev*. 1946;69:37-38.
4. Hahn EL. Spin echoes. *Phys Rev*. 1950;80:580-594.
5. Lauterbur PC. Image formation by induced local interactions: examples employing nuclear magnetic resonance. *Nature*. 1973;242:190-191.
6. Lauterbur PC. Magnetic resonance zeugmatography. *Pure Appl Chem*. 1974;40:149-157.
7. Garroway AN, Grannell PK, Mansfield P. Image formation in NMR by a selective irradiative process. *J Phys C*. 1974;7:L457-L462.
8. Mansfield P, Maudsley AA. Medical imaging by NMR. *Br J Radiol*. 1977;50:188-194.
9. Twieg DB. The k-trajectory formulation of the NMR imaging process with applications in analysis and synthesis of imaging methods. *Med Phys*. 1983;10:610-621.
10. Zhu DC, Penn RD. Full-brain T_1 mapping through inversion recovery fast spin echo imaging with time-efficient slice ordering. *Magn Reson Med*. 2005;54:725-731.
11. Zaharchuk G, Martin AJ, Rosenthal G, Manley GT, Dillon WP Measurement of cerebrospinal fluid oxygen partial pressure in humans using MRI. *Magn Reson Med*. 2005;54:113-121.
12. Wright PJ, Mougin OE, Totman JJ, et al. Water proton T_1 measurements in brain tissue at 7, 3, and 1.5 T using IR-EPI, IR-TSE, and MPRAGE: results and optimization. *Magn Reson Mater Phy*. 2008;21:121-130.
13. Schmitt P, Griswold MA, Jakob PM, et al. Inversion recovery true FISP: quantification of T_1, Y_2, and spin density. *Magn Reson Med*. 2004;51:661-667.
14. Lin C, Bernstein M, Huston J, Fain S. Measurements of T_1 relaxation times at 3.0 T: implications for clinical MRA. Proc Intl Soc. *Magn Reson Med*. 2001;9:1391.
15. Stanisz GJ, Odrobina EE, Pun J et al. T_1, T_2 Relaxation and magnetization transfer in tissue at 3 T. *Magn Reson Med*. 2005;54:507-512.
16. Deoni SCL. Transverse relaxation time (T_2) mapping in the brain with off-resonance correction using phase-cycled steady-state free precession imaging. *Magn Reson Imag*. 2009;30:411-417.
17. Deoni SCL, Ward HA, Peters TM, Rutt BK. Rapid T_2 estimation with phase-cycled variable nutation steady-state free precession. *Magn Reson Med*. 2004;52:435-439.
18. Madler B, Harris T, MacKay AL. 3D-Relaxometry – quantitative T_1 and T_2 brain mapping at 3 T. *Proc Intl Soc Magn Reson Med*. 2006;14:958.
19. Moran PR. A flow velocity zeugmatographic interlace for NMR imaging in humans. *Magn Reson Imag*. 1982;1:197-203.
20. Underwood SR, Firmin DN, Klipstein RH, Rees RS, Longmore DB. Magnetic resonance velocity mapping: clinical application of a new technique. *Br Heart J*. 1987;57:404-412.
21. Ahn CB, Kim JH, Cho ZH. High-speed spiral-scan echo planar NMR imaging. *IEEE Trans Med Imag*. 1986;5:2-7.
22. Meyer CH, Hu BS, Nishimura DG, Macovski A. Fast spiral coronary artery imaging. *Magn Reson Med*. 1992;28:202-213.
23. Mugler JP, Brookeman JR. Three-dimensional magnetization-prepared rapid gradient-echo imaging (3D MP RAGE). *Magn Reson Med*. 1990;15:152-157.
24. Sodickson DK, Manning WJ. Simultaneous acquisition of spatial harmonics (SMASH): fast imaging with radiofrequency coil arrays. *Magn Reson Med*. 1997;38:591-603.
25. Pruessmann KP, Weiger M, Scheidegger MB, Boesiger P. SENSE: sensitivity encoding for fast MRI. *Magn Reson Med*. 1999;42:952-962.
26. Madore B, Glover GH, Pelc NJ. Unaliasing by Fourier-encoding the overlaps using the temporal dimension (UNFOLD), applied to cardiac imaging and fMRI. *Magn Reson Med*. 1999;42:813-828.
27. Griswold MA, Jakob PM, Heidemann RM, et al. Generalized autocalibrating partially parallel acquisitions (GRAPPA). *Magn Reson Med*. 2002;47:1202-1210.

Chapter 3
Functional Magnetic Resonance Imaging

Lawrence H. Sweet

Introduction

Functional magnetic resonance imaging (FMRI) is a noninvasive neuroimaging technique that enables quantification of brain function over time with an unprecedented balance of temporal and spatial resolution. FMRI has shown great utility in cognitive neuroscience and clinical research. Targets of FMRI investigations usually involve the neural networks associated with discrete *cognitive* challenges (broadly defined to include all brain processes, such as emotional, motivational, sensory, and motor challenges).

Although now firmly established as a valuable tool, FMRI is a relatively young and rapidly advancing technique with a great deal of yet untapped potential, particularly when combined with other magnetic resonance imaging (MRI) techniques. Over the past two decades FMRI researchers have made substantial contributions in localizing and understanding normal human brain functions. FMRI has also been effective in the detection and understanding of abnormal brain function. Interesting recent clinical developments include presurgical brain mapping and the use of FMRI to predict and assess treatment outcomes.

With the rapid growth of FMRI research and efforts to develop clinical applications, it has become critical to identify potential strengths and limitations of this technology. This chapter provides an overview of blood oxygen level dependent (BOLD) FMRI, summarizing underlying assumptions, basic methods, strengths, and limitations, and suggesting future directions, particularly those relevant to clinical research in behavioral medicine and clinical neuroscience.

Historical Overview

FMRI research has grown rapidly in the two decades following the discovery of BOLD contrast.[51] Since the first reports of BOLD employed in human experiments in the early 1990s,[42,52] FMRI has rapidly diversified in terms of cognitive domains and populations studied. The growth of FMRI research is reflected in the number of publications indexed on the National Institutes of Health PubMed search engine with "FMRI" in the title or abstract. This number has increased from just two in 1993, the first year they appear, to 1,883 in the year 2008 alone (see Fig. 3.1). Although title and abstract searches underestimate the total number of publications on FMRI, they demonstrate the dramatic increase over time.

The early BOLD FMRI experiments used subtraction and cross-correlation analyses of blocked designs to demonstrate task-associated BOLD response in primary motor or visual processing areas among healthy participants. For example, Bandetini and colleagues[6] identified brain voxels most-synchronized with the on/off time course of a self-paced finger-tapping task. FMRI studies of higher-order cognitive processes, such as language[7] and executive functions,[21] began to appear soon after using similar cross-correlation methods. Early studies typically did not examine the whole brain and tended to include small sample sizes. However, the technique was soon applied to whole-brain imaging experiments investigating higher-order

L.H. Sweet (✉)
Department of Psychiatry and Human Behavior,
Warren Alpert Medical School of Brown University,
Providence, RI 02912, USA
e-mail: lawrence_sweet@brown.edu

R.A. Cohen and L.H. Sweet (eds.), *Brain Imaging in Behavioral Medicine and Clinical Neuroscience*,
DOI 10.1007/978-1-4419-6373-4_3, © Springer Science+Business Media, LLC 2011

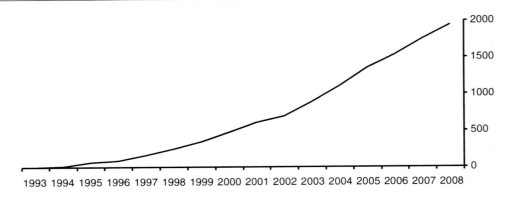

Fig. 3.1 Annual totals of Medline indexed publications with "FMRI" in title or abstract

functions of every major cognitive domain (e.g., memory, language, attention, and emotional functioning). For example, Rao and colleagues[59] reported a whole-brain network of cortical and subcortical brain structures that exhibited activity associated with a conceptual reasoning paradigm among 11 healthy adults. The goal of many of the early FMRI studies was localization of brain function that was associated with a particular cognitive domain, which was elicited by an experimental challenge. Localization of function could be readily demonstrated using small samples, particularly using statistically powerful blocked designs and assessment of robust visual and motor responses (for a discussion of statistical power and sample size in FMRI see[23]). Other considerations, such as FMRI cost, availability of MRI scanners capable of FMRI, and technical complexity in data acquisition and analysis also favored studies with lower sample sizes.

Within a decade FMRI investigators had directed their attention to participants of all ages and a variety of psychiatric and neurologic populations. It is noteworthy that the predominant functional neuroimaging techniques of the time employed radioactive tracers, which could not be administered to children for research purposes and had limitations on repeated exposures that were required for longitudinal experiments. By the early 2000s healthy cognitive functioning (e.g.,[1,4,15,26,27,34,54]), as well as developmental disorders, such as epilepsy (e.g.,[10,30,35,49,70]), dyslexia (e.g.,[5,20,29,66,77]), and ADHD (e.g.,[3,16,25]) had been studied among children. Psychiatric disorders studied included substance abuse (cocaine [e.g.,[12,44,48,80]], nicotine [e.g.,[9,24,36,41]], alcohol [e.g.,[28,45,64,76]]), anxiety disorders (phobias [e.g.,[8,53,62]], obsessive–compulsive disorder [e.g.,[2,46]]), schizophrenia (e.g.,[17,33,37,43,65,78]), and personality disorders (e.g.,[63]).

Neurological populations studied included Multiple Sclerosis,[56,69,71] Parkinson's disease,[31,32,47,57,60,61] and Alzheimer's disease patients.[38,40,58,67,68]

Major advances in FMRI methodology occurred in the late 1990s with the development event-related experimental designs and application of multiple regression analyses. Multiple regression enabled more sophisticated analyses of blocked design experiments with multiple experimental conditions and covariates. More ground-breaking was regression in combination with event-related designs to identify activity associated with rapid presentations of stimulus trials.[13,22,39,81] Therefore, despite a time lag and slow return to baseline that are characteristic of BOLD hemodynamics, multiple overlapping responses to rapid events could be modeled and effects from different conditions could be quantified. This advance grew out of the findings that BOLD responses could be detected following very brief stimuli[6] (<1 s) and that responses to such stimuli were additive and approximately linear (Dale, and Buckner 1997).[11] These were significant advances because event-related designs could be developed which did not require long interstimulus intervals in order to allow the hemodynamic response to return to baseline after each stimulus presentation. Event-related designs also provided more flexibility in stimulus presentation than the blocked design, which had been the neuroimaging paradigm used in positron emission tomography (PET) and FMRI research. Oddball paradigms and randomization of events became possible. Other advantages of rapid event-related designs include observation of the evolution of activity over short periods of time[19] (e.g., 10 s) and the ability to retrospectively categorize stimulus events into different conditions based upon performance.[79]

BOLD FMRI Signal Quantification and Experimental Design

While the goal of traditional MRI is typically to acquire high-resolution images of brain anatomy to identify structural abnormalities, the primary goal of FMRI is to detect variations in MRI signal that occur over time to infer neural demands for oxygen-rich blood. BOLD FMRI uses the magnetic properties of hemoglobin as an endogenous contrast agent to follow task-associated changes in oxygen. This method takes advantage of the fact that deoxyhemoglobin is paramagnetic while oxyhemoglobin is not, and the observation that neural activity reliably leads to the delivery of an excess of oxyhemoglobin. A smaller deoxyhemoglobin to oxyhemoglobin ratio in the capillary beds surrounding active neurons yields a more homogenous magnetic field and a greater MR signal. While it is known that increased neural activity results in vasodilation and greater delivery of an excess of oxygen-rich blood, the intervening mechanisms have not been well established.

When rapid MRI acquisitions using echoplanar T2* sequences sensitive to paramagnetic distortions of deoxyhemoglobin are repeated, a time series including both spatial and temporal information is obtained. When this is coupled with precise experimental challenges that enable this variation to be fractionated by different cognitive conditions, it is possible to obtain data that reflects changes in brain function associated with specific processes. Although FMRI is used to infer brain activity temporally associated with a cognitive paradigm, this is accomplished indirectly by tracking hemodynamic functions. In short, relative cerebrovascular changes in oxygenation are quantified in response to neural activity elicited by cognitive challenges. Therefore, FMRI relies on quantification of cerebrovascular responses that are under normal circumstances spatially and temporally coupled with the underlying neural activity.

FMRI data acquisition sessions involve stimulus presentation and usually some type of behavioral response. BOLD signal is sampled per voxel (i.e., three-dimensional pixels) in repeated acquisitions of a larger brain volume during a carefully designed stimulus presentation protocol. Brain volumes may include the whole brain or selected slices in any plane. For example, one whole-brain volume of 48 contiguous 3 mm thick axial slices with 3 mm^2 in-plane resolution (i.e., 3 mm^3 voxels) might be acquired every 3 s. Partial brain imaging allows increased spatial resolution and temporal sampling rates. Resulting raw data undergo several preprocessing steps to yield a motion-corrected time-dependent signal course for each voxel in the acquired volume.

The raw BOLD signal obtained from each voxel of an individual is typically converted to a standardized metric to allow comparison across subjects or time. For example, a simple method is subtracting an individual's mean baseline signal (e.g., during rest) from mean signal during an experimental condition (e.g., finger tapping; see Fig. 3.2). This is done in each brain voxel. Since BOLD signal changes usually fall well below 10% compared to baseline, stimulus/rest cycles are repeated to increase sampling rates and therefore reliability. Mean difference scores calculated for each cycle may be compared to a hypothetical mean of zero (i.e., the null hypothesis) using a one-sample student's t-test for each voxel. Other methods such as cross-correlation and multiple regression can be used to determine how closely each voxel's time course is synchronized with the time course of the stimulation. In multiple regression analyses individual voxels are assigned a value for each condition (i.e., predictor). Each value corresponds to the variance in that voxel's BOLD signal (i.e., criterion) that is associated with each condition. These values, often called parameter estimates, are typically assigned a statistical value based on sampling rates and multiple comparisons to determine significance thresholds. The term *activation* is used to denote clusters of voxels in which the association of the BOLD signal to the task condition exceeds a significance threshold. *Deactivation* usually denotes significant decreases in activity relative to a resting or active baseline.

Group level statistical tests may be performed once the dependent variable is calculated for each individual (i.e., task-related effects are calculated per voxel). However, these *activation maps* must first be spatially transformed into a standard stereotaxic space and they are usually spatially blurred to compensate for individual differences in functional anatomy. Examples of dependent variables used in these analyses include mean difference scores (e.g., percent signal change), parameter estimates (e.g., coefficients representing attributed variance), and statistical effects (e.g., z and t statistics).

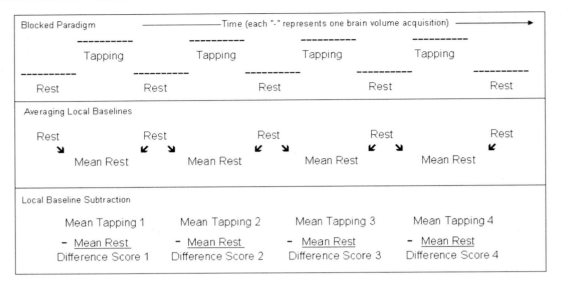

Fig. 3.2 Local baseline subtraction of activity during a blocked finger-tapping paradigm

Major types of group level analyses are voxel-wise and ROI analyses. In voxel-wise analyses a statistical test (e.g., *t*-tests, ANOVAs) is performed for each brain voxel to examine the effects of group or condition. The results are then thresholded per voxel (typically corrected for multiple comparisons) and a cluster size threshold is usually applied. This method is ideal for localization of brain response and exploration of the effects of group or condition; however, it has limitations in use for hypothesis testing, since a refutable hypothesis also requires a precise prediction about spatial location and extent. ROI analyses typically average the dependent variable (i.e., task or condition-related effects) in predetermined regions, although other descriptive statistics such as medians may be used. Examples of ROIs include anatomical boundaries, clusters reported in previous literature, and regions defined empirically within the same study. These methods allow straightforward hypothesis testing using standard statistical packages, since each ROI is typically represented by one value per individual.

Associated behavioral data, if recorded, are used to validate that participants appropriately respond to the challenge, and to examine performance or self-report measures related to the experimental hypotheses. This is important for those paradigms in which behavioral measures may be calculated because changes in brain activity that are simply temporally associated with the paradigm do not necessarily indicate that the level of activity relates to the level of the behavior. Moreover, assessment of behavioral performance is critical in the interpretation of the brain response. For example, lower brain activity in a group exhibiting similar performance as a control group has very different implications than relatively lower activity associated with worse performance. At a more basic level, gathering responses from participants in the scanner offers validity that they are actually doing what they are expected during the paradigm (e.g., above chance performance and not sleeping or daydreaming).

Strengths and Limitations of BOLD FMRI

Prior to the development of FMRI, PET and single photon emission computed tomography (SPECT) were the primary functional imaging methods available for localization of brain function. These methods rely on the detection of radioactive contrast agents usually administered through intravenous infusion. BOLD FMRI, on the other hand, relies on endogenous contrast created by changes in the ratio of oxygenated to deoxygenated hemoglobin induced by the increased oxygen demands of firing neurons. Thus, while FMRI, PET, and SPECT offer some overlap in the information they provide, they also offer unique profiles of advantages and disadvantages, and each allows quantification of unique information about brain function and cerebral hemodynamics. Table 3.1 summarizes key advantages and limitations of common functional neuroimaging techniques.

Table 3.1 Functional techniques used to measure brain response to experimental challenges over time

	Resolution	Cost		Advantages	Disadvantages
SPECT	cm	min	High	Absolute blood flow, specific molecules, out of scanner paradigms possible	Radioactive tracers, invasive, design limits, cyclotron availability
PET	mm	min	Higher		
EEG	Poor	ms	Low	Noninvasive, flexible designs	Spatial resolution, especially subcortical structures, availability (MEG), strong magnetic field (MEG)
MEG	mm	ms	Higher		
BOLD FMRI	mm	s	High	Noninvasive, availability, multisequence imaging, flexible designs, absolute blood flow (ASL)	Movement and susceptibility artifact, noise, confined space, strong magnetic field and radio waves, response lag, partial brain (ASL)
ASL FMRI	mm	s	High		
NIRS	Poor	s	Low	Noninvasive, portable, flexible	Limited to small areas of cortex

SPECT single photon emission computed tomography, *PET* positron emission tomography, *EEG* electroencephalography, *MEG* magnetoencephalography, *BOLD* blood oxygen dependent, *FMRI* functional magnetic resonance imaging, *ASL* perfusion imaging using arterial spin labeling, *NIRS* near infrared spectroscopy, *min* minutes, *s* seconds, *ms* milliseconds

Although other FMRI techniques are available using perfusion MRI, BOLD echoplanar is the most common. For instance a promising alternative is arterial spin labeling (ASL), which tags blood electromagnetically to determine absolute levels of cerebral blood flow in units of milliliters/milligrams/second. Like BOLD FMRI, ASL may be acquired sequentially during cognitive challenges to track task-related changes in blood flow. The major advantage of this technique over BOLD is the ability to measure perfusion changes in absolute terms; however, several relative limitations make BOLD the more practical alternative for most research applications. These include lower availability, and more complexity in acquisition and data analyses, including lower signal-to-noise ratios and limitations on whole-brain imaging.

BOLD FMRI has several advantages over other non-MRI functional neuroimaging techniques. These include an excellent balance of increased spatial resolution, faster temporal sampling, greater design flexibility, and availability. BOLD FMRI, as typically performed, already offers the advantages of investigating concurrent relationships between brain response, behavioral response, and structural morphometry as observed on routinely acquired high-resolution T1-weighted images. Moreover, additional MRI scans may be acquired during the FMRI session (e.g., T2, perfusion, and diffusion weighted scans, fluid-attenuated inversion recovery [FLAIR], and magnetic resonance spectroscopy [MRS]) with only relatively little additional inconvenience to the examinee (i.e., additional time). BOLD FMRI is noninvasive, repeatable, and less expensive than PET, allowing more design flexibility. While *typical* FMRI spatial resolution is 3–5 mm³ for whole-brain studies with *typical* temporal resolution of 2–4 s, spatial resolution < 1 mm³ and temporal resolution below 1 s can be achieved with specialized sequences. A good balance of spatial and temporal resolution is chosen based upon the study questions, with an inherent trade-off between these two parameters and the extent of brain coverage. Thus, smaller regions of interest and more transient cognitive processes can be reliably observed using FMRI compared to other functional neuroimaging techniques. FMRI designs have been evolving, providing greater flexibility, especially after the introduction of rapid event-related designs in the late 1990s. Finally, FMRI has the advantage of the proliferation of MRI systems in most large medical settings. Standard clinical MRI scanners are technically capable of running FMRI sequences; however, an additional contract with the scanner manufacturer is usually necessary to enable this capability.

At the same time, there are several special considerations for FMRI experimental design, study implementation, and data analysis. Unique participant screening procedures are needed compared to the non-MRI-based techniques, particularly in clinical samples. When studying any population using FMRI, investigators must be particularly sensitive to participant safety and comfort. MR contraindications include surgical implants such as some cardiac stents and magnetically activated devices such as pacemakers, some injuries involving metal, pregnancy (for research purposes), and claustrophobia. Women are typically excluded from research if they test positive for pregnancy and participants endorsing possible injuries involving metal, particularly to the eyes, are either excluded or examined for embedded metal fragments (e.g., Water's veiw x-ray). Also, patients who require oxygen tanks, wheelchairs, and other assistive devices require special provisions for assessment in the scanner. Patients with claustrophobia cannot be administered anxiolytic medication due to confounding effects on the cognitive and emotional processes under investigation. Safety is also a special consideration with cognitively impaired patients who may be unable to follow instructions or may forget to disclose important information.

Other comfort issues include screening for body morphometry (size and shape), the loud scanner noise produced by the scanner during BOLD sequences, and ability to lie still during the exam, which may last more than an hour. Scanner noise in conjunction with hearing difficulties may make verbal responding difficult, and may require more sophisticated responding and stimulus presentation paradigms. These paradigms may be more confusing to patients with cognitive problems than standard behavioral or neuropsychological assessment. FMRI is particularly sensitive to movement artifact. Therefore patients who cannot lie still during the exam may not yield reliable data.

Other technical issues include stimulus presentation, response collection, reliability, and artifact. All equipment must be MRI-compatible equipment (safe and functional in a strong magnetic field) and capable of presenting stimuli to participants who are lying with their head in the center of a narrow MRI bore (i.e., an approximately 55 cm diameter, 2 m long tube). Major complications related to data analysis include generalizability of findings, movement artifacts, and susceptibility artifacts (distortions in the magnetic fields due to rapid transitions between space, bone, and parenchyma). Generalizability of findings may be a problem because acquisition equipment and parameters, preprocessing methods, statistical analyses, thresholding of significant effects, and technology differ across sites and studies. Susceptibility artifact occurs in orbitofrontal regions near the nasal sinuses and inferior temporal regions near the ear canal, which limits FMRI of functions associated with these areas. Depending upon the spatial resolution of the scan, head movement of only 3 mm may be enough to shift the data acquisition from the original voxel to an adjacent voxel. Movement is a particular problem if it is associated with one of the experimental conditions (e.g., more vigorous button presses during the experimental condition compared to the baseline condition).

An additional factor that complicates interpretation of BOLD FMRI lies in the necessity for a relative baseline. Since BOLD signal is compared to a control condition, it cannot be scaled to an absolute across groups, or even individuals. Therefore, group differences in BOLD signal actually represent a group by task level interactions, where task level includes an uncontrolled baseline. Unfortunately, without additional and infrequently used scanning techniques such as ASL, it is not possible to determine if groups are equated on the control condition. There is a need for neuroimaging studies that combine methods such as FMRI, DTI, and MRS to characterize the interactions between the structural, functional, and metabolic disturbances over time.

Finally, FMRI research with patient populations is expensive. With few exceptions, FMRI is not currently available for routine clinical testing, nor is it reimbursed by insurance companies. FMRI requires sophisticated infrastructure and considerable expertise. It depends upon specialized equipment and highly trained personnel from several different disciplines, such as clinicians, radiologists, engineers, physicists, statisticians, neuroscientists, programmers, computer technologists, and scanner technologists.

Future Directions

Functional neuroimaging has proven useful in localization of neural functions and in the investigation of neural and cerebrovascular dysfunction among clinical populations. It has also been useful in understanding behavioral manifestations of neural and psychophysiological abnormalities. Functional neuroimaging has great potential in several fields of inquiry, including the assessment of severity, prognosis, and disease course in patients, the search for effective treatments, and a better understanding of neural mechanisms in general as they begin to fail. The great utility of functional neuroimaging in clinical research is only beginning to extend into clinical practice. An excellent example of this is the use of BOLD FMRI in presurgical mapping of brain function.[18] Language, memory, and motor systems are mapped with selective behavioral challenges and avoided during neurosurgery. As other functional MRI techniques such as ASL FMRI become more practical numerous new applications await.

Technical advances such as non-echoplanar sequences to reduce susceptibility artifacts, higher field-strength magnets, and more powerful preprocessing and statistical analysis techniques will continue to produce significant advances in FMRI research. With the finding that BOLD effects decline among older healthy adults, it is crucial to understand how much of this decline is related to similar factors in patients with disorders directly affecting hemodynamics. Understanding of these intervening hemodynamic mechanisms will be crucial to interpreting BOLD data from patients with compromised cerebrovascular systems.

Another future direction relates to the fact that standardized tests are not available for FMRI. For example, FMRI studies have employed paradigms derived from a wide range of different cognitive tasks, but for the most part have employed relatively small sample sizes. Most of these studies were not conducted with goal of developing normative data on behavioral performance or on how the brain normally responds during particular paradigms. With only limited efforts to date to establish normative databases, with reliability and validity data for people across different age groups, it is very difficult to interpret findings from a single patient. Statistically significant group differences in brain activity may reflect relatively subtle effects that are not readily apparent in the results from a single patient. Accordingly, before most techniques can become clinically useful, there is much standardization that needs to be accomplished for each of the functional brain imaging methods.

In contrast to active FMRI challenges, several research groups have also been investigating resting BOLD activity and the default mode network. The default network is set of brain regions that are most active when there are no external cognitive demands. The greatest activity is observed in this system during unstructured rest and the least activity is observed during tasks that require concerted external focus. It has been proposed that the default network is related to one's internal stream of consciousness and that may serve as an imagery simulator for creative thinking.[14] There has been a rapid shift and growth in research on the default network since it was first recognized as being more than simply uncontrolled baseline processing. Relative deactivation of the default network during active cognitive challenges appear to represent relative suppression of task-unrelated cognitive processes.[50] We have observed further suppression default

network activity after increasing difficulty level in working memory paradigms. These include introducing rhyming interference in healthy groups,[73] and following clinical challenges, such as nicotine withdrawal,[74] suspension of treatment for sleep apnea,[75] and concurrent with compensatory activity in MS patients.[55,72] These findings suggest that the degree of suppression of the default network may be an objectively quantifiable reflection of increased difficulty, and may be useful as an endophenotypic marker of brain dysfunction, even when behavioral signs have not yet manifested.

In addition to the factors described above and in Table 3.1, MRI has a major advantage over electroencephalograpic, radiological, and optical functional neuroimaging techniques, in that multiple MRI sequences are available for use in the same imaging session. Each of these MRI sequences can be used in combination to gather structural (e.g., T1, T2, FLAIR, DTI), functional (BOLD, ASL), and metabolic (MRS) information during the same exam. As some of these exciting complimentary techniques are combined with functional neuroimaging in clinical research, substantial leaps in our understanding of brain disorders are certain to follow. The revolutionary impact of T1, T2, and FLAIR MRI on diagnostics in disorders such as multiple sclerosis and stroke is clear. However, we are now able to further capitalize on these advances by precisely mapping function and dysfunction in relation to proximal and distal structural pathology.

A good example of multisequence FMRI research has evolved from our efforts to characterize the relationships between systemic vascular disease, cerebrovascular perfusion, and associated brain function. With rapidly growing experimental and clinical applications, it is important to demonstrate the validity and reliability of the BOLD FMRI technique among groups where cerebral hemodynamics may be altered. This is crucial among populations with known alterations of vascular integrity and subsequent hemodynamic responsivity (e.g., older adults and patients with cardiovascular and cerebrovascular diseases). Cardiovascular disease without large vessel stroke is a model system for studying such hemodynamic functions.

We have been examining the relationship between the neural, cognitive, and hemodynamic consequences of severe cardiovascular disease and their impact on our ability to assess cardiovascular disease patients using FMRI. We have proposed a model in which systemic

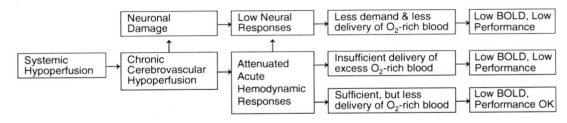

Fig. 3.3 Effects of cardiovascular disease on relationships between hemodynamic and cognitive functions

hypoperfusion secondary to severe cardiovascular disease leads to cerebrovascular hypoperfusion (Fig. 3.3). We predict that cerebrovascular hypoperfusion then leads to an altered BOLD response to cognitive challenges via two mechanisms. The *first* is a neural mechanism by which chronic hypoperfusion leads to neuronal damage and dysfunction. This, in turn, results in cognitive impairment as observed by lower cognitive performance and lower BOLD response to cognitive challenges. This is the typical model of coupled neural and hemodynamic response assumed when results of FMRI studies of patients are reported (top of Fig. 3.3). The *second*, alternative mechanism can be tested by measuring how acute hemodynamic response is altered (BOLD reactivity and cerebrovascular hypoperfusion) independent of cognitive performance, or even cognitive demands (bottom of Fig. 3.3). Central to the assumed vs. alternative distinction is the differentiation between chronic and acute effects of hypoperfusion, followed by the determination if normally excessive acute hemodynamic responses are sufficient to support neural demands. Thus, we expect significant decoupling of the normal task-related BOLD response among subsamples of cardiovascular disease patients that extends beyond the chronic effects of hypoperfusion on neuronal integrity. In this group, oxygen delivery is likely to decrease but remain sufficient for normal cognitive function.

Investigation of this model requires multisequence MRI including functional ASL, BOLD FMRI, and consideration of structural impact of the disease via high-resolution FLAIR and T1 imaging. These sequences, when combined with targeted cognitive and physiological challenges (e.g., hypercapnia) yield the necessary information to calculate baseline perfusion rates, BOLD and perfusion response to the challenges, oxygen consumption rates, white and gray matter structural integrity, and concurrent cognitive performance. While experimental design, data analysis and integration of results pose substantial challenges, this invaluable set of information may be acquired in a single scanning session.

In sum, only two decades since its discovery, FMRI has become a firmly established and rapidly developing technique that continues to hold great potential to further contribute substantially to research in behavioral medicine and clinical neuroscience. FMRI possesses unprecedented utility as a method to evaluate models of brain dysfunction, detect abnormalities, and assess outcomes. With an unprecedented balance of technical advantages, flexibility, feasibility, and potential for multisequence imaging, clinical applications of FMRI are also likely to become more common in the near future. Multisequence imaging including BOLD and perfusion MRI, and assessment of default network function in patient populations are particularly promising areas for clinical development. However, in addition to the standard MRI contraindications routinely used in clinical scanning (e.g., for MS and stroke), other complications may limit the development of clinical FMRI. Verification of the validity of BOLD studies among clinical populations is particularly important given the compromise of cerebrovasculature in some patients. Validation of this technique among clinical samples requires a better understanding the effects of aging on BOLD signal, basic clarification of the meaning of greater or less task-related signal compared to healthy control participants, and better control for confounding differences in the relative baselines used in FMRI.

References

1. Adleman NE, Menon V, Blasey CM, et al. A developmental fMRI study of the Stroop color-word task. *Neuroimage*. 2002;16(1):61–75.

2. Adler CM, McDonough-Ryan P, Sax KW, Holland SK, Arndt S, Strakowski SM. fMRI of neuronal activation with symptom provocation in unmedicated patients with obsessive compulsive disorder. *J Psychiatr Res.* 2000;34(4–5): 317–324.
3. Anderson CM, Polcari A, Lowen SB, Renshaw PF, Teicher MH. Effects of methylphenidate on functional magnetic resonance relaxometry of the cerebellar vermis in boys with ADHD. *Am J Psychiatry.* 2002;159(8):1322–1328.
4. Ahmad Z, Balsamo LM, Sachs BC, Xu B, Gaillard WD. Auditory comprehension of language in young children: neural networks identified with fMRI. *Neurology.* 2003; 60(10):1598–1605.
5. Aylward EH, Richards TL, Berninger VW, et al. Instructional treatment associated with changes in brain activation in children with dyslexia. *Neurology.* 2003;61(2):212–219.
6. Bandettini PA, Jesmanowicz A, Wong EC, Hyde JS. Processing strategies for time-course data sets in functional MRI of the human brain. *Magn Reson Med.* 1993;30(2):161–173.
7. Binder JR, Rao SM, Hammeke TA, et al. Functional magnetic resonance imaging of human auditory cortex. *Ann Neurol.* 1994;35(6):662–672.
8. Birbaumer N, Grodd W, Diedrich O, et al. fMRI reveals amygdala activation to human faces in social phobics. *Neuroreport.* 1998;9(6):1223–1226.
9. Bloom AS, Hoffmann RG, Fuller SA, Pankiewicz J, Harsch HH, Stein EA. Determination of drug-induced changes in functional MRI signal using a pharmacokinetic model. *Hum Brain Mapp.* 1999;8(4):235–244.
10. Boor S, Vucurevic G, Pfleiderer C, Stoeter P, Kutschke G, Boor R. EEG-related functional MRI in benign childhood epilepsy with centrotemporal spikes. *Epilepsia.* 2003;44(5): 688–692.
11. Boynton GM, Engel SA, Glover GH, Heeger DJ. Linear systems analysis of functional magnetic resonance imaging in human V1. *J Neurosci.* 1996;16(13):4207–4221.
12. Breiter HC, Gollub RL, Weisskoff RM, et al. Acute effects of cocaine on human brain activity and emotion. *Neuron.* 1997;19(3):591–611.
13. Buckner RL, Bandettini PA, O'Craven KM, et al. Detection of cortical activation during averaged single trials of a cognitive task using functional magnetic resonance imaging. *Proc Natl Acad Sci U S A.* 1996;93(25):14878–14883.
14. Buckner RL, Andrews-Hanna JR, Schacter DL. The brain's default network: anatomy, function, and relevance to disease. *Ann N Y Acad Sci.* 2008;1124:1–38.
15. Bunge SA, Dudukovic NM, Thomason ME, Vaidya CJ, Gabrieli JD. Immature frontal lobe contributions to cognitive control in children: evidence from fMRI. *Neuron.* 2002;33(2):301–311.
16. Bush G, Frazier JA, Rauch SL, et al. Anterior cingulate cortex dysfunction in attention-deficit/hyperactivity disorder revealed by fMRI and the counting Stroop. *Biol Psychiatry.* 1999;45(12):1542–1552.
17. Callicott JH, Ramsey NF, Tallent K, et al. Functional magnetic resonance imaging brain mapping in psychiatry: methodological issues illustrated in a study of working memory in schizophrenia. *Neuropsychopharmacology.* 1998;18(3): 186–196.
18. Chakraborty A, McEvoy AW. Presurgical functional mapping with functional MRI. *Curr Opin Neurol.* 2008;21(4): 446–451.

19. Cohen JD, Perlstein WM, Braver TS, et al. Temporal dynamics of brain activation during a working memory task. *Nature.* 1997;386:604–607.
20. Corina DP, Richards TL, Serafini S, et al. fMRI auditory language differences between dyslexic and able reading children. *Neuroreport.* 2001;12(6):1195–1201.
21. D'Esposito M, Detre JA, Alsop DC, et al. The neural basis of the central executive system of working memory. *Nature.* 1995;378:279–281.
22. Dale AM, Buckner RL. Selective averaging of rapidly presented individual trials using fMRI. *Hum Brain Mapp.* 1997; 5(5):329–340.
23. Desmond JE, Glover GH. Estimating sample size in functional MRI (fMRI) neuroimaging studies: statistical power analyses. *J Neurosci Methods.* 2002;118(2):115–128.
24. Due DL, Huettel SA, Hall WG, Rubin DC. Activation in mesolimbic and visuospatial neural circuits elicited by smoking cues: evidence from functional magnetic resonance imaging. *Am J Psychiatry.* 2002;159(6):954–960.
25. Durston S, Tottenham NT, Thomas KM, et al. Differential patterns of striatal activation in young children with and without ADHD. *Biol Psychiatry.* 2003;53(10):871–878.
26. Gaillard WD, Balsamo LM, Ibrahim Z, Sachs BC, Xu B. fMRI identifies regional specialization of neural networks for reading in young children. *Neurology.* 2003;60(1):94–100.
27. Gaillard WD, Pugliese M, Grandin CB, et al. Cortical localization of reading in normal children: an fMRI language study. *Neurology.* 2001;57(1):47–54.
28. George MS, Anton RF, Bloomer C, et al. Activation of prefrontal cortex and anterior thalamus in alcoholic subjects on exposure to alcohol-specific cues. *Arch Gen Psychiatry.* 2001;58(4):345–352.
29. Georgiewa P, Rzanny R, Hopf JM, et al. fMRI during word processing in dyslexic and normal reading children. *Neuroreport.* 1999;10(16):3459–3465.
30. Graveline CJ, Mikulis DJ, Crawley AP, Hwang PA. Regionalized sensorimotor plasticity after hemispherectomy fMRI evaluation. *Pediatr Neurol.* 1998;19(5):337–342.
31. Grossman M, Cooke A, DeVita C, et al. Grammatical and resource components of sentence processing in Parkinson's disease: an fMRI study. *Neurology.* 2003;60(5):775–781.
32. Haslinger B, Erhard P, Kampfe N, et al. Event-related functional magnetic resonance imaging in Parkinson's disease before and after levodopa. *Brain.* 2001;124(Pt 3):558–570.
33. Hofer A, Weiss EM, Golaszewski SM, et al. An FMRI study of episodic encoding and recognition of words in patients with schizophrenia in remission. *Am J Psychiatry.* 2003;160(5):911–918.
34. Holland SK, Plante E, Weber Byars A, Strawsburg RH, Schmithorst VJ, Ball WS Jr. Normal fMRI brain activation patterns in children performing a verb generation task. *Neuroimage.* 2001;14(4):837–843.
35. Holloway V, Gadian DG, Vargha-Khadem F, Porter DA, Boyd SG, Connelly A. The reorganization of sensorimotor function in children after hemispherectomy. A functional MRI and somatosensory evoked potential study. *Brain.* 2000;123(Pt 12):2432–2444.
36. Jacobsen LK, Gore JC, Skudlarski P, Lacadie CM, Jatlow P, Krystal JH. Impact of intravenous nicotine on BOLD signal response to photic stimulation. *Magn Reson Imaging.* 2002;20(2):141–145.

37. Jessen F, Scheef L, Germeshausen L, et al. Reduced hippocampal activation during encoding and recognition of words in schizophrenia patients. *Am J Psychiatry*. 2003; 160(7):1305–1312.

38. Johnson SC, Saykin AJ, Baxter LC, et al. The relationship between fMRI activation and cerebral atrophy: comparison of normal aging and alzheimer disease. *Neuroimage*. 2000; 11(3):179–187.

39. Josephs O, Turner R, Friston K. Event-related fMRI. *Hum Brain Mapp*. 1997;5:243–248.

40. Kato T, Knopman D, Liu H. Dissociation of regional activation in mild AD during visual encoding: a functional MRI study. *Neurology*. 2001;57(5):812–816.

41. Kumari V, Gray JA, Ffytche DH, et al. Cognitive effects of nicotine in humans: an fMRI study. *Neuroimage*. 2003;19(3): 1002–1013.

42. Kwong KK, Belliveau JW, Chesler DA, et al. Dynamic magnetic resonance imaging of human brain activity during primary sensory stimulation. *Proc Natl Acad Sci U S A*. 1992; 89:5675–5679.

43. Lawrie SM, Whalley HC, Job DE, Johnstone EC. Structural and functional abnormalities of the amygdala in schizophrenia. *Ann N Y Acad Sci*. 2003;985:445–460.

44. Lee JH, Telang FW, Springer CS Jr, Volkow ND. Abnormal brain activation to visual stimulation in cocaine abusers. *Life Sci*. 2003;73(15):1953–1961.

45. Levin JM, Ross MH, Mendelson JH, et al. Reduction in BOLD fMRI response to primary visual stimulation following alcohol ingestion. *Psychiatry Res*. 1998;82(3):135–146.

46. Levine JB, Gruber SA, Baird AA, Yurgelun-Todd D. Obsessive–compulsive disorder among schizophrenic patients: an exploratory study using functional magnetic resonance imaging data. *Compr Psychiatry*. 1998;39(5):308–311.

47. Lewis SJ, Dove A, Robbins TW, Barker RA, Owen AM. Cognitive impairments in early Parkinson's disease are accompanied by reductions in activity in frontostriatal neural circuitry. *J Neurosci*. 2003;23(15):6351–6356.

48. Li SJ, Biswal B, Li Z, et al. Cocaine administration decreases functional connectivity in human primary visual and motor cortex as detected by functional MRI. *Magn Reson Med*. 2000;43(1):45–51.

49. Liegeois F, Connelly A, Salmond CH, Gadian DG, Vargha-Khadem F, Baldeweg T. A direct test for lateralization of language activation using fMRI: comparison with invasive assessments in children with epilepsy. *Neuroimage*. 2002; 17(4):1861–1867.

50. McKiernan KA, Kaufman JN, Kucera-Thompson J, Binder JR. A parametric manipulation of factors affecting task-induced deactivation in functional neuroimaging. *J Cogn Neurosci*. 2003;15(3):394–408.

51. Ogawa S, Lee TM, Kay AR, Tank DW. Brain magnetic resonance imaging with contrast dependent on blood oxygenation. *Proc Natl Acad Sci U S A*. 1990;87(24):9868–9872.

52. Ogawa S, Tank DW, Menon R, et al. Intrinsic signal changes accompanying sensory stimulation: functional brain mapping with magnetic resonance imaging. *Proc Natl Acad Sci U S A*. 1992;89:5951–5955.

53. Paquette V, Levesque J, Mensour B, et al. "Change the mind and you change the brain": effects of cognitive–behavioral therapy on the neural correlates of spider phobia. *Neuroimage*. 2003;18(2):401–409.

54. Paskavitz J, Sweet LH, Wellen J, Cohen R. Recruitment and stabilization of brain activation within a working memory task; an FMRI study. *Brain Imaging Behav*. 2010;4(1):5–21.

55. Paskavitz J, Sweet LH, Samuel J. Deactivations during working memory distinguishes multiple sclerosis patients from controls. Presented at the 14th annual meeting of the Organization for Human Brain Mapping, Melbourne, Australia, June, 2008. *Neuroimage*. 2008;41(S1):S5 [abstract].

56. Penner IK, Rausch M, Kappos L, Opwis K, Radu EW. Analysis of impairment related functional architecture in MS patients during performance of different attention tasks. *J Neurol*. 2003;250(4):461–472.

57. Peters S, Suchan B, Rusin J, et al. Apomorphine reduces BOLD signal in fMRI during voluntary movement in Parkinsonian patients. *Neuroreport*. 2003;14(6):809–812.

58. Prvulovic D, Hubl D, Sack AT, et al. Functional imaging of visuospatial processing in Alzheimer's disease. *Neuroimage*. 2002;17(3):1403–1414.

59. Rao SM, Bobholz JA, Hammeke TA, et al. Functional evidence for subcortical participation in conceptual reasoning skills. *Neuroreport*. 1997;8:1987–1993.

60. Rowe J, Stephan KE, Friston K, Frackowiak R, Lees A, Passingham R. Attention to action in Parkinson's disease: impaired effective connectivity among frontal cortical regions. *Brain*. 2002;125(Pt 2):276–289.

61. Sabatini U, Boulanouar K, Fabre N, et al. Cortical motor reorganization in akinetic patients with Parkinson's disease: a functional MRI study. *Brain*. 2000;123(Pt 2):394–403.

62. Schneider F, Weiss U, Kessler C, et al. Subcortical correlates of differential classical conditioning of aversive emotional reactions in social phobia. *Biol Psychiatry*. 1999;45(7): 863–871.

63. Schneider F, Habel U, Kessler C, Posse S, Grodd W, Muller-Gartner HW. Functional imaging of conditioned aversive emotional responses in antisocial personality disorder. *Neuropsychobiology*. 2000;42(4):192–201.

64. Schneider F, Habel U, Wagner M, et al. Subcortical correlates of craving in recently abstinent alcoholic patients. *Am J Psychiatry*. 2001;158(7):1075–1083.

65. Schlosser R, Gesierich T, Kaufmann B, et al. Altered effective connectivity during working memory performance in schizophrenia: a study with fMRI and structural equation modeling. *Neuroimage*. 2003;19(3):751–763.

66. Shaywitz BA, Shaywitz SE, Pugh KR, et al. Disruption of posterior brain systems for reading in children with developmental dyslexia. *Biol Psychiatry*. 2002;52(2):101–110.

67. Small SA, Nava AS, Perera GM, Delapaz R, Stern Y. Evaluating the function of hippocampal subregions with high-resolution MRI in Alzheimer's disease and aging. *Microsc Res Tech*. 2000;51(1):101–108.

68. Sperling RA, Bates JF, Chua EF, et al. fMRI studies of associative encoding in young and elderly controls and mild Alzheimer's disease. *J Neurol Neurosurg Psychiatry*. 2003;74(1):44–50.

69. Staffen W, Mair A, Zauner H, et al. Cognitive function and fMRI in patients with multiple sclerosis: evidence for compensatory cortical activation during an attention task. *Brain*. 2002;125(Pt 6):1275–1282.

70. Stapleton SR, Kiriakopoulos E, Mikulis D, et al. Combined utility of functional MRI, cortical mapping, and frameless stereotaxy in the resection of lesions in eloquent areas of brain in children. *Pediatr Neurosurg*. 1997;26(2):68–82.

71. Sweet L, Rao S, Primeau P, Mayer A, Cohen R. Functional magnetic resonance imaging of working memory among multiple sclerosis patients. *J Neuroimaging*. 2004;14(2): 150–157.

72. Sweet L, Rao S, Primeau P, Durgerian S, Cohen R. FMRI response to increased verbal working memory demands among patients with multiple sclerosis. *Hum Brain Mapp*. 2006;27(1):28–36.

73. Sweet LH, Paskavitz JF, Haley AP, Gunstad JJ, Nyalakanti PK, Cohen RA. Imaging phonological similarity effects in verbal working memory. *Neuropsychologia*. 2008;46(4): 1114–1123.

74. Sweet LH, Mulligan RC, Finnerty CE, Jerskey BA, David SP, Cohen RA, Niaura RS. Effects of nicotine withdrawal on verbal working memory and associated brain response. *Psychiatry Res*. 2010 Jul 30;183(1):69–74.

75. Sweet LH, Jerskey BA, Aloia MS. Default network response to a working memory challenge after withdrawal of continuous positive airway pressure treatment for obstructive sleep apnea. *Brain Imaging Behav*. 2010;4(2):155–163.

76. Tapert SF, Brown GG, Kindermann SS, Cheung EH, Frank LR, Brown SA. fMRI measurement of brain dysfunction in alcohol-dependent young women. *Alcohol Clin Exp Res*. 2001;25(2):236–245.

77. Temple E, Poldrack RA, Salidis J, et al. Disrupted neural responses to phonological and orthographic processing in dyslexic children: an fMRI study. *Neuroreport*. 2001;12(2): 299–307.

78. Volz HP, Gaser C, Hager F, et al. Brain activation during cognitive stimulation with the Wisconsin card sorting test – a functional MRI study on healthy volunteers and schizophrenics. *Psychiatry Res*. 1997;75(3):145–157.

79. Wagner AD, Schacter DL, Rotte M, et al. Building memories: remembering and forgetting of verbal experiences as predicted by brain activity. *Science*. 1998;281(5380):1188–1191.

80. Wexler BE, Gottschalk CH, Fulbright RK, et al. Functional magnetic resonance imaging of cocaine craving. *Am J Psychiatry*. 2001;158(1):86–95.

81. Zahran E, Aguire G, D'Esposito M. A trial-based experimental design for fMRI. *Neuroimage*. 1997;6:122–138.

Chapter 4
Diffusion-Tensor Imaging and Behavioral Medicine*

Stephen Correia and Assawin Gongvatana

Historically, the role of white matter in human cognition and behavior has received less attention than that of gray matter.[1] It was not until the 1960s that Geschwind (1926–1984) firmly established the importance of white matter in supporting normal mental activity in his classic work on disconnection syndromes.[2-4] Since then, interest in the role of white matter in cognition, emotion, and behavior has grown. By the late 1980s, magnetic resonance imaging (MRI) was widely adopted for detecting brain disorders. The introduction of diffusion-tensor imaging (DTI) in the mid-1990s[5-7] provided a new *in vivo* MRI tool for gaining unprecedented insight into the structure of white matter and its functional correlates. DTI provides information about the structural coherence and topography of biological tissue based on measurement of the rate and direction of water diffusion. DTI is particularly useful in fibrous tissue such as cerebral white matter or muscle where the linear arrangement of cell structures constrains water to diffuse faster along the fibers than in other directions.

This chapter provides ia primer about DTI and its reviews application to behavioral medicine. Part I briefly reviews the physical underpinnings, data acquisition schemes, and methods of visualizing and quantifying DTI data. A full treatment of the relevant MRI physics and other technical topics is beyond the scope of this chapter, and readers are advised to consult the references for more detailed information. Part II reviews the literature on the use of DTI to study cerebral white matter in clinical conditions relevant to behavioral medicine.

Part I: Basic Concepts

Diffusion in the Brain

Diffusion is the naturally occurring physical process in which particles mix in the absence of bulk motion and under thermodynamic equilibrium.[8] The phenomenon can be illustrated by placing a drop if ink in a large container of water. The ink will gradually spread out about equally in all directions until eventually becoming evenly distributed within the container. Robert Brown's report of the random motion of pollen particles under a microscope (i.e., Brownian motion) provides a framework for describing the phenomenon of diffusion.[9] It is now known that this movement of particles in water is caused by collisions from the constant random thermal movement of the water molecules.

The squared displacement $\langle x^2 \rangle$ of water molecules in three dimensions over a period of time t can be described by Einstein's equation.[10]

$$\langle x^2 \rangle = 6Dt. \tag{4.1}$$

The constant D is the diffusion coefficient, which varies according to the properties of the diffusing molecules, the temperature, and the microstructural features of the medium. It is the sensitivity of D to the microstructural environment of the medium that makes it a useful quantity for probing the structure of biological tissue.[8,11].

---

*Dr. Correia's work on this chapter was partly supported by the US Department of Veterans Affairs. The contents of this chapter do not represent the views of the Department of Veterans Affairs or the USA.

S. Correia (✉)
Department of Psychiatry and Human Behavior, Brown University, Providence, RI, USA
e-mail: SCorreia@Butler.org

R.A. Cohen and L.H. Sweet (eds.), *Brain Imaging in Behavioral Medicine and Clinical Neuroscience*,
DOI 10.1007/978-1-4419-6373-4_4, © Springer Science+Business Media, LLC 2011

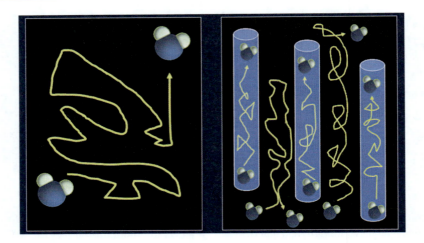

Fig. 4.1 Schematic depiction of water diffusion in the brain in intra- and extracellular compartments. (*Left*) Isotropic diffusion of water is not orientationally specific. (*Right*) Directions of anisotropic diffusion depend on the microstructural environment. Based on http://www.cim.mcgill.ca/~shape/projects/tractography/tractography.html

Biological tissue contains membranes of cell bodies, organelles, and other macromolecular structures that constrain the diffusion of water molecules.[12,13] In free water, diffusion is *isotropic*. That is, the probabilistic displacement of a water molecule over a period of time is equal in all directions. Water diffusion in biological structures such as the ventricles of the brain is mainly unrestricted and, accordingly, is highly isotropic. Diffusion is also largely isotropic in gray matter where cell bodies and organelles restrict diffusion in an orientationally nonspecific manner. White matter, consisting of axons and their associated microtubules and myelin, has an orientationally specific arrangement resulting in *anisotropic* water diffusion. That is, diffusion is faster along the direction of the axons than in other directions[1] (see Fig. 4.1).

Measuring Diffusion in the Brain

The extent to which water diffusion in the brain is isotropic or anisotropic and the direction of anisotropic diffusion can be measured using MRI. The MRI method used for these measurements is based on a spin echo acquisition[15] in which two brief magnetic

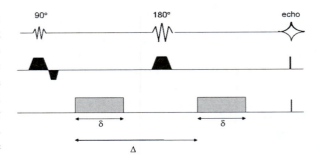

Fig. 4.2 Schematic representation of the Stejskal-Tanner pulsed gradient spin echo acquisition. The two diffusion-encoding gradients (*bottom line*) in this example are of equal strength (G) and duration (δ)

field gradient pulses (*diffusion-encoding gradient*) are applied on either side of the 180° refocusing radiofrequency pulse of the spin echo sequence[8] (Fig. 4.2).

The first diffusion-encoding gradient pulse causes dephasing of proton (^{1}H) spins. The gradient is turned off, and a brief interval transpires before the application of a second diffusion-encoding gradient pulse. Protons bound to macromolecules such as proteins comprising cell membranes are stationary. Since dephasing is related to magnetic field strength and since the gradients are applied in opposite directions, the dephasing of these stationary protons caused by the first gradient is reversed by the second one. That is, these protons experience the same magnetic field

---

[1] In cerebral white matter, diffusion is about four to seven times faster along axons than across due to the axonal membrane and microtubules and to myelin.[12,14]

strength during both gradients because their physical location relative to the gradient has not changed. As a result, they regain their initial phase and there is no (or minimal) net signal loss compared to the signal present before the application of the diffusion-encoding gradients. The situation is different for protons bound in water molecules. These molecules and their dephased protons will diffuse to a new location during the interval between the first and second diffusion-encoding gradient. As a result, they will likely experience a different magnetic field strength when the second gradient is applied. Therefore, unlike the stationary protons, these protons in water molecules will not regain their phase and, as a result, there will be signal loss in comparison to the signal prior to the application of the diffusion-encoding gradients[2]. Stated differently, voxels with displaced protons due to diffusion will show attenuated signal (S) after the application of diffusion gradients when compared with nondiffusion-weighted signals (S_0) acquired at the same voxels. Voxels with greater diffusion will have greater signal attenuation than voxels with less diffusion. It has been shown that the degree of signal attenuation can be expressed as:

$$\frac{S}{S_0} = e^{-\gamma^2 G^2 \delta^2 (\Delta - (\delta/3))D} = e^{-bD},$$

$$b = \gamma^2 G^2 \delta^2 \left(\Delta - \frac{\delta}{3}\right). \qquad (4.2)$$

The diffusion weighting factor b, sometimes referred to simply as the b-value or b-factor, depends on the strength of the diffusion-encoding gradient (G), its duration (δ), the time interval between the gradient pair (Δ), and the gyromagnetic ratio (γ). Given these known acquisition parameters, and the measured S and S_0, the diffusion coefficient D can be computed.

This measurement scheme has long been utilized clinically in the form of diffusion-weighted imaging (DWI). Typically, diffusion-encoding gradients are applied in three orthogonal directions producing three corresponding diffusion-weighted images. A diffusion coefficient can then be computed separately for each image to reflect the diffusion magnitude along that direction in each voxel. This value is typically referred to as *apparent* diffusion coefficient (ADC), reflecting the fact that D is not directly measured. DWI has been widely used clinically in the detection of acute

ischemia, which causes reduction in water diffusion.[17-19] This results in less signal attenuation on the diffusion-weighted images and a lower ADC, thus the ischemic region appears hyperintense on the diffusion-weighted image and hypointense on the ADC image.[20] [3] This makes it easy to detect acute ischemia even when conventional T2-weighted and T1-weighted conventional images appear essentially normal (see Fig. 4.3).

In isotropic tissues, D can be represented by a single value that is invariant regardless of applied gradient direction. However, in tissues where diffusion is orientationally specific, a scalar index of diffusion is inadequate for describing water diffusion within a voxel. This is because the diffusion-weighted signal is dependent on the correspondence between the direction of the applied gradient and the direction of water diffusion, such that signal is most attenuated when the gradient direction overlaps with the diffusion direction. DWI is thus of limited utility for accurately characterizing anisotropic tissues such as white matter.

The Diffusion Tensor

DTI addresses this limitation by using a tensor model to describe water diffusion in three-dimensional space. A tensor is a mathematical construct used to represent multidirectional vector forces such as strain and/or diffusion.[21,22] The diffusion tensor D is a 3×3 symmetric matrix.

$$D = \begin{bmatrix} D_{xx} & D_{xy} & D_{xz} \\ D_{yx} & D_{yy} & D_{yz} \\ D_{zx} & D_{zy} & D_{zz} \end{bmatrix}. \qquad (4.3)$$

A minimum of six diffusion-weighted images with unique gradient-encoding directions, in nique tensor parameters ($D_{xy} = D_{yx}$, $D_{xz} = D_{zx}$, $D_{yz} = D_{zy}$).[6]

The diffusion tensor[4] for each imaging voxel can be decomposed into three orthogonal principal eigenvectors ε_1, ε_2, and ε_3, ordered by the magnitudes of their

---

[2] Diffusion occurs during the application of gradients as well.

[3] Ischemia appears hyperintense on the DWI and hypointense on the ADC image during the acute phase of stroke. These signal characteristics gradually return to normal or near normal in the weeks and months following the injury. See Chap. 18.

[4] The diffusion tensor is usually estimated using linear regression model based on log-transformed diffusion signals.[6]

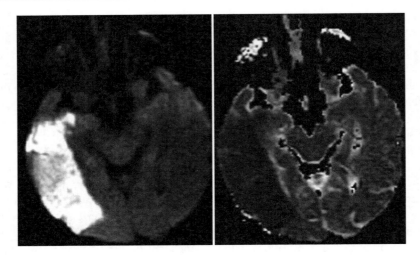

Fig. 4.3 (*Left*) An axial slice of a diffusion weighted image showing a large hyperintense region in the inferior temporal lobe due to ischemia acquired about 35 minutes after symptom onset. (*Right*) The same slice on an ADC map showing the same region as hypointense. (http://emedicine.medscape.com/article/1155506-diagnosis)

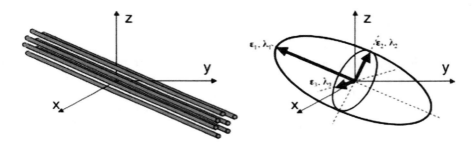

Fig. 4.4 Schematic representation of white matter fibers (left) and a diffusion ellipsoid showing the probabilistic displacement of a water molecule diffusing in the fiber environment. The direction of the orientation of greatest diffusion is assumed to be parallel to the fiber orientation[23]

corresponding eigenvalues, i.e., $\lambda_1 > \lambda_2 > \lambda_3$. These quantities reflect the direction and magnitude of diffusivity in the reference frame of the underlying biological tissue, independent of the scanner axes. Thus, ε_1 represents the dominant fiber direction (i.e., the one with the largest diffusion magnitude) in each voxel.

A diffusion tensor can be visualized by an ellipsoid where the axes are defined by the eigenvectors (Fig. 4.4). When diffusion is isotropic, that is, the magnitude of diffusion is equal in all directions ($\lambda_1 = \lambda_2 = \lambda_3$), the diffusion ellipsoid is reduced to a sphere. Depending on the relative magnitudes of the three eigenvalues, anisotropic tissues can yield a number of ellipsoid shapes (Fig. 4.5).

A notable limitation of the tensor model of water diffusion should be considered in interpreting such data. DTI data are typically acquired at the scale of millimeters, whereas axon diameters are at the micron scale. Thus, each imaging voxel may contain a large number of axons. Since the diffusion tensor is computed using the signal from each voxel, the data represents the bulk diffusion characteristics of the whole voxel regardless of intravoxel tissue composition. Therefore, in brain regions containing multiple populations of crossing, merging, or diverging fibers (e.g., the internal capsule), the diffusion tensor may not provide an ideal representation of diffusion characteristics. More advanced acquisition and computation schemes for diffusion-weighted MRI data have been proposed that take into consideration the contributions from multiple intravoxel tissue compartments.[25] At this time, such techniques are typically limited by long acquisition time and computational complexity, and have not been widely adopted in human studies.

Considerations for Acquisition of DTI Data

Some key factors to consider in DTI acquisitions include image resolution, the number of diffusion-encoding directions, selection of *b*-values, and the number of

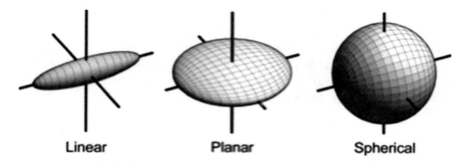

Fig. 4.5 Diffusion tensors depicted as *ellipsoids* with various relative magnitudes of their eigenvalues (adapted from Malloy et al.[24])

repeated acquisitions (i.e., the number of times diffusion is measured in each direction). These factorss are weighed against several constraints including the hardware limitations of the MRI scanner, the total scanning time, and signal-to-noise ratio (SNR) of the acquired images. SNR increase can be achieved by repeated acquisitions of both diffusion-weighted and non-weighted images (i.e., the images acquired with $b=0$). However, this requires longer scan duration, which increases subject burden, risk of subject movement, and scan cost.

Increasing the resolution of the acquired image (i.e., smaller voxel dimensions) permits more spatially detailed analysis of white matter coherence but often results in decreased SNR. An optimal tradeoff between image resolution and SNR is determined based on the purpose of the DTI acquisition.

Increasing the number of diffusion-encoding directions improves the estimates of the diffusion-tensor parameters at the cost of scan time. Jones[26] showed that the benefit of additional directions diminishes at around 30 directions, although incrementally greater precision in characterizing white matter can still be obtained with more directions.

Higher *b*-values improve sensitivity to diffusion but require longer echo times. This has the effect of both increasing transverse relaxation thereby reducing SNR and increasing acquisition time. According to Jones,[16] *b*-values in the range of 900–1,200 s/mm² are generally optimal for most applications. Acquiring the data using multiple non-zero *b*-values also improves diffusion measurement.[27] Optimization of DTI data acquisition is an active area of investigation and depends on factors such as the magnetic field strength of the scanner and gradient performance as well as the intended usages of the data.[28] For example, DTI tractography (described below) typically benefits from smaller isotropic voxels acquired with greater number of gradient directions.[29] Readers interested in more thorough treatment of these and other issues related to DTI data acquisition are referred to recent reviews by Pipe[30] and Mukherjee et al.[28]

Utilization of DTI Data

There are two broad methods for utilizing the tensor information obtained from DTI. Scalar metrics can be derived from the tensor eigenvalues to reflect the degree of diffusivity and isotropy within each voxel. In addition, three-dimensional tractography models can be created based on the dominant fiber direction (ε_1) to represent white matter tract topology.

Scalar Metrics

Scalar metrics are calculated for each voxel based on the eigenvalues of the diffusion tensor. These metrics can be parsed into two broad groups: diffusivity metrics and anisotropy metrics. A widely reported diffusivity metric is mean diffusivity (MD), which is the average of the three eigenvalues, and represents the average magnitude of water diffusion in a voxel.[13] MD can also be computed from the trace (i.e., sum of the diagonal elements) of the tensor matrix, another commonly used metric of diffusivity.

$$\mathrm{MD} = \frac{\lambda_1 + \lambda_2 + \lambda_3}{3} = \frac{D_{xx} + D_{yy} + D_{zz}}{3} = \frac{\mathrm{Trace}}{3}. \quad (4.5)$$

Other commonly reported diffusivity metrics include axial diffusivity (AD, also referred to as parallel diffusivity), which corresponds to the direction with the highest rate of diffusion ($AD = \lambda_1$) and is typically considered to be a marker of axon integrity.[31] Radial diffusivity (RD) is a complementary metric that characterizes diffusion along the two minor axes ($RD = (\lambda_2 + \lambda_3)/2$) and is often interpreted as a marker of myelin integrity.

Perhaps the most widely used scalar metric for quantifying anisotropic diffusion is fractional anisotropy (FA), which represents the variance of the three eigenvalues normalized for the overall magnitude of diffusion in each voxel.[13] FA ranges from 0 for perfect isotropy to 1 for perfect anisotropy.

$$FA = \sqrt{\frac{3}{2}} \sqrt{\frac{(\lambda_1 - \overline{\lambda})^2 + (\lambda_2 - \overline{\lambda})^2 + (\lambda_3 - \overline{\lambda})^2}{\lambda_1^2 + \lambda_2^2 + \lambda_3^2}},$$

$$\overline{\lambda} = \frac{\lambda_1 + \lambda_2 + \lambda_3}{3} = MD. \qquad (4.6)$$

A related metric, *relative anisotropy* (RA), is the ratio of isotropic to anisotropic diffusion.[21] Like FA, RA also increases from 0 to 1 with increasing anisotropy.

$$RA = \frac{1}{\sqrt{3}} \sqrt{\frac{(\lambda_1 - \overline{\lambda})^2 + (\lambda_2 - \overline{\lambda})^2 + (\lambda_3 - \overline{\lambda})^2}{\overline{\lambda}}}. \qquad (4.7)$$

Diffusivity and anisotropy metrics differ in terms of consistency across different white matter regions. In a sample of eight healthy young adults, Pierpaoli et al[33] found that diffusivity was relatively consistent across regions of interest in the pyramidal tract, optic radiation, splenium of corpus callosum, centrum semiovale, and other white matter regions (Trace $\approx 2.1 \times 10^{-3}$ mm²/s). In contrast, the degrees of anisotropy across these ("the same" sound like homogeneity within each region) regions were far more variable, likely attributable to differences in the directional coherence of white matter.

Understanding the biological underpinnings of white matter diffusion anisotropy is critically important for interpreting the results of DTI studies. It has been shown that axonal membranes provide the primary contribution to diffusion anisotropy. Myelin makes a secondary contribution, whereas neurofilaments, microtubules, and fast axonal transport make limited contributions to diffusion anisotropy.(REF 32).[32]

Diffusivity measures (e.g., MD, AD, and RD) provide additional information about the underlying microstructural environment than FA or RA in isolation. In many pathological conditions, decreased structural integrity of cerebral white matter is characterized by increased diffusivity and decreased anisotropy. However, this might not always be the case. For example, cerebral edema has been shown to be related to both increases and decreases in FA.[34] Decreased FA could reflect either decreased diffusion along the primary axis (i.e., along the axons) or increased diffusion along the secondary or tertiary axes (i.e., perpendicular to the axons).[32] Such differences in diffusion changes along the parallel or secondary and tertiary axes could reflect different underlying pathological processes, for example, axon loss vs. demyelination. Accordingly, optimal interpretation of DTI data requires examining measures of anisotropy and diffusivity in all axes as reflected by the individual eigenvalues from the diffusion tensor.

Visualizing Scalar DTI Metrics

Scalar metrics can be visualized as grayscale maps, in which provide image contrast images based on the scalar value. For example, brighter regions on MD maps reflect higher MD values, and brighter areas on FA maps reflect higher FA values, and so on for other scalar values. This can be helpful in distinguishing between tissue types or brain regions based on these characteristics (Fig. 4.6). For example, the ventricles typically exhibit high diffusivity relative to gray or white matter and appear bright on an MD map. Similarly, large cohesive fiber bundles such as the corpus callosum typically exhibit high anisotropy, and appear brighter on an FA map than smaller and less cohesive fibers such as those in the corona radiata.

To enhance the utility of these scalar maps, directional information from the diffusion tensor can be embedded to indicate the primary diffusion direction in each voxel. This is shown in the rightmost image in Fig. 4.6, in which the colors represent the direction of the principal eigenvector (ε_1), with red corresponding to the left–right axis, green to the anterior–posterior axis, and blue to the superior–inferior axis. The color hues are modulated by the angular distance between ε_1 and these axes, and the intensities are modulated by FA.[35] Note the predominance of red voxels in the corpus callosum, is comprised of left-right oriented contains commissural fibers.

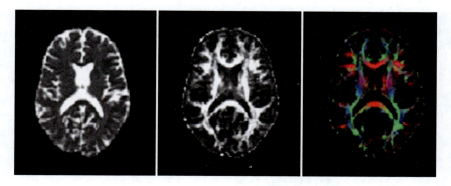

Fig. 4.6 A single axial slice showing maps of MD (*left*) and FA (*middle*) and a color-coded map of the principal diffusion direction (ε_1) modulated by FA (*right*)

Fig. 4.7 (*Left*) FA-modulated principal diffusion direction map. (*Right*) *Expanded view* showing tensor *ellipsoids* in the genu of the corpus callosum

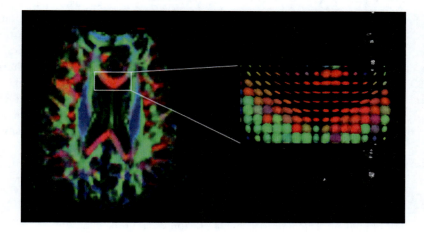

An alternative to scalar metric maps for visualizing DTI data is to create image maps of the the diffusion ellipsoid to each image voxel in order to directly visualize both the direction and magnitude of diffusion in all three axes (Fig. 4.7).

Tractography

DTI tractography is a general term that can be applied to any method that computes three-dimensional models of white matter pathways based on directional information obtained from the diffusion tensor. Tractography models provide information about the topography of cerebral white matter, including the shape and trajectory of white matter tracts. Such models have been shown to bear a close resemblance to known white matter structure, although. Currently, there is no widely accepted gold standard method for validating the anatomic accuracy of tractography models.[36] One study[37] showed very good correspondence between streamline tractography models of healthy controls and postmortem dissection of a different set of brains in select tracts including occipitofrontal, temporoparietal, and temporo-occipital connections. Also, high correspondence among tractography results, histology, and MR-visible tracers have been obtained in porcine brain, at least in major pathways.[38]

A variety of computational algorithms have been developed for generating tractography models. Our focus here will be on the widely-used diffusion tensor-based streamline method. We will also provide a brief overview of a more recent probabilistic tractography method.

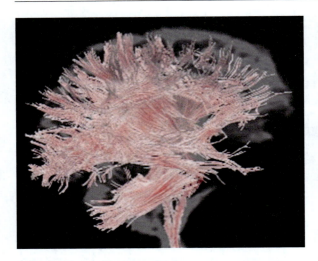

Fig. 4.8 A whole-brain streamline tractography model overlaid on a sagittal slice of non-diffusion weighted ($b=0$) image

Streamline Methods

Streamline methods[39-43] involve propagating three-dimensional space curves (or *streamlines*) from a seed point through the tensor field such that the curve follows the orientation of the principle eigenvector across voxels[43] (Fig. 4.8). The propagation terminates when prespecified thresholds are met for minimum anisotropy (typically around FA of 0.2) and maximum curvature (typically 90° or greater). The minimum anisotropy threshold limits the likelihood of streamlines being propagated into regions that are less likely to be white matter. Curvature thresholds limit the likelihood of a streamline taking an abrupt high angle turn. Such turns are more likely to reflect fiber-tracking errors rather than true underlying white matter structure. Figure 4.8 shows a three-dimensional reconstruction of a whole-brain streamline tractography model generated using an algorithm described in Correia et al.[49]

Probabilistic Tractography

In traditional streamline algorithms, the direction of fiber tract propagation is driven solely by the direction of the principal eigenvector. This does not take into consideration the degree of uncertainty involved in tensor estimation. Probabilistic tractography provides a framework to integrate this uncertainty into the fiber tract streamlining process.[44] Rather than setting predetermined cutoffs for stopping a streamline in regions of high uncertainty (e.g., regions of low anisotropy due to fiber crossings), probabilistic tractography incorporates uncertainty into the fiber tract streamlining process.[44] That is, it tries to answer the question of how much confidence one can have in a given dataset that a path originating at a specified seed point passes through a particular region. Probabilistic tractography estimates uncertainty in the data based on prior information and assumptions about the data (e.g., a characteristics of parameters thought to represent the underlying fiber structure) in combination with some assumption about the noise distribution in the data. These assumptions are then used to generate probability distributions of the diffusion parameters of interest including the primary diffusion direction. These probability distributions are then used to estimate the likelihood of connectivity between brain regions. This general model has been extended to address multiple intravoxel tissue compartments (e.g., crossing fibers in multiple directions) by estimating additional parameters that reflect the relative contributions of the individual compartments to the measured diffusion-weighted signal.[45]

Quantitative Analysis of DTI Data

A key advantage of DTI is its sensitivity to white matter change that is too subtle to be detected by conventional MRI techniques such as T2-weighted images.[46] However, in many situations, these changes are apparent only after quantitative analysis, as they are not obvious on visual inspection of scalar metric maps or tractography models.[5] Some of the more commonly used quantitative analytical approaches are outlined below.

Region of Interest Approach

The region of interest (ROI) approach involves segmentation of specific brain regions under investigation for quantitative analysis. DTI metrics such as FA and MD can then be extracted to reflect diffusion

---

[5] In certain applications, tractography models may provide useful qualitative information that is apparent on visual inspection, such as deflection in the normal trajectory of fiber pathways due to a space occupying lesion, developmental anomalies, subcortical ischemic vascular disease, and other processes.

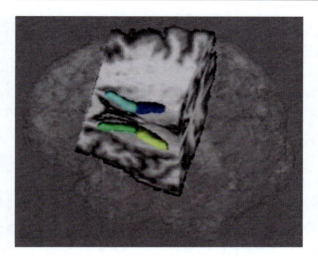

Fig. 4.9 A three-dimensional reconstruction of ROIs in the bilateral anterior and posterior internal capsules drawn on four consecutive axial slices

characteristics within the segmented regions. ROI is appropriate when there is an *a priori* hypothesis pertaining to particular white matter pathways or regions. ROI approaches provide a high degree of control over the region being measured. The method can be performed with minimal initial data manipulation such as spatial registration, which can be computationally intensive and may produce errors. However, the ROI approach, when implemented manually, suffers from a number of limitations. Reliable implementation can be time-consuming and requires trained raters with good knowledge of brain anatomy. Establishing high inter-rater and intrarater reliability can be challenging and raters can be subject to bias. Moreover, error may result from inadvertent inclusion of unwanted voxels in the ROI (i.e., partial volume effect). Thoughtfully developed criteria that clearly and replicably define region placement, the use of ROI exemplar images showing the placement of the region, frequent checks for rater drift, and careful blinding can minimize these problems (Fig. 4.9).

Voxel-Based Morphometry

In contrast to the ROI approach, voxel-based morphometry (VBM)[47] permits voxelwise examination of the whole-brain volume without regionally specific *a priori* hypotheses. VBM is a collection of mostly automated image processing and statistical analysis methods. The typical steps include registration of all images to a common template, and spatial smoothing (i.e., deliberate blurring) of the data to remove high spatial frequency information that may compromise the analysis. In addition, VBM often involves a segmentation step that produces maps of gray matter, white matter, and CSF that can be used for separate analyses of these tissue classes. The spatial alignment permits between-subject data analysis on a voxel-by-voxel basis. A hypothetical example involving comparison of whole brain FA between a group of 30 patients and 30 controls can help illustrate the general principle for readers unfamiliar with this approach. In this example, after spatial alignment to a common template, 60 FA values (one for each subject) are mapped on to each image voxel of the template . This spatial correspondence permits each voxel in one group to be compared with the same voxel in the other group. Statistical analyses in VBM can involve group comparisons or correlation between voxels and some continuous cognitive or behavioral measure on a voxel-by-voxel basis.

As in other voxel-wise techniques, statistical analysis of VBM results is complicated by Type I error inflation due to multiple comparisons. A number of statistical approaches, such as Gaussian random field theory, have been proposed to address such issue.

A strength of using VBM for DTI data analysis include its consideration of all voxels in the dataset, which allows examination of the whole brain without *a priori* hypotheses regarding specific white matter regions. In addition, the approach is largely automated, which reduces errors related to rater reliability. Drawbacks of VBM include its reliance on a high degree of accuracy in spatial registration between brain volumes, which usually require computationally intensive non-linear transformations. Relatively minor compromise in registration accuracy can lead to incorrect results. In addition, the extent of spatial smoothing can strongly affect the conclusions of the analysis, and there is no clear consensus on the optimal amount of smoothing.[48]

Quantitative Tractography

A variety of methods have been developed to quantify the coherence of white matter pathways using both the geometric information of the generated tractography model and the scalar metrics within the tracts. The most commonly used approaches to generating tractography models include those that produce a whole-brain model which can be segmented for tracts of interest (TOI) and those that produce TOI based on regional seed points (e.g., from a cortical region to a subcortical nuclei). Like ROI approaches, quantitative tractography is generally used to test *a priori* hypotheses pertaining to a particularly white matter pathway. Scalar diffusion metrics can be extracted from voxels within the TOI to characterize its diffusion characteristics. In addition, geometric measures such as the density or length of fibers have been shown to be sensitive to white matter changes (e.g., Correia et al[49]).

Quantitative tractography permits selection of white matter pathways, which in many cases is impossible with scalar metric maps, particularly for pathways with complex trajectories such as the superior longitudinal fasciculus. Disadvantages of quantitative tractography include the need for highly trained raters for manual TOI selection and the challenges of establishing intra-rater and inter-rater reliability and minimizing rater bias. Also, generating tractography models can be computationally expensive, and segmentation of tracts can be time-consuming. Small pathways are prone to errors in tract generation and may be difficult to locate. In addition, even some large pathways, such as the superior longitudinal fasciculus can be very difficult to accurately segment and there is no consensus gold standard for judging accuracy. TOI selection is also vulnerable to error due to partial volume effects (i.e., inclusion of incorrect fibers).

Tract-Based Spatial Statistics

Tract-based spatial statistics (TBSS) allows a voxelwise examination of large white matter tracts in the whole brain.[48] This approach operates on the assumptions that maximum FA is found at the center of white matter tracts and that a three-dimensional skeleton model can be reliably generated from these FA values in large tracts. The procedure involves non-linear registrations of FA volumes between subjects, which are then averaged and used to generate the three-dimensional skeleton. Imperfect registration is accounted for in individual brains by a spatial search algorithm to map FA values onto the skeleton. A similar mapping can be applied to other DTI metrics such as MD. The procedures yield DTI indices mapped onto skeletons

that are geometrically identical between subjects, which allow direct voxelwise analysis without the need for additional spatial registration. Due to the lack of spatial smoothing and the non-linear data transformation, nonparametric statistical approaches to address multiple comparisons (e.g., permutation-based approaches with cluster thresholding) are generally used (Fig. 4.10).

Imaging Artifacts

Diffusion-weighted images suffer from a number of potential imaging artifacts. See Jones[16] for more extensive treatment of these issues.

Subject Motion

Movement during image acquisition can cause ghosting artifacts and inaccurate anatomic location of the signal.[51] Moreover, such movement causes the tissue to move relative to the prescribed diffusion-encoding gradient, thereby exposing it to a different gradient strength, which, in turn, can result in errors in measured diffusion. Several approaches have been used to minimize head motion during scanning such as placing a strap across the forehead and filling the space around the head with padding or other comfortable material. Physiological motion due to cardiac pulsation and eye movements can be minimized by rapid data acquisition or by timing the acquisition to the participant's heart rate (i.e., *cardiac gating*). Post-scan corrections for head movement can be accomplished using rigid-body adjustments of the brain image.

Eddy Currents

The rapidly switching and relatively long-duration magnetic field gradients used in DTI acquisition interact with electrically conductive components of the scanner to produce unintended slowly decaying magnetic fields.[16,52] These unwanted magnetic fields alter the prescribed diffusion-encoding gradients, which can lead to errors in measured diffusion and geometric distortions in the diffusion-weighted images.[53-55] Eddy current artifact typically manifests as a rim of high intensity at the edges of the brain (i.e., cortical gray matter rim) on FA images. Several methods have

4 Diffusion-Tensor Imaging and Behavioral Medicine

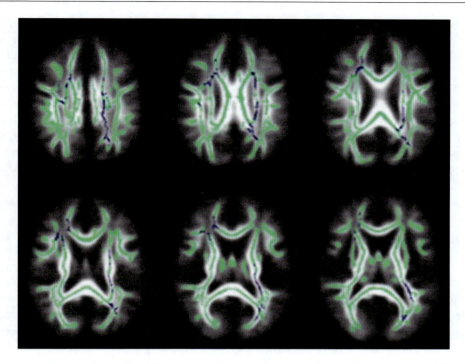

Fig. 4.10 Sample consecutive 5-mm slices showing voxels with significant difference in MD (*blue*) between two subject groups, overlaid on white matter tract skeleton (*green*), and average FA image (*grayscale*) used to generate the skeleton[50]

been proposed for controlling eddy current effects during signal acquisition such as the use of bipolar diffusion gradients on either side of the 180° refocusing pulse[53] and adding a second refocusing pulse to the spin echo sequence.[56] Post-processing methods are numerous and include rigid body or affine registration of the diffusion-weighted images to the nonweighted image, use of a model of the eddy currents collected separately to correct for distortions,[57] and various methods for image alignment and distortion modeling.[54,55,58,59] More sophisticated corrections take into account the temporal evolution of eddy currents and subject motion over the course of data acquisition.[60,61]

Magnetic Susceptibility Artifacts

Tissue and air have different susceptibility to magnetization. These differences can produce unintended local magnetic field gradients at tissue–air boundaries, which can cause severe degradation of the diffusion signal and geometric distortion.[16,51] Methods to minimize magnetic susceptibility artifacts include changes to the acquisition scheme (e.g., parallel imaging[62-65] and post-hoc corrections[58,60,66]).

Image Noise

External noise, including radio frequency and electrical interference, can cause a wide range of imaging errors.[51,67] Approaches to minimizing the effects of noise include repeated acquisitions, increasing the number of diffusion-encoding directions,[51] constraining the tensor estimation algorithm to produce only non-negative principal diffusivities, smoothing the diffusion-weighted images prior to tensor fitting,[68-71] and post hoc statistical adjustments.

Part II: Clinical Application

The number of published DTI studies has blossomed over the past 10 years. An online search of the phrase "diffusion tensor imaging" on PubMed yields 19 articles published in 1998, compared with 689 published in 2008. The breadth of patient populations studied with DTI has increased across the lifespan from infancy to old age and in the variety of clinical populations including numerous neurological and psychiatric disorders. The sensitivity of DTI to subtle white matter changes that fall below the threshold of detection on conventional MRI makes it relevant to behavioral medicine. However, the number of studies in this area is relatively small in comparison with other populations. Many of these behavioral health conditions such as hypertension, alcohol and substance abuse, diabetes mellitus, and human immunodeficiency virus infection have potential direct or indirect effects on cerebral white matter that may impact cognitive and behavioral function. This section provides a review of the recent DTI literature in some of these conditions.

Hypertension

Hypertension is a major public health concern affecting at least 65 million Americans.[72] Behavioral interventions – including adherence to healthy diets, exercise regimens, and compliance with pharmacological treatments – can be implemented to prevent and control hypertension. Among the elderly, hypertension is the second strongest risk factor after age for subcortical hyperintense white matter lesions (WML) on T2-weighted images.[73] These WML are thought to represent incomplete infarction due to hypoperfusion.[74] These lesions give rise to a partial disconnection syndrome that contributes to cognitive decline particularly in speed of mental processing and certain aspects of executive function.[75]

DTI has been shown to provide greater sensitivity to subtle hypertensive white matter injury than traditional T2-weighted images,[76] making it a potentially useful modality for detecting the early effects of hypertension. O'Sullivan et al[77] demonstrated that subtle changes in white matter even in regions that appear normal on T2-weighted images can have cognitive effects in patients with hypertension. They used DTI to examine the effect of white matter coherence on cognition in 36 patients with hypertension and WML on T2-weighted images and in 19 healthy controls. Increased MD was found both within lesions and in normal-appearing white matter. In addition, increased MD in normal-appearing white matter was related to lower full scale IQ and lower performance on measures of executive function.

A clear relationship between systolic blood pressure and white matter coherence was demonstrated by Maclullich et al.[78] These researchers found that systolic blood pressure was positively correlated with MD in

ROIs in the frontal, occipital, parietal, and temporal white matter and in the center of the genu and splenium of the corpus callosum. MD was also correlated with diastolic blood pressure in the genu of the corpus callosum. There is evidence that treatment for hypertension moderates its impact on white matter function. Hannesdottir et al[79] examined 40 patients with medically treated hypertension, 10 patients with untreated hypertension, and 30 normotensive controls. Untreated hypertensive subjects exhibited positive correlations between MD and performances on tests of executive functioning and attention, but no significant correlations were not found in the normotensive or treated hypertensive groups.

These hypertensive white matter changes have been shown to be associated with changes in brain metabolism. For example, Nitkunan et al[80] examined 29 individuals with cerebral small vessel disease (SVD) with evidence of lacunar stroke, 63 individuals with hypertension without stroke, and 42 normotensive controls. DTI and magnetic resonance spectroscopy (MRS) data were collected in an ROI in the centrum semiovale. SVD patients exhibited a significant correlation between increased MD and decreased N-acetylaspartate (NAA), a marker of axonal damage. This association was also present in the hypertensive group, but the magnitude of correlation was not significantly different from that of the control group.

Taken together, these studies indicate that hypertension has an adverse impact on cerebral white matter that is detectable using DTI and that the white matter changes correlate with cognitive function and a marker of neuronal integrity. There is also evidence that adequate treatment for hypertension moderates its impact on white matter. Thus, there appears to be a role for DTI in quantifying the early effects of hypertension on the brain, which may be potentially useful as an outcome measure of the impact of pharmacological and behavioral interventions for hypertension on cerebral white matter integrity.

Diabetes and Metabolic Syndrome

Diabetes and metabolic syndrome also present major public health concerns. An estimated 23.6 million Americans have diabetes[81] and an estimated 47 million have metabolic syndrome.[82] Behavioral interventions can play a major role in preventing and managing these conditions. Diabetes is a risk factor for WML[83] possibly due to its impact on microvascular endothelium.[84] Some studies have demonstrated an association between diabetes (mostly type 2) and WML,[85] while others have failed to find the association.[73,86] Limited sensitivity of T2-weighted imaging to subtle white matter changes may help explain these inconsistencies, which underscores the potental role of DT for assessing white matter integrity in diabetes and metabolic syndrome I.

Type 1 diabetes can provide a model for understanding the impact of type 2 diabetes on white matter and is itself a focus of behavioral medicine in terms of promoting treatment compliance. Kodl et al[87] used TBSS to examine major white matter tracts via TBSS in 25 individuals with extensive histories of type 1 diabetes and 25 controls. Diabetic subjects exhibited lower reduced FA in the posterior corona radiata and the optic radiation. Reduced FA also correlated with poorer performance on the copy portion of the Rey–Osterreith Complex Figure Drawing Test and the Grooved Pegboard Test, and with the duration of diabetes and increased hemoglobin A1C level. These effects appear to extend to type 2 diabetes. Yau et al[88] conducted a study of 24 individuals with type 2 diabetes and 17 controls. They reported diffuse FA and MD abnormalities in diabetic subjects, predominantly in the frontal and temporal white matter. Reduced FA in the temporal stem was related to decreased performance on a test of emotional memory Segura et al[89] used a voxelwise analysis of DTI to examine white matter coherence in 19 patients with metabolic syndrome and 19 age-matched controls. Patients with metabolic syndrome showed an anterior–posterior pattern of deterioration in white matter, reflected by decreased FA and increased MD. As with hypertension, these studies highlight the potential of DTI as a marker of early white matter injury in patients with diabetes and metabolic syndrome. To date, however, no studies have used DTI to examine the impact of treatment of these conditions.

Alcohol Abuse

It has long been known that long-term heavy alcohol exposure is associated with the degradation of white matter (Pfefferbaum 2000). Moreover, there is a clear role for behavioral interventions in alcohol-use disorders. Several studies have demonstrated the utility of DTI for investigating these changes. Using TBSS and probabilistic tractography, Yeh et al[90] examined 11 recovering alcoholics during their first week of abstinence and 10 light-drinking controls. Relative to the controls, the recovering alcoholics showed decreased FA and increased MD in the cortico-striatal and limbic pathways and in frontal white matter. Diffusion abnormalities were also found in commissural fibers and were associated with greater drinking severity. Decreased FA in frontal and limbic fiber tracts was associated with lower visuospatial memory performance. This study by Yeh et al aligns with several studies published by Sullivan and colleagues showing a negative impact of alcohol abuse on white matter coherence using DTI.[91-94] In a recent study, Pfefferbaum et al[95] utilized quantitative fiber tracking to examine 87 alcoholics and 88 controls. Decreased FA and increased RD were found in alcoholic subjects primarily in the frontal forceps, internal and external capsules, fornix, superior cingulate bundle, and superior longitudinal fasciculus. Posterior and inferior bundles were relatively spared. In men, but not women, lifetime alcohol consumption was associated with adverse changes in DTI indices in a number of brain regions examined. However, as a group, men showed greater lifetime alcohol exposure than women. In a second analysis with a subgroup of men who were matched to the women for lifetime alcohol exposure, women showed more DTI evidence of white matter degradation in several fiber bundles, suggesting that women may have greater vulnerability to the adverse effects of alcohol on white matter. Among all alcoholics, poorer performance on speeded tests correlated with DTI markers of regional white matter degradation.

Nicotine and Substance Use

Nicotine addiction and substance abuse have major impacts on public health. These conditions are clearly excellent targets for behavioral interventions. Paul et al[96] examined ten chronic smokers and ten nonsmokers. Compared with nonsmokers, chronic smokers actually exhibited significantly increased FA in the corpus callosum as a whole although this effect approached, but did not reach significance in the splenium. In addition, subjects with lower cigarette use exhibited significantly increased FA in the body of the corpus callosum compared with subjects with higher cigarette use and nonsmokers. This latter finding is counterintuitive as it suggests that low cigarette use is actually associated with improved coherence of white matter in the corpus callosum. The authors speculate that this effect could potentially be related to neurogenic properties of nicotine possibly in combination with an interaction between severity of cigarette use and age of onset of smoking.

White matter abnormalities have been found in structural MRI and MRS in methamphetamine (METH) abusers.[97-99] A number of studies have examined METH-related brain changes using DTI. In a study of 30 adult METH users and 30 control subjects, Alicata et al[100] found that METH users exhibited decreased FA in right frontal white matter and increased MD in left caudate and bilateral putamen. Increased MD in the left putamen was associated with earlier initiation of METH use, greater daily amounts, and a higher cumulative lifetime dose. Increased MD in the right putamen was associated with greater daily amounts and a higher cumulative lifetime dose. Salo et al[101] examined 37 abstinent METH abusers and 17 controls. METH users, but not control subjects, exhibited significant correlations between FA in the genu of the corpus callosum and performance on measures of cognitive control. Kim et al[102] found decreased FA in the genu of the corpus callosum in 11 abstinent METH abusers compared with 13 controls.

Cocaine abuse has also been shown to have an adverse impact of cerebral white matter.[103] In a study of 21 individuals with chronic cocaine dependence and 21 controls, Lim et al[104] found that cocaine users exhibited decreased FA in the inferior frontal white matter that was associated with the duration of cocaine abuse. The FA changes were not found in other brain regions. This result extends a previous finding of decreased FA in the same region in cocaine abusers.[105] Ma et al[106] examined 19 individuals with cocaine dependence and 18 controls. Cocaine users exhibited changes in subregions of the corpus callosum including decreased FA, increased RD, and increased MD in the isthmus; increased RD and MD in the rostral body; and decreased FA in the splenium. Moeller et al[107] showed that cocaine abusers have reduced FA in the genu and rostral body of the corpus callosum. These changes were significantly correlated with a measure of impulse control and target discrimination, which provides support for the hypothesis that decreased inhibitory control in cocaine abusers is related to degradation of frontal regulatory systems. Romero et al[108] found a similar impact of cocaine use on frontal white matter including reduced FA in the anterior cingulate white matter.

Heroin abuse can result in the development of spongiform encephalopathy particularly after inhaled use.[109] One study used DTI to examine white matter change in 16 heroin-dependent individuals and 16 controls using a voxelwise approach.[110] Reduced FA related to heroin use was found in the bilateral frontal subgyral regions, right precentral gyrus, and left cingulate gyrus. FA in the right frontal subgyral was negatively correlated with the duration of heroin use.

Across these DTI studies of methamphetamine, cocaine, and heroin, there is general evidence for greater involvement of frontal white matter circuits than more posterior regions. Results such as these highlight the ability of DTI to detect white matter changes that have implications for real-world cognitive and behavioral function.

HIV Infection

More than one million individuals are living with HIV/AIDS in the USA. HIV infection is frequently accompanied by cognitive deficits, which in some cases can progress to HIV-associated dementia, a debilitating condition involving severe cognitive and functional impairment.[111] Behavioral interventions can play major roles both in preventing the infection such as education regarding HIV transmission and in disease management such as interventions aimed at promoting medication adherence, promoting behavioral health and healthy immune system, and preventing coinfections such as pneumonia and hepatitis.

HIV-related white matter abnormalities have been reported in numerous structural MRI studies, magnetic resonance spectroscopystudies, and postmortem studies. DTI provides a method for obtaining more information regarding HIV-related white matter changes.[112] Gongvatana et al[50] examined major white matter tracts using TBSS in 39 HIV-infected individuals and 25 seronegative controls. HIV-infected subjects as a whole exhibited abnormal white matter in the internal capsule, inferior longitudinal fasciculus, and optic radiation, while subjects with AIDS exhibited more widespread damage, including in the internal capsule and the corpus callosum. Cognitive impairment in the HIV-infected group was related to white matter injury in the internal capsule, corpus callosum, and superior longitudinal fasciculus. Pfefferbaum et al[95] used quantitative fiber tracking to examine 42 HIV-infected individuals and 88 seronegative controls. HIV-infected subjects exhibited increased AD in the internal and external capsules, superior cingulate bundles, and posterior sectors of the corpus callosum, while subjects with AIDS exhibited more extensively increased AD in posterior callosal sectors, fornix, and superior cingulate bundle. HIV-infected subjects, patients not on antiretroviral treatment, exhibited higher RD in the occipital forceps, inferior cingulate bundle, and superior longitudinal fasciculus.

Part III: Conclusion

DTI is a relatively novel and rapidly developing MRI technique that provides indirect information about the microstructural coherence of biological tissue based on measurement of water diffusion in three dimensions. The most common measures derived from DTI are the scalar indices of water diffusivity and diffusion anisotropy, which remain useful especially in examining white matter changes that are not easily detected using other neuroimaging modalities. A more advanced application of DTI involves using directional information from the diffusion tensor to estimate the primary direction of water diffusion in each imaging voxel. The brain tractography model derived from such information is the only currently available tool for *in vivo* examination of structural brain connectivity.

Optimal acquisition and utilization of DTI data poses a number of technical challenges, including the various potential imaging artifacts, the intrinsically low level of acquired signal relative to noise, and the computation complexity involved in deriving clinically meaningful information from the data. However, through careful planning and fine-tuning of image acquisition procedures, excellent image quality can be obtained from a relatively brief scanning session. In addition, a number of user-friendly computation tools for DTI data have become available, many of them cab be found on the internet at no cost. The availability of these tools has resulted in the rapid increase in the application of DTI in

various clinical populations. These investigations have demonstrated the utility of DTI in behavioral health conditions, both in its role as a potentially more sensitive measure of white matter change and in its ability to provide information regarding *in vivo* brain structural connectivity not obtainable by other means. It also provides additional avenues for investigating the relationship between brain structures and function, through cognitive, emotional, and behavioral correlates.

Acknowledgment The authors would like to thank Kathryn Devlin for her help in preparing the manuscript. The views expressed in this chapter are not those of the Department of Veterans Affairs.

References

1. Filley CM. The neurologic background. In *The Behavioral Neurology of White Matter*. New York: Oxford University Press; 2001:3-18.
2. Geschwind N. Disconnexion syndromes in animals and man. II. *Brain*. 1965;88:585-644.
3. Geschwind N. Disconnexion syndromes in animals and man. I. *Brain*. 1965;88:237-294.
4. Geschwind N, Kaplan E. A human cerebral deconnection syndrome. A preliminary report. *Neurology*. 1962;12:675-685.
5. Basser PJ. Inferring microstructural features and the physiological state of tissues from diffusion-weighted images. *NMR Biomed*. 1995;8:333-344.
6. Basser PJ, Mattiello J, LeBihan D. Estimation of the effective self-diffusion tensor from the NMR spin echo. *J Magn Reson B*. 1994;103:247-254.
7. Basser PJ, Mattiello J, LeBihan D. MR diffusion tensor spectroscopy and imaging. *Biophys J*. 1994;66:259-267.
8. Basser PJ, Ozarslan E. Introduction to diffusion MR. In: Johansen-Berg H, Behrens TEJ, eds. *Diffusion MRI*. London: Academic; 2009:3-10.
9. Brown R. A brief account of microscoplal observations made in the months of June, July, and August, 1827, on the particles contained in pollen of plants; and on the general existence of active molecules in organic and inorganic bodies. *Edinb New Philos J*. 1828;4:161-173.
10. Einstein A. Uber die von der molekularkinetischen Theorie der warme gefordete Bewegung von in rubenden Flussigkeiten suspendierten Teilchen. *Annalen der Physik*. 1905;4:549-560.
11. Alexander AL, Lee JE, Lazar M, Field AS. Diffusion tensor imaging of the brain. *Neurotherapeutics*. 2007;4:316-329.
12. Beaulieu C. The basis of anisotropic water diffusion in the nervous system – a technical review. *NMR Biomed*. 2002;15:435-455.
13. Le Bihan D, Mangin JF, Poupon C, et al. Diffusion tensor imaging: concepts and applications. *J Magn Reson Imaging*. 2001;13:534-546.
14. Basser PJ, Pierpaoli C. Microstructural and physiological features of tissues elucidated by quantitative-diffusion-tensor MRI. *J Magn Reson B*. 1996;111:209-219.

15. Stejskal EO, Tanner JE. Spin diffusion measurements: spin echoes in teh presence of a time-dependent field gradient. *J Chem Phys*. 1965;42:288-292.
16. Jones DK. Gaussian modeling of the diffusion signal. In: Johansen-Berg H, Behrens TEJ, eds. *Diffusion MRI*. London: Academic; 2009:37-54.
17. Dardzinski BJ, Sotak CH, Fisher M, Hasegawa Y, Li L, Minematsu K. Apparent diffusion coefficient mapping of experimental focal cerebral ischemia using diffusion-weighted echo-planar imaging. *Magn Reson Med*. 1993; 30:318-325.
18. Li TQ, Chen ZG, Hindmarsh T. Diffusion-weighted MR imaging of acute cerebral ischemia. *Acta Radiol*. 1998;39:460-473.
19. Pierpaoli C, Righini A, Linfante I, Tao-Cheng JH, Alger JR, Di Chiro G. Histopathologic correlates of abnormal water diffusion in cerebral ischemia: diffusion-weighted MR imaging and light and electron microscopic study. *Radiology*. 1993;189:439-448.
20. Warach S, Gaa J, Siewert B, Wielopolski P, Edelman RR. Acute human stroke studied by whole brain echo planar diffusion-weighted magnetic resonance imaging. *Ann Neurol*. 1995;37:231-241.
21. Park HJ. Quantification of white matter using diffusion-tensor imaging. *Int Rev Neurobiol*. 2005;66:167-212.
22. Strandberg, J. Introduction to tensors. <http://medlem.spray.se/gogelo/tensors.pdf/>; 2005.
23. Jellison BJ, Field AS, Medow J, Lazar M, Salamat MS, Alexander AL. Diffusion tensor imaging of cerebral white matter: a pictorial review of physics, fiber tract anatomy, and tumor imaging patterns. *AJNR Am J Neuroradiol*. 2004;25:356-369.
24. Malloy P, Correia S, Stebbins G, Laidlaw DH. Neuroimaging of white matter in aging and dementia. *Clin Neuropsychol*. 2007;21:73-109.
25. Frank LR. Characterization of anisotropy in high angular resolution diffusion-weighted MRI. *Magn Reson Med*. 2002;47:1083-1099.
26. Jones DK. The effect of gradient sampling schemes on measures derived from diffusion tensor MRI: a Monte Carlo study. *Magn Reson Med*. 2004;51:807-815.
27. Brihuega-Moreno O, Heese FP, Hall LD. Optimization of diffusion measurements using Cramer-Rao lower bound theory and its application to articular cartilage. *Magn Reson Med*. 2003;50:1069-1076.
28. Mukherjee P, Chung SW, Berman JI, Hess CP, Henry RG. Diffusion tensor MR imaging and fiber tractography: technical considerations. *AJNR Am J Neuroradiol*. 2008;29:843-852.
29. Mukherjee P, Berman JI, Chung SW, Hess CP, Henry RG. Diffusion tensor MR imaging and fiber tractography: theoretic underpinnings. *AJNR Am J Neuroradiol*. 2008;29:632-641.
30. Pipe J. Pulse sequences for diffusion-weighted MRI. In: Johansen-Berg H, Behrens TEJ, eds. *Diffusion MRI*. London: Academic; 2009:11-35.
31. Song SK, Sun SW, Ramsbottom MJ, Chang C, Russell J, Cross A. Dysmyelination revealed through MRI as increased radial (but unchanged axial) diffusion of water. *Neuroimage*. 2002;17:1429-1436.
32. Beaulieu C. The biological basis of diffusion anisotropy. In: Johansen-Berg H, Behrens TEJ, eds. *Diffusion MRI*. London: Academic; 2009:105-126.

33. Pierpaoli C, Jezzard P, Basser PJ, Barnett A, Di Chiro G. Diffusion tensor MR imaging of the human brain. *Radiology*. 1996;201:637-648.
34. Assaf Y, Pasternak O. Diffusion tensor imaging (DTI)-based white matter mapping in brain research: a review. *J Mol Neurosci*. 2008;34:51-61.
35. Pajevic S, Pierpaoli C. Color schemes to represent the orientation of anisotropic tissues from diffusion tensor data: application to white matter fiber tract mapping in the human brain. *Magn Reson Med*. 1999;42:526-540.
36. Hubbard PL, Parker GJM. Validation of tractography. In: Johansen-Berg H, Behrens TEJ, eds. *Diffusion MRI*. London: Academic; 2009:353-375.
37. Lawes IN, Barrick TR, Murugam V, et al. Atlas-based segmentation of white matter tracts of the human brain using diffusion tensor tractography and comparison with classical dissection. *Neuroimage*. 2008;39:62-79.
38. Dyrby TB, Sogaard LV, Parker GJ, et al. Validation of in vitro probabilistic tractography. *Neuroimage*. 2007;37:1267-1277.
39. Parker GJ, Wheeler-Kingshott CA, Barker GJ. Estimating distributed anatomical connectivity using fast marching methods and diffusion tensor imaging. *IEEE Trans Med Imaging*. 2002;21:505-512.
40. Mori S, Crain BJ, Chacko VP, van Zijl PC. Three-dimensional tracking of axonal projections in the brain by magnetic resonance imaging. *Ann Neurol*. 1999;45:265-269.
41. Lazar M, Weinstein DM, Tsuruda JS, et al. White matter tractography using diffusion tensor deflection. *Hum Brain Mapp*. 2003;18:306-321.
42. Zhang S, Demiralp C, Laidlaw D. Visualizing diffusion tensor MR images using streamtubes and streamsurfaces. *IEEE Trans Vis Comput Graph*. 2003;9:454-462.
43. Basser PJ, Pajevic S, Pierpaoli C, Duda J, Aldroubi A. In vivo fiber tractography using DT-MRI data. *Magn Reson Med*. 2000;44:625-632.
44. Behrens TE, Woolrich MW, Jenkinson M, et al. Characterization and propagation of uncertainty in diffusion-weighted MR imaging. *Magn Reson Med*. 2003;50:1077-1088.
45. Behrens TE, Berg HJ, Jbabdi S, Rushworth MF, Woolrich MW. Probabilistic diffusion tractography with multiple fibre orientations: What can we gain? *Neuroimage*. 2007;34:144-155.
46. Moseley M. Diffusion tensor imaging and aging – a review. *NMR Biomed*. 2002;15:553-560.
47. Ashburner J, Friston KJ. Voxel-based morphometry – the methods. *Neuroimage*. 2000;11:805-821.
48. Smith SM, Jenkinson M, Johansen-Berg H, et al. Tract-based spatial statistics: voxelwise analysis of multi-subject diffusion data. *Neuroimage*. 2006;31:1487-1505.
49. Correia S, Lee SY, Voorn T, et al. Quantitative tractography metrics of white matter integrity in diffusion-tensor MRI. *Neuroimage*. 2008;42:568-581.
50. Gongvatana A, Schweinsburg BC, Taylor MJ, et al. White matter tract injury and cognitive impairment in human immunodeficiency virus-infected individuals. *J Neurovirol*. 2009;15:187-195.
51. Basser PJ, Jones DK. Diffusion-tensor MRI: theory, experimental design and data analysis – a technical review. *NMR Biomed*. 2002;15:456-467.

52. Patton JA. MR imaging instrumentation and image artifacts. *Radiographics*. 1994;14:1083-1096. quiz 1097-1088.
53. Alexander AL, Tsuruda JS, Parker DL. Elimination of eddy current artifacts in diffusion-weighted echo-planar images: the use of bipolar gradients. *Magn Reson Med*. 1997;38:1016-1021.
54. Bastin ME. Correction of eddy current-induced artefacts in diffusion tensor imaging using iterative cross-correlation. *Magn Reson Imaging*. 1999;17:1011-1024.
55. Techavipoo U, Lackey J, Shi J, Guan X, Lai S. Estimation of mutual information objective function based on Fourier shift theorem: an application to eddy current distortion correction in diffusion tensor imaging. *Magn Reson Imaging*. 2009;27:1281-1292.
56. Reese TG, Heid O, Weisskoff RM, Wedeen VJ. Reduction of eddy-current-induced distortion in diffusion MRI using a twice-refocused spin echo. *Magn Reson Med*. 2003;49:177-182.
57. Jezzard P, Barnett AS, Pierpaoli C. Characterization of and correction for eddy current artifacts in echo planar diffusion imaging. *Magn Reson Med*. 1998;39:801-812.
58. Ardekani S, Sinha U. Geometric distortion correction of high-resolution 3 T diffusion tensor brain images. *Magn Reson Med*. 2005;54:1163-1171.
59. Zhuang J, Hrabe J, Kangarlu A, et al. Correction of eddy-current distortions in diffusion tensor images using the known directions and strengths of diffu-sion gradients. *J Magn Reson Imaging*. 2006;24:1188-1193.
60. Andersson JL, Skare S. A model-based method for retro-spective correction of geometric distortions in diffusion-weighted EPI. *Neuroimage*. 2002;16:177-199.
61. Rohde GK, Barnett AS, Basser PJ, Marenco S, Pierpaoli C. Comprehensive approach for correction of motion and dis-tortion in diffusion-weighted MRI. *Magn Reson Med*. 2004;51:103-114.
62. Bammer R, Auer M, Keeling SL, et al. Diffusion tensor imaging using single-shot SENSE-EPI. *Magn Reson Med*. 2002;48:128-136.
63. Andersson JL, Skare S, Ashburner J. How to correct suscep-tibility distortions in spin-echo echo-planar images: applica-tion to diffusion tensor imaging. *Neuroimage*. 2003;20:870-888.
64. Morgan PS, Bowtell RW, McIntyre DJ, Worthington BS. Correction of spatial distortion in EPI due to inhomogeneous static magnetic fields using the reversed gradient method. *J Magn Reson Imaging*. 2004;19:499-507.
65. Wang FN, Huang TY, Lin FH, et al. PROPELLER EPI: an MRI technique suitable for diffusion tensor imaging at high field strength with reduced geometric distortions. *Magn Reson Med*. 2005;54:1232-1240.
66. Merhof D, Soza G, Stadlbauer A, Greiner G, Nimsky C. Correction of susceptibility artifacts in diffusion tensor data using non-linear registration. *Med Image Anal*. 2007;11:588-603.
67. Chavez S, Storey P, Graham SJ. Robust correction of spike noise: application to diffusion tensor imaging. *Magn Reson Med*. 2009;62:510-519.
68. Ding Z, Gore JC, Anderson AW. Reduction of noise in diffu-sion tensor images using anisotropic smoothing. *Magn Reson Med*. 2005;53:485-490.
69. McGraw T, Vemuri BC, Chen Y, Rao M, Mareci T. DT-MRI denoising and neuronal fiber tracking. *Med Image Anal*. 2004;8:95-111.
70. Parker GJ, Schnabel JA, Symms MR, Werring DJ, Barker GJ. Nonlinear smoothing for reduction of systematic and random errors in diffusion tensor imaging. *J Magn Reson Imaging*. 2000;11:702-710.
71. Tabelow K, Polzehl J, Spokoiny V, Voss HU. Diffusion ten-sor imaging: structural adaptive smoothing. *Neuroimage*. 2008;39:1763-1773.
72. Fields LE, Burt VL, Cutler JA, Hughes J, Roccella EJ, Sorlie P. The burden of adult hypertension in the United States 1999 to 2000: a rising tide. *Hypertension*. 2004;44:398-404.
73. de Leeuw FE, de Groot JC, Breteler MMB. White matter changes: frequency and risk factors. In: Pantoni L, Intzitari D, Wallin A, eds. *The Matter of White Matter: Clinical and Pathophysiological Aspects of White Matter Disease Related to Cognitive Decline and Vascular Dementia*, vol. 10. Utrecht, the Netherlands: Academic Pharmaceutical Productions; 2000:19-33.
74. Englund E. Neuropathology of white matter disease: paren-chymal changes. In: Pantoni L, Inzitari D, Wallin A, eds. *The Matter of White Matter: Clinical and Pathophysiological Aspects of White Matter Disease Related to Cognitive Decline and Vascular Dementia*, vol. 10. Utrecht, the Netherlands: Academic Pharmaceutical Productions; 2000:223-246.
75. Gunning-Dixon FM, Raz N. The cognitive correlates of white matter abnormalities in normal aging: a quantitative review. *Neuropsychology*. 2000;14:224-232.
76. Filippi M, Cercignani M, Inglese M, Horsfield MA, Comi G. Diffusion tensor magnetic resonance imaging in multiple sclerosis. *Neurology*. 2001;56:304-311.
77. O'Sullivan M, Morris RG, Huckstep B, Jones DK, Williams SC, Markus HS. Diffusion tensor MRI correlates with executive dysfunction in patients with ischaemic leu-koaraiosis. *J Neurol Neurosurg Psychiatry*. 2004;75:441-447.
78. Maclullich AM, Ferguson KJ, Reid LM, et al. Higher sys-tolic blood pressure is associated with increased water dif-fusivity in normal-appearing white matter. *Stroke*. 2009;40(12):3869-3871.
79. Hannesdottir K, Nitkunan A, Charlton RA, Barrick TR, MacGregor GA, Markus HS. Cognitive impairment and white matter damage in hypertension: a pilot study. *Acta Neurol Scand*. 2009;119:261-268.
80. Nitkunan A, Charlton RA, McIntyre DJ, Barrick TR, Howe FA, Markus HS. Diffusion tensor imaging and MR spectroscopy in hypertension and presumed cerebral small vessel disease. *Magn Reson Med*. 2008;59:528-534.
81. National Diabetes Information Clearinghouse, N.D.I. *National Diabetes Statistics*. Bethesda, MD: National Institute of Diabetes and Digestive and Kidney Diseases; 2007.
82. Diseases and Conditions Index, D.A.C. *Metabolic Syndrome*. Bethesda, MD: National Heart Lung and Blood Institute; 2007.
83. Biessels GJ, Koffeman A, Scheltens P. Diabetes and cognitive impairment. Clinical diagnosis and brain imaging in patients attending a memory clinic. *J Neurol*. 2006;253:477-482.

84. Hassan A, Hunt BJ, O'Sullivan M. et al. Markers of endothelial dysfunction in lacunar infarction and ischaemic leukoaraiosis. *Brain*. 2003;126:424-432.

85. Murray AD, Staff RT, Shenkin SD, Deary IJ, Starr JM, Whalley LJ. Brain white matter hyperintensities: relative importance of vascular risk factors in nondemented elderly people. *Radiology*. 2005;237:251-257.

86. Schmidt R, Launer LJ, Nilsson LG, et al. Magnetic resonance imaging of the brain in diabetes: the Cardiovascular Determinants of Dementia (CASCADE) Study. *Diabetes*. 2004;53:687-692.

87. Kodl CT, Franc DT, Rao JP, et al.Diffusion tensor imaging identifies deficits in white matter microstructure in subjects with type 1 diabetes that correlate with reduced neurocognitive function. *Diabetes*. 2008;57:3083-3089.

88. Yau PL, Javier D, Tsui W, et al. Emotional and neutral declarative memory impairments and associated white matter microstructural abnormalities in adults with type 2 diabetes. *Psychiatry Res*. 2009;174(3):223-230.

89. Segura B, Jurado MA, Freixenet N, Falcon C, Junque C, Arboix A. Microstructural white matter changes in metabolic syndrome: a diffusion tensor imaging study. *Neurology*. 2009;73:438-444.

90. Yeh PH, Simpson K, Durazzo TC, Gazdzinski S, Meyerhoff DJ. Tract-Based Spatial Statistics (TBSS) of diffusion tensor imaging data in alcohol dependence: abnormalities of the motivational neurocircuitry. *Psychiatry Res*. 2009; 173:22-30.

91. Pfefferbaum A, Adalsteinsson E, Sullivan EV. Supratentorial profile of white matter microstructural integrity in recovering alcoholic men and women. *Biol Psychiatry*. 2006;59: 364-372.

92. Pfefferbaum A, Sullivan EV, Hedehus M, Adalsteinsson E, Lim KO, Moseley M. In vivo detection and functional correlates of white matter microstructural disruption in chronic alcoholism. *Alcohol Clin Exp Res*. 2000;24:1214-1221.

93. Sullivan EV, Pfefferbaum A. Neurocircuitry in alcoholism: a substrate of disruption and repair. *Psychopharmacology*. 2005;180:583-594.

94. Pfefferbaum A, Sullivan EV. Microstructural but not macrostructural disruption of white matter in women with chronic alcoholism. *Neuroimage*. 2002;15:708-718.

95. Pfefferbaum A, Rosenbloom M, Rohlfing T, Sullivan EV. Degradation of association and projection white matter systems in alcoholism detected with quantitative fiber tracking. *Biol Psychiatry*. 2009;65:680-690.

96. Paul RH, Grieve SM, Niaura R, et al. Chronic cigarette smoking and the microstructural integrity of white matter in healthy adults: a diffusion tensor imaging study. *Nicotine Tob Res*. 2008;10:137-147.

97. Bae SC, Lyoo IK, Sung YH, et al. Increased white matter hyperintensities in male methamphetamine abusers. *Drug Alcohol Depend*. 2006;81:83-88.

98. Ernst T, Chang L, Leonido-Yee M, Speck O. Evidence for long-term neurotoxicity associated with methamphetamine abuse: A 1H MRS study. *Neurology*. 2000;54:1344-1349.

99. Thompson PM, Hayashi KM, Simon SL, et al. Structural abnormalities in the brains of human subjects who use methamphetamine. *J Neurosci*. 2004;24:6028-6036.

100. Alicata D, Chang L, Cloak C, Abe K, Ernst T. Higher diffusion in striatum and lower fractional anisotropy in white matter of methamphetamine users. *Psychiatry Res*. 2009;174: 1-8.

101. Salo R, Nordahl TE, Buonocore MH, et al. Cognitive control and white matter callosal microstructure in methamphetamine-dependent subjects: a diffusion tensor imaging study. *Biol Psychiatry*. 2009;65:122-128.

102. Kim IS, Kim YT, Song HJ, et al. Reduced corpus callosum white matter microstructural integrity revealed by diffusion tensor eigenvalues in abstinent methamphetamine addicts. *Neurotoxicology*. 2009;30:209-213.

103. Lyoo IK, Streeter CC, Ahn KH, et al. White matter hyperintensities in subjects with cocaine and opiate dependence and healthy comparison subjects. *Psychiatry Res*. 2004; 131:135-145.

104. Lim KO, Wozniak JR, Mueller BA, et al. Brain macrostructural and microstructural abnormalities in cocaine dependence. *Drug Alcohol Depend*. 2008;92:164-172.

105. Lim KO, Choi SJ, Pomara N, Wolkin A, Rotrosen JP. Reduced frontal white matter integrity in cocaine dependence: a controlled diffusion tensor imaging study. *Biol Psychiatry*. 2002;51:890-895.

106. Ma L, Hasan KM, Steinberg JL, et al. Diffusion tensor imaging in cocaine dependence: regional effects of cocaine on corpus callosum and effect of cocaine administration route. *Drug Alcohol Depend*. 2009;104: 262-267.

107. Moeller FG, Hasan KM, Steinberg JL, et al. Reduced anterior corpus callosum white matter integrity is related to increased impulsivity and reduced discriminability in cocaine-dependent subjects: diffusion tensor imaging. *Neuropsychopharmacology*. 2005;30:610-617.

108. Romero MJ, Asensio S, Palau C, Sanchez A, Romero FJ. Cocaine addiction: diffusion tensor imaging study of the inferior frontal and anterior cingulate white matter. *Psychiatry Res*. 2010;181(1):57-63.

109. Bega DS, McDaniel LM, Jhaveri MD, Lee VH. Diffusion weighted imaging in heroin-associated spongiform leukoencephalopathy. *Neurocrit Care*. 2009;10:352-354.

110. Liu H, Li L, Hao Y, et al. Disrupted white matter integrity in heroin dependence: a controlled study utilizing diffusion tensor imaging. *Am J Drug Alcohol Abuse*. 2008;34: 562-575.

111. McArthur JC, Brew BJ, Nath A. Neurological complications of HIV infection. *Lancet Neurol*. 2005;4: 543-555.

112. Woods SP, Carey CL, Iudicello JE, Letendre SL, Fennema-Notestine C, Grant I. Neuropsychological aspects of HIV infection. In: Grant I, Adams KM, eds. *Neuropsychological Assessment of Neuropsychiatric and Neuromedical Disorders*. 3rd ed. New York, NY: Oxford University Press; 2009.

Chapter 5
Perfusion MRI

Richard Hoge

Introduction

Magnetic resonance imaging is notable for offering a broad array of both anatomic and functional image contrast types. Although the term "functional MRI" has become nearly synonymous with blood oxygenation level-dependent (BOLD) contrast, there exist in fact many other mechanisms whereby functional or physiological signal variations may be observed using MRI. Of particular interest, and the topic of this chapter, is the rich set of methods available for imaging tissue perfusion and other aspects of vascular function in the brain.

Perfusion, defined as the rate at which blood is delivered to tissue and commonly expressed in units of milliliters of blood delivered per 100 ml of brain tissue per minute, is a useful marker for brain activity and viability due to its critical role in supporting neuronal (and glial) function. Variations in tissue perfusion rate can reflect increased energy demand during increased neuronal workload or deficits related to a pathological incident such as a stroke. The resting rate of brain perfusion in an individual is believed to decline gradually with age, [1,2] and the ability of the brain's vasculature to supply rapid increases in blood flow to meet sudden changes in energy demand may also be degraded by vascular or other health problems.[3,4]

Perfusion MRI techniques can be broadly categorized based on the following characteristics:

1. The physical process is used to create image contrast: This may be via an injected contrast agent, or spatially selective RF tagging. The latter case is known as *arterial spin labeling* (ASL), and we will refer to the RF and gradient pulses used to generate flow contrast as the *tagging module* of the pulse sequence (note that the terms "tag" and "label" will be used interchangeably in this text; the hydrogen nuclei detected on most clinical MRI systems may be equivalently referred to as *spins* or *protons*).
2. The approach used to capture the image (e.g., spin-echo vs. gradient-echo, echo-planar imaging vs. spiral or other imaging method, sequential multi-slice vs. 3D acquisition), is referred to below as the *image readout module* (or simply readout module). In the case of an ASL acquisition, the tagging module is first applied to generate flow-dependent contrast in the brain, after which the image readout module is applied to capture an image of this.
3. The specific physiological parameter represented by the image signal [e.g., perfusion, cerebral blood volume (CBV), time-to-peak (TTP), mean transit time (MTT)], is determined by point 1, but may also be influenced by point 2.

As indicated above, perfusion MRI techniques can be grouped into those based on injection of a blood-borne contrast agent versus ASL methods in which the MRI system applies additional radio frequency (RF) pulses to achieve image contrast related to blood flow through spatially selective tagging of blood flowing in the major arteries supplying the brain. The methods based on contrast agents are often referred to as susceptibility contrast techniques, since the injected

R. Hoge (✉)
Department of Physiology and Institute of Biomedical Engineering, Université de Montréal, Centre de recherche de l'institut universitaire de gériatrie de Montréal, Montréal, QC, Canada
e-mail: r.hoge@umontreal.ca

R.A. Cohen and L.H. Sweet (eds.), *Brain Imaging in Behavioral Medicine and Clinical Neuroscience*,
DOI 10.1007/978-1-4419-6373-4_5, © Springer Science+Business Media, LLC 2011

agent alters the magnetic susceptibility of the blood. Perturbation of blood susceptibility leads to dramatic changes in the T2 and T2* of tissues (see Chap. 2 for a discussion of basic MRI physics). Thus, a fundamental difference between these two approaches is that contrast based on injected agents is observed via fairly robust alterations of the pattern of transverse magnetization created by the excitation pulse in the image readout module, while techniques using spatially selective RF tagging create a much more subtle pattern of contrast in the longitudinal magnetization that is available for subsequent excitation in the image readout module. For this reason, the inherent sensitivity of the susceptibility method for a *single* measurement of blood flow in the brain is much higher than that of ASL. However, as we will see below, the two techniques are applied in very different ways that render each of them appropriate for specific purposes. Currently, susceptibility-based methods are widely used in the clinic to assess resting brain perfusion in stroke patients, while ASL techniques are more widely adopted in research studies of dynamic perfusion responses during functional tasks. In the following sections, we will discuss the various approaches used in more detail.

Susceptibility Methods

Susceptibility methods for imaging brain perfusion depend on changes in transverse relaxation rates (T2, T2*) caused by injection of a paramagnetic contrast agent. As we shall see, perfusion imaging techniques based on injected contrast agents can be further categorized depending on whether the agent is injected as a rapid bolus or as a standard intravenous injection with the goal of obtaining a stable concentration of the compound distributed throughout the blood.

Dynamic Susceptibility Contrast Methods

For making a single measurement of resting brain perfusion, particularly in patients who may suffer from acute and focal impairments in blood flow (i.e., stroke), susceptibility methods based on rapid, intravenous bolus injections of rare earth compounds incorporating gadolinium or dysprosium have become the clinical option of choice. Rapid bolus passage creates a brief but pronounced darkening in T2*-weighted images, yielding a well-defined signal curve that can be modeled to extract several hemodynamic parameters including TTP, MTT, cerebral blood flow, and CBV. In the vast majority of bolus passage studies, the paramagnetic element gadolinium (atomic symbol Gd) is used as the contrast agent to create the required disruption of magnetic susceptibility and subsequent shortening of T2* (dysprosium, atomic symbol Dy, is also used but less commonly). Since rare earth elements such as gadolinium and dysprosium are moderately toxic, they are administered with a chelating agent such as diethylene triamine pentaacetic acid (DTPA) to reduce biological interaction and to accelerate clearance of the agent from the body via the kidneys. Typical elimination half-life for the contrast agent Gd-DTPA in humans is approximately 90 min (based on information in product monograph for several commercial Gd-DTPA products).

The pulse sequences used to measure MRI signal changes during bolus passage studies are typically single-shot echo-planar imaging (EPI) acquisitions with either gradient or spin-echo readouts. The main requirement is that the image contrast be sensitive to changes in T2 or T2* (achieved using spin-echo or gradient-echo, respectively). Spin-echo sequences are believed to emphasize microvascular (capillary) effects, which are more representative of parenchymal perfusion, while gradient-echo sequences may be biased toward signals arising in larger blood vessels.[5,6] The pulse sequences used with contrast agents are simpler than those used with ASL methods, since contrast is provided by the agent and only a suitably (T2 or T2*) weighted image readout module is needed. Typically, a sequence of a hundred or more images is acquired over a period of 1–2 min while the bolus of agent is injected. The resultant image sequence depicts the abrupt signal drop caused by the contrast agent which can be over 50% of the initial signal (see Fig. 5.1).

The change in T2*-weighted signal created by the bolus passage can be converted to a relative change in contrast agent concentration by expressing the signal change as the change in R2* (1/T2*). The resultant time–concentration curve is assumed to be equal to the convolution of the *arterial input function* (AIF), which can be measured by sampling the bolus passage curve from an artery entering the brain, with an

5 Perfusion MRI

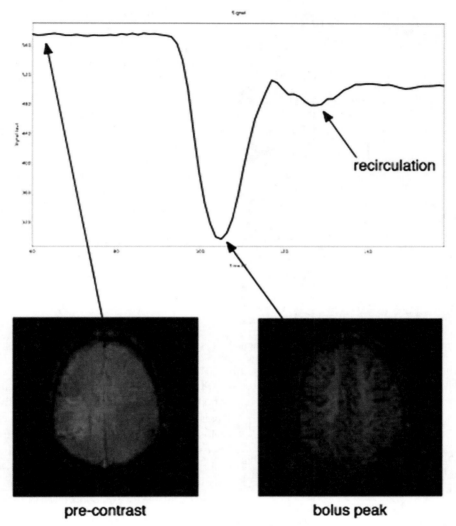

Fig. 5.1 Bolus passage curve in brain (gray matter) following injection of Gadolinium-DTPA contrast agent. The initial signal drop as well as a subsequent curve showing recirculation of the bolus can be seen. Duration of the bolus passage is approximately 20 s in this example. Raw (unprocessed) MR images are shown before the arrival of the bolus and at moment of peak contrast agent concentration upon arrival

impulse response function representing additional delay and dispersion between the point where the AIF is measured and a given location in the brain. Mathematical deconvolution of the AIF from the signal observed at each image voxel is then performed to produce an estimate of cerebral blood flow at each location (Fig. 5.2).[7] Other parameters that can be extracted from the bolus passage curve include the TTP, MTT, and CBV. The TTP is simply the time at which the peak signal change occurred, while the MTT is the average time over which a unit volume of blood occupies the capillary bed (equal to CBV divided by cerebral blood flow). CBV can be computed as the integral of the time–concentration curve. It should be noted that all of these parameter estimates represent the average value over the period during which the bolus passage is measured. The requirement to measure the entire bolus passage curve for a single estimate of blood flow means that this approach is not suitable for procedures such as functional studies in which transient variations in blood flow must be continually monitored.

Maps of TTP and cerebral blood flow typically show regional alterations associated with stroke with

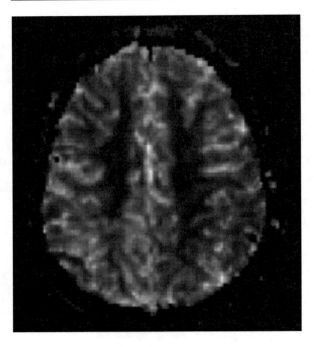

Fig. 5.2 Image of cerebral blood flow computed from dynamic bolus passage curve. The raw images were acquired using a spin-echo sequence, and the in-plane spatial resolution is 1.7 mm. Slice thickness was 5 mm

great sensitivity, making them extremely useful for assessing clinical prognosis in such cases.

With the ongoing proliferation of higher field magnets, it should be mentioned that while susceptibility-based contrast is generally amplified at higher field, the effects produced by exogenous agents such as Gd-DTPA or USPIOs are so pronounced that even at 1.5 T these methods are highly effective. This is in contrast with BOLD imaging, where the faint signal modulations associated with brain activation are much more readily detected at higher field strengths. The reliability of dynamic susceptibility contrast (DSC) methods at 1.5 T is another reason for their extremely wide clinical adoption.

Steady-State Techniques

The relatively rapid elimination of chelated rare earth agents such as Gd-DTPA results in a continually varying concentration of the agent in the blood, which would confound any attempts to perform continual monitoring of contrast agent distribution over a time scale of minutes. A second class of agents, based on ultrasmall superparamagnetic iron oxide (USPIO) particles is used as a contrast agent for imaging blood volume for the specific reason that its elimination half-life is considerably longer (over 5 h),[8] resulting in relatively stable blood concentration levels. When such agents are in steady state in the blood, changes in CBV result in linearly proportional changes in the T2*-weighted signal of perfused tissues. Such agents can, therefore, be used to detect and quantify changes in CBV in functional experiments.[9] Since the hemodynamic measures available are restricted to dynamic measures of CBV in functional experiments, USPIOs have been less prominent in clinical applications for measuring brain perfusion. These compounds have, however, found clinical application for studying immune responses in multiple sclerosis, stroke, and cancer, since they are taken up in macrophages and can therefore be used to track macrophage infiltration.[10-12]

Arterial Spin Labeling

ASL methods are those in which the image readout module is preceded by additional, spatially selective RF pulses, which are used to invert the magnetic polarity of blood flowing toward the brain (a 180° RF pulse is used; see Chap. 2 on basic MR physics). Arrival of such tagged blood at an image voxel causes the local value of longitudinal magnetization, which determines the imaging signal available for excitation, to vary in a flow-dependent manner (delivery of the inverted blood magnetization causes the brain signal to decrease slightly). This tagging originates purely through the intrinsic nuclear magnetization of the blood, and no injected contrast agent is required. One advantage of ASL is, therefore, that it can be considered completely noninvasive. Since the actual MR image intensity of a tagged voxel depends on many other factors besides delivery of the blood-borne tag, control acquisitions (identical except without tagging) are generally interleaved between tagged acquisitions in an ASL image series. The flow-dependent signal component can then be isolated through subtraction of adjacent image pairs (an example of ASL images before and after subtraction is shown in Fig. 5.3). Since an image depicting regional perfusion can be obtained in a single subtraction pair (which can be acquired in 4 s), the ASL approach is much more suitable to the continuous measurement of blood flow in functional studies than gadolinium bolus studies. However, the contrast-to-noise

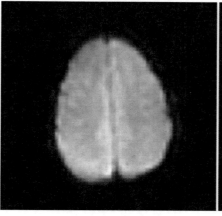

| Raw EPI | Mean difference image |

Fig. 5.3 Example of ASL images before and after subtraction and averaging. The weak ASL tagging signal is not visible to the naked eye, but after pairwise subtraction and averaging the pattern of perfusion contrast between gray and white matter can be clearly seen. Note that the in-plane spatial resolution of the ASL perfusion image (3.75 mm) is much lower than that of the DSC image shown in Fig. 5.2. A slice thickness of 6 mm was used

ratio of a single ASL subtraction image is much lower than that of a flow map derived from bolus passage data. This shortcoming can be overcome by averaging many ASL subtraction images acquired over a period of several minutes.

The pulse sequences used for ASL are more complex than those used for susceptibility methods, due to the need for additional RF and gradient pulses in the tagging module. The classification of ASL sequence variants is, therefore, rather more involved, but a given sequence can be described based on the following attributes:

1. The geometry and timing with which the tagging region, typically a band covering the arteries of the neck, is inverted: This can be done using either continuous or pulsed application of RF energy. In addition to geometric selection of blood for tagging, blood flow velocity may also be used.
2. The application of additional measures used to control the duration of tag delivery, important to ensure quantitative accuracy in pulsed ASL (PASL).
3. The technique used in the imaging readout module to capture the pattern of contrast in the longitudinal magnetization created by the first two steps.

In the following sections, we discuss these aspects in more detail and see that they have important consequences for the sensitivity and accuracy of ASL methods.

Creation of the Spin Label

As noted above, ASL can be divided into several broad categories based on how selective tagging of blood is performed. We discuss here pulsed and continuous ASL (CASL) methods and, briefly, a newer class of velocity-selective techniques. The tagging scheme used plays an important role in determining the range of flow conditions under which the pulse sequence will yield accurate measures, and also the degree to which confounding factors such as magnetization transfer effects are controlled. We first consider PASL, which is currently the most widely used approach.

Pulsed ASL

Pulsed techniques have formed the most popular class of ASL methods for several years, largely due to the fact that solutions have been available to control potentially confounding effects associated with magnetization transfer and uncontrolled tag duration. PASL methods are also generally practicable on a broad range of clinical MRI systems, which has not always been the case for continuous labeling techniques.

The first step in a typical PASL sequence is to apply a 180° RF pulse to invert the magnetization in a region that includes the major arteries supplying blood to the brain.

The tag region, which may be a band of approximately transverse orientation covering the neck and positioned parallel to the stack of imaging slices covering the brain, is selected using a shaped RF pulse and selection gradient as described in Chap. 2. All soft tissues and blood within the defined region are inverted, and the blood thus labeled continues to flow toward the brain. A delay of 1 to 1.5 s is typically inserted between this inversion prepulse and the imaging module to allow the tagged blood to flow to the brain regions that are to be imaged.

Although we discuss variants of this in detail below, a typical tagging module might invert a band of blood 10 cm thick separated from the most inferior image slice by a gap of 1 cm. Remember that the tag carried by the blood consists of its inverted nuclear magnetic polarization, which is not affected by displacement during flow but does decay with a time constant of T1 as it flows to the brain.

Two limitations associated with PASL, compared with other techniques described below, relate to its sensitivity and its accuracy under varying flow conditions. The sensitivity of ASL is impaired by the fact that all of the blood inverted for labeling is created effectively at a single instant (the RF pulse used is very short). The label, therefore, decays exponentially with time constant T1 during the entire interval (typically 1–1.5 s as noted above) between the inversion pulse of the labeling module and the excitation pulse of the image readout module. The effect of the tagged blood is to create a small reduction of the image signal in brain tissues once it is delivered; the potential signal reduction would be a maximum immediately following inversion (when the strong blood magnetization signal is negated) but is much weaker by the time the blood is actually delivered and the image captured. This is part of the reason why ASL signal changes observed in functional experiments are considered typically to be about an order of magnitude smaller (relative to the raw, presubtraction EPI signal) than signals observed during the changes seen during an equivalent BOLD fMRI experiment (the weak signal is also due to the low blood volume fraction in gray matter). It has also limited the clinical application of both PASL and CASL in patients with stroke, since the prolonged label delivery times associated with ischemic stroke may result in complete decay of any tagging signal.

The second limitation, relating to accuracy, is due to the fact that the complete delivery of a bolus of inverted blood defined solely by the spatial extent of a tagging band may result in an ASL subtraction signal that "saturates" for very high global blood flow changes. This would result in an inability to detect flow changes during global manipulations such as hypercapnia induction. While there is no way to recover the ASL signal lost due to T1 decay, we see that there are approaches that can be used to ensure that the ASL difference signal is always a linear function of blood flow, even during very large global flow increases.

It is important to note that, in both DSC and ASL methods, there exists a bolus passage curve in the brain tissues (see Fig. 5.4 for an example of an ASL bolus passage curve). An important difference is that, in the case of a DSC study, this curve may last 20 s and that it is repeatedly sampled by the acquired image series. This is the optimal situation for quantitative tracer kinetic modeling and allows fairly straightforward methods to be used to quantify blood flow. In the case of ASL, the bolus passage curve is much shorter (2–3 s), and it is generally only sampled once, typically well after the bolus has finished flowing through the brain. It is this latter characteristic that can lead to errors in ASL signal if the bolus duration is defined through a fixed width rather than using a fixed time duration.[13]

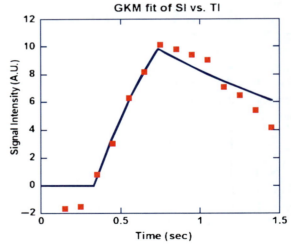

Fig. 5.4 Bolus passage curve for ASL experiment, obtained by systematically varying the postlabel inversion delay time (TI) during repeated measurements. Measured subtraction signal intensity (SI) values are shown in *red*, together with a general kinetic model (GKM) fit to the data. Arrival of both the leading and trailing edges of the bolus of tagged blood can be seen. Duration of the bolus passage is approximately 0.5 s. Image acquisition is typically performed at around 1.5 s, during the period of label clearance

Another challenge that affects both PASL and CASL methods is the control of magnetization transfer (MT) effects. Magnetization transfer is a phenomenon in which off-resonance RF energy, which would not normally affect water protons in tissue, is nonetheless able to excite other hydrogen nuclei associated with large biological molecules (proteins, lipids), due to the latter having a much broader resonance peak. Although such macromolecular protons are generally not visible in MRI due to their very short T2 relaxation times, reduction of the macromolecular proton signal by off-resonance RF energy can result in an indirect reduction of the water signal due to the transfer of longitudinal magnetization (hence the term MT) between these two populations of nuclei. Thus, even though a spatially selective inversion pulse targeting the neck is "off resonance" with respect to the head (and therefore should not affect its protons), there may still be a small signal reduction in the water proton signal from the head due to magnetization transfer. Because isolation of the flow-dependent portion of the total MRI signal requires subtraction of a control acquisition, which is identical to the label acquisition in every respect except for the presence of labeled blood, simply turning off the RF pulse in the control acquisition may lead to an unbalanced MT effect that could be erroneously attributed to blood flow. For this reason, most pulsed labeling schemes currently in use include an RF pulse in the control phase whose purpose is to balance MT effects from the labeling pulse (but which tags no blood).

Here, we describe several of the most popular PASL labeling schemes (shown in Fig. 5.5), for the purpose of illustrating their relative merits under different applications. We see that much of the variation relates to the approach taken to control for MT effects.

Echo-Planar Imaging and Signal Targeting with Alternating Radio Frequency

Echo-planar imaging and signal targeting with alternating radio frequency (EPISTAR) is the earliest reported PASL technique.[14] In this approach, the label phase consists of a slice-selective inversion band targeting the region inferior to the slices to be imaged which will result in delivery of labeled blood to the brain. The control phase consists of an inversion band identical to that used in the label phase, but placed *above* the imaged slices separated by an equal gap (presumably not overlapping with any arterial vessels). In spite of the symmetry of this arrangement, off-resonance MT effects are only truly controlled along a single slice, and any additional image slices acquired above or below this central location could potentially still suffer uncontrolled MT effects. More complex variants were proposed which included multiple inversion pulses at reduced power in the control phase, but other more recent tagging variants discussed below are likely to offer improved MT control in multislice acquisitions. It is also possible

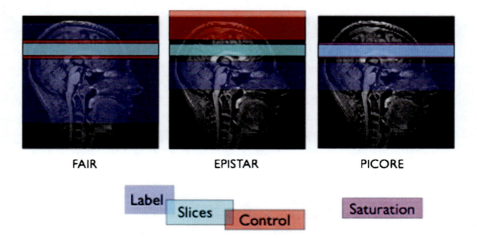

Fig. 5.5 Tagging geometry variants of arterial spin labeling. The label and control regions targeted by spatially selective tagging pulses are shown respectively in *dark blue* and *red*. The slices acquired by the image readout module are shown in *light blue*. The additional saturation band used in PICORE, which overlaps with the image slices, is shown in *purple*

that blood entering the imaged volume from above may result in an erroneously inverted flow signal (i.e., negative instead of positive).

One advantage of tagging schemes such as EPISTAR, in which the tagging pulses do not overlap with the imaged slices, is that the control images can be used to measure BOLD effects in a functional experiment. In approaches such as FAIR (discussed below), where the longitudinal magnetization of the imaged slices may be greatly reduced, or where background suppression techniques are used, this is not an option. A disadvantage of having this high background signal is that spontaneous or task-related BOLD signal changes may increase levels of physiological noise or result in subtraction errors if the BOLD signal is systematically changing (i.e., at the onset or cessation of a stimulus). Subtraction errors from BOLD contamination can be controlled using surround subtraction methods (tag images are subtracted from the average of their two neighbors), by using the shortest possible echo time and/or using a spin-echo readout, or by acquiring multi-TE data and extrapolating the signal at TE = 0.

An additional concern in EPISTAR and other PASL variants is that if the spatial profile of the tagging pulse is not sharply square, then subtraction errors may be introduced simply due to overlap of an unintentionally broad tag boundary with some of the most inferior image slices. Previously, this situation was avoided by using a large spatial gap (greater than 1 cm) between the upper edge of the tag volume and the nearest image slice, at the expense of increased transit delay. Today, this concern has largely been addressed through the use of inversion pulse designs such as FOCI[15] or BASSI,[16,17] which produce very sharp slice profiles even for relatively broad inversion bands (20 cm).

Within limits imposed by T1 decay, the amount of ASL signal available depends partly on the width of the tagging band selected. Historically, thicknesses on the order of 10 cm have been popular due to restrictions imposed by transmit–receive head coils used in early publications (these smaller coils did not extend very far over the neck). With the increasing use of receive-only phased array coils for detection, inversion and excitation are now typically performed using the body coil integrated into the bore of most clinical MRI systems (at 3 T and below; this may be more rare at 7 T). This makes broader tagging bands feasible, of

20 cm or more in thickness. It should be noted that to retain sharp edges in such broad inversion bands may require longer pulses and/or higher energy deposition, but 20 cm appears to be readily attainable at 3 T using BASSI pulses.[17] Broader tagging bands may also improve the efficacy of strategies such as QUIPSS II (discussed below) for controlling tag duration to ensure quantitative accuracy.

Flow Alternating Inversion Recovery

In flow alternating inversion recovery (FAIR), the label phase consists of a nonselective inversion pulse and the control phase is a selective pulse that covers the slice or slices to be imaged. Since both label and control prepulses are "on resonance" for the imaged slices, magnetization transfer effects are not an issue. Inversion band profile is still a concern, since "rounding" of the profile of the control band near its edges results in subtraction errors in the top and bottom slices. To avoid this, the control band usually extends some distance above and below the outermost slices (analogous to the gap used in EPISTAR and PICORE), and sharp profiles can be ensured through the use of FOCI or BASSI pulses. FAIR performed with body coil inversion may offer the largest possible amount of ASL signal at high flow rates, if the spatial profile of the transmit coil allows inversion over a very large region (in practice, this will vary and must be assessed on a given MRI system).

A distinguishing characteristic of FAIR is that the inversion pulses for both the label and control phases overlap with the image slices. With typical delay times between inversion and excitation ranging from 1 to 1.5 s, the image intensity in the acquired slices (determined by T1 recovery from inversion) is substantially reduced below the value that would be observed with the more fully relaxed longitudinal magnetization typical of EPISTAR or PICORE. This may be an advantage due to the reduction of signal fluctuation associated with BOLD effects or subject motion, but it precludes the use of image data for analysis of BOLD signals (since the sensitivity is likely to be reduced to an unacceptable degree).

In terms of the quantity and sophistication of RF and gradient pulses used, FAIR is probably the simplest PASL variant. This may render it less vulnerable to system hardware instabilities than sequences requiring extensive RF and/or gradient activity.

It should be noted that FAIR may tag blood arriving from either above or below the imaged volume.

Proximal Inversion with a Control for Off-Resonance Effects

As of this writing, Proximal inversion with a control for off-resonance effects (PICORE)[13] is perhaps the most widely used PASL tagging variant since it offers control of MT effects in multislice acquisitions and leaves the image slice magnetization untouched for analysis of BOLD signals in the control image series if required.

The PICORE tagging variant uses a simple but elegant means to eliminate MT errors in subtraction images. Since magnetization transfer involves the alteration of *longitudinal* magnetization in the imaged slices by the inversion prepulse, the effect cannot happen if the longitudinal magnetization is already zero. This situation is achieved in PICORE by applying one or more 90° pulses selective for the imaged volume immediately prior to application of the selective inversion pulse used for tagging, as well as before the corresponding pulse used in the control phase. The control-phase counterpart to the inversion tagging pulse is an identical RF pulse that is played out with no gradient. This will not result in the inversion or excitation of any tissue, but should exert similar off-resonance effects on the imaged volume (which having just been saturated should not experience any MT effects anyhow).

As with EPISTAR, PICORE allows use of the sequence of control images for analysis of BOLD signals in functional studies. The same considerations with respect to tag band profiles apply.

Continuous ASL

The earliest methods proposed for ASL[18,19] were based on continuous application of a sinusoidal RF waveform, in conjunction with a field gradient oriented along the direction of blood flow, during a period of several seconds. Because the resonant frequency of blood protons varies as they flow through the magnetic field gradient, they experience an apparent "sweep" of the applied frequency relative to their instantaneous resonant frequency. If the amplitude of the RF waveform is sufficiently high, the protons undergo what is termed adiabatic inversion as they flow through the labeling plane, which is the

point along the gradient at which the resonant frequency is equal to the frequency of the continuously applied RF. Other static tissues simply have their net magnetization reduced to zero by the combination of prolonged RF radiation and magnetic field gradient. At the end of the labeling period, an additional gap of 1–2 s is inserted prior to the image readout module to allow all labeled blood to flow to the brain tissues.

Relative to the PASL methods described above, the continuous labeling approach has two main advantages. The first is that the amount of tagged blood available for delivery to a given brain voxel is defined solely by the duration of the RF tagging waveform (rather than the geometric extent of the tag band created by an inversion pulse). This has the important consequence that the ASL difference signal is always a linear function of tissue perfusion, which may not be the case when tag duration is determined by the width of an inversion band as in PASL (although techniques such as QUIPSS II, described below, address this). The second advantage is that while the blood tagged in PASL is only fully inverted (and therefore capable of providing maximum contrast) at the instant the inversion pulse is applied, in CASL the brain is supplied with fully inverted blood during the entire tagging interval. This greatly reduces the loss of tag signal through T1 decay during the delivery period, resulting in increased image sensitivity.

CASL is subject to the same magnetization transfer concerns as PASL, since the prolonged application of high-amplitude RF can generate a significant MT effect in brain tissues. In a single-slice acquisition, the effect could easily be cancelled in the control phase by inverting the polarity of the tagging gradient, creating a labeling plane on the opposite side of the slice.[18,19] However, this approach would not be effective in a multislice acquisition, since the MT phenomenon would only be cancelled in a single central slice. This limitation has been overcome using schemes in which the control phase creates two closely spaced inversion planes, resulting in a 360° rotation of the magnetization and elimination of any potential tagging effect.[20,21] With appropriate adjustment of RF amplitude, this allows closer matching of the MT effects caused by the tag phase.

In spite of the obvious advantages of CASL, it has been less widely adopted than PASL. This is likely due to the fact that many clinical MRI systems include RF amplifiers that are not optimized for the generation of prolonged pulses. The required waveforms may be impossible to generate due to software restrictions or hardware limits. At higher field strengths, the amount of RF energy deposition caused by such sequences may also exceed permissible limits (the risks are primarily related to heating, which may be a problem in clinical populations with impaired thermal regulation). This has been addressed more recently through the development of what are known as pseudocontinuous ASL methods, in which a long series of RF pulses are concatenated to produce a similar effect to a truly continuous pulse. The length of gap required between pulses, relative to the length of the pulses, is determined by the MRI system's hardware and software limitations. Results comparable to those obtained using true continuous methods have been reported on standard clinical MRI systems.[22]

An additional approach which has been demonstrated for CASL is the use of a small, dedicated external coil that is placed against the neck and used specifically for labeling of blood in the neck arteries.[23] This technique reduces energy deposition, due to the small size of the coil. In some cases, an entire external RF amplifier and coil system is used, triggered by logic pulses emitted by the scanner at the appropriate time. Although this approach can be used to bypass technical limitations of the RF transmit system on clinical scanners for long RF pulses, the need for additional hardware have limited the adoption of this approach. It should be noted that such methods permit demonstration of the perfusion territories associated with specific arteries in the neck,[24] which may be of interest for investigating the impact of vascular disease.

Another concern with CASL methods is that the labeling efficiency depends on the velocity of blood flow perpendicular to the labeling plane defined by the RF/gradient pairing. If the labeling plane intersects several arteries (e.g., carotid and vertebral) such that they cross at different angles, it is possible that the degree of labeling may vary in the different vessels (i.e., the blood may not be fully inverted in vessels more oblique to the labeling plane). This could potentially create spurious differences in the apparent pattern of regional blood flow, since brain regions whose perfusion territory is primarily served by a poorly labeled vessel will have reduced ASL signal. It is therefore probably wise to place the labeling plane at a location where the vessel geometry is uniformly perpendicular to the labeling plane. It is possible that mixing of blood in the circle of Willis may alleviate the above effect, but this is likely to vary widely between individuals.

Velocity-Sensitive ASL

As noted above, there are several concerns which may arise when blood is selected for labeling based on spatial location, either in a tagging band below the brain as in PASL, or as it passes through a labeling plane as in CASL. The time required for labeled blood to travel between the tagging region and brain tissue may be so prolonged in the case of ischemic stroke that the tag is completely eliminated through T1 decay (resulting in a lower limit to the dynamic range). Very large gaps between the top of a PASL tag band and the top slices of a whole-brain acquisition may also result in excessive label decay. To address these concerns, a class of ASL methods based on velocity selectivity rather than spatial selectivity has been introduced. This approach is called velocity-selective arterial spin labeling (VSASL).[25]

VSASL makes use of the fact that it is possible to selectively manipulate the longitudinal magnetization of flowing blood based on its flow velocity. This is achieved using special RF and gradient pulse combinations that can saturate (reduce to zero) the magnetization of blood that is flowing above some cutoff velocity that is specified by selecting the appropriate pulse parameters. Note that, in VSASL, the blood is saturated rather than inverted, due to the limitations of velocity selective pulses currently available. This decreases to the potential contrast available compared with PASL and CASL, but in special cases, the other characteristics of VSASL may offset this limitation.

In a VSASL acquisition, blood flowing above a certain cutoff velocity is first tagged. This cutoff velocity is typically selected to be sufficiently high that blood in the major arteries supplying the brain will be selected (note that this may also include blood in large veins). The spatial boundary of the resultant tagging "front" are arbitrary, and do not influence the results obtained. After a delay time to allow the tagged blood to flow into the brain, an image is acquired in which a second set of velocity selective pulses is used to include only those spins that are below the cutoff velocity. This ensures that, in the tag image, only spins that are initially flowing above the cutoff velocity and which subsequently decelerated are included. Venous blood, which typically accelerates as it progresses along the venous tree, is thus excluded. The control acquisition, required to isolate the flow-dependent component, is identical to the tagging acquisition except that the initial velocity-selective pulses (for high-velocity spins) are excluded.

Concerns in VSASL include confounding effects associated with diffusion, subject motion, and pulsatile CSF flow. These issues have been largely addressed through careful selection of VS pulse parameters.[25] Although the contrast-to-noise ratio of the flow signal in VSASL has been reported to be somewhat lower than that obtained using current PASL methods, VSASL remains promising due to the fact that it should in theory remain effective even in the presence of slow or collateral blood flow. It is also the only ASL method that guarantees that only arterial, and not venous, blood is tagged. Due to the complexity of implementation and ongoing requirements to improve immunity to motion and diffusion effects, VSASL has not surpassed PASL methods in frequency of use at this writing.

Methods Used to Control Duration of ASL Tagging

Now that we have examined in detail the various methods used to label arterial blood, we briefly consider the problem of how to ensure that the resultant ASL signal can be used as a quantitative indicator of cerebral blood flow. As noted above, defining an ASL tag bolus based purely on geometric extent is not sufficient to ensure quantitative accuracy of the ASL subtraction signal. In particular, we wish to ensure that the ASL difference signal is a linear function of cerebral blood flow under all conditions. Under conditions of extremely slow flow, there is of course the risk that complete T1 decay of the tag will prevail, in which case it is not possible to measure blood flow below a certain level. However, a greater concern is that, at high flow rates, a compression of the tag duration occurs which leads to a spurious reduction of the apparent flow signal.[13,26] This can lead to a paradoxical situation where large increases in blood flow, particularly if they are global in nature, are underestimated or even completely undetected during a PASL measurement. The problem is of particular concern for global effects such as hypercapnic manipulations (used to measure vascular reactivity[27] or in calibrated MRI methods[28,29]) since increase of blood flow throughout the brain can substantially accelerate flow in the major arteries lower down in the neck, leading to large shifts in the times at which the tag enters and clears a given brain location.

To avoid the scenario described above, it is necessary that the duration during which tagged blood flows into a brain voxel be constant regardless of the flow rate. A number of approaches have been proposed to ensure this, all of them variants of a method originally termed quantitative imaging of perfusion using a single subtraction (QUIPSS).[13] In the approach known as QUIPSS II (a second version of QUIPSS[30]), additional RF saturation pulses that are selective for the tag band are applied at some predetermined time after the initial inversion. The effect of these pulses, which are applied in both the label and control phases, is to eliminate the ASL signal in any tagged blood that remains in the tagging band when that saturation pulse is applied. If these pulses are applied before the distal end of the labeled bolus exits the tagging region (as they must be for this approach to be effective), then the duration of bolus delivery will be completely determined by the time between inversion and saturation (usually denoted TI1; the interval between inversion and excitation is denoted TI2). Under such conditions, the ASL signal can be treated as a quantitative index of cerebral blood flow.

Variants of the QUIPSS II approach that have been widely adopted include Q2TIPS (QUIPSS II with thin-slice TI1 periodic saturation), in which a thin sheet along the top edge of the labeling region is continually saturated with a series of closely spaced $90°$ pulses after TI1.[31] This approach avoids errors related to nonuniform slab profiles that may arise when a thick slab is saturated using a single $90°$ pulse.

It should be noted that methods such as QUIPSS II are not required for CASL, since the tag duration is explicitly defined by the length of time during which the continuous labeling pulse is applied.

Absolute Perfusion Quantification with ASL

The discussion above has addressed the question of how to achieve flow-dependent contrast and ensure that the resultant signal is a linear function of cerebral blood flow. We now consider how ASL measures can be translated into absolute units of perfusion, commonly expressed as milliliters of blood per 100 ml of brain tissue per minute (ml/100 ml/min).

If QUIPSS II or an equivalent variant has been used, the ASL difference signal ΔM can be approximated as

$$\Delta M = 2M_{0B} f \tau e^{-TI_2/T_{1B}}$$

where M_{0B} is the fully relaxed magnetization of blood (in the arbitrary intensity units of the MRI scanner), f is cerebral blood flow in ml/ml/s, τ is the time duration of the tag (equal to TI1), TI2 is the interval between inversion and excitation, and T_{1B} is the T1 recovery time constant for blood (see ref. [26] for an extensive analysis). Here, we have omitted an additional correction factor, often denoted q, which is generally close to one and which accounts for exchange of tagged water from blood to tissue and the associated small departure from the blood T1 as well as tag clearance via reverse exchange and subsequent venous outflow. It is also possible to include an additional term for T2 decay, but for steady-state measurements, we can assume T2 to be constant. The value for M_{0B} can be estimated by a variety of means, but most commonly a separate EPI scan of fully relaxed magnetization (i.e., a single scan with no preceding RF pulses) is acquired and the value for blood is estimated by multiplying the average value in a region of interest covering cerebrospinal fluid (CSF) by a known proportionality constant.[32] It is, then, possible to solve the above equation for the flow f, which will have units of inverse time (dimensionally equivalent to ml/ml/s, the reciprocal of units for MTT).

Image Readout for Arterial Spin Labeling

As noted above, the sequence components used to achieve flow-dependent contrast are separate from that part of the sequence used to actually acquire the image. Although the labeling module plays a predominant role in determining the characteristics of the resultant image, the image readout module can also have an impact. Here, we describe some of the implications of the various methods available.

Spin-Echo Vs. Gradient Echo

The use of a spin-echo (SE) readout can result in improved signal-to-noise ratio (SNR), due to the reduced signal decay (T2 applies instead of T2*). Spin-echo acquisitions also exhibit little or no signal dropout in areas near air-filled sinuses, an effect which can be pronounced in gradient-echo (GE) acquisitions (particularly with the thick slices and otherwise large voxels used to boost SNR in ASL studies). While gradient-echo readouts are considered mandatory for BOLD fMRI at common clinical field strengths (1.5 and 3 T at this time), there is no requirement for susceptibility contrast in a pure ASL acquisition so SE may be a viable alternative. If one intends to use the untagged sequence of control images for BOLD analysis however, a GE acquisition is required.

Fast Imaging Techniques

Virtually all of the perfusion imaging methods described require a means of acquiring an image in a near instantaneous fashion. This allows rapid alternation between tag and control states, giving the best possible matching of any uncontrolled imaging variables that may fluctuate during the procedure. It is also essential in functional imaging applications where the perfusion signal is to be continuously monitored during some experimental manipulation. The vast majority of published work has been based on EPI, in which the Fourier transform of the object is rapidly scanned along a rectilinear grid following a single RF excitation. While EPI offers very fast image capture and relatively good image quality (it is also the standard approach for functional BOLD imaging), there are a number of limitations that have led to the exploration of other fast imaging variants.

One limitation is the relatively long readout durations required in EPI, which can result in a fairly long effective echo time. This can result in reduced SNR due to T2* decay, as well as contamination from BOLD signal fluctuations. Shorter echo times can be achieved using partial Fourier techniques in EPI (only a portion of the Fourier transform is collected) but have also been obtained using spiral imaging readouts (the effective TE can be made very short, almost zero)[33] and single-shot fast spin-echo readouts (a sequence of 180° refocusing pulses are used to greatly reduce T2* decay and otherwise eliminate susceptibility effects).[34] Spiral imaging may have the additional advantage that physiological and/or instrumental fluctuations result in less degradation of image stability than in EPI.[35] However, spiral sequences can be complex to implement and reconstruct, and they exhibit their own class of distinctive artifacts in areas of perturbed magnetic susceptibility.

Volumetric Acquisition

Many of the initial demonstrations of ASL techniques were performed using a single imaging slice, and it is often much simpler to control for confounding effects such as magnetization transfer or timing errors under such conditions. In the majority of studies, however, it is desirable to acquire coverage of most or all of the brain. This entails acquisition of multiple image slices, which is most commonly performed using a rapid sequence of 2D acquisitions. This approach is simple and generally effective, and whole-brain coverage using ten or more slices of 5–8 mm thickness is readily attainable.

One drawback with sequential 2D acquisition of volumetric imaging data is that the postlabel delay increases successively for each additional slice acquired. This introduces regional variations in the degree of T1 decay experienced by the tag, and may bias results and limit the number of slices that can be acquired. One way around this is the use of a single-shot 3D readout, which results in the instantaneous capture of the entire 3D distribution of longitudinal magnetization throughout the brain. In theory, 3D acquisitions also offer a signal-to-noise benefit since the additional phase-encodes required are equivalent to additional signal averaging. However, the long read-out times required to record the 3D Fourier transform make such approaches challenging, even with the use of hybrid gradient and spin-echo approaches.[34] Nonetheless, additional work on hybrid fast imaging sequences (spirals, parallel imaging) may render this approach feasible for widespread adoption.

Suppression of Macrovascular Signal

As in BOLD fMRI, a common concern in ASL is the possible contamination of parenchymal perfusion signal with much larger signals due to large vessels. In ASL, the presence of larger arteries containing tagged blood can lead to very high subtraction signals. One method for alleviating this is the use of flow crusher gradients,[36] which dephase the signal in blood vessels flowing above a cutoff velocity determined by the amplitude and timing of a bipolar gradient pair. Another approach is to set the delay between inversion and imaging to be sufficiently long that the intravascular tag will have exited the imaged volume before excitation (hence the common use of TI1 values in the order of 1.5 s).

Background Suppression

As mentioned above in the section on FAIR labeling, reducing the level of signal in the static brain tissues (i.e., the signal common to both label and control phases) can greatly reduce unwanted signal fluctuations associated with subject movement and uncontrolled BOLD effects due to respiration or other physiological sources. When FAIR labeling is used, this may happen fortuitously depending on the postlabel delay time selected. In labeling schemes such as EPISTAR and PICORE, however, the background signal intensity is normally high. This can be reduced through the addition of one or more inversion prepulses,[37,38] which are independent of the labeling pulses, and spatially selective for the imaged slices (this approach is known as ASSIST, for *attenuating the static signal in arterial spin tagging*). A single inversion prepulse can be used to nullify the signal from a particular tissue type if the appropriate inversion delay is chosen, based on the T1 value for the tissue to be suppressed. Two inversion pulses can be used to eliminate two tissues types and will greatly reduce signal intensity for a range of T1 values. While such background suppression techniques also reduce the label signal slightly, this is more than offset by the reduction in physiological variation and the overall contrast-to-noise ratio is typically improved.

Implications of Magnetic Field Strength

It has been noted that ASL methods suffer from an inherently low SNR, due to the weakness of the tagging signal and compounded by the fact that this signal decays rapidly during delivery to brain tissues. These concerns make ASL a technique that is particularly likely to benefit from increased magnetic field strength, since the longitudinal magnetic polarization, the induced RF signal, and T1 recovery time for blood all increase with field. It has indeed been found that the contrast-to-noise ratio of steady-state perfusion images is higher at 4 than 1.5 T, although the same report did not conclude there was improved sensitivity in activation data at higher field.[39] The improvements at high field may be partly offset by greater signal fluctuation due to susceptibility effects and subject motion (the use of background suppression techniques may alleviate these to some extent, but this was not explored).

Conclusion

The above discussion should serve as a foundation for further reading of the MRI perfusion imaging literature and help provide an intuitive grasp of the central concepts required to plan a study using this class of techniques. Although the present chapter has focused on imaging of cerebral blood flow, the reader should be aware of other emerging techniques that can be used to image related hemodynamic parameters. Notable methods include VASO[40] and VERVE[41] which have been used to measure total and venous CBV. The role of these methods, like ASL, has been largely to investigate in more detail the biophysical mechanisms underlying the much more sensitive but physiologically ambiguous BOLD signal.

Functional neuroimaging methods are increasingly applied in populations of clinical relevance such as the elderly or patients suffering from cardiovascular or neurodegenerative disease. Due to the complex interaction between neuronal, metabolic, and vascular factors involved in such studies, the ability to perform detailed and specific measurements of hemodynamic and metabolic variables are likely to become extremely important.

References

1. Campbell AM, Beaulieu C. Pulsed arterial spin labeling parameter optimization for an elderly population. *J Magn Reson Imaging*. 2006;23(3):398–403.
2. Parkes LM, Rashid W, Chard DT, Tofts PS. Normal cerebral perfusion measurements using arterial spin labeling: reproducibility, stability, and age and gender effects. *Magn Reson Med*. 2004;51(4):736–743.
3. Mandell DM, Han JS, Poublanc J, Crawley AP, Kassner A, Fisher JA, Mikulis DJ. Selective reduction of blood flow to white matter during hypercapnia corresponds with leukoaraiosis. *Stroke*. 2008;39(7):1993–1998.
4. Ances, Liang, Leontiev, Perthen, Fleisher, Lansing, Buxton. Effects of aging on cerebral blood flow, oxygen metabolism, and blood oxygenation level dependent responses to visual stimulation. *Hum Brain Mapp*. 2008;39(7):(null).

5. Weisskoff RM, Zuo CS, Boxerman JL, Rosen BR. Microscopic susceptibility variation and transverse relaxation: theory and experiment. *Magn Reson Med*. 1994;31(6): 601–610.
6. Boxerman JL, Bandettini PA, Kwong KK, et al. The intravascular contribution to fMRI signal change: Monte Carlo modeling and diffusion-weighted studies in vivo. *Magn Reson Med*.1995;34(1):4–10.
7. Yamada K, Wu O, Gonzalez RG, et al. Magnetic resonance perfusion-weighted imaging of acute cerebral infarction: effect of the calculation methods and underlying vasculopathy. *Stroke*. 2002;33(1):87–94.
8. Shen T, Weissleder R, Papisov M, Bogdanov A, Brady TJ. Monocrystalline iron oxide nanocompounds (MION): physicochemical properties. *Magn Reson Med*. 1993;29(5); 599–604.
9. Leite FP, Tsao D, Vanduffel W, et al. Repeated fMRI using iron oxide contrast agent in awake, behaving macaques at 3 Tesla. *Neuroimage*. 2002;16(2):283–294.
10. Stoll, Bendszus. Imaging of inflammation in the peripheral and central nervous system by magnetic resonance imaging. *Neuroscience*. 2008;16(2):1151–1160.
11. Bellin MF, Beigelman C, Precetti-Morel S. Iron oxide-enhanced MR lymphography: initial experience. *Eur J Radiol*. 2000;34(3):257–264.
12. Saleh A, Schroeter M, Jonkmanns C, Hartung HP, Mödder U, Jander S. In vivo MRI of brain inflammation in human ischaemic stroke. *Brain*. 2004;127(Pt 7):1670–1677.
13. Wong EC, Buxton RB, Frank LR. Implementation of quantitative perfusion imaging techniques for functional brain mapping using pulsed arterial spin labeling. *NMR Biomed*. 1997;10(4–5):237–249.
14. Edelman RR, Siewert B, Darby DG, et al. Qualitative mapping of cerebral blood flow and functional localization with echoplanar MR imaging and signal targeting with alternating radio frequency. *Radiology*. 1994;192(2):513–520.
15. Ordidge RJ, Wylezinska M, Hugg JW, Butterworth E, Franconi F. Frequency offset corrected inversion (FOCI) pulses for use in localized spectroscopy. *Magn Reson Med*. 1996;36(4): 562–566.
16. Warnking JM, Pike GB. Bandwidth-modulated adiabatic RF pulses for uniform selective saturation and inversion. *Magn Reson Med*. 2004;52(5):1190–1199.
17. Warnking JM, Pike GB. Reducing contamination while closing the gap: BASSI RF pulses in PASL. *Magn Reson Med*. 2006;55(4):865–873.
18. Williams DS, Detre JA, Leigh JS, Koretsky AP. Magnetic resonance imaging of perfusion using spin inversion of arterial water. *Proc Natl Acad Sci U S A*. 1992;89(1):212–216.
19. Detre JA, Leigh JS, Williams DS, Koretsky AP. Perfusion imaging. *Magn Reson Med*. 1992;23(1):37–45.
20. Wang J, Zhang Y, Wolf RL, Roc AC, Alsop DC, Detre JA. Amplitude-modulated continuous arterial spin-labeling 3.0-T perfusion MR imaging with a single coil: feasibility study. *Radiology*. 2005;235(1):218–228.
21. Alsop DC, Detre JA. Multisection cerebral blood flow MR imaging with continuous arterial spin labeling. *Radiology*. 1998;208(2):410–416.
22. Fernández-Seara M, Edlow, Hoang, Wang J, Feinberg, Detre JA. Minimizing acquisition time of arterial spin labeling at 3T. *Magn Reson Med*. 2008;59(6):1467–1471.

23. Zhang W, Silva AC, Williams DS, Koretsky AP. NMR measurement of perfusion using arterial spin labeling without saturation of macromolecular spins. *Magn Reson Med.* 1995;33(3):370–376.

24. Zaharchuk G, Ledden PJ, Kwong KK, Reese TG, Rosen BR, Wald LL. Multislice perfusion and perfusion territory imaging in humans with separate label and image coils. *Magn Reson Med.* 1999;41(6):1093–1098.

25. Wong EC, Cronin M, Wu WC, Inglis LR, Frank LR, Liu TT. Velocity-selective arterial spin labeling. *Magn Reson Med.* 2006;55(6):1334–1341.

26. Buxton RB, Frank LR, Wong EC, Siewert B, Warach S, Edelman RR. A general kinetic model for quantitative perfusion imaging with arterial spin labeling. *Magn Reson Med.* 1998;40(3):383–396.

27. Mandell DM, Han JS, Poublanc J, et al. Mapping cerebrovascular reactivity using blood oxygen level-dependent MRI in patients with arterial steno-occlusive disease: comparison with arterial spin labeling MRI. *Stroke.* 2008;39(7): 2021–2028.

28. Davis TL, Kwong KK, Weisskoff RM, Rosen BR. Calibrated functional MRI: mapping the dynamics of oxidative metabolism. *Proc Natl Acad Sci U S A.* 1998;95(4):1834–1839.

29. Hoge RD, Atkinson J, Gill B, Crelier GR, Marrett S, Pike GB. Investigation of BOLD signal dependence on cerebral blood flow and oxygen consumption: the deoxyhemoglobin dilution model. *Magn Reson Med.* 1999;42(5):849–863.

30. Wong EC, Buxton RB, Frank LR. Quantitative imaging of perfusion using a single subtraction (QUIPSS and QUIPSS II). *Magn Reson Med.* 1998;39(5):702–708.

31. Luh WM, Wong EC, Bandettini PA, Hyde JS. QUIPSS II with thin-slice TI1 periodic saturation: a method for improving accuracy of quantitative perfusion imaging using pulsed arterial spin labeling. *Magn Reson Med.* 1999;41(6):1246–1254.

32. Floyd TF, Ratcliffe SJ, Wang J, Resch B, Detre JA. Precision of the CASL-perfusion MRI technique for the measurement of cerebral blood flow in whole brain and vascular territories. *J Magn Reson Imaging.* 2003;18(6):649–655.

33. Li TQ, Moseley ME, Glover G. A FAIR study of motor cortex activation under normo- and hypercapnia induced by breath challenge. *Neuroimage.* 1999;10(5):562–569.

34. Crelier GR, Hoge RD, Munger P, Pike GB. Perfusion-based functional magnetic resonance imaging with single-shot RARE and GRASE acquisitions. *Magn Reson Med.* 1999;41(1):132–136.

35. Krüger G, Glover GH. Physiological noise in oxygenation-sensitive magnetic resonance imaging. *Magn Reson Med.* 2001;46(4):631–637.

36. Ye FQ, Mattay VS, Jezzard P, Frank JA, Weinberger DR, McLaughlin AC. Correction for vascular artifacts in cerebral blood flow values measured by using arterial spin tagging techniques. *Magn Reson Med.* 1997;37(2):226–235.

37. St Lawrence KS, Frank JA, Bandettini PA, Ye FQ. Noise reduction in multi-slice arterial spin tagging imaging. *Magn Reson Med.* 2005;53(3):735–738.

38. Ye FQ, Frank JA, Weinberger DR, McLaughlin AC. Noise reduction in 3D perfusion imaging by attenuating the static signal in arterial spin tagging (ASSIST). *Magn Reson Med.* 2000;44(1):92–100.

39. Wang J, Alsop DC, Li L, et al. Comparison of quantitative perfusion imaging using arterial spin labeling at 1.5 and 4.0 Tesla. *Magn Reson Med.* 2002;48(2):242–254.

40. Lu H, Golay X, Pekar JJ, Van Zijl PCM. Functional magnetic resonance imaging based on changes in vascular space occupancy. *Magn Reson Med.* 2003;50(2):263–274.

41. Stefanovic B, Pike GB. Venous refocusing for volume estimation: VERVE functional magnetic resonance imaging. *Magn Reson Med.* 2005;53(2):339–347.

Chapter 6
Proton Magnetic Resonance Spectroscopy (^{1}H MRS): A Practical Guide for the Clinical Neuroscientist

Andreana P. Haley and Jack Knight-Scott

The Basic Principles of Magnetic Resonance Spectroscopy

Nuclear magnetic resonance emerged in the early 1970s as a tool for elucidating the structure of organic molecules. Since that time, its applications have expanded into multiple other areas. In 1995, magnetic resonance spectroscopy (MRS) was approved by the US Food and Drug Administration for clinical use including differential diagnosis and treatment monitoring in medical conditions such as cancer and multiple sclerosis. The principles of MRS are very similar to those of MRI (see Chap. 2 for details on basic MR physics). Briefly, MRS is founded on the observation that the nuclei of atoms with odd atomic numbers possess a small detectable magnetic field. According to the laws of electromagnetism, all moving charges constitute electrical currents, which generate magnetic fields in their neighborhoods, and thus cause the individual nuclei to possess a "magnetic moment." In other words, the individual nuclei behave like magnetic dipoles and rotate around their axes or oscillate much like the Earth around its axis (Fig. 6.1). The strength of this magnetic moment and oscillation frequency are unique to each nuclear species. The nuclei themselves are often referred to as "spins." Under normal conditions, spins are randomly arranged (Fig. 6.2a); however, when exposed to a strong external magnetic field, such as the one created by the magnet of a magnetic resonance imaging (MRI) scanner, the spins align along the axis of the external field (Fig. 6.2b). While the spins are aligned with the external magnetic field, a radio frequency pulse at their resonance frequency can excite or "flip" the spins. After the pulse is discontinued, the nuclei relax or return to their original state, but in doing so, these oscillating spins generate a weak magnetic field that is detected by special coils. The signal detected by these coils is called the free induction decay or FID. In the case of MRI, the signal from the highly abundant water molecules in the brain is reconstructed into an image, providing structural information about the tissue sample using a mathematical process called Fast Fourier Transformation. The location of various water molecules is spatially encoded through an imposed frequency distribution with the help of additional magnetic gradients (Fig. 6.3a).

MRS, on the other hand, utilizes the inherent frequency distribution that exists between different chemicals. As mentioned earlier, the rotational frequency of atomic nuclei is unique for each nucleus. This unique frequency is called the Larmor frequency and it is governed by the local magnetic field at the site of the proton(s) that make up that particular chemical group. The local magnetic fields are generated by the electrons surrounding the nucleus. If the surrounding magnetic fields were absent, all the nuclei for a given atom would have the same Larmor frequency when placed in a homogeneous magnetic field. Spectroscopically, this would yield a single sharp peak. However, the inherent variation in the local magnetic frequencies results in a spread of multiple peaks. The term used for this phenomenon is "chemical shift." Scientists can identify different molecules through differences in chemical shift. Because the Larmor frequency is directly proportional to the magnetic field strength, the chemical shift is typically expressed in units of parts

---

A.P. Haley (✉)
Department of Psychology, The University
of Texas at Austin, Austin, TX, USA
e-mail: haley@psy.utexas.edu

R.A. Cohen and L.H. Sweet (eds.), *Brain Imaging in Behavioral Medicine and Clinical Neuroscience*,
DOI 10.1007/978-1-4419-6373-4_6, © Springer Science+Business Media, LLC 2011

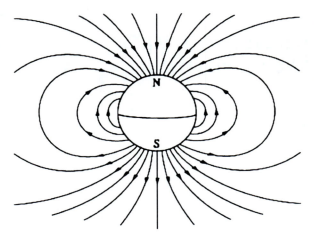

Fig. 6.1 Magnetic dipole

per million (ppm) to allow standardization between magnets of differing field strengths. Thus, the output of any spectroscopy examination constitutes a plot of spectral peaks superimposed on a baseline (Fig. 6.3b). The information about the chemical composition of the sample is imbedded in the characteristics of the peaks in the spectrum. The peak position along the horizontal axis (frequency axis) identifies the metabolite yielding the signal. The area under each peak is directly proportional to the concentration of the metabolite within the sample volume. The area can be measured using curve-fitting techniques (see Section "Quantification").

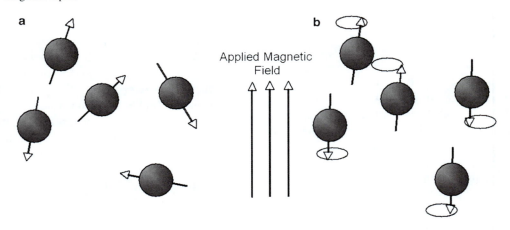

Fig. 6.2 (a) Randomly oriented spins outside magnetic field. (b) Spins inside (aligned with) magnetic field

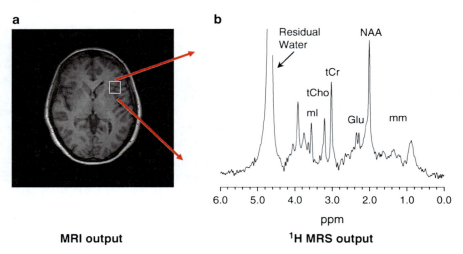

Fig. 6.3 (a, b) A representation of the output generated by an MRI scan at 3 T (a) and a short echo time ¹H MRS examination at 3 T (b). While an MRI image provides structural information about the brain, a ¹H MRS exam provides information about the chemical composition of a tissue sample. *mI* myo-inositol, *tCho* total choline, *tCr* total creatine, *NAA* N-acetyl-aspartate, *Glu* glutamate, *mm* macromolecules

Required Hardware

The basic hardware required to undertake clinical MRS studies is a strong, homogeneous magnet (≥1.5 T, preferably 3 T or greater) and an appropriately tuned radiofrequency coil for the excitation and subsequent detection of the MR signal. For studies of the brain, the patient typically is asked to lie in the center of a 50 cm bore superconducting magnet with a birdcage style coil placed over the head. Initially, a set of conventional MR images are acquired in different planes to ascertain the desired neuroanatomical location for the subsequent volume-localized MRS.

Important MRS Terms

Localization and Volume-of-Interest

The process of selecting a specific region from which to collect neurochemical information in spectroscopy is called localization. There are two classifications of localization: multi-voxel and single-voxel. Currently, single-voxel techniques are the most widely employed technique for human spectroscopy studies. In single-voxel spectroscopy, localization of the volume-of-interest (VOI) or voxel-of-interest (typically in the shape of a cuboid), is achieved through a "crossfire" technique using a series of three radiofrequency pulses and rapidly switching small magnetic field gradients to excite three orthogonal slices (white regions in Fig. 6.4a).

The intersection of these three slices gives the VOI. Additional magnetic gradients are employed to suppress any signal from the slice regions outside the VOI. The detected signal is usually in the form of an "echo." This signal is then mathematically transformed using the Fast Fourier Transform to yield a spectrum with frequency on the horizontal axis and signal intensity on the vertical axis.

Echo Time

The waiting period before sampling the MR signal following an excitation pulse is called echo time (TE). Studies can be conducted in either short (i.e., TE < 35 ms) or long (i.e., TE > 135 ms) echo time; however, short echo times are crucial for detecting metabolites with complex multiple peaks or j-coupling effects, such as glutamate and glucose. Since the signal decays in time, the longer the echo time, the lower the number of detectable metabolites and the weaker their peak intensities. For example, on a 1.5 T MR system, at TE = 144 ms (long echo time), there are only three visible metabolite peaks: N-acetyl-aspartate, creatine, and free choline (Fig. 6.5c). The intensity of these remaining peaks is

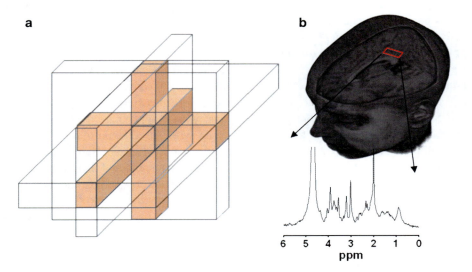

Fig. 6.4 (**a**, **b**) Volume-of-Interest (VOI) localization. Orthogonal slice excitation scheme employed for exciting the VOI to be sampled (**a**) and typical results (**b**)

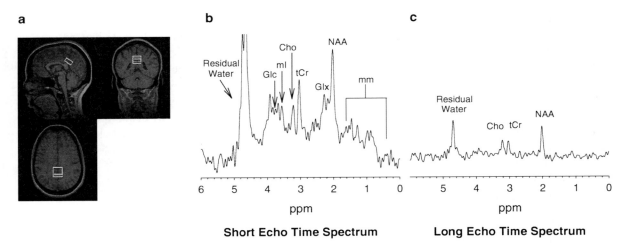

Fig. 6.5 (**a, b, c**) Volume-Of-Interest (VOI) in the posterior cingulate gyrus (**a**) and representative spectra generated by short echo time (TE=10 ms (**b**)) and long echo time (TE=144 ms (**c**)) ¹H MRS examinations at 1.5 T

reduced by approximately two-thirds when compared to the data if sampled at TE=10 ms (short echo time, Fig 6.5b). Complex multiplets, such as glutamate and glutamine (Glx), are completely absent in the long echo time spectrum, greatly reducing the information content of the spectrum.

Shimming

Shimming is the term used to describe adjustments made to the homogeneity of the magnetic field after a person or an object is placed in the scanner. *Establishing a good shim is the single-most important aspect of performing a good spectroscopy study.* The quality of a spectrum can basically be defined by three quantities: water suppression efficiency, resolution, and signal-to-noise ratio; all three are greatly affected by the shim. Water suppression is easier if the shim is good; the ability to identify and separate overlapping peaks, i.e., resolution, is improved by a good shim; and the signal-to-noise ratio is increased, and subsequently the minimum number of averages reduced, when the shim is good. Preliminary assessment of the shim can be employed to determine whether or not an acquisition should be attempted. In any case, some measure of the shim should always be known before collecting a spectrum (Fig. 6.6).

Water Suppression

Because of the high abundance of water in the human brain, the detectable water signal in ¹H MRS is approximately 10,000 times stronger than the signal for any other metabolite (Fig. 6.7). Suppressing the water signal allows peaks from other metabolites to become visible. Some residual water signal is usually visible around 4.7 ppm. Poor water suppression can significantly degrade the quality of MRS data, particularly at lower field strengths.

Spin–Lattice (T_1) and Spin–Spin (T_2) Relaxation Times

As mentioned earlier, exposure to a strong external magnetic field causes the magnetic spins to align along the axis of the external field. In this state, a radio frequency pulse applied at their resonance frequency can excite them. After the pulse is discontinued, the nuclei relax, returning to their original state. The rate of relaxation is exponential and therefore defined by the constants $1/T_1$ and $1/T_2$. T_1 defines the time it takes to transfer approximately two-third of the energy from the nucleus to the surrounding molecules as thermal motion (heat). The process is known as spin–lattice or longitudinal relaxation. T_2, on the other hand, involves energy transfer between nuclei and is referred to as spin–spin or transverse relaxation.

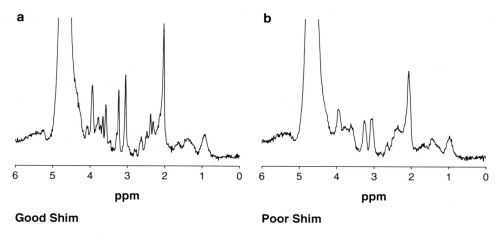

Fig. 6.6 (**a, b**) Effect of shimming on spectral quality at 3 T: good shim = 10 Hz (**a**), and poor shim = 19 Hz (**b**). Both the resolution and signal–noise ratio are reduced by the poor shim

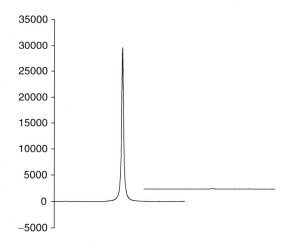

Fig. 6.7 MR signal from unsuppressed water (concentration ~110 M) compared to signal from neurochemicals (concentration ~1–20 mM)

Quantification

Quantification of metabolite concentrations is an important issue in MRS that is yet to be resolved despite the fact that important advances have been made. Scientists moved through several stages of peak characterization including weighing paper cut outs of spectral peaks for relative peak area estimates and using rulers to measure peak heights. Currently, the two primary quantification software packages for ^{1}H MRS are LCModel[30] and jMRUI.[26] While both software packages use sophisticated curve-fitting techniques, LCModel is a software package with the single task of fitting *in vivo* spectra. In comparison, jMRUI is a multifunction software package, capable of user-tailored data processing and includes several methods for fitting the data. In the area of data quantification, LCModel is very user-friendly, does not require a background or training in spectroscopy, and hence can be largely treated as a black box by novice users. In comparison, as currently implemented, jMRUI usage requires detailed understanding of spectroscopy processing methods and thus appears largely limited to spectroscopists.

Another important issue in MRS is how spectral peaks should be referenced for standardization. Both internal (e.g., water or another metabolite) and external (e.g., a test tube of a certain chemical placed next to the subject's body) references have been employed. Thus, metabolite concentrations are usually reported as either ratios to creatine or absolute concentrations. A problem with using creatine ratios is that a disease-induced change in creatine concentrations may obscure true changes in the metabolite concentrations reported as ratios to creatine. To avoid the assumption that creatine concentrations remain unchanged by disease processes or age, absolute concentrations may be used. With the use of an internal water reference, metabolite concentrations can be reported as millimoles per kilogram of brain water as described by Knight-Scott et al.[19]

¹H MRS Visible Metabolites of Neurobiological Significance

A variety of chemicals can be selectively identified along the frequency axis according to their unique resonance frequencies. The most visible neurochemicals in ¹H MRS are discussed below.

2.02 ppm: N-Acetyl-Aspartate (NAA)

N-acetyl-aspartate (NAA) is exclusively found in neurons and oligodendrocyte-type-2 astrocyte progenitor cells[3,35] and is widely regarded as a marker of neuronal viability, synaptic health, and metabolism.[9] During development, paralleling myelination, NAA levels increase dramatically during the first years of life, and then gradually plateau in early adulthood.[17,20,37] Alternatively, reductions in NAA concentrations have been reported in traumatic brain injury and seem to reflect diffuse axonal injury and metabolic changes significantly related to clinical outcome.[6] Lower NAA concentrations in patients relative to healthy controls have also been reported in a number of neurodegenerative disorders such as Alzheimer's disease,[36] Parkinson's disease and parkinsonian syndromes.[8] Reports of age-related declines in NAA concentrations have been less consistent. Studies utilizing ratios have reported age-related declines in NAA,[33] while others, utilizing absolute concentrations or employing atrophy corrections have found stable gray matter NAA concentrations across the age spectrum.[29,32] NAA also appears to reflect mitochondrial health and, thus decreases with oxidative phosphorylation dysfunction.[10] Thus, while reduced NAA can reflect neuronal death, as in stroke,[14,31] it may also reflect transient mitochondrial impairment that is at least partially reversible.[11,12]

3.26 ppm: Choline (Cho), Phosphocholine (PCh), and Glycerophosphocholine (GPC)

The Cho peak, with contributions from several membrane-bound choline compounds, primarily PCh and GPC, is usually considered a marker of membrane

health and turn over.[9] Paralleling myelination, levels of Cho decrease with age during the first 3 years of life.[37] Changes in Cho with increasing age in adulthood have been reported, but the findings show regional variability that is difficult to interpret. For example, choline-containing compounds have been reported to increase with age in frontal gray and parietal white matter[7,21] and whole brain gray matter,[29] but not in occipital gray matter[32] and the hippocampus.[1] In disease conditions, substantial increases in Cho levels have been reported in conditions associated with tissue repair, breakdown, or inflammation such as malignant tumors,[18] multiple sclerosis,[4,11] and HIV infection.[28]

3.03 ppm: Creatine (Cr) and Phosphocreatine (PCr)

The Cr peak, with contributions from creatine and phosphocreatine, is usually considered a marker of energy metabolism. In both clinical and research settings, Cr is often assumed to be stable and used as an internal reference for the calculation of metabolite ratios such as NAA/Cr or Cho/Cr.[9] However, alterations in cerebral Cr and PCr concentrations have been demonstrated in conditions of altered cerebral energy metabolism such as brain tumors.[22] Therefore, metabolite ratios should be interpreted with caution. Age-related changes in Cr have also been reported in the literature, but the findings vary across studies and are difficult to interpret. For example, both Cr and PCr have been reported to increase with age in frontal gray and parietal white matter[7,21] and whole brain gray matter.[29] Others have found Cr to be stable with age in parietal white, occipital gray matter[32] and the hippocampus.[1] Another important fact to bear in mind is that Cr is not synthesized in the brain; therefore, cerebral Cr concentrations can be substantially affected by systemic disease and peripheral Cr administration.[9]

3.56 ppm: Myo-Inositol

Although the role of myo-inositol (mI) is not well understood, it has been proposed to be a glial marker[5] and elevations of mI levels in conditions associated with neuronal loss have been interpreted as a sign of gliosis.[7] However, mI concentrations also may be unrelated to gliosis. mI is an organic osmolite[9] and a precursor for the synthesis of the second messenger inositol tri-phosphate.[13] Therefore, changes in mI concentrations may reflect changes in osmolality or second messenger cascades rather than glial proliferation. Elevations in mI concentrations have been found in conditions associated with cognitive impairment such as Down's syndrome[2,25] and Alzheimer's disease.[23,24,27] Age-related elevations in mI concentrations have been reported in frontal gray[7] but not in parietal white or occipital gray matter,[21,32] possibly reflecting regional differences in the aging process.

3.44 and 3.8 ppm: Glucose

Glucose (Glc) is the main energy source for the brain, continuously delivered from the periphery.[34] At 1.5 T, Glc produces a complex multiplet spectrum centered at 3.4 and 3.8 ppm.[15] At high field strengths of 4.0 T and greater, a singlet at 5.23 ppm is also observable.[16] As noted by Gruetter et al,[16] quantification of glucose from this resonance is preferable as glucose is clearly resolved at this frequency on a 4 T

MR system. However, on lower-field clinical MR systems, this resonance overlaps with the broad wings of the 4.7 ppm water peak and is undetectable after water suppression. At 1.5 T, it is preferable to quantify glucose from the peak at 3.44 ppm because it is less likely than the 3.8 ppm to be influenced by the water suppression or exhibit distortions from the residual water peak. A consideration with quantifying glucose concentration from the resonance at 3.44 ppm is the overlap with other resonances such as myo-inositol, choline, and taurine.

2.34 and 2.36 ppm: Glutamate

Glutamate (Glu) is the primary excitatory neurotransmitter in the brain. At 1.5 T, Glu and glutamine (Gln) are overlapping complex multiplets that are impossible to separate without resorting to specialized spectroscopy techniques called spectral editing. The combination of the overlapping peaks is generally represented as Glx. With standard sequences, Glu is only visible at short echo times. At 3.0 T, the 2.34 and 2.36 Glu resonances are adequately separated from the Gln resonance to provide unequivocally identification of Glu.

Researcher's checklist for setting up a ¹H MRS experiment

General considerations
- Is the required hardware available for MRS data collection?
- MRI scanner (1.5 T or greater, preferably 3 T or greater)
- Is the required software available for MRS data processing?
- Data processing computer equipped with LCModel or jMRUI

Hypothesis
- Does your hypothesis have a chemical basis?
- Are any of the chemicals NMR visible?
- Do you have a specific anatomical region of interest?
- Is your anatomical region of interest "spectroscopy friendly," i.e., can a good shim be achieved with minimal adjustments and within a reasonable period of scan time?

Study design
- Acquisition method (Spectroscopy sequence)
- Multi-voxel vs. single-voxel
- Long echo time vs. short echo time (TE)
- Internal vs. external reference

Data processing method
- Quantification/Identification method
- Absolute quantification vs. ratios
- Data presentation

Other Chemicals in the ^{1}H MRS Spectrum

Other chemicals, such as glutamine, alanine, and macromolecules also contribute to the ^{1}H MRS spectra, but are not well resolved in the typical 1.5 T clinical MRI scanners. Lactate is visible in proton spectra under anaerobic conditions.[9]

Imaging Other Nuclei

The proton nucleus (^{1}H) in the hydrogen atom is the most commonly observed nucleus in spectroscopy studies. However, similar methods can be applied to collect information from other endogenous nuclei such as ^{31}P, or labeled probes such as ^{7}Li, ^{13}C, and ^{19}F. These other types of spectroscopy generally require the purchase of specialized coils and are not readily available on clinical scanners. Another disadvantage is their relatively low sensitivity requiring longer collection times or sampling of very large regions.

References

1. Angelie E, Bonmartin A, Boudraa A, Gonnaud PM, Mallet JJ, Sappey-Marinier D. Regional differences and metabolic changes in normal aging of the human brain: proton MR spectroscopic imaging study. *AJNR Am J Neuroradiol.* 2001;22:119–127.
2. Berry GT, Wang ZJ, Dreha SF, Finucane BM, Zimmerman RA. In vivo brain myo-inositol levels in children with Down syndrome. *J Pediatr.* 1999;135:94–97.
3. Birken DL, Oldendorf WH. N-acetyl-l-aspartic acid: a literature review of a compound prominent in ^{1}H-NMR spectroscopic studies of brain. *Neurosci Biobehav Rev.* 1989;13:23–31.
4. Bitsch A, Bruhn H, Vougioukas V, et al. Inflammatory CNS demyelination: histopathologic correlation with in vivo quantitative proton MR spectroscopy. *AJNR Am J Neuroradiol.* 1999;20:1619–1627.
5. Brand A, Engelmann J, Leibfritz D. A ^{13}C NMR study on fluxes into the TCA cycle of neuronal and glial tumor cell lines and primary cells. *Biochimie.* 1992;74:941–948.
6. Brooks WM, Friedman SD, Gasparovic C. Magnetic resonance spectroscopy in traumatic brain injury. *J Head Trauma Rehabil.* 2001;16:149–164.
7. Chang L, Ernst T, Poland RE, Jenden DJ. In vivo proton magnetic resonance spectroscopy of the normal aging human brain. *Life Sci.* 1996;58:2049–2056.
8. Clarke CE, Lowry M. Systematic review of proton magnetic resonance spectroscopy of the striatum in Parkinsonian syndromes. *Eur J Neurol.* 2001;8:573–577.
9. Danielsen ER, Ross B. *Magnetic Resonance Spectroscopy Diagnosis of Neurological Diseases.* New York, NY: Marcel Dekker; 1999.
10. Dautry C, Vaufrey F, Brouillet E, et al. Early N-acetylaspartate depletion is a marker of neuronal dysfunction in rats and primates chronically treated with the mitochondrial toxin 3-nitropropionic acid. *J Cereb Blood Flow Metab.* 2000;20:789–799.
11. Davie CA, Hawkins CP, Barker GJ, et al. Serial proton magnetic resonance spectroscopy in acute multiple sclerosis lesions. *Brain.* 1994;117(Pt 1):49–58.
12. De Stefano N, Matthews PM, Arnold DL. Reversible decreases in N-acetylaspartate after acute brain injury. *Magn Reson Med.* 1995;34:721–727.
13. Fisher SK, Heacock AM, Agranoff BW. Inositol lipids and signal transduction in the nervous system: an update. *J Neurochem.* 1992;58:18–38.
14. Gillard JH, Barker PB, van Zijl PC, Bryan RN, Oppenheimer SM. Proton MR spectroscopy in acute middle cerebral artery stroke. *AJNR Am J Neuroradiol.* 1996;17:873–886.
15. Govindaraju V, Young K, Maudsley AA. Proton NMR chemical shifts and coupling constants for brain metabolites. *NMR Biomed.* 2000;13:129–153.
16. Gruetter R, Garwood M, Ugurbil K, Seaquist ER. Observation of resolved glucose signals in ^{1}H NMR spectra of the human brain at 4 Tesla. *Magn Reson Med.* 1996;36:1–6.
17. Huppi PS, Posse S, Lazeyras F, Burri R, Bossi E, Herschkowitz N. Magnetic resonance in preterm and term newborns: ^{1}H-spectroscopy in developing human brain. *Pediatr Res.* 1991;30:574–578.
18. Katz-Brull R, Lavin PT, Lenkinski RE. Clinical utility of proton magnetic resonance spectroscopy in characterizing breast lesions. *J Natl Cancer Inst.* 2002;94:1197–1203.
19. Knight-Scott J, Haley AP, Rossmiller SR, et al. Molality as a unit of measure for expressing ^{1}H MRS brain metabolite concentrations in vivo. *Magn Reson Imaging.* 2003;21:787–797.
20. Kreis R, Ernst T, Ross BD. Development of the human brain: in vivo quantification of metabolite and water content with proton magnetic resonance spectroscopy. *Magn Reson Med.* 1993;30:424–437.
21. Leary SM, Brex PA, MacManus DG, et al. A (1)H magnetic resonance spectroscopy study of aging in parietal white matter: implications for trials in multiple sclerosis. *Magn Reson Imaging.* 2000;18:455–459.
22. Li X, Lu Y, Pirzkall A, McKnight T, Nelson SJ. Analysis of the spatial characteristics of metabolic abnormalities in newly diagnosed glioma patients. *J Magn Reson Imaging.* 2002;16:229–237.
23. Miller BL, Moats RA, Shonk T, Ernst T, Woolley S, Ross BD. Alzheimer disease: depiction of increased cerebral myo-inositol with proton MR spectroscopy. *Radiology.* 1993;187:433–437.
24. Moats RA, Ernst T, Shonk TK, Ross BD. Abnormal cerebral metabolite concentrations in patients with probable Alzheimer disease. *Magn Reson Med.* 1994;32:110–115.

25. Murata T, Koshino Y, Omori M, et al. In vivo proton magnetic resonance spectroscopy study on premature aging in adult Down's syndrome. *Biol Psychiatry*. 1993;34:290–297.
26. Naressi A, Couturier C, Devos JM, et al. Java-based graphical user interface for the MRUI quantitation package. *MAGMA*. 2001;12:141–152.
27. Parnetti L, Tarducci R, Presciutti O, et al. Proton magnetic resonance spectroscopy can differentiate Alzheimer's disease from normal aging. *Mech Ageing Dev*. 1997;97:9–14.
28. Paul RH, Ernst T, Brickman AM, et al. Relative sensitivity of magnetic resonance spectroscopy and quantitative magnetic resonance imaging to cognitive function among nondemented individuals infected with HIV. *J Int Neuropsychol Soc*. 2008;14:725–733.
29. Pfefferbaum A, Adalsteinsson E, Spielman D, Sullivan EV, Lim KO. In vivo spectroscopic quantification of the *N*-acetyl moiety, creatine, and choline from large volumes of brain gray and white matter: effects of normal aging. *Magn Reson Med*. 1999;41:276–284.
30. Provencher SW. Estimation of metabolite concentrations from localized in vivo proton NMR spectra. *Magn Reson Med*. 1993;30:672–679.
31. Sappey-Marinier D, Calabrese G, Hetherington HP, et al. Proton magnetic resonance spectroscopy of human brain: applications to normal white matter, chronic infarction, and MRI white matter signal hyperintensities. *Magn Reson Med*. 1992;26:313–327.
32. Saunders DE, Howe FA, van den Boogaart A, Griffiths JR, Brown MM. Aging of the adult human brain: in vivo quantitation of metabolite content with proton magnetic resonance spectroscopy. *J Magn Reson Imaging*. 1999;9:711–716.
33. Schuff N, Amend DL, Knowlton R, Norman D, Fein G, Weiner MW. Age-related metabolite changes and volume loss in the hippocampus by magnetic resonance spectroscopy and imaging. *Neurobiol Aging*. 1999;20:279–285.
34. Stryer L. *Basic Neurochemistry: Molecular, Cellular, and Medical Aspects*. New York: Raven; 1988.
35. Urenjak J, Williams SR, Gadian DG, Noble M. Specific expression of *N*-acetylaspartate in neurons, oligodendrocyte-type-2 astrocyte progenitors, and immature oligodendrocytes in vitro. *J Neurochem*. 1992;59:55–61.
36. Valenzuela MJ, Sachdev P. Magnetic resonance spectroscopy in AD. *Neurology*. 2001;56:592–598.
37. van der Knaap MS, van der Grond J, van Rijen PC, Faber JA, Valk J, Willemse K. Age-dependent changes in localized proton and phosphorus MR spectroscopy of the brain. *Radiology*. 1990;176:509–515.

Chapter 7
Functional Near-Infrared Spectroscopy

Farzin Irani

Introduction

Functional near-infrared spectroscopy (fNIRS) is an emerging brain-imaging technology that capitalizes on the changing optical properties of brain tissue and uses light in the near-infrared range of the visible spectrum to measure hemodynamic responses to sensory, motor, and other cognitive activity. fNIRS offers relatively non-invasive, safe, potentially portable, low-cost methods of both direct and indirect monitoring of brain activity.[16,26,50,54,55,58,59] It has potential for more ecologically valid measures of brain function and has many attributes necessary to translate laboratory work into more realistic, everyday settings and clinical environments. Despite the potential benefits of fNIRS and its availability for several years, it has not achieved significant clinical use. This hesitation may be due to relative unfamiliarity with fNIRS in the field. In addition, the research published to date has been relatively conservative, focusing on establishing fNIRS as a valid and reliable neuroimaging technology when compared to established technologies such as functional magnetic resonance imaging (fMRI). Furthermore, as outlined below, currently there are several limitations to fNIRS, yet recently extending the scope of fNIRS to examine a variety of cognitive, behavioral, neurological, and neurorehabilitation applications has been emphasized.[1,26] This chapter is a reflection of our prior review and hopes to continue to familiarize researchers and clinicians with fNIRS, its potential, and limitations.

F. Irani (✉)
Department of Psychiatry, Neuropsychiatry Division, University of Pennsylvania, 3400 Spruce Street, Gates Building – 10th Floor, Philadelphia, PA 19104, USA
e-mail: firani@upenn.edu

Principles

Brain activity is associated with a number of physiological events, two of which can be assessed using optical techniques. During neuronal activity, ionic fluxes for sodium and potassium influence the cell's membrane potential. Neuronal activity is fueled by glucose metabolism. Increases in neural activity result in increased glucose and oxygen consumption from the local capillary bed. A reduction in local glucose and oxygen stimulates the brain to increase local arteriolar vasodilation, which increases local cerebral blood flow (CBF) and cerebral blood volume (CBV). This mechanism is known as neurovascular coupling.[17] Over a period of several seconds, the increased CBF carries both glucose and oxygen to the area. Oxygen is transported via hemoglobin in the blood. The increased oxygen transported to the area typically exceeds the local neuronal rate of oxygen utilization, resulting in an overabundance of cerebral blood oxygenation in active area.[12] The initial increase in neural activity is thought to result in a focal increase in deoxygenated hemoglobin in the capillary bed as oxygen is withdrawn from the hemoglobin for use in the metabolization of glucose. Yet, this feature of the vascular response has been much more difficult to measure and more controversial than hyperoxygenation (see *NeuroImage 13*, 953–1015, 2001 and ref.[38] for a more detailed discussion).

Oxygenated (oxy-Hb) and deoxygenated hemoglobin (deoxy-Hb) have characteristic optical properties in the visible and near-infrared light range. The change in concentration of these molecules during neurovascular coupling can be measured using optical methods.[6,55] The measurement of changes in the ratio of oxy-Hb to deoxy-Hb is the most commonly used method for near-infrared spectroscopy. Most biological tissues are

---

R.A. Cohen and L.H. Sweet (eds.), *Brain Imaging in Behavioral Medicine and Clinical Neuroscience*,
DOI 10.1007/978-1-4419-6373-4_7, © Springer Science+Business Media, LLC 2011

relatively transparent to light in the near-infrared range between 700 and 1,000 nm, largely because hemoglobin absorption and water absorption is limited at these wavelengths. However, the chromophores oxy-Hb and deoxy-Hb reflect specific wavelengths in this range. Thus, this spectral band is known as the "optical window" for non-invasive assessment of brain activation.[30]

Photons introduced at the scalp pass through the tissue, and are absorbed, scattered, or reflected back from oxy-Hb and deoxy-Hb. Because relatively predictable quantities of photons follow a banana-shaped path back to the surface of the skin, these can be measured using photodetectors.[18] Changes in the chromophore's concentrations cause changes in the reflected light intensity, and are quantified using a modified Beer–Lambert law. The Beer–Lambert law is an empirical description of optical attenuation in a highly scattering medium.[8,9] By measuring absorbance/reflectance changes at two or more wavelengths, one of which is more sensitive to oxy-Hb and the other to deoxy-Hb, changes in the relative concentration of these chromophores can be calculated.

Using these principles, it is possible to assess brain activity through the intact skull in adult human subjects using fNIRS.[6,16,23,32,56] In addition to hemoglobin, other chromophores, including cytochrome-c oxidase can be also be assessed using optical techniques. Cytochrome-c oxidase, a marker of metabolic demands, holds the potential to provide more direct information about neuronal activity than hemoglobin.[21,30] However, cytochrome-c oxidase is used much less frequently than the hemoglobin-based measures (see ref. [21] for more detail).

A more controversial method known as *Event-Related Optical Signal (EROS)* capitalizes on the changes in the optical properties of the cell membranes that occur as a function of ionic fluxes during firing.[16] Optical properties of cell membranes change in the depolarized state relative to its resting state.[38,46,49] Optical methods can be used to detect these changes. The ability to measure the actual depolarization state of neuronal tissue is advantageous since it is a direct measure of neural activity and has millisecond-level time resolution similar to EEG and MEG), but with more superior spatial resolution.

However, there are a number of limitations to the non-invasive use of the EROS signal in humans. A primary disadvantage of the fast optical signal is the high signal-to-noise ratio resulting from the need to image through skin, skull, and cerebrospinal fluid. Basic sensory and motor movements such as tactile stimulation and finger tapping require between 500 and 1,000 trials to establish a reliable signal.[14] There has also been a failure to replicate the results of experiments reporting the "fast optical signal" in response to a visual stimulus.[52] The low signal-to-noise ratio may play a role in current difficulties with experimental replication and more cross-validation work is warranted. These methods also require a more expensive and cumbersome laser-based light source (versus an LED-based light source), are not portable, and have an increased risk of inadvertent eye damage. In contrast, LED-based near-infrared sources pose very little, if any, risk upon eye exposure.[4] In spite of these current limitations, the fast optical signal continues to be an important area of investigation since it offers glimpses of the ideal in neuroimaging—the direct measurement of neuronal activity with millisecond time resolution and superior spatial resolution.

Apparatus

A functional near-infrared apparatus is typically comprised of: (1) a simple headpiece that contains:(a) the *light source or optode* consisting of either light-emitting diodes (LEDs) or fiber-optical bundles and (b) *light detectors or photodetector* that receive the light after it has been reflected from the tissue; (2) a data acquisition board that hosts the electronic system to control the light sources and collect the reflected light; and (3) the host server or computer. Figure 7.1 demonstrates the portable CW-fNIRs system that was originally described by Dr. Briton Chance's laboratory and has been in use by our biomedical engineering and psychology group at Drexel University.[38]

Since light is scattered after entering the tissue, a photodetector placed 2–7 cm away from the optode can collect light after it has passed through the tissue. When the distance between the source and photodetector is set at 4 cm, the fNIRS signal becomes sensitive to hemodynamic changes within the top 2–3 mm of the cortex, extending laterally 1 cm on either sides and perpendicular to the axis of source-detector spacing.[5,40] Studies have shown that at inter-optode distances as short as 2–2.5 cm, gray matter is part of the sample volume.[5,11]

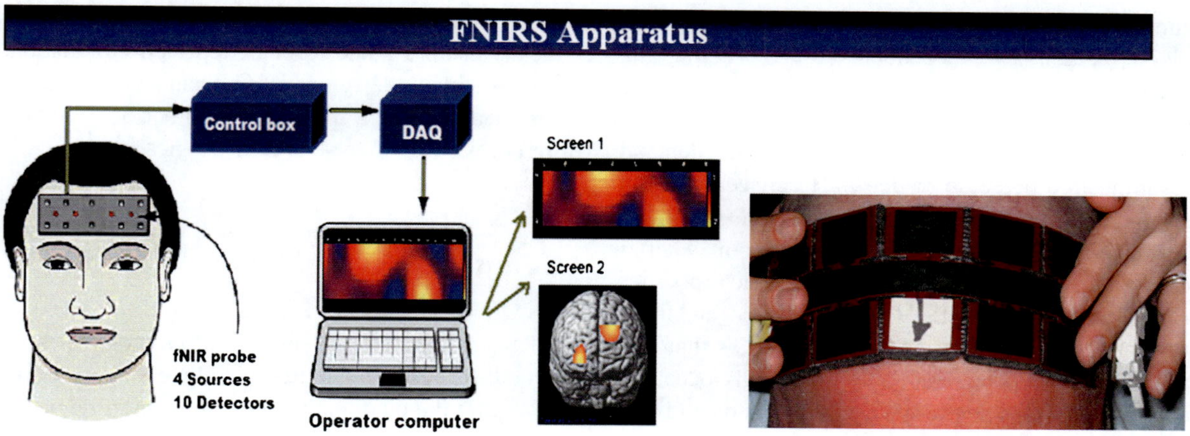

Fig. 7.1 An example of a CW-fNIRS system

A wide variety of both commercial and custom-built fNIRS instruments are currently in use.[50] These systems differ with respect to their system engineering, with tradeoffs between light sources, detectors, and instrument electronics. Three distinct types of fNIRS implementations have been developed. These are (1) time domain systems, (2) frequency domain systems, and (3) continuous wave spectroscopy measurements. Others have provided more detail discussions of differences between these systems,[22,27,38] but briefly, *in time domain systems*, extremely short incident pulses of light are applied to the tissue and the temporal distribution of photons that carry the information about tissue scattering and absorption is measured. In *frequency domain systems*, the light source is amplitude modulated to the frequencies in the order of tens to hundreds Megahertz. The amplitude decay and phase shift of the detected signal with respect to the incident light are measured to characterize the optical properties of tissue. In continuous *wave fNIRS systems* (CW), apply light to tissue at a constant amplitude and measure the attenuation of amplitude of the incident light.[22,27,38] Although CW systems provide somewhat less information than time or frequency domain systems, they also have several advantages for certain applications. First, they can use LEDs rather than lasers, making them safe with respect to their effects on the eyes, including the retina. Second, they are cheaper to manufacture than time-resolved and frequency domain systems, which increases likelihood of deploying these systems in clinical settings. Third, these systems can be designed to be very small, making them practical for use in educational or clinical settings.

Comparison with Other Neuroimaging Technologies

Methods that directly measure summation of neural function, such as electroencephalography (EEG), event-related brain potentials (ERPs), and magnetoencephalography (MEG) allow monitoring of direct consequences of brain electromagnetic activity with excellent temporal resolution (milliseconds). However, these technologies have limited spatial resolution since there is spatial smearing related to the skull and there is difficulty in localizing activated sources due to multiple dipole fitting solutions (but see refs. [24,48] for advances in dipole localization).

Indirect methods of neural function such as positron emission tomography (PET), single-positron emission computed tomography (SPECT), and fMRI monitor hemodynamic and metabolic changes associated with neuronal activity with impressive spatial resolution. However, temporal resolution is usually limited, and these techniques are associated with neuronal activity based on a poorly understood neurovascular coupling function.[6,50] PET and SPECT are also limited in their ability to perform continuous or repeated measurements since there are concerns regarding their use of radioactive isotopes.

fMRI is currently considered the "gold standard" for measuring functional brain activation since it offers safe, non-invasive, functional brain imaging with high spatial resolution. It is therefore useful to focus on comparing these two technologies in further detail. More complete descriptions of the principles of fMRI are available at length elsewhere (e.g.,[15,29] but briefly summarized, the primary measure used for fMRI is the blood oxygen level–dependent (BOLD) signal that accompanies neuronal activation in the brain. As discussed previously, increased CBF to an active area exceeds the additional neuronal metabolic demand, resulting in a decrease of deoxy-Hb concentration in the local tissue. The magnetic susceptibility of blood containing oxy-Hb differs very little from water or other tissues, which have low paramagnetic properties. However, deoxy-Hb is highly paramagnetic, and therefore has very different magnetic properties than surrounding tissues, and can act as a naturally occurring contrast agent.[42] The presence of deoxygenated blood in a given area results in a less uniform magnetic field. Because the MRI signal depends on the uniformity of the magnetic field experienced by water molecules, less uniformity (i.e., when more deoxy-Hb is present) results in a greater mixture of signal frequencies, and therefore a more rapid decay of the overall signal. In contrast, as deoxygenated blood in a given area is replaced by oxygenated blood, the local magnetic environment becomes more uniform, and the MRI signal lasts longer, and is therefore stronger during image acquisition. The signal change is typically between 1 and 5%, depending on the strength of the magnetic field and sensitivity of the cognitive process being examined. Therefore, fMRI, like fNIRS, is an indirect measure of neuronal activity, assessing changes in the relative concentration of deoxy-Hb in local tissue. There is no simple relationship between the magnitude of the signal change and any single physiological parameter, as it relies on changes in blood flow, blood volume, and local oxygen tension. There is also a time delay between when the local neurons are activated and begin to use oxygen and when vasodilatation occurs allowing an increased blood flow and the transport of oxy-Hb to the area. Labeled the hemodynamic response, this process occurs over several seconds following the initiation of neuronal activity.

The more commonly used fNIRS technology (i.e., utilizing the measurement of hemoglobin-based chromophores) shares much in common with the BOLD-based signal. It measures relative changes in concentrations of deoxy-Hb that are dependent on the hemodynamic response, making both indirect measures of neural activity with temporal resolution on the order of seconds due to limitations of the hemodynamic response. Both technologies are also safe, non-invasive, and can be used repeatedly with the same individuals.

Due to their signal to noise ratios, both technologies typically require some level of repeated stimulation, either in a block design or in an event-related design. From there, however, there are a number of important differences between the two technologies.

Strengths

FNIRS has a number of unique properties that hold potential for research studies and clinical applications that require the quantitative measurement of hemodynamic changes in the cortex. The limitations of fMRI relative to fNIRS include the fact that participants must lie within the confines of the magnet bore, which limits its use for many applications including imaging of many patients with severe symptoms. The refrigerant systems used to cool the magnets also produce loud noises, which can interfere with certain protocols. fMRI is also sensitive to movement artifact where subject movements on the order of a few millimeters can invalidate the data (although more accurate and robust motion correction algorithms are available; see refs. [2,3]). Also, the intense strength of the magnets necessary to create the MRI signal precludes the use of any ferrous metals in or around the magnet. Finally, fMRI systems are quite expensive, with an initial cost of between 1.5 and 7 million dollars, depending on the strength of the magnet, and individual participant runs can cost several hundred dollars per subject.

In contrast to fMRI, fNIRS measures relative changes in oxy-Hb as well as deoxy-Hb, and total blood flow, which can be calculated from the differential equation. Participants can sit upright and work on a computer,[27] watch televisions or movies, and even walk on a treadmill. Its compact, portable, and potentially wireless design can allow for more ecologically valid investigations of brain function. FNIRS systems are not as susceptible to movement artifact as fMRI, and algorithms for the removal of motion artifact during desktop as well as ambulatory use have been created ([28]). These attributes also allow fNIRS to be used with children and with patient populations that may find confinement to an fMRI magnet overwhelming or painful. A number of sensor applications exist, depending on their use, including caps, tension straps, and medical grade adhesive applications. FNIRS is quiet and comfortable, and is therefore amenable to sensitive protocols such as the induction of positive moods. It is readily amenable to integration with a number of other technologies, including EEG and transcranial magnetic stimulation (TMS). Portable systems that operate from a laptop computer and a control box approximately $2'' \times 6'' \times 8''$ are available. Finally, fNIRS is relatively inexpensive with available systems ranging between $25,000 and $200,000.

Limitations

Despite its advantages, fNIRS is unlikely to supplant fMRI for basic research on the neurophysiological underpinnings of various cognitive, emotional, and motivational processes for two important reasons. First, fMRI has better spatial resolution, on the order of 1 mm^3, although the fast imaging of fMRI reduces its spatial resolution somewhat to a few millimeters relative to conventional MRI. By contrast, due to the scatter of photons in a diverse medium, current fNIRS systems have a spatial resolution on the order of 1 cm^2. Second, fMRI has the capacity to image the entire brain, whereas fNIRS is limited to the outer cortex. Although a large hemorrhage could be imaged as deep as the thalamus with fNIRS, more subtle signals, such as those induced by a cognitive or an emotional event, are limited to a depth of approximately 2–4 mm of the cortex. Other inherent limitations of fNIRS technology include the use of cranial reference points, attenuation of the light signal by extracerebral matter, comparisons of fNIRS data between subjects, the impact of skin pigmentation on signal detection, and difficulties obtaining absolute baseline concentrations of oxy-Hb and deoxy-Hb.[37,59] Current bioengineering efforts at several institutions (e.g., Drexel University, University of Pennsylvania, University of Illinois, Harvard Medical School) are addressing many of these issues, as well as the use of portable handheld computing devices that can download data. Efforts also continue to improve comfort and flexibility for the participant, through the use of improved flexibility in sensor designs and wireless systems.

However, despite being around for several years, the technology is still considered to be in its infancy, and there may be continued beliefs that an emerging technology, though useful in the future, is yet not ready for practical clinical delivery.[7] Finally, the advent of a portable technology that is able to provide continuous measurements of neurobiological signals within variable environmental conditions heightens the need for systematic, informatics-driven modifications of clinical databases based on standardized and normative data.[7] This need has yet to be fulfilled for fNIRS and will require extensive research commitments in the future.

Validation Efforts

Much research effort has been focused on concurrent validation of fNIRS with more established functional neuroimaging technologies such as fMRI. This includes establishing the sensitivity, accuracy, and reliability of fNIRS under a variety of experimental and clinical conditions.[39,55,59] Toronov et al (2001)[53] found high temporal correlations between the BOLD signal in fMRI and the deoxy-Hb concentration in fNIRS on a motor task. Using another simple motor task, Strangman et al[51] attempted to characterize the amplitude correspondences between the two modalities by simultaneously acquiring fNIRS and BOLD fMRI data and comparing Delta (1/BOLD) (approximately R(2) (*)) to changes in deoxy-Hb, oxy-Hb, and total hemoglobin (TotHb) concentrations derived from fNIRS. After accounting for systematic errors associated with each of the signals, they found strong correlations between fMRI changes and all optical measures, with oxy-Hb providing the strongest correlation. This finding held even when including scalp, skull, and inactive brain tissue in the average BOLD signal. Similarly, cross-validative comparisons have also been made on patients with a hemiparetic stroke,[31] cerebral ischemia,[36] as well as young and elderly subjects.[35] These studies have suggested that on motor tasks, fNIRS is able to provide direct information about neuronal activity–associated changes in cerebral parameters that are partly reflected in the BOLD signal.[57]

Other investigations suggest greater correspondence between the BOLD response and deoxy-Hb. Huppert et al (2006)[25] utilized a short-duration event-related finger tapping task while conducting simultaneous fMRI and fNIRS measurements. The task evoked activity in the primary motor and sensory cortices, and there was a significant correlation across all participants between Δ (1/BOLD) and deoxy-Hb responses. Similar results were obtained for a study that employed a simple visual stimulation task (Schroeter et al. 2006).[47] Hemodynamic activity was invoked in the visual cortex bilaterally, and changes in the BOLD signal were highly correlated with deoxy-Hb, while lower correlations were obtained for oxy-Hb and total Hb. There is also emerging evidence of within-subjects stability of fNIRS signals (Plichta et al. 2006).[45] Three-week test–retest reliability was examined in 12 participants using simple visual stimuli. Channel-wise intraclass correlation coefficients at the group level revealed good reliability and excellent reproducibility with respect to the quantity of activated channels and the location of the detected activation. Results at the level of the participant, however, were less reliable.

There are also data implicating concurrent validation of fNIRS with fMRI using a variety of tasks. Obrig et al[39] demonstrated concordance between fNIRS and fMRI signals using visual stimulation and a response inhibition task. They demonstrated the ability of fNIRS to discriminate between motor and premotor responses of a Go/No-Go task, additionally demonstrating that the biological signals detected by the two devices were largely consistent. Similarly, in a study examining breath holding using fMRI and fNIRS, MacIntosh et al (2003)[33] observed a generally concordant relationship between fMRI and fNIRS signals, but there were significant differences in measurement sensitivity between BOLD and fNIRS when utilizing this task. Platek et al[43,44] have also indirectly shown concordance between fNIRS and fMRI in a face-recognition task.

An attempt at examining the ecological validity of fNIRS was carried out in a study examining the correspondence of fMRI and fNIRS during an apple-peeling task.[41] The investigators found congruity between fNIRS and fMRI for those brain areas subserving the motoric, visual, and cognitive components of the apple-peeling task. There were, however, discrepancies in the spatial localization data, whereby the mock apple-peeling task, as performed during fMRI scanning, did not invoke the same activation observed by fNIRS in the prefrontal cortex during actual apple peeling. Albeit still requiring further research, these findings highlight the potential for fNIRS to elucidate brain–behavior relationships during ecologically valid paradigms, particularly in cases where data across simulated and ecologically valid paradigms are dissimilar. Further cross-validation efforts are needed to compare fNIRS with other functional neuroimaging modalities in laboratory and real-world environments.

Thus, preliminary evidence appears to be generally consistent in implicating the concordance of fMRI and fNIRS signals, even in paradigms requiring more complex cognitive and physiological activities than simple motoric responses. The scarcity of such data, coupled with occasional disparities, however, suggests a need for further research on the congruence between fNIRS and fMRI. Despite the current limitations, studies that have ventured to use fNIRS to investigate various clinical populations have highlighted the potential for its application in examining various neurological and psychiatric disorders.

Applications

FNIRS has been employed as a measure of cognitive workload in complex, "realistic" tasks and holds promise as an aid for creating symbiotic relationships between operators and operational environments.[27] It has been deployed by the medical community in settings including pediatrics and has played an important role in the study of neonatal cerebral hemodynamics in hypoxic–ischemic brain injury in small preterm babies.[10] In breast cancer research, fNIRS optical imaging has offered unique advantages for diagnostic imaging of solid tumors.[19,20] The ability of fNIRS to detect intracranial hematomas has also been examined in patients admitted to hospitals with head trauma, demonstrating a greater absorption at 760 nm over the affected hemisphere than the contralateral side.[14] Additionally, in patients with normotensive acute congestive heart failure, dual-wavelength fNIRS has helped determine critically low oxygen levels resulting in improved cerebral oxygen saturation during treatment of acute heart failure.[34] It has also been used to measure sensory, motor, and cognitive demands of tasks administered to a variety of neurological (Alzheimer's disease, Parkinson's disease, epilepsy, traumatic brain injury) and psychiatric (schizophrenia, mood disorders, anxiety disorders) populations.[26] Applications of fNIRS to neurorehabilitation of cognitive disabilities has also been reviewed previously.[1]

The versatility of the technology is also apparent in its ease of customizability. For instance, the Hematoscope or Hematoma detector (InfraScan, Inc., Philadelphia, PA) is being marketed for field deployment to the military for army medics to make quick assessments on the spot for critical cost/benefit analyses. This future application is particularly relevant in clinical neuropsychology due to its potential for immediate on-site clinical assessment, for example during a motor vehicle accident. This malleability of the technology to clinical as well as research applications is perhaps one of the most exciting aspects of fNIRS.

Conclusions and Future Implications

fNIRS is able to offer a non-invasive, potentially portable, safe, low-cost method of both direct and indirect monitoring of brain activity over extended time periods. It makes it possible to design translational research and clinical studies that possess ecological validity, which is currently not possible with the constraints of other functional neuroimaging technologies. It offers the potential to provide unique insights into the etiology and treatment of various brain disorders. Yet, as an emerging technology, it is still limited in several ways. These include limited spatial resolution, use of cranial reference points, attenuation of the light signal by extracerebral matter, comparisons of fNIRS data between subjects, the impact of skin pigmentation on signal detection, difficulties obtaining absolute baseline concentrations of oxy-Hb and deoxy-Hb, failures to replicate, high signal-to-noise ratios in EROS signals, its early developmental stage, and the need for informatics-driven modifications of clinical databases based on standardized and normative data.

Despite its current limitations, it is an FDA-approved emergent technology that for certain applications offers several advantages over currently available functional neuroimaging techniques, such as fMRI, PET, and EEG. Although it is unlikely to immediately replace these techniques, it can permit non-invasive and continuous monitoring of cortical activity within a comfortable setting that may provide good ecological validity. Its application extends beyond the confines of traditional neuroimaging laboratory settings to clinical application. The versatility of this technology is also apparent in studies that have utilized fNIRS with children as young as 1.5 years of age to study various epileptic seizures. Its usefulness is further highlighted in its application to acute care settings including pediatric intensive care units. This malleability of fNIRS to clinical as well as research applications is perhaps one of the most exciting aspects of fNIRS.

Acknowledgments The author would like to thank members of Drexel University's Department of Psychology and School of Biomedical Engineering, Science and Health Systems for their continual support. In particular, this chapter is a reflection of the work from the laboratories of Drs. Banu Onaral, Britton Chance, Maria Schulthesis, Scott Bunce, and Douglas Chute.

References

1. Arenth PM, Ricker JH, Schultheis MT. Applications of functional near-infrared spectroscopy (fNIRS) to neurorehabilitation of cognitive disabilities. *Clin Neuropsychol.* 2007;21(1):38–57.
2. Ashburner J, Friston KJ. Nonlinear spatial normalization using basis functions. *Hum Brain Mapp.* 1999;7(4):254–266.
3. Ashburner J, Friston KJ. Unified segmentation. *Neuroimage.* 2005;26(3):839–851.
4. Bozkurt A, Onaral B. Safety assessment of near infrared light emitting diodes for diffuse optical measurements. *Biomed Eng Online.* 2004;3(1):9.
5. Chance B, Leigh JS, Miyake H, et al. Comparison of time-resolved and -unresolved measurements of deoxyhemoglobin in brain. *Proc Natl Acad Sci USA.* 1988;85(14): 4971–4975.
6. Chance B, Zhuang Z, UnAh C, Alter C, Lipton L. Cognition-activated low-frequency modulation of light absorption in human brain. *Proc Natl Acad Sci USA.* 1993;90(8):3770–3774.
7. Chute DL. Neuropsychological technologies in rehabilitation. *J Head Trauma Rehabil.* 2002;17(5):369–377.
8. Cope M. *The Development of a Near-Infrared Spectroscopy System and Its Application for Noninvasive Monitoring of Cerebral Blood and Tissue Oxygenation in the Newborn Infant.* London: Univ. College London; 1991.
9. Cope M, Delpy DT. System for long-term measurement of cerebral blood and tissue oxygenation on newborn infants by near infra-red transillumination. *Med Biol Eng Comput.* 1988;26(3):289–294.
10. Crowe JH, Rea PA, Wickramasinghe Y, Rolfe P. Towards non-invasive optical monitoring of cerebral metabolism. In: Rolfe P, ed. *Paper presented at the Proc. Int. Conf. Fetal Neonatal Physiol. Meas.*, Oxford, England; 1984.
11. Firbank M, Okada E, Delpy DT. A theoretical study of the signal contribution of regions of the adult head to near-infrared spectroscopy studies of visual evoked responses. *Neuroimage.* 1998;8(1):69–78.
12. Fox PT, Raichle ME, Mintun MA, Dence C. Nonoxidative glucose consumption during focal physiologic neural activity. *Science.* 1988;241(4864):462–464.
13. Franceschini MA, Boas DA. Noninvasive measurement of neuronal activity with near-infrared optical imaging. *Neuroimage.* 2004;21(1):372–386.
14. Gopinath SP, Robertson CS, Grossman RG, Chance B. Near-infrared spectroscopic localization of intracranial hematomas. *J Neurosurg.* 1993;79(1):43–47.

15. Gore J. Out of the shadows – MRI and the Nobel Prize. *N Engl J Med.* 2003;349(24):2290–2292.

16. Gratton G, Corballis PM, Cho E, Fabiani M, Hood DC. Shades of gray matter: noninvasive optical images of human brain responses during visual stimulation. *Psychophysiology.* 1995;32(5):505–509.

17. Gratton G, Goodman-Wood MR, Fabiani M. Comparison of neuronal and hemodynamic measures of the brain response to visual stimulation: an optical imaging study. *Hum Brain Mapp.* 2001;13(1):13–25.

18. Gratton G, Maier JS, Fabiani M, Mantulin WW, Gratton E. Feasibility of intracranial near-infrared optical scanning. *Psychophysiology.* 1994;31(2):211–215.

19. Gurfinkel M, Ke S, Wen X, Li C, Sevick-Muraca EM. Near-infrared fluorescence optical imaging and tomography. *Dis Markers.* 2003;19(2–3):107–121.

20. Hawrysz DJ, Sevick-Muraca EM. Developments toward diagnostic breast cancer imaging using near-infrared optical measurements and fluorescent contrast agents. *Neoplasia.* 2000;2(5):388–417.

21. Heekeren HR, Kohl M, Obrig H, et al. Noninvasive assessment of changes in cytochrome-c oxidase oxidation in human subjects during visual stimulation. *J Cereb Blood Flow Metab.* 1999;19(6):592–603.

22. Hoshi Y. Functional near-infrared optical imaging: utility and limitations in human brain mapping. *Psychophysiology.* 2003;40(4):511–520.

23. Hoshi Y, Tamura M. Dynamic multichannel near-infrared optical imaging of human brain activity. *J Appl Physiol.* 1993;75(4):1842–1846.

24. Hughes JR, John ER. Conventional and quantitative electro-encephalography in psychiatry. *J Neuropsychiatry Clin Neurosci.* 1999;11(2):190–208.

25. Huppert J, Hoge RD, Diamond SG, Franceschini MA, Boas A. A temporal comparison of BOLD, ASL, and NIRS hemodynamic responses to motor stimuli in adult humans, *Neuroimage.* 2006;29:368–382.

26. Irani F, Platek SM, Bunce S, Ruocco AC, Chute D. Functional near infrared spectroscopy (fNIRS): an emerging neuroimaging technology with important applications for the study of brain disorders. *Clin Neuropsychol.* 2007;21(1):9–37.

27. Izzetoglu K, Bunce S, Onaral B, Pourrezaei K, Chance B. Functional optical brain imaging using NIR during cognitive tasks. *Int J Hum Comput Interact Spec Issue Augmented Cogn.* 2004;17:211–227.

28. Izzetoglu M, Devaraj A, Bunce S, Onaral B. Motion artifact cancellation in NIR spectroscopy using Wiener filtering. *IEEE Trans Biomed Eng.* 2005;52(5):934–938.

29. Jezzard P, Mathews PM, Smith SM. *Functional MRI: An Introduction to Methods.* New York: Oxford University Press; 2001.

30. Jobsis FF. Noninvasive, infrared monitoring of cerebral and myocardial oxygen sufficiency and circulatory parameters. *Science.* 1977;198(4323):1264–1267.

31. Kato H, Izumiyama M, Koizumi H, Takahashi A, Itoyama Y. Near-infrared spectroscopic topography as a tool to monitor motor reorganization after hemiparetic stroke: a comparison with functional MRI. *Stroke.* 2002;33(8):2032–2036.

32. Kato T, Kamei A, Takashima S, Ozaki T. Human visual cortical function during photic stimulation monitoring by means

of near-infrared spectroscopy. *J Cereb Blood Flow Metab.* 1993;13(3):516–520.

33. MacIntosh BJ, Klassen ML, Menon RS. Transient hemo-dynamics during a breath hold challenge in a two part functional imaging study with simultaneous near-infrared spectroscopy in adult humans, *NeuroImage.* 2003;20:246–1252.

34. Madsen PL, Nielsen HB, Christiansen P. Well-being and cerebral oxygen saturation during acute heart failure in humans. *Clin Physiol.* 2000;20(2):158–164.

35. Mehagnoul-Schipper DJ, van der Kallen BF, Colier WN, et al. Simultaneous measurements of cerebral oxygenation changes during brain activation by near-infrared spectroscopy and functional magnetic resonance imaging in healthy young and elderly subjects. *Hum Brain Mapp.* 2002;16(1):14–23.

36. Murata Y, Sakatani K, Katayama Y, Fukaya C. Increase in focal concentration of deoxyhaemoglobin during neuronal activity in cerebral ischaemic patients. *J Neurol Neurosurg Psychiatry.* 2002;73(2):182–184.

37. Obrig H, Villringer A. Near-infrared spectroscopy in functional activation studies. Can NIRS demonstrate cortical activation? *Adv Exp Med Biol.* 1997;413:113–127.

38. Obrig H, Villringer A. Beyond the visible – imaging the human brain with light. *J Cereb Blood Flow Metab.* 2003;23(1):1–18.

39. Obrig H, Wenzel R, Kohl M, et al. Near-infrared spectroscopy: does it function in functional activation studies of the adult brain? *Int J Psychophysiol.* 2000;35(2–3):125–142.

40. Okada F, Firbank M, Schweiger M, Arridge SR, Cope M, Delpy DT. Theoretical and experimental investigation of near-infrared light propagation in a model of the adult head. *Appl Opt.* 1997;36:21–31.

41. Okamoto M, Dan H, Shimizu K, et al. Multimodal assessment of cortical activation during apple peeling by NIRS and fMRI. *Neuroimage.* 2004;21(4):1275–1288.

42. Pauling L. Magnetic properties and structure of oxyhemo-globin. *Proc Natl Acad Sci USA.* 1977;74(7):2612–2613.

43. Platek S, Fonteyn L, Myers TE, et al. Functional near infra-red spectroscopy (fNIRS) reveals differences in self – other processing as a function of schizotypal personality traits. *Schizophr Res.* 2005;73(1):125–127.

44. Platek SM, Keenan JP, Gallup GG Jr, Mohamed FB. Where am I? The neurological correlates of self and other. *Brain Res Cogn Brain Res.* 2004;19(2):114–122.

45. Plichta M, Herrmann MJ, Baehne CJ, Ehlis A, Richter MM, Pauli P, Fallgatter AJ. Event-related functional near-infrared spectroscopy (fNIRS): Are the measurements reliable?, *NeuroImage.* 2006;31:116–124.

46. Rector DM, Poe GR, Kristensen MP, Harper RM. Light scattering changes follow evoked potentials from hippocampal Schaeffer collateral stimulation. *J Neurophysiol.* 1997;78(3):1707–1713.

47. Schroeter ML, Kupka T, Mildner T, Uludag K, Yves von Cramon D. Investigating the post-stimulus undershoot of the BOLD signal–a simultaneous fMRI and fNIRS study, *Neuroimage.* 2006;30:349–358.

48. Srinivasan R, Tucker DM, Murias M. Estimating the spatial Nyquist of the human EEG. *Behav Res Methods Instrum Comput.* 1998;30:8–19.

49. Stepnoski RA, LaPorta A, Raccuia-Behling F, Blonder GE, Slusher RE, Kleinfeld D. Noninvasive detection of changes

in membrane potential in cultured neurons by light scattering. *Proc Natl Acad Sci USA*. 1991;88(21):9382–9386.

50. Strangman G, Boas DA, Sutton JP. Non-invasive neuroimaging using near-infrared light. *Biol Psychiatry*. 2002;52(7): 679–693.

51. Strangman G, Culver JP, Thompson JH, Boas DA. A quantitative comparison of simultaneous BOLD fMRI and NIRS recordings during functional brain activation. *Neuroimage*. 2002;17(2):719–731.

52. Syre F, Obrig H, Steinbrink J, Kohl M, Wenzel R, Villringer A. Are VEP correlated fast optical signals detectable in the human adult by non-invasive near infrared spectroscopy (NIRS)? *Adv Exp Med Biol*. 2003;530:421–431.

53. Toronov V, Webb A, Choi JH, Wolf M, Safonova L, Wolf U, Gratton E. Study of local cerebral hemodynamics by frequency-domain near-infrared spectroscopy and correlation with simultaneously acquired functional magnetic resonance imaging. *Opt Express*. 2001;9:417–427.

54. Totaro R, Barattelli G, Quaresima V, Carolei A, Ferrari M. Evaluation of potential factors affecting the measurement of cerebrovascular reactivity by near-infrared spectroscopy. *Clin Sci (Lond)*. 1998;95(4):497–504.

55. Villringer A, Chance B. Non-invasive optical spectroscopy and imaging of human brain function. *Trends Neurosci*. 1997;20(10):435–442.

56. Villringer A, Planck J, Hock C, Schleinkofer L, Dirnagl U. Near infrared spectroscopy (NIRS): a new tool to study hemodynamic changes during activation of brain function in human adults. *Neurosci Lett*. 1993;154(1–2): 101–104.

57. Wobst P, Wenzel R, Kohl M, Obrig H, Villringer A. Linear aspects of changes in deoxygenated hemoglobin concentration and cytochrome oxidase oxidation during brain activation. *Neuroimage*. 2001;13(3):520–530.

58. Wolf M, Wolf U, Choi JH, et al. Functional frequency-domain near-infrared spectroscopy detects fast neuronal signal in the motor cortex. *Neuroimage*. 2002;17(4):1868–1875.

59. Zabel TA, Chute DL. Educational neuroimaging: a proposed neuropsychological application of near-infrared spectroscopy (nIRS). *J Head Trauma Rehabil*. 2002;17(5): 477–488.

Chapter 8
Methodological Considerations for Using BOLD fMRI in the Clinical Neurosciences

Kathy S. Chiou and Frank G. Hillary

The BOLD fMRI Affect

The advancement of MRI methods has provided researchers with unique opportunities to examine human brain function in vivo. Since the introduction of blood oxygen level dependent functional magnetic resonance imaging (BOLD fMRI or BOLD) in the early 1990s, the number of published studies using this method to examine cognitive, motor, and sensory functioning has increased each year. In the year 2000, roughly 1,000 articles were published using fMRI, and this number topped 2,500 in the year 2006 with no clear sign of asymptote.[1]

fMRI maintains several important advantages over other imaging techniques, including its non-invasiveness, its availability, and the attractive tradeoff it offers between reasonably high temporal and spatial resolution. Even given the popularity of fMRI, its incredible flexibility, and usefulness for examining brain–behavior relationships, there are important methodological considerations when used in clinical samples. This chapter addresses methodological issues that arise with the use of fMRI in clinical research, with particular emphasis on considerations for data acquisition, data processing and analysis, and interpretation of fMRI results in clinical populations.

Data Acquisition

The MRI Environment

Although the requirement of lying still in the magnet for extended durations is reasonably well tolerated by healthy participants, this is not the case in all clinical populations. The confining nature of the MRI environment leads to a number of potential problems. For example, in some circumstances, it may be difficult to achieve ideal head placement within the magnetic field; in pediatric populations, differences in head circumference, neck length, and shoulder width may affect head positioning.[41] Moreover, there are inherent difficulties using fMRI methods to examine individuals with larger heads and bodies (e.g., studies of obesity, male athletes). It is also important to note that physiology may also be influenced by posture; depending on head tilt, cortical arousal (as measured by EEG) and perfusion pressure may all be affected, ultimately resulting in a change in the hemodynamic reference function.[67]

The physical and psychological consequences of lying in a scanner for sustained periods of time are not trivial; Raz et al[67] found that these circumstances may influence cognitive performance as well as hemodynamics. There are several factors associated with the MRI environment that may cause anxiety for participants. The lengthy procedure of preparation for entrance into the scanner (screening, paradigm training, reviewing consent forms) and the physical sensation of being confined in the bore can lead to a feeling of anxiety including claustrophobia and panic.[7,55]

F.G. Hillary (✉)
Department of Psychology, Pennsylvania State University, 223 Moore Building, University Park, PA 16802, USA
e-mail: fhillary@psu.edu

R.A. Cohen and L.H. Sweet (eds.), *Brain Imaging in Behavioral Medicine and Clinical Neuroscience*,
DOI 10.1007/978-1-4419-6373-4_8, © Springer Science+Business Media, LLC 2011

This anxiety may cause not only emotional discomfort and changes in cognitive performance but also physiological changes (changes in heart rate, blood pressure) that might affect blood flow and, subsequently, the fMRI signal.

Head Motion and Sources of Noise in fMRI Data

Whether it is due to subject discomfort or it is intrinsic to a specific behavioral paradigm, some measureable degree of head movement is inevitable in MRI; even healthy individuals who are highly tolerant of the scanning environment demonstrate movement up to a millimeter.[23] Furthermore, it has been found that greater head movement is typical in special samples; for example, work by D'Esposito et al[15] demonstrated that during a visual reaction time paradigm, older participants showed greater translational movement than younger participants. These data were corroborated in a study of stroke recovery, where significantly greater head movement was observed in both the clinical and age-match "control" sample compared to a younger healthy adult.[71] Head movement during scanning may result in misalignment of the images, artifacts, and signal loss[78] that have important implications for data quality and interpretation.

Because head movement is nearly universal to fMRI experiments and problematic for the integrity of MRI data, techniques have been developed to reduce physical head movement and correct for movement that does occur. To reduce head movement, some investigators have advocated the use of a bite bar or mouth piece attached to the head coil and have demonstrated that its use significantly reduces drift around the X and Z axes.[57] There is less information about the effectiveness of using a bite bar in clinical samples, in particular those with attentional difficulties and/or who are prone to anxiety/claustrophobia. Sedation has been used to control motion when imaging young infants; however, it typically requires nursing or other staff to be present and introduces potential medical risks, including hypothermia. Examiners have recommended that fitting the child to a special neonatal head coil in a MR-compatible incubator is a safer way to obtain more accurate imaging data.[21]

Separately, subject preparation and experimental designs have been shown to influence motion. Prior to entering the scanner, researchers may coach the participant to remain still and offer reminders between data acquisition periods. Researchers may also attempt to reduce motion by increasing comfort in the MRI environment by including padding and blanketing, and frequent "check-in" periods with the participant. A practice session in a mock scanner may also be helpful for participants (especially children and adolescents), to become accustomed to the MRI setting.[20] Experimental designs can be manipulated to minimize the effects of movement; for example, Birn et al[2] found that single trial or event-related designs contained significantly less artifact due to motion when compared to a block design.

While reducing movement on the front end (i.e., during data collection) is critical, complete elimination of motion is rarely achieved. For this reason, examiners have worked to develop analytic procedures for the identification and/or removal of the effects of head movement on functional imaging data. Traditionally, data preprocessing includes a step rigid body registration in which a set of images is transformed according to specific parameters to match an identified source image in order to reduce movement artifact.

Early methods for motion correction have been met with mixed success. Investigators citing problems with image registration based upon voxelwise signal intensity developed a contour-based registration technique, emphasizing edges of the skull and brain, capable of differentiating motion-related activation from stimulus-induced activation.[3] More recently, investigators have successfully demonstrated the usefulness of nonrigid body registration to better account for motion-induced artifact[80] while others have separated motion-induced and stimulus-induced signal variability via independent component analysis.[48] A number of additional methods have been developed to deal with motion correction including modifications to rigid body motion correction[56] and correction of geometric distortions that occur through the use of a "map-slice-to-volume" method (for details see ref.[81]). Ultimately, some form of motion correction is essential prior to any image analysis and the exact nature of motion correction may depend upon the research question. In most cases, slow incremental translational movement (in the x or y plane) is more easily accounted for than larger movement or movement in the z-plane or during the "phase encoding" period of MRI data acquisition (see Chap. 1 of this volume). In the case of the latter, the trial may need to be aborted and reacquired if significant motion is observed during data collection. If motion is not observed until data preprocessing and cannot be eliminated with motion correction, the affected volumes may need to be removed, or at worst, the entire trial may need to be eliminated from analysis.

Finally, while it is not head motion strictly speaking, other investigators have developed methods to deal with motion in the fMRI signal due to vascular fluctuations and respiration. These two sources of physiological noise are critical to account for in fMRI, and this becomes increasingly evident at high field strengths.[36] One commonly used method to account for physiological fluctuations is RETROspective Image CORrection (RETROICOR).[25] Recent work has refined the application of RETROICOR, so that it is optimized with regard to slice timing correction and volume registration (see ref. [36]); this modification of the RETROICOR method has been used to correct for physiological noise by introducing new regressors into the model that would account for errors caused by traditional registration.

Data Processing and Analyzing the BOLD fMRI Signal

Data Preparation

Following data acquisition, there are multiple intermediary steps involved in order to convert the data from raw image data to a format that can be analyzed and interpreted; these stages of "preprocessing" vary to some degree depending upon the purpose of the research. Typically, the processes of realignment, coregistration, spatial normalization, and smoothing are commonly used to consolidate and align the volumes of time series data. Realignment is initially used to "line up" images and reduce motion artifact, and coregistration permits co-localization of functional and structural image data. In normalization, or image standardization, data are transferred into standardized space, so that each voxel is assigned to a coordinate system and can be identified and compared between subjects and between groups of subjects. Normalization algorithms can be quite different between imaging softwares (e.g., AFNI vs. SPM) and the assumptions made by these analytic procedures should be known prior to use, particularly in clinical cases.

Of note, preprocessing procedures, and in particular normalization, are based upon the assumption that anatomical structures and their localized functions are identical for all groups; in the case that there are structural abnormalities in the brain (e.g., stroke, tumor, traumatic brain injury), images may be misaligned and misrepresented. There is emerging literature on different methods of normalization that will account for lesions or abnormalities in the structure of the brain including the use of affine-only or linear transformation of the data. Because nonlinear warping is often preferred, methods such as cost-function lesion masking can be used, which essentially assigns zero values to areas of lesion, so that nonlinear algorithms do not attempt to minimize voxelwise differences between the data and the template in areas of abnormality (see refs.[8] Crinion et al. 2007, and Friston[14]).

Activation Detection and Statistical Considerations

Voxel based and region of interest (ROI) are two general categories of analytic methods used to examine fMRI data. A voxel-based approach is a comparison of hemodynamic response change on a voxelwise basis throughout the brain. In this approach, a statistical threshold is chosen and activation and significant activation is determined by the extent that the number of voxels that exceed the set threshold. There is no rule for determining the threshold for a dataset, and as a consequence determining what is and what is not "active" is often arbitrary. By setting conservative thresholds, researchers risk increase in Type II errors; that is, genuine activation that remains sub-threshold due to correction would be missed. For example, Cohen and DuBois[13] found an increase in Type II errors and inconsistencies in assessing activation magnitude when using voxel counting approaches to analyze a motor and visual task; they suggest the use of a linear systems approach for more stable assessment of activation across trials (for full details please refer to ref. [12]).

Several methods are now available that permit corrections for multiple comparisons without eliminating relevant activation due to conservative thresholding that is the result of traditional Bonferroni correction. These techniques include family wise correction and random field theory (see refs. [24,73]) and a method that relies on examining the false discovery rate (FDR) (Genovese, Lazar, Nichols, 2002[82]). Ultimately, achieving the "correct" threshold is a controversial issue with novel methods still being developed (see Pendse et al. 2009[83]) and some investigators moving away from absolute thresholds to more continuous measurements of activation, providing the opportunity to examine change in the BOLD signal in a pre-specified region regardless of if the signal, is statistically suprathreshold in that region.

In a ROI approach, whole-brain voxelwise analyses of the BOLD response are not conducted, instead anatomical regions that are of particular interest to the researcher are first identified and isolated for analysis. By examining only the signal change in discrete locations, the number of statistical comparisons that needs to be made is reduced, resulting in increased statistical power.[61] The ROI approach has also been suggested for use of exploring data and testing specific brain areas that already have functional definitions (see ref. [62]). An assumption of this method is that researchers will be able to precisely and reliably identify ROIs; for example, choosing ROI that are too large or unrelated to the task may result in dilution of signal detection. While greater anatomical specificity may be provided via ROI analysis, identification of regions can be labor intensive and require reliability checks in order to guarantee anatomical accuracy within and between raters. In the case of the latter, reliability of ROI identification has been increased through the use of data analytic softwares that facilitate identification of specific neuroanatomy as it exists in "normalized" space.

Test–Retest Reliability and Reproducibility in fMRI

Variability in cortical activity may occur within and across participants, scan sessions, and time. Findings regarding the reproducibility of measures of cortical activity have been mixed depending on the population, how activation is measured (e.g., percent signal change or active voxel count), and modality of the task (i.e., sensory, motor, or cognitive task). For example, in studies of motor activity, Havel et al[27] found that reproducibility of activation was dependent upon the motor units involved; it was the highest for movements in the primary motor–sensory areas (e.g., hand and foot movements) and lowest for mouth movements. In a separate study, when engaged in a visual motor drawing task, survivors of stroke were found to be more reliable in within-session scans compared to between-session scans, and measurements of signal change were more reliable than voxel counting methods.[43]

Recent work in multiple sclerosis (MS) examining motor activation using a hand tapping task was conducted across five European imaging centers, using scanners from different manufacturers.[5] Data derived within participants were more consistent than between participants and, again, "activation" determined as maximum signal change had higher reproducibility than using ROI voxel counts.[5] Importantly, they also found that there was greater variability in the runs of the individuals with MS compared to the healthy individuals[5]; these findings are consistent with what has been repeatedly observed in behavioral data (e.g., clinical samples demonstrate greater variability).

Studies investigating reproducibility of results of fMRI activation during cognitive stimulation have been met with mixed results. In a study of working memory in healthy individuals, activation data collected from four different imaging institutions demonstrated comparable findings for the spatial location and distribution of cortical activity across participants.[11] Similar to results in motor and sensory studies, functional imaging results in individuals with schizophrenia engaged in a working memory task demonstrated greater variability compared to healthy participants.[51]

In the study of language recovery, there has been reasonable convergence of findings in stroke patients recovering from aphasia,[45] but consistency is at least partially dependent upon task selection and complexity.[19] Thus, the reliability observed in fMRI studies of clinical samples have been at least partially dependent upon the task, the domain, and the clinical population, which has important implications for the generalizability of clinical fMRI studies. Past difficulty with replication suggests that tight control over task stimulation is paramount and results require conservative interpretation regarding implications for any clinical population. Overall, similar to studies of behavioral deficit, it should be anticipated that there is greater variability in functional imaging data in clinical samples compared to "control" samples. As is the case with behavioral data, this requires researchers to address the heterogeneity in their sample, integration of behavioral data and functional data, larger sample sizes, and replication of findings.

The Basis of the BOLD Signal

As noted elsewhere in this volume (see Chap. 1), the BOLD signal is a surrogate for neuronal firing that has no inherent quantity. For a comprehensive review of the biophysics of the BOLD signal, please refer to Logothetis.[49] Because the BOLD fMRI signal is a surrogate for neuronal firing, research using these methods must be careful to account for factors that could potentially change the basic relationship between neuronal firing and the BOLD response. These factors, outlined below, range from natural between-subject differences in the cerebrovasculature to the effects of neurodevelopment or pathophysiology on blood flow.

Natural Heterogeneity in the Brain

Studies examining variability in the BOLD signal reveal that its basic shape and timing is relatively stable for similar regions across subjects; however, differences in the shape of the BOLD signal across regions within individuals have been documented.[9,69] Much of this difference may be assigned to differential metabolism between anatomical regions within the brain. For example, it has been observed in animal studies that compared to the cortex, basal ganglia, and white matter, the rat hippocampus showed a decreased sensitivity to changes in oxygenation as measured by BOLD.[18] In humans, Siesjo[74] found that metabolic activity in the white matter can be differentiated with that observed in cortical gray matter. The differences in the BOLD signal between white and gray matter have been attributed to differences in metabolic rates, vascular regulation, and vascular architecture.[63]

Taken together, these studies suggest that at least part of the differences in signal intensity throughout the brain may be due to vascular differences and natural variation in the metabolism rather than differences in underlying neuronal activity. These fundamental differences in neurometabolism between neuroanatomical regions have important implications for study design and require methods sensitive to spatially distinct signal-to-noise ratio (SNR).

Effects of Normal Development on the BOLD Signal

The process of normal aging in humans is invariably accompanied by some degree of change in cerebral vasculature. These changes in the vasculature may cause age-dependent differences in the BOLD signal. There is a growing literature demonstrating that normal aging results in diminished cerebral blood flow throughout the brain.[15,37] Work in older adults by D'Esposito et al[15] revealed that reduction in baseline cerebral blood flow (CBF0 values reduced SNR, making it more difficult to detect stimulus-induced signal alterations. The increased SNR found in younger populations and higher levels of noise in older populations was also found by Huettel et al.[35] In their investigation of mean hemodynamic response functions, both groups had similar onset times, rate of rise, and peak amplitude; however, the peak of the hemodynamic response function was reached earlier by the population of elderly participants, and there was more variability across subjects.[35] These data are consistent with what is known about normal brain development, where CBF values peaking early in life and decrease consistently over the life course.[76] An important analysis of the hemodynamic response function in younger adults, older healthy adults, and older adults with Alzheimer's disease demonstrated distinct latencies between groups (see ref. [10]). Moreover, these latencies were greater in visual cortex compared to motor cortex (see Fig. 8.1), which have important implications for modeling the hemodynamic response function in even-related designs.

Changes in neurovasculature and blood flow do not only affect the elderly, populations at the other end of the age spectrum are likely to have altered cerebral blood flow and hemodynamic response functions as well. Differences in the BOLD signal seen in children may occur because circulatory and respiratory system development is not yet complete. In childhood, myelination

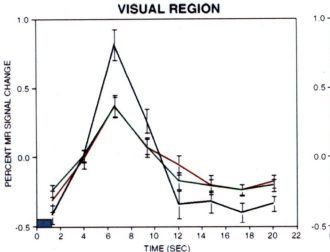
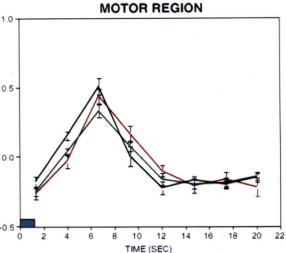

Fig. 8.1 The selectively averaged hemodynamic responses are shown for visual (*left panel*) and motor (*right panel*) regions. Each panel displays mean data from each subject group with the *line color* indicating group: *black* = young adults, *green* = nondemented older adults, and *red* = demented older adults. Error bars indicate standard error of the mean. The *blue mark* at the *bottom* of each panel represents when the visual stimulus was presented. Permission sought for Buckner et al,[10] JoCN

in the brain is also going under development, and it remains unclear if and how the amount of myelination may affect blood flow.[4] In a review investigating studies that document differences seen in the hemodynamic response of children, the findings have been mixed; some studies have found that the shape of the hemodynamic response function is dependent upon age, while others have not been able to confirm this finding.[41]

In infants, changes in regional cerebral blood flow and oxygenation that affect the fMRI signal may be due to environmental circumstances; infants are less likely to maintain their own body temperatures and will often have physiological responses to hypothermia caused by the cold and low humidity environment of imaging rooms.[21] However, this limitation may be addressed by using a specially designed MR-compatible incubator to provide more hospitable conditions for the infant.[21]

Age is not the only variable that may cause changes in cerebral vasculature gender and gender-specific hormones may also influence the velocity of cerebral blood flow as well. In a study comparing aging women and men, it was found that for women more than men, blood flow velocity declines significantly in the 4th and 5th decades of life.[39] Further, for women who were treated with hormone replacement therapy, their pattern of blood flow velocity reflected that found in premenopausal women.[39] Taken together, these factors make it important to consider both gender and age when comparing clinical and healthy populations.

Effects of Injury and Pathology on the BOLD Signal

There is also evidence that diseases affecting the central nervous system may also result in alterations in baseline cerebrovascular parameters. In MS, average CBF values are reduced in areas adjacent to lesion sites and normal appearing white matter (NAWM).[47] Similarly, investigations in HIV have documented altered cerebral blood flow in both symptomatic and asymptomatic participants[79] and even in cases where clinical neuroimaging was negative.[50]

In the study of the effects of brain tumor, it has been found that distance of a mass or lesion from the motor region, edema, and age have strong influences on measured signal change; the larger the distance between the mass and motor region, the higher the measured signal change, and increases in edema lead to decreases in measured signal change.[44] The type of mass that is present may also affect signal change; a trend was found that high-grade gliomas and infiltrating tumors were more likely than benign or extra axial tumors to be associated with lower signal change.[44] The relationship between the severity of the grade of tumor and activation has been confirmed by Holodny et al[34]; their findings suggest that especially in glioblastomas, the side contralateral to the tumor will demonstrate a greater volume of activation. It is hypothesized that the tumor causes a loss of autoregulation of blood flow; if the ability to autoregulate is lost, increased neural activity is not responded to by a corresponding increase in blood flow.[34] Another explanation for the differences in blood flow is that the tumor mass may be positioned, so that it compresses the veins, causing changes in blood pressure that make it difficult to pick up on signal change.[34]

Both traumatic and non-traumatic brain injury have important influences on blood flow in areas near sites of lesion as well as global affects. By definition, cerebrovascular accident represents an alteration in blood flow and perfusion. For example, it was found that after suffering from a lacunar stroke, the BOLD signal is lower in both the unaffected and affected hemispheres suggesting that the vascular disease is diffuse in its influence.[60] Moreover, overt stroke or aneurysm is not required for there to be measurable disruption in blood flow that could affect the BOLD signal. Studies in chronic hypertension, without evidence of ischemia, have shown reduced cerebral blood flow.[72] Animal studies in TBI have repeated demonstrated baseline alterations cerebrovascular parameters.[6,22,26,40,52,70] These changes may exist long after injury.[40] In humans, these findings have been corroborated; using PET-reduced CBF has been noted in perilesional areas following TBI.[28,29] Most recently, the influence of local brain lesions on BOLD fMRI signal was directly measured using a breath hold and arterial spin-labeling methodology.[32] Findings in this study revealed that TBI influences the basic components comprising the fMRI signal, including cerebral blood flow, oxygen extraction fraction, and blood flow transit time, and these effects were particularly salient in peri-lesional areas.

In sum, there are measurable affects of brain injury, brain disease, and even normal aging on cerebrovascular parameters that have direct implications for the resulting BOLD signal. The influences of cerebrovascular change on the BOLD signal are critical to consider for appropriate fMRI data interpretation. Without methodological manipulations permitting documentation of these influences, activation changes secondary to *vascular* changes could be incorrectly interpreted as activation

change secondary to *neuronal* changes reflecting, for example, neural compensation mechanisms. Methods now exist that permit "standardization" of the BOLD signal, thus removing, or at least reducing, the influence of group-related changes in cerebrovascular reactivity on the fMRI data (see Kannurpatti and Biswal 2007[38]). Such considerations are critical when making between-group comparisons.

Effects of Exogenous Substances/ Medication on BOLD

Aside from aging or pathology, there may be treatment factors that affect blood flow and the BOLD signal. The use of pharmacological drugs for treatment is common in clinical populations; although these may include medications that are used to alter physiology in the body and to manage subjective symptoms, they may also have profound effects on cerebral blood flow. Some medications have been found to decrease activation. For example, mannitol is a drug that is often used to reduce intracranial pressure in the brain as well as a sugar substitute for patients with diabetes. Mannitol has been found to affect plasma osmolarity and alters cerebral blood flow. In a study using rats, cerebral blood flow decreased to 81% of baseline after 10 min of a mannitol injection and decreased further to only 65% after 20 min.[17] Interestingly enough, during the time after injection, there were also spontaneous, transient increases in cerebral blood flow, of which the cause remains unclear.[17] Another drug that has been linked with decrease of blood flow after use is lorazepam, most commonly used to treat symptoms of anxiety. The use of this medication has been linked to significant decreases in activation of the hippocampus, fusiform gyrus, and inferior prefrontal cortex; furthermore, this decrease in activation was associated with poor performance on memory tasks.[75]

While the use of some drugs decrease cerebral blood flow, others are linked with increases. One such drug is fluoxetine. Used as a treatment for motor hemiparesis, patients recovering from lacunar stroke using fluoxetine demonstrated an increase in activation in the primary motor cortex ipsilateral to the lesion from their stroke.[59] Another drug, Rivastigamine, a cholinesterase inhibitor, has been used to decrease the rate of deterioration in Alzheimer's disease. The use of this medication has been found to increase bilateral activation of the fusiform gyrus during facial encoding tasks; on simple working memory tasks, signal increases were noted in the frontal lobes; however, the activation became more variable when the task load increased.[68]

Medical and psychiatric pharmacological treatments are not the only substances that may influence blood flow; certain substances found in common day use may also have an effect. Caffeine is a substance used daily by many people for its stimulating effects. Caffeine not only has an excitatory effect on the neurons in the adenosine receptors but also acts as a vasoconstrictor. Studies regarding caffeine and brain activation have been mixed. Some findings report that caffeine can cause as much as a 13.2% decrease in cerebral perfusion, and a decrease of 4.4% in resting BOLD signals, however, respond normally during activation.[58] Due to the low levels at resting baseline, a response results in a seemingly large increase in BOLD signal; while these findings suggest that caffeine may be used as a booster to enhance the detection of activation,[58] to those that are not aware of the effect of caffeine on the BOLD signal, this could give a false sense of the magnitude of activation. The amount of caffeine consumed regularly also influences the signal. Individuals who consume higher amounts of caffeine have been noted to upregulate more adenosine receptors, which leads to the excitatory effects having precedence over vasoconstrictive effects. The magnitude of the BOLD signals has been found to be correlated to caffeine consumption, with those who ingest greater amounts of caffeine showing greater signal changes.[46]

Both pharmacological medications and substances that may be ingested as part of dietary intake have the ability to alter blood flow; depending on the drug and the study, these alterations may be correlated with either improved or worsened performance. It is important then for the researcher conducting studies in clinical populations to note what medications his/her participants may be using, and to be aware what implications that has for the interpretation of brain activation. Researchers may also want to consider advising their participants to follow certain dietary guidelines prior to scanning to control for potential changes in blood flow due to substance consumption.

fMRI Data Interpretation

An Infinite Number of Explanations for "Activation"

Interpretation of functional imaging data is often difficult and highly dependent upon the methodological control and how closely a priori hypotheses are guided by existing theory. Early functional MRI work of cognitive, sensory, and motor functioning in clinical samples was loosely integrated to theory, and interpretations were often based upon already known functional neuroanatomy. This type of work is not isolated to the clinical imaging research. In a paper discussing the opportunities made available to the neurosciences by imaging, one researcher laments the current state of data interpretation in the cognitive neurosciences:

> It is unfortunate that most discussion sections in functional imaging papers simply list a number of post- hoc interpretations of the findings.
>
> –Richard Henson, 2005

The following section focuses on those factors that influence the reliability of imaging data and permit conservative, hypothesis data interpretations. Factors of focus here include paradigm development and control, data analysis, and the influence of additional factors such as affect.

Post hoc analyses in the absence of methodological constraint may result in virtually limitless explanations for any dataset. For this reason, it has been argued that functional imaging data may be more difficult to interpret than behavioral data.[42] It should, therefore, be the goal to use specific study designs that aid in eliminating possible explanations and there are two important manipulations that increase control: (1) choose tasks that can be performed with proficiency by the clinical sample, (2) manipulate task load and directly examine performance vs. fMRI signal relationships.

Tasks that Can Be Performed

In order to constrain the infinite number of possible explanations for any fMRI dataset, one basic requirement is to ensure that the participant is capable of performing the task and this is particularly important to control for in participants demonstrating cognitive deficits.[65,66] As noted by Price and Friston,[64] this mandate, at first glance, appears a bit counterintuitive, given that the traditional motivation in neuropsychology to characterize the nature and magnitude of behavioral "deficit." However, if a behavior is absent (e.g., aphasia) and a task cannot be performed by the patient group, the reason for any resulting between-group differences in the data is very difficult to ascertain. For example, if a patient group cannot perform a task and demonstrates "under-activity" or the inability to engage relevant neural networks compared to healthy adults, then the failure to bring "online" the relevant neuroanatomical substrate(s) may be either the cause or the consequence of the performance deficit (see ref.[64]). Moreover, if the subject is not responding reliably, experimental control is lost; the examiner has no real way of identifying what the subject is doing during the task, making the data uninterpretable.[33,64] Because of this, clinical samples must be able to perform the task they are given and behavior must be integrated with functional imaging data to permit meaningful data interpretation.

In order to facilitate designing tasks that may be universally performed, Price and Friston[65] have identified two types of manipulations that may be applied: (1) task manipulations and (2) stimulus manipulations. A task manipulation, also referred to as an explicit processing paradigm, is a manipulation of the task (and therefore the cognitive processes that are involved) in order to observe any corresponding changes in performance and activation. These types of manipulations may be used when populations are already capable of performing a task and can help to distinguish between the use of typical or atypical neuronal processes.

A stimulus manipulation, or implicit processing paradigm, refers to a change in the stimuli used, but there is no change in the actual task; performance is not expected to change in this type of manipulation. Stimulus manipulations may be used when participants have marked deficits and the imaging is being utilized to assess implicit processes that otherwise cannot be detected by other means (e.g., behavioral testing).

Once a researcher guarantees that a task can be performed by the clinical sample, interpretation of between-group differences depends upon the nature of the difference (e.g., "over" or "under" activity) and the relationship between this difference and performance (more on the latter below). With regard to the former, Fig. 8.2 is adapted from Price and Friston[65] that outlines the possible interpretations to altered functional activity. An important goal is to determine the components of the network that are necessary and/or sufficient for a task to be performed. Figure 8.2 may serve as a heuristic for making interpretations regarding between-group differences in task-related activation when clinical samples can adequately perform the task.

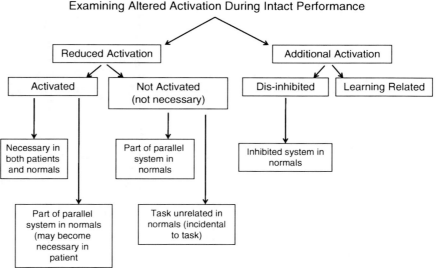

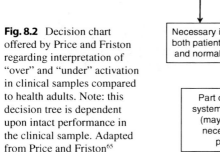

Fig. 8.2 Decision chart offered by Price and Friston regarding interpretation of "over" and "under" activation in clinical samples compared to health adults. Note: this decision tree is dependent upon intact performance in the clinical sample. Adapted from Price and Friston[65]

Directly Examine Performance and Activation Relationships

A second method for eliminating alternative hypotheses when interpreting functional imaging data is to directly manipulate task load in order to alter task difficulty and performance. In doing so, this direct manipulation allows one to observe subsequent changes in the BOLD response that are directly linked to changing performance levels. Having multiple levels of task difficulty also allows factorial modeling of the BOLD signal and the examination of interaction effects between levels (see refs. [30], Rypma & D'Esposito, 1999[84]). Changes in the BOLD response can be therefore linked directly to a manipulation in the paradigm as the investigator directly influences performance level.

Related to task load manipulation, examiners can use performance (e.g., accuracy, reaction time) as a regressor to predict the BOLD signal, thus allowing for the BOLD signal to be measured only as it changes as a function of performance. Figure 8.3 below shows results of a speeded information-processing task in individuals sustaining traumatic brain injury. The analysis here demonstrates the separation of baseline changes in the BOLD signal (or sensory/motor) from those that are rate limiting (e.g., directly related to reaction time). Direct examination of the activation x performance relationships is critical in clinical fMRI, where performance decrements are likely to occur (even with careful subject selection). Thus, manipulating task load, multi-factorial designs, and directly examining performance vs. activation may help to eliminate alternative explanations for fMRI findings.[15,31]

Clinical fMRI and the Trouble with Subtraction

The limitations inherent in cognitive subtraction have generally been acknowledged but permitted within the larger cognitive neuroscience literature (Friston et al., 1996[85]). However, such limitations are amplified in clinical studies. The reason is that not only does subtraction presuppose some linearity in the contribution of subordinate cognitive processes (i.e., pure insertion), but in creating contrast images via cognitive subtraction, this method also presumes that what is "subtracted" is reliably equivalent between groups. Remarkably, the necessity for control task equivalency may threaten the viability of tasks requiring even very simplistic response scenarios. For example, in one of the few clinical studies to provide activation maps of the control task—in this case, a simple reaction time task requiring a button press to indicate detection of a stimulus—a study by Chang et al. (2001[86]) demonstrated that individuals with HIV activated a more elaborate neural network in the control task (see ref. [33]).

Because the cache of neural resources that may be dedicated to process any given task is finite, if critical support networks come "online" at lower task load that serve as a control for higher task load (e.g., 2-back – 1-back),

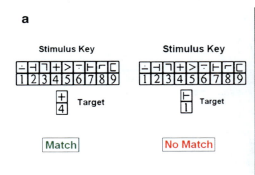
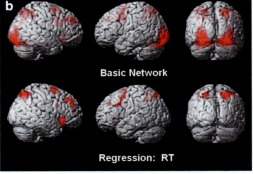
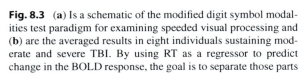

Fig. 8.3 (**a**) Is a schematic of the modified digit symbol modalities test paradigm for examining speeded visual processing and (**b**) are the averaged results in eight individuals sustaining moderate and severe TBI. By using RT as a regressor to predict change in the BOLD response, the goal is to separate those parts of the neural network involved in basic stimulus processing (e.g., visual perception) (*top*), from those that are more closely tied to "decision making" (*bottom*). *Source*: reprinted with permission from Frank G. Hillary, Department of Psychology, Penn State, University Park, PA

these neural resources will be effectively eliminated while creating contrast images. This effect was observed in work by Sweet et al[77] who noted that individuals with MS failed to demonstrate continued increase in PFC involvement as task demand increased (e.g., 2-back vs. 3-back) and that it was assignable to early recruitment of the same PFC resources at lower task loads that might be essentially eliminated via cognitive subtraction at higher task loads (e.g., 3-back – 2-back). Similar effects, if not similar interpretations, have been observed in TBI.[53,54] Thus, the use of "on/off" block designs and demanding control tasks may: (1) create spurious between-group inequalities in activation or (2) hide those differences that do exist. As noted above, this problem is ameliorated by guaranteeing that the clinical sample can easily tolerate and perform well on the control task.

Influence of Mood/Affect on Data Interpretation

In clinical populations, mood and affect often account for differences in cognitive functioning compared to healthy populations. Perhaps not surprisingly then, affect may also contribute to alterations in cerebral blood flow. Mood disorders such as major depressive disorder and bipolar disorder have been linked to structural abnormalities in the prefrontal cortex, cingulate, temporal lobe, reduced gray matter in the left anterior cingulate, and reductions in hippocampal volume.[16] These areas of abnormal structure formation have also been linked to alterations in cerebral blood flow and glucose metabolism; for example, Drevets et al[16] found that initially, metabolic activity appeared to be reduced in the anterior cingulate, however, when the deficits in structural volume were controlled for, the metabolic activity turned out to be increased during phases of depression and reduced during phases where patients were medicated. This increase in metabolic activity during depressive phases of pathology has also been observed in the amygdala, anterior cingulate, and the ventromedial prefrontal cortex.[16] Abnormal hemodynamic response patterns were also observed in the amygdala when emotional stimuli were presented to patients with depression.[16] Taken together, this literature indicates that altered mood has consequences for brain, imaging and examiners should consider the influence of mood/affect on the data.

Controlling for influence of affect on data interpretation is an important obstacle in fMRI studies of cognitive deficit, in particular given the potential relationship between poor performance and emotional changes (e.g., increased anxiety with each incorrect response). Investigators hoping to determine the degree of anxiousness should assess "state" anxiety before and after scanning; emphasis should also be given, so that participants understand task demands and the importance of best effort instead of the expectation of perfect performance.

Conclusions

Functional magnetic resonance imaging provides a unique opportunity to observe the neural networks associated with cognitive, motor, and sensory deficit. Early work using fMRI in the clinical neurosciences has established its utility and advanced its methods; yet, there are inherent limitations to fMRI that must be considered in clinical imaging studies. Both the nature of the scanning process and the pathology present in clinical populations contribute to methodological difficulty in the acquisition, processing, and interpretation of imaging data. An understanding of these limitations and careful implementation of novel methods for controlling unwanted error will help to advance the use of fMRI methods for understanding of brain function in neurological and medical disorders.

References

1. Bandettini P. Functional MRI today. *Int J Psychophysiol.* 2007;63:138–145.
2. Birn RM, Bandettini PA, Cox RW, Shaker R. Event-related fMRI of tasks involving brief motion. *Hum Brain Mapp.* 1999;7:106–114.
3. Biswal BB, Hyde JS. Contour-based registration technique to differentiate between task activated and head motion induced signal variations in fMRI. *Magn Reson Med.* 1997;38(3):470–476.
4. Bookheimer SY. Methodological issues in pediatric neuroimaging. *Ment Retard Dev Disabil Res Rev.* 2000;6:161–165.
5. Bosnell R, Wegner C, Kincses ZT, et al. Reproducibility of fMRI in the clinical setting: implications for trial designs. *Neuroimage.* 2008;42:603–610.
6. Bouma GJ, Muizelaar JP, Choi SC, Newlon PG, Young HF. Cerebral circulation and metabolism after severe traumatic brain injury: the elusive role of ischemia. *J Neurosurg.* 1991;75(5):685–693.

7. Brennan SC, Redd WH, Schorr PB, et al. Anxiety and panic during magnetic resonance scans. *Lancet*. 1988;2(8609):512.

8. Brett M, Leff AP, Rorden C, Ashburner J. Spatial normalization of brain images with focal lesions using cost function masking. *Neuroimage*. 2001;14:486–500.

9. Buckner RL, Koutstaal W, Schacter DL, Dale AM, Rotte MR, Rosen BR. Functional-anatomic study of episodic retrieval: II. Selective averaging of event-related fMRI trials to test the retrieval success hypothesis. *Neuroimage*. 1998;7:163–175.

10. Buckner RL, Snyder AZ, Sanders AL, Raichle ME, Morris JC. Functional brain imaging of young, nondemented, and demented older adults. *J Cogn Neurosci*. 2000;12(suppl 2):24–34.

11. Casey BJ, Cohen JD, O'Craven K, et al. Reproducibility of fMRI results across four institutions using a spatial working memory task. *Neuroimage*. 1998;8:249–261.

12. Cohen MS. Parametric analysis of fMRI data using linear systems methods. *Neuroimage*. 1997;6:93–103.

13. Cohen MS, DuBois RM. Stability, repeatibility, and the expression of signal magnitude in functional magnetic resonance imaging. *J Magn Reson Imaging*. 1999;10:33–40.

14. Crinion J, Ashburner J, Leff A, Brett M, Price C, Friston K. Spatial normalization of lesioned brains: performance evaluation and impact on fMRI analyses. *Neuroimage*. 2007;37:866–875.

15. D'Esposito M, Zarahn E, Aguirre GK, Rypma B. The effect of normal aging on the coupling of neural activity to the bold hemodynamic response. *Neuroimage*. 1999;10:6–14.

16. Drevets WC, Price JL, Furey ML. Brain structural and functional abnormalities in mood disorders: implications for neurocircuitry models of depression. *Brain Struct Funct*. 2008;213:93–118.

17. Duckrow RB. Decreased cerebral blood flow during acute hyperglycemia. *Brain Res*. 1995;703:145–150.

18. Dunn JF, Wadghiri YZ, Meyerand ME. Regional heterogeneity in the brain's response to hypoxia measured using BOLD MR imaging. *Magn Reson Med*. 1999;41:850–854.

19. Eaton KP, Szaflarski JP, Altaye M, et al. Reliability of fMRI for studies of language in post-stroke aphasia subjects. *Neuroimage*. 2008;41:311–322.

20. Epstein JN, Casey BJ, Tonev ST, et al. Assessment and prevention of head motion during imaging of patients with attention deficit hyperactivity disorder. *Psychiatry Res*. 2007;155(1):75–82.

21. Erberich SG, Friedlich P, Seri I, Nelson MD Jr, Blüml S. Functional MRI in neonates using neonatal head coil and MR compatible incubator. *Neuroimage*. 2003;20:683–692.

22. Forbes ML, Hendrich KS, Kochanek PM, et al. Assessment of cerebral blood flow and CO_2 reactivity after controlled cortical impact by perfusion magnetic resonance imaging using arterial spin labeling in rats. *J Cereb Blood Flow Metab*. 1997;17(8):865–874.

23. Friston KJ, Williams S, Howard R, Frackowiak RSJ, Turner R. Movement related effects in fMRI time series. *Magn Reson Med*. 1996;35:346–355.

24. Friston KJ, Worsley KJ, Frackowiak RSJ, et al. Assessing the significance of local activation using their spatial extent. *Hum Brain Mapp*. 1994;1:214–220.

25. Glover GH, Li TQ, Ress D. Image-based method for retrospective correction of physiological motion effects in fMRI: RETROICOR. *Magn Reson Med*. 2000;44(1):162–167.

26. Golding EM. Sequelae following traumatic brain injury, The cerebrovascular perspective. *Brain Res Rev*. 2002;38(3):377–388.

27. Havel T, Braun B, Rau A, et al. Reproducibility of activation in four motor paradigms: an fMRI study. *J Neurol*. 2006;253:471–476.

28. Hattori N, Huang SC, Wu HM, et al. PET investigation of post-traumatic cerebral blood volume and blood flow. *Acta Neurochir Suppl*. 2003;86:49–52.

29. Hattori N, Huang SC, Wu HM, et al. Acute changes in regional cerebral (18)f-FDG kinetics in patients with traumatic brain injury. *J Nucl Med*. 2004;45(5):775–783.

30. Henson R. What can functional neuroimaging tell the experimental psychologist? *Q J Exp Psychol*. 2005;58A(2):193–233.

31. Hillary FG, Genova HM, Chiaravalloti ND, Rypma B, DeLuca J. Prefrontal modulation of working memory performance in brain injury and disease. *Hum Brain Mapp*. 2006;27(11):837–847.

32. Hillary FG, Biswal B. The influence of neuropathology on the fMRI signal: a measurement of brain or vein? *Clin Neuropsychol*. 2007;21:58–72.

33. Hillary FG. Neuroimaging of working memory dysfunction and the dilemma with brain reorganization hypothesis. *J Int Neuropsychol Soc*. 2008;14(4):526–534.

34. Holodny AI, Schulder M, Liu W, Wolko J, Maldjian JA, Kalnin AJ. The effect of brain tumors on BOLD functional MR imaging activation in the adjacent motor cortex: implications for image-guided neurosurgery. *Am J Neuroradiol*. 2000;21:1415–1422.

35. Huettel SA, Singerman JD, McCarthy G. The effects of aging upon the hemodynamic response measured by functional MRI. *Neuroimage*. 2001;13:161–175.

36. Jones TB, Bandettini PA, Birn RM. Integration of motion correction and physiological noise regression in fMRI. *Neuroimage*. 2008;42:582–590.

37. Kamper AM, Spilt A, de Craen AJM, van Buchem MA, Westendorp RGJ, Blauw GJ. Basal cerebral blood flow is dependent on the nitric oxide pathway in elderly but not in young healthy men. *Exp Gerontol*. 2004;39:1245–1248.

38. Kannurpatti SS, Biswal BB. Detection and scaling of task-induced fMRI-BOLD response using resting state fluctuations. *Neuroimage*. 2008;40(4):1567–1574.

39. Katstrup A, Dichgans J, Niemeier M, Schabet M. Changes of cerebrovascular CO2 reactivity during normal aging. *Stroke*. 1998;29:1311–1314.

40. Kochanek PM, Hendrich KS, Dixon CE, Schiding JK, Williams DS, Ho C. Cerebral blood flow at one year after controlled cortical impact in rats; assessment by magnetic resonance imaging. *J Neurotrauma*. 2002;19(9):1029–1037.

41. Kotsoni E, Byrd D, Casey BJ. Special considerations for functional magnetic resonance imaging of pediatric populations. *J Magn Reson Imaging*. 2006;23:877–886.

42. Kosslyn SM. If neuroimaging is the answer, what is the question? *Phil Trans R Soc Lond B*. 1999;354:1283–1294.

43. Kimberley TJ, Khandekar G, Borich M. fMRI reliability in subjects with stroke. *Exp Brain Res*. 2008;186:183–190.

44. Krings T, Reinges MHT, Willmes K, et al. Factors related to the magnitude of T2* MR signal changes during functional imaging. *Neuroradiology*. 2002;44:459–466.

8 Methodological Considerations for Using BOLD fMRI in the Clinical Neurosciences

45. Kurland J, Naeser MA, Baker EH, et al. Test-retest reliability of fMRI during nonverbal semantic decisions in moderate-severe nonfluent aphasia patients. *Behav Neurol.* 2004;15(3–4): 87–97.
46. Laurienti PJ, Field AS, Burdette JH, et al. Dietary caffeine consumption modulates fMRI measures. *Neuroimage.* 2002;17:751–757.
47. Law M, Saindane AM, Ge Y, et al. Microvascular abnormality in relapsing-remitting multiple sclerosis: perfusion MR imaging findings in normal-appearing white matter. *Radiology.* 2004;231(3):645–652.
48. Liao R, McKeown MJ, Krolik JL. Isolation and minimalization of head motion- induced signal variation in fMRI data using independent component analysis. *Magn Reson Med.* 2006;55:1396–1413.
49. Logothetis NK. The neural basis of the blood-oxygen-level-dependent functional magnetic resonance imaging signal. *Phil Trans R Soc Lond B.* 2002;357:1003–1037.
50. Maini CL, Pigorini F, Pau FM, et al. Cortical cerebral blood flow in HIV-1-related dementia complex. *Nucl Med Commun.* 1990;11(9):639–648.
51. Manoach DS, Halpern EF, Kramer TS, et al. Test-retest reliability of a functional MRI working memory paradigm in normal and schizophrenic subjects. *Am J Psychiatry.* 2001;158: 955–958.
52. Martin NA, Patwardhan RV, Alexander M, et al. Characterization of cerebral hemodynamic phases following severe head trauma: hypoperfusion, hyperemia, and vasospasm. *J Neurosurg.* 1997; 87(1):9–19.
53. McAllister TW, Saykin AJ, Flashman LA, et al. Brain activation during working memory 1 month after mild traumatic brain injury. *Neurology.* 1999;53(6):1300–13008.
54. McAllister TW, Sparling MB, Flashman LA, Guerin SJ, Mamourian AC, Saykin AJ. Differential working memory load effects after mild traumatic brain injury. *Neuroimage.* 2001;14:1004–1012.
55. McIsaac HK, Thordarson DS, Shafran R, Rachman S, Poole G. Claustrophobia and the magnetic imaging procedure. *J Behav Med.* 1998;21(3):255–268.
56. Mendes J, Kholmovski E, Parker DL. Rigid-body motion correction with self-navigation MRI. *Magn Reson Med.* 2009;61(3):739–747.
57. Menon V, Lim KO. Design and efficacy of a head-coil bite bar for reducing movement-related artifacts during functional MRI scanning. *Behav Res Methods Instrum Comput.* 1997;29(4):589–594.
58. Mulderink TA, Gitelman DR, Mesulam M, Parrish TB. On the use of caffeine as a contrast booster for BOLD fMRI studies. *Neuroimage.* 2002;15:37–44.
59. Pariente J, Loubinoux I, Carel C, et al. Fluoxetine modulates motor performance and cerebral activation of patients recovering from stroke. *Ann Neurol.* 2001;50:718–729.
60. Pineiro R, Pendlebury S, Johansen-Berg H, Matthews PM. Altered hemodynamic responses in patients after subcortical stroke measured by functional MRI. *Stroke.* 2002;33: 103–109.
61. Poldrack RA. Can cognitive processes be inferred from neuroimaging data? *Trends Cogn Sci.* 2006;10(2):59–63.
62. Poldrack RA. Tools of the trade: region of interest analysis for fMRI. *SCAN.* 2007;2:67–70.
63. Posse S, Olthoff U, Weckesser M, Jäncke L, Müller-Gäartner H, Dager SR. Regional dynamic signal changes during controlled hyperventilation assessed with blood oxygen level-dependent functional MR imaging. *AJNR Am J Neuroradiol.* 1997;18:1763–1770.
64. Price CJ, Friston KJ. Scanning patients with tasks they can perform. *Hum Brain Mapp.* 1999;8:102–108.
65. Price CJ, Friston KJ. Functional imaging studies of neuropsychological patients: applications and limitations. *Neurocase.* 2002;8:345–354.
66. Price CJ, Friston KJ. Functional imaging in cognitive neuroscience II: imaging patients. In: Farah MJ, Feinberg TE, eds. *Patient-Based Approaches to Cognitive Neuroscience.* 2nd ed. Cambridge, MA: MIT Press; 2006:47–54.
67. Raz A, Lieber B, Soliman F, et al. Ecological nuances in functional magnetic resonance imaging (fMRI): psychological stressors, posture, and hydrostatics. *Neuroimage.* 2005; 25:1–7.
68. Rombouts SARB, Barkhof F, van Meel CS, Scheltens P. Alterations in brain activation during cholinergic enhancement with rivastigmine in Alzheimer's disease. *J Neurol Neurosurg Psychiatry.* 2002;73:665–671.
69. Schacter DL, Buckner RL, Koutstaal W, Dale AM, Rosen BR. Late onset of anterior prefrontal activity during true and false recognition: an event-related fMRI study. *Neuroimage.* 1997;6:259–269.
70. Schroder ML, Muizelaar JP, Kuta AJ, Choi SC. Thresholds for cerebral ischemia after severe head injury: relationship with late CT findings and outcome. *J Neurotrauma.* 1996;13(1): 17–23.
71. Seto E, Sela G, McIlroy WE, et al. Quantifying head motion associated with motor tasks used in fMRI. *Neuroimage.* 2001;14:284–297.
72. Sierra C, de la Sierra A, Chamorro A, Larrousse M, Domenech M, Coca A. Cerebral hemodynamics and silent cerebral white matter lesions in middle-aged essential hypertensive patients. *Blood Press.* 2004;13(5):304–309.
73. Siegmund DO, Worsley KJ. Testing for a signal with unknown location and scale in a stationary Gaussian random field. *Ann Stat.* 1994;23:608–639.
74. Siejö BK. *Brain Energy Metabolism.* New York: Wiley; 1978.
75. Sperling R, Greve D, Dale A, et al. Functional MRI detection of pharmacologically induced memory impairment. *Proc Natl Acad Sci USA.* 2002;99(1):455–460.
76. Swank RL, Roth JG, Woody DC Jr. Cerebral blood flow and red cell delivery in normal subjects and in multiple sclerosis. *Neurol Res.* 1983;5(1):37–59.
77. Sweet LH, Rao SM, Primeau M, Mayer AR, Cohen RA. Functional magnetic resonance imaging of working memory among multiple sclerosis. *J Neuroimaging.* 2004;14(2): 150–157.
78. Thacker NA, Burton E, Lacey AJ, Jackson A. The effects of motion on parametric fMRI analysis techniques. *Physiol Meas.* 1999;20:251–263.
79. Tran Dinh YR, Mamo H, Cervoni J, Caulin C, Saimot AC. Disturbances in the cerebral perfusion of human immune deficiency virus-1 seropositive asymptomatic subjects: a quantitative tomography study of 18 cases. *J Nucl Med.* 1990;31(10):1601–1607.

80. Wu DH, Guo Y, Lu CC, Suri J. Improvement to functional magnetic resonance imaging (fMRI) methods using non-rigid body image registration methods for correction in the presence of susceptibility artifact effects. In: *Proceedings of the 28th IEEE EMBS Annual International Conference*. New York, 2006:1018–1020.

81. Yeo DT, Fessler JA, Kim B. Concurrent correction of geometric distortion and motion using the map-slice-to-volume method in echo-planar imaging. *Magn Reson Imaging*. 2008;26(5):703–714.

82. Genovese CR, Lazar NA, Nichols T. Thresholding of statistical maps in functional neuroimaging using the false discovery rate. *Neuroimage*. 2002;15(4):870–878.

83. Pendse G, Borsook D, Becerra L. Enhanced false discovery rate using Gaussian mixture models for thresholding fMRI statistical maps. *Neuroimage*. 2009;47(1):231–261.

84. Rypma B, D'Esposito M. The roles of prefrontal brain regions in components of working memory: effects of memory load and individual differences. Proc Natl Acad Sci. 1999;96(11):6558–6563.

85. Friston KJ, Price CJ, Fletcher P, Moore C, Frackowiak RSJ, Dolan RJ. The Trouble with Cognitive Subtraction. *Neuroimage*. 1996;4(2):97–104.

86. Chang L, Speck O, Miller EN, Braun J, Jovicich J, Koch C, Itti L, Ernst T. Neural correlates of attention and working memory deficits in HIV patients. *Neurology*. 2001;57(6):1001–1007.

Chapter 9
Application of Functional Neuroimaging to Examination of Nicotine Dependence

Sean P. David, Lawrence H. Sweet, Ronald A. Cohen, James MacKillop, Richard C. Mulligan, and Raymond Niaura

Overview

Functional neuroimaging methods have provided cognitive neuroscientists with a way of studying brain activity associated with cognitive and behavioral processes that underlie addiction to nicotine and tobacco, and there has been a trend of markedly increasing numbers of functional neuroimaging studies of nicotine dependence, using multiple imaging approaches, over the last 15 years.[1,2]

This chapter is intended to provide an introduction to investigators interested in utilizing the wide array of neuroimaging approaches and behavioral paradigms available for assessment of neurobiological mechanisms associated with nicotine and tobacco use. As the chapter is an overview, it barely touches the surface of the rich biobehavioral data available from this rapidly growing corpus of literature.

Following a brief primer on the neurobiology of nicotine addiction in Sect. 2, each of the major functional neuroimaging approaches utilized in nicotine dependence research is discussed in Sect. 3, and illustrations of the applications of neuroimaging approaches in nicotine dependence research are described in Sect. 4. As will become evident, there are many types and subtypes of functional neuroimaging modalities utilized in nicotine and tobacco research. However, the most dominant func-

tional neuroimaging approach utilized to date has been functional magnetic resonance imaging (fMRI) in terms of the number of published studies (see Table 9.2). Even so, many other neuroimaging modalities have been applied in nicotine dependence research, and depending on the hypotheses being explored, each method has distinct advantages or disadvantages for investigators exploring the neurobiology of nicotine dependence.

Neurobiology of Nicotine Dependence

The development and maintenance of nicotine dependence is complex and involves multiple brain regions and neurotransmitter systems. Approximately 85–90% of the nicotine absorbed by smoking is metabolized by the liver, while 10–15% is excreted as cotinine in the urine.[3] Approximately 80% of nicotine is metabolized into the major metabolite cotinine with CYP2A6 mediating 85–100% of this reaction.[3] The mesocorticolimbic dopamine system is a primary brain region of interest in the study of pharmacodynamic effects of drugs of abuse, in general,[4] and nicotine specifically.[5] The mesocorticolimbic system consists of cell bodies in the midbrain which project to the amygdala, nucleus accumbens, and prefrontal cortex. Nicotine binds to nicotinic acetylcholine receptors (nAChRs) in the ventral tegmental area, stimulating burst firing of dopamine in the nucleus accumbens and a complex cascade of events involving multiple neurotransmitter systems, also including alterations in other catecholamine pathways including serotonin and norepinephrine, as well as opioid, GABA, and glutamate pathways.[6] With repetitive exposure to nicotine (and other constituents of tobacco smoke), neuroadaptive changes take place that are theorized to result in escalating incentive

S.P. David (✉)
Division of Family & Community Medicine,
Department of Medicine, Stanford University School
of Medicine, Stanford, CA, USA
and
Policy, SRI International, Menlo Park, CA, USA
and
Family Medicine, Alpert Medical School of Brown University,
Providence, RI, USA
e-mail: spdavid@stanford.edu

R.A. Cohen and L.H. Sweet (eds.), *Brain Imaging in Behavioral Medicine and Clinical Neuroscience*,
DOI 10.1007/978-1-4419-6373-4_9, © Springer Science+Business Media, LLC 2011

Functional Neuroimaging Approaches

The range of neuroimaging approaches applied to nicotine dependence research is wide, and incorporates fMRI and structural MRI, positron emission tomography (PET), single-photon emission computed tomography (SPECT), magnetoencephalography (MEG), and magnetic resonance spectroscopy (MRS), and a growing number of studies are incorporating genotype as a predictive independent variable whereby neuroimaging data serve as highly specific neurobiological measures, or, in some cases, phenotypes for genetic association studies.

Functional Magnetic Resonance Imaging

FMRI has become a widely used technology for neurophysiological nicotine dependence studies because of its high spatial and temporal resolution, relative to some (i.e., PET and single-photon emission tomography), but not all of the other functional neuroimaging methods, its noninvasiveness and lack of radioactive tracers, and its ability to be used for repeated measures. Moreover, the use of MRI for research is extremely versatile, permitting examination of blood-oxygen-level-dependent-signal (BOLD) response, regional cerebral blood flow (rCBF), arterial spin labeling (ASL) perfusion, diffusion tensor imaging (DTI), and interregional connectivity. Other approaches contribute different types of data that may be complementary to fMRI, and each approach has unique advantages and disadvantages based on the research questions posed as discussed below. Each of these MRI approaches permits assessment of very different functional domains.

Positron Emission Tomography

PET involves the use of intravenously administered radioactive ligands labeled with short-lived positron-emitting isotopes of carbon, oxygen, nitrogen, or fluorine attached to molecules. When ligands are administered systemically they cross the blood–brain barrier and bind to specific molecular targets such as neurotransmitter receptors or transporters. The ligands emit positrons, which collide with electrons and release gamma rays. Serial blood sampling of arterial concentrations of the ligand and the detection of gamma rays indicate the location of the receptor targets. When combined with the established pharmacokinetic properties of each ligand, investigators can estimate the binding potential (BP) of receptors, and affinity for specific endogenous ligands using established mathematical models. The BP is directly proportional to the availability of ligand binding sites and thus provides an estimation of the concentration or density of the receptor of interest in specified brain ROIs.

Thus, PET provides the ability to trace the binding and distribution of specific ligands such as nicotine (e.g., [^{11}C]-labelled nicotine). PET is therefore useful for the examination of quantity and distribution of specific molecular targets with direct relevance to nicotine dependence such as the DA D_2 receptor ([^{11}C]raclopride)[10] and others. Table 9.1 provides examples of radioactive ligands used in PET and single-photon emission tomography studies (described below), specific to particular receptor subtypes, which are being used increasingly in studies of nicotine dependence.

As many of the ligands are competitive antagonists of receptors of interest, PET also provides information on endogenous neurotransmitter release in response to pharmacological challenges. Combined with fMRI and other imaging techniques described below, PET functional imaging can therefore provide a rich array of data in vivo once only available in invasive animal studies.

Single-Photon Emission Computed Tomography

Similar to PET, SPECT utilizes radioactive isotopes but with much longer half-lives than those used in PET. The longer half-life of isotopes limits the temporal resolution of SPECT and, as such, SPECT has not been used extensively in nicotine dependence research in recent years.

9 Application of Functional Neuroimaging to Examination of Nicotine Dependence

Table 9.1 Radioligands commonly used in nicotine dependence research

Ligand	Molecular target	Permits evaluation of
[¹¹C]SCH-23390	D1 receptors	D1 receptor occupancy
[¹¹C]raclopride	D2 receptors	D2 receptor occupancy
[⁹⁹ᵐTx]TRODAT-1[¹²³I]β-CIT	Dopamine transporter	Dopamine transporter availability
[¹¹C]WAY-100635	5-HT$_{1A}$	5-HT$_{1A}$ receptor occupancy
[¹⁸F]altanserin	5-HT$_{2A}$	5-HT$_{2A}$ receptor occupancy
[¹¹C]McN-5652[¹²³I]β-CIT	Serotonin transporter	Serotonin transporter availability
[¹¹C]nicotine2-[¹⁸F]-A-85380 5-[¹²³I]-iodo-A-85380 ([¹²³I]5-IA)	Nicotinic acetylcholine	Nicotinic acetylcholine receptor distribution
[¹¹C]clorgyline	MAO-A	MAO-A activity
[¹¹C]^L-deprynyl-D2	MAO-B	MAO-B activity
[¹⁸F]DOPA	All DA receptors	Dopamine activity
[¹¹C]carfentanil	μ-opioid receptors	μ-opioid receptor occupancy
[¹⁵O]H$_2$O	Nonspecific	Global and regional cerebral blood flow
[¹⁸F]-fluorodeoxyglucose (FDG)	Nonspecific	Glucose metabolism

The table lists radioligands used in positron emission tomography studies with relevance to nicotine dependence

SCH-23390 = ((R)-(+)-7-chloro-8-hydroxy-3-methyl-1-phenyl-2,3,4,5-tetrahydro-1H-3-benzazepine hydrochloride); TRODAT-1 = Tc99m Tropane; McN-5652 = Pyrrolo[2,1-a]isoquinoline, 1,2,3,5,6,10b-hexahydro-6-[4-(methylthio)phenyl]-, (6S,10bR)-, (2R,3R)-2,3-di-(O-4-methylphenyloxy)butanedioate; FDG = 2-fluoro-2-deoxy-d-glucose

Electroencephalography, Event-Related Potentials, and Magnetoencephalography

Electroencephalography (EEG) measures the difference in emitted voltage between a site located on the scalp and a reference site where no EEG activity is expected. EEG waveforms are thought to represent the summed postsynaptic activity of cortical pyramidal cells.[11] EEG activity in the frequency of different waveforms has been associated with functional outcomes such as working memory and with emotional traits and states and, as such, can be useful in nicotine addiction research.

Event-related potentials (ERP) are useful in providing information on cortical responses to discrete stimuli and differ from EEG in the high temporal resolution of responses to stimuli (within ms). The spatial resolution of EEG and ERP is relatively low when compared to fMRI. However, spatial resolution is proportional to the number of electrodes and has improved with the development of high-density electrode arrays. A promising feature of EEG and ERP is that they can be used with fMRI and PET and could therefore complement these methods by providing additional information on large distributions of neurons. EEG and ERP modalities are not necessarily considered neuroimaging procedures but are discussed here because these approaches do provide functional data localized to specific brain regions and have been excellent complements to neuroimaging approaches such as MEG.

MEG, similar to EEG and ERP, measures changes in electrical activity in the brain, but unlike EEG and ERP, MEG also measures changes in magnetic fields generated by such activity. MEG has better spatial resolution than EEG or ERP but has not been used extensively in nicotine dependence research.

Magnetic Resonance Spectroscopy

Although used less frequently, MRS can also be used to study biochemistry of the brain, including measurements of concentrations of some key neurotransmitters such as GABA and glutamate.

Imaging Genomics

"Imaging genomics" is a type of genetic association study but differs from conventional association studies by defining phenotypes as discrete, physiological responses to behavioral tasks, environmental, or pharmacological stimuli. Such phenotypes, more biologically proximal to the gene product, are considered more reliable, high-level phenotypes – or so-called "endophenotypes". As such, candidate genes ideal for imaging genomic studies are those with well-characterized functional effects as demonstrated in vitro and/or in vivo. At the time of this writing, to our knowledge, there are only four published imaging genomic studies specifically focused on nicotine dependence;[12-15] however, there are manifold more imaging genomic studies in the literature with relevance to nicotine dependence (e.g., examining genetic influences on striatal D2 receptor binding),[16] and the field of imaging genomics for nicotine dependence and smoking cessation research is expected to grow rapidly in coming years. For an excellent review, see Ray et al., 2008.[2]

Advantages and Disadvantages of Different Neuroimaging Approaches for Nicotine Dependence Research

FMRI and PET/SPECT each have advantages and disadvantages depending on the research questions posed. If one is examining activation patterns responding to specific stimuli, fMRI is clearly advantageous compared with PET and SPECT because of its (fMRI) higher spatial and temporal resolution. The noninvasive nature of fMRI also permits investigators to maximize statistical power with the employment of multiple measures to evaluate the effect of specific stimuli on neural activation. Furthermore, fMRI permits greater flexibility and versatility in experimental design than in vivo molecular imaging approaches. For example, PET requires block designs and repeated-measures studies are difficult given the health risks associated with repetitive exposure to radioactive ligands. PET, SPECT, and MRS have advantages in terms of ability to provide functional data on specific neurochemical substrates. The major disadvantages of PET and SPECT are the radiation exposure and invasiveness involved, limiting the number of scans a subject may have, the cost, the need to prepare appropriate radioligands, and the lower spatial and temporal resolution.[17,18] As previously mentioned, ERP has very high temporal resolution and thus may have advantages over MRI for measurement of responses to stimuli in the millisecond range. MRS and fMRI have obvious advantages in providing statistical activation maps overlaid upon high-resolution structural brain images and the ability to conveniently acquire additional types of images during the same session – such as clinical scans. However, MRS has a distinct disadvantage by not necessarily providing whole-brain coverage using currently available methods.

Functional Neuroimaging Studies of Nicotine Dependence

The range of neuroimaging approaches utilized in nicotine dependence research is broad, with utilization of nearly all imaging modalities, stimuli cue exposure and cognitive/affective task paradigms, and dependent variables (e.g., regional blood flow (cerebral perfusion), BOLD, receptor binding, brain structure and connectivity). Therefore, the discussion of specific neuroimaging studies of nicotine dependence in Sect. 4 is organized by experimental manipulation typologies. At the time of this writing, at least 58 functional neuroimaging studies of nicotine dependence in humans using radiological (e.g., magnetic resonance, PET, SPECT) methods have been published and/or presented over the last 15 years, and this number includes neither radiological studies relevant to but not involving nicotine or nicotine dependence tasks using radioligands for receptors within neurological pathways implicated in nicotine dependence (Table 9.1) or assessments nor studies using nonradiological neuroimaging (e.g., ERP, EEG). Of the 58 studies reviewed and described in Table 9.2, there were 10 studies examining smoking or emotional cue exposure, attention, or affect without contrasts between abstinence, smoking satiation, or nicotine administration contrasts, 15 studies examining effects of nicotine on cue reactivity or task performance contrasts, and/or receptor binding, 26 studies examining abstinence effects on cue reactivity or task performance, cue reactivity or task performance contrasts, and seven studies using task-free approaches.

Cue Exposure Effects and Cognitive, Affective, or Working Memory Tasks

Cue exposure paradigms frequently used in neuroimaging studies of nicotine dependence include smoking cue reactivity (often comparing smoking-related to nonsmoking images), or presentation of images such

Table 9.2 Functional neuroimaging studies of nicotine dependence

Study	Subjects	Design	Experimental conditions	Paradigm	Measures	Modality
Cue, emotional, or cognitive/working memory paradigms (no drug administration or nicotine abstinence-effects contrasts)						
Brody et al. (2002) USA[25]	*Experimental group:* 20 smokers Mean 33 cig/day 70% male Mean age 43 years *Comparison group:* 20 non-smokers 55% male Mean age 37 years	2×2 repeated-measures ANOVA Cue (smoking, neutral) Smoking status (smoker, non-smoker)	*Experimental group:* Prescan tobacco abstinence status not reported Mean CO 23.1 ppm smoking cue scan 24.1 ppm neutral scan *Comparison group:* Mean CO 1.7 ppm smoking cue scan 1.5 ppm neutral scan	Pictorial cues Video Smoking-related Neutral	Self-reported craving, depression, anxiety, smoking quantity	[18F]-FDG PET (regional glucose metabolism)
David et al. (2005) UK[27]	*Experimental group:* 9 smokers Mean 18 cig/day 44% male Mean age 34 years *Comparison group:* 11 never-smokers Never smoked regularly 37% male Mean age 28 years	2×2×2 repeated-measures ANOVA Cue (smoking, neutral) Hemisphere (right, left) Smoking status (smoker, non-smoker)	*Experimental group:* Overnight abstinence prescan Mean CO 2.9 ppm No nicotine *Comparison group:* No nicotine	Pictorial cues Photos Smoking-related Neutral Gender discrimination task for reaction times Keypress	Self-reported craving, withdrawal, smoking quantity Reaction times	fMRI BOLD
Due et al. (2002) USA[24]	*Experimental group:* 12 smokers Mean 24 cig/day 67% male Mean age 22 years *Comparison group:* 6 never-smokers Never smoked regularly 67% male Mean age 25 years	2×2×4 repeated-measures ANOVA Cue (smoking, neutral) Hemisphere (right, left) Time (4, 6, 8, 10 s) Post-hoc comparison of smokers and never-smokers	*Experimental group:* 10 h abstinence prescan Mean CO 13.2 ppm No nicotine *Comparison group:* No nicotine	Pictorial cues Photos Smoking-related Neutral Target (animals) Keypress	Self-reported craving, mood, smoking quantity	fMRI BOLD
Finnerty et al. (2009) USA[40]	*Experimental group:* 9 smokers Mean cig/day not reported 22% male Mean age 34 years *Comparison group:* No comparison group	2×3 repeated-measures ANOVA Task (active, rest) Emotional valence (neutral, positive, negative) Post-hoc Correlation of BOLD signal with affect and withdrawal symptoms	*Experimental group:* International Affective Picture Series (IAPS) Mean CO not reported *Comparison group:* None	Pictorial cues Photos IAPS Positive Negative Neutral	Self-reported affect, withdrawal	fMRI BOLD

(continued)

Table 9.2 (continued)

Study	Subjects	Design	Experimental conditions	Paradigm	Measures	Modality
Franklin et al. (2007) USA[28]	*Experimental group:* 21 smokers Mean 20 cig/day 43% male Mean age 34 years *Comparison group:* None	2×2×6 repeated-measures ANOVA Cue (smoking, neutral) Hemisphere (right, left) Region (6 regions)	*Experimental group:* 2 separate, counterbalanced scanning sessions for smoking cues and neutral cues, respectively Ad libitum smoking before each session Mean CO not reported Comparison group: None	Pictorial cues Photos Smoking-related Neutral	Self-reported nicotine dependence, withdrawal, craving, smoking quantity	ASL MRI
[a]Franklin et al. (2009) USA[12]	*Experimental group:* 10 smokers with [b]DAT 9/9 or 9/10 genotype Mean 20 cig/day 60% male Mean age 38 years *Comparison group:* 9 smokers with DAT 10/10 genotype Mean 23 cig/day 44% male Mean age 34 years	2×2×2 repeated-measures ANOVA: voxelwise analyses rather than region of interest analyses Cue (smoking, neutral) Hemisphere (right, left) Genotype (DAT: 9/9 or 9/10, 10/10)	*Experimental group:* Same paradigm as Franklin et al. (2007) Mean CO not reported *Comparison group:* All participants in both genotype strata underwent same cue exposure paradigm Mean CO not reported	Pictorial cues Photos Smoking-related Neutral	Self-reported nicotine dependence, withdrawal, craving, smoking quantity	ASL MRI
Jacobsen et al. (2007a) USA[67]	*Experimental group:* 33 participants with prenatal nicotine exposure: 26 smokers Mean 13 cig/day 27% male Mean 13 cig/day Mean age 16 years 7 non-smokers 57% male Mean age 17 years *Comparison group:* 30 participants without prenatal nicotine exposure: 14 smokers	2×2×2 repeated-measures ANOVA Attention task (simple, selective) Prenatal nicotine exposure (exposed, nonexposed) Smoking status (smoker, non-smoker)	*Experimental group:* Visual & auditory word & nonword cues; lexical discrimination Smokers: Ad libitum smoking Mean CO not reported, however, saliva & plasma cotinine reported *Comparison group:* Non-smokers Same paradigm	Auditory & visual selective & divided attention task	Prenatal environmental exposures, self-reported nicotine dependence, mood, withdrawal, craving, smoking quantity Accuracy Keypress Reaction times	fMRI BOLD

	Mean 12 cig/day 43% male Mean age 17 years 16 non-smokers 56% male Mean age 16 years					
Lee et al. (2005) South Korea[29]	*Experimental group:* 8 smokers Mean 15 cig/day 100% male Mean age 17 years *Comparison group:* No comparison group	2×2 repeated-measures ANOVA Cue (smoking, neutral) Presentation (2D, 3D virtual reality)	*Experimental group:* 7 h abstinence prescan Mean CO not reported	Pictorial cues Virtual environment Smoking-related Neutral	Self-reported nicotine dependence, craving, smoking situations, smoking quantity	fMRI BOLD
McBride et al. (2006) Canada[30]	*Experimental group:* 10 expectant smokers Mean cig/day not reported per group 50% male Mean age 30 years *Comparison group:* 9 nonexpectant smokers Mean cig/day not reported per group 56% male Mean age 24 years	$2 \times 2 \times 2$ repeated-measures ANOVA Cue (smoking, neutral) Smoking (satiated, abstinent) Expectancy (expectant, nonexpectant)	*Experimental group:* Informed they were permitted to smoke after scan Mean CO not reported separately according to expectancy group *Comparison group:* Asked not to smoke for at least 4 h postscan Within-subjects comparison Abstinent day: 12 h abstinence prescan Mean CO 6.3 ppm Smoking day: Ad libitum smoking Mean CO 10.39 ppm	Pictorial cues Video smoking-related Neutral	Self-reported craving, mood, nicotine dependence, smoking quantity	fMRI BOLD
Okuyemi et al. (2006) USA[34]	*Experimental group:* 17 smokers: 8 African-American (AA) smokers Mean 8 cig/day 25% male Mean age 39 years 9 European-American (EA) smokers Mean 8 cig/day 44% male	$3 \times 2 \times 2$ repeated-measures ANOVA Cue (smoking, neutral, baseline) Ethnicity (AA, EA) Smoking status (smoker, non-smoker)	*Experimental group:* Smokers 12 h abstinence prescan AA smokers Mean CO 6.0 ppm EA smokers Mean CO 8.0 ppm *Comparison group:* AA non-smokers Mean CO 0.3 ppm EA non-smokers Mean CO 0.8 ppm	Pictorial cues Photos Smoking-related Neutral	Self-reported nicotine dependence, smoking urges depression, anxiety, stress, smoking quantity	fMRI BOLD

(continued)

Table 9.2 (continued)

Study	Subjects	Design	Experimental conditions	Paradigm	Measures	Modality
	Mean age 37 years Comparison group: 17 non-smokers 8 AA non-smokers 25% male Mean age 37 years 9 EA non-smokers 33% male Mean age 35 years		All participants in both groups underwent the same paradigm			
Smolka et al. (2006) Germany[35]	*Experimental group:* 10 smokers Mean 16 cig/day Mean age 32 years 100% male *Comparison group:* No comparison group	Repeated-measures ANOVA Cue (smoking, neutral)	*Experimental group:* Prescan abstinence not reported Mean CO not reported *Comparison group:* None	Pictorial cues Photos Smoking-related Neutral	Self-reported craving, nicotine dependence	fMRI BOLD
Sweet et al. (2009) USA[36]	*Experimental group:* 15 smokers Mean 21 cig/day 67% male Mean age not reported *Comparison group:* Within-subjects comparison	2 × 2 repeated-measures ANOVA Cue (smoking, neutral) Smoking (satiated, abstinent)	*Experimental group:* Overnight abstinent Mean CO not reported *Comparison group:* None	Pictorial cues Photos Smoking-related Neutral	Self-reported nicotine dependence & smoking quantity	fMRI BOLD
Nicotine and/or tobacco effects						
Brody et al. (2004) USA[43]	*Experimental group:* 10 smokers randomized to smoke prescan Mean 30 cig/day 80% male Mean age 37 years *Comparison group:* 10 smokers randomized to not smoke prescan Mean 24 cig/day 70% male Mean age 35 years	2 × 2 repeated-measures ANOVA Drug (cigarette, no cigarette) Smoking status (smoker, non-smoker)	*Experimental group:* Smoking group Mean CO 13.4 ppm *Comparison group:* Non-smoking group Mean CO 12.4 ppm	No behavioral task	Self-reported craving, smoking urges, anxiety, depressed mood, smoking quantity	[^{11}C]raclopride PET (D2 receptor BP)

Bloom et al. (1999) USA[44]	*Experimental group:* 10 smokers Mean cig/day and %male not described Mean age 26 years *Comparison group:* Within-subjects comparison	1-way ANOVA Nicotine (nicotine, saline)	*Experimental group:* i.v. saline vs. 1.5 mg nicotine Mean CO not reported	Nicotine No behavioral task	Self-reported or observed behavioral measures not reported	fMRI Wave Action Protocol (proportion of active voxels)
Ernst et al. (2001) USA[57]	*Experimental group:* 11 smokers Mean 33.9 cig/day 45% male Mean age 32 years *Comparison group:* 11 ex-smokers Mean 3.2 cig/day (prior to quitting) 55% male Mean age 30 years	$2 \times 2 \times 2$ repeated-measures ANOVA Smoking status (smokers, ex-smokers) Drug (nicotine gum, placebo gum) Task (2-back, control)	*Experimental group:* 12 h abstinence Nicotine gum (2 pieces of 2 mg gum) and placebo gum on separate sessions CO not reported *Comparison group:* Nicotine gum (2 pieces of 2 mg gum) and placebo gum on separate sessions CO not reported	Nicotine N-back test Keypress	Self-reported nicotine dependence, withdrawal and anxiety, smoking quantity Error rate Reaction times	$H_2^{15}O$ PET (regional cerebral blood flow)
Geissing et al. (2007) Germany[50]	*Experimental group:* 15 non-smokers 80% male Mean age 27 years *Comparison group:* Within-subjects comparison	2×2 repeated-measures ANOVA Drug (nicotine gum, placebo gum) Cued target (valid cue, invalid cue)	*Experimental group:* Nicotine gum 2 mg Mean CO not reported No nicotine *Comparison group:* Placebo gum Mean CO not reported	NicotineCued target detection task Keypress	No self-reported behavioral measures Error rate Reaction times	fMRI BOLD
Jacobsen et al. (2002) USA[45]	*Experimental group:* 9 smokers Mean 25 cig/day 44% male Mean age 29 years *Comparison group:* None	Impact of nicotine infusion on signal change in occipital cortex Task: none	*Experimental group:* Overnight abstinence Mean CO <10 ppm 2× saline infusion 3× nicotine infusion *Comparison group:* n/a	Nicotine Photic stimulation: black and white checked pattern Flashing at 8 Hz for 30 s alternating with rest	Self-reported craving, withdrawal, smoking urges, smoking quantity	fMRI BOLD

(continued)

Table 9.2 (continued)

Study	Subjects	Design	Experimental conditions	Paradigm	Measures	Modality
Jacobsen et al. (2004) USA[58]	*Experimental group:* 13 smokers with schizophrenia Mean 26 cig/day 85% male Mean age 43 years *Comparison group:* 13 smokers without schizophrenia Mean 28 cig/day 69% male Mean age 42 years Scanned twice: after placement nicotine	2×2×2×2 repeated-measures ANOVA Schizophrenia (schizophrenic, nonschizophrenic) Working memory (high load, low load) Attention (high load, low load) Drug (nicotine, placebo)	*Experimental group:* Counterbalanced sessions for nicotine patch (weight-based dose: 28 mg or 35 mg) 2 levels working memory (*1*-back, 2-back) 2 levels selective attention load (binaural & dichotic stimuli) Mean CO not reported but plasma nicotine levels reported *Comparison group:* Same paradigm	Nicotine Auditory *N*-back Keypress	Self-reported nicotine dependence, withdrawal, craving, depression, schizophrenic symptoms (schizophrenics only), smoking quantity Response accuracy Reaction times	fMRI functional connectivity
Kumari et al. (2003) UK[46]	*Experimental group:* 11 never-smokers "Never" not defined 100% male Mean age not stated *Comparison group:* None	2×2×4 mixed-design ANOVA Drug (nicotine, placebo) Order (1st, 2nd) Load (*0, 1, 2, 3*-back) Separate analyses for accuracy and latency	*Experimental group:* 1× saline infusion 1× nicotine (12 μg/kg body weight) infusion Double-blind crossover 2 weeks apart *Comparison group:* n/a	Nicotine Parametric *N*-back working memory task Keypress	Accuracy (% correct) Latency (ms)	fMRI BOLD
Lawrence et al. (2002) USA[51]	*Experimental group:* 15 smokers Mean 22 cig/day 47% male Mean age 22 years *Comparison group:* 14 non-smokers "Non" not defined 50% male Mean age 22 years	2×2 repeated-measures ANOVA Drug (nicotine, placebo) Task (RVIP, control) Group (smoker, non) Task (RVIP, control)	*Experimental group:* 1× 21 mg nicotine patch 1× placebo patch Single-blind crossover Separation not stated *Comparison group:* No nicotine	Nicotine Rapid visual information processing task Keypress	Self-reported mood scale, smoking quantity Number of targets detected Latency to target stimuli (ms)	fMRI BOLD
Stein et al. (1998) USA[47]	*Experimental group:* 16 smokers Mean cig/day not reported 56% male Mean age 26 years *Comparison group:* None	Dose–response effect on regional brain activity Task: None	*Experimental group:* 3× nicotine infusion Mean CO not reported *Comparison group:* n/a	Nicotine No behavioral task	Likert scale self-reported feelings	fMRI rCBF

						[^{11}C]raclopride PET (D2 receptor BP)
Takahashi et al. (2008) Japan[49]	*Experimental group:* 12 smokers Mean cig/day not reported 100% male Mean age 26 years *Comparison group:* 6 non-smokers Mean age 24 years	2 × 2 repeated-measures ANOVA Drug (nicotine, placebo) Session (1st, 2nd)	*Experimental group:* 24 h abstinence prescan Mean CO not reported *Comparison group:* 2 mg gum or placebo on in 2 sessions, respectively Mean CO not reported Participants randomized to receive either nicotine or placebo gum first	Nicotine No behavioral task	Self-reported nicotine dependence, craving, smoking quantity	
Thiel et al. (2005) Germany[54]	*Experimental group:* 15 non-smokers Mean cig/day not reported 42% male Mean age 24 years *Comparison group:* Within-subjects comparison	3 × 2 mixed-design ANOVA Drug (nicotine 1 mg gum, nicotine 2 mg gum, placebo gum) Cue (alerting contrast: neutral –no cue, reorienting contrast: invalid – valid cue)	*Experimental group:* Nicotine 1 mg gum *Comparison groups:* Nicotine 2 mg gum Placebo gum Mean CO not reported Counterbalanced design applied with participants scanned on 3 sessions receiving placebo, 1 mg, 2 mg gum	Visual cued-target attention task Keypress	Reaction times for each task Subjective drug effects Reaction times	fMRI BOLD
Thiel et al. (2007a) Germany[52]	*Experimental group:* 16 smokers Mean cig/day not reported 69% male Mean age 28 years *Comparison group:* Within-subjects comparison	3 × 2 × 2 repeated-measures ANOVA Cue (no cue, visual cue, auditory cue) Target stimuli (visual target, auditory target) Drug (nicotine 2 mg gum, placebo gum)	*Experimental group:* Mean CO not reported Nicotine 2 mg gum *Comparison groups:* Placebo gum Counterbalanced design applied with participants scanned on 2 sessions receiving placebo, 2 mg gum	Visual & auditory cued-target attention task Keypress	Self-reported alertness, contentedness, calmness Reaction times	fMRI BOLD
Thiel et al. (2008) Germany[53]	*Experimental group:* 15 smokers Mean cig/day not reported 80% male Mean age 27 years *Comparison group:* Within-subjects comparison	2 × 2 × 2 repeated-measures ANOVA Cue validity (valid, invalid) Cue magnitude (long, short) Side/hemifield (left, right) Drug (nicotine, placebo)	*Experimental group:* Nicotine 2 mg gum *Comparison groups:* Placebo gum Counterbalanced design applied with participants scanned on 2 sessions receiving placebo, 2 mg gum Mean CO not reported for any participants	Modified visual cued-target detection task Keypress	Cue validity Reaction times	fMRI BOLD

(continued)

Table 9.2 (continued)

Study	Subjects	Design	Experimental conditions	Paradigm	Measures	Modality
Tregellas et al. (2005) USA[54]	*Experimental group:* 5 smokers and 4 non-smokers with schizophrenia. Mean cig/day not reported. 78% male. Mean age 34 years. *Comparison group:* Within-subjects comparison	2×2 repeated-measures ANOVA Drug (nicotine gum, placebo) Task (pursuit task, control)	*Experimental group:* Smokers. Nicotine 6 mg gum or placebo gum. *Comparison group:* Nicotine 4 mg gum or placebo gum. Smokers and non-smokers were not compared statistically	Smooth pursuit eye movement task	Pursuit task performance	fMRI BOLD
Vossel et al. (2008) Germany[56]	*Experimental group:* (nicotine group) 12 non-smokers. Mean age 24 years. 58% male. *Comparison group:* (placebo group) 12 non-smokers. Mean age 26 years. 50% male	2×2×2 mixed ANOVA with the Within-subject factors cueing (valid, invalid) Cue validity (90; 60%) Between-subject factor drug (placebo; nicotine)	*Experimental group:* Nicotine 2 mg gum. *Comparison group:* Placebo gum. Randomized controlled trial	Location-cueing task	Self-reported drug effects: alertness, contentedness, calmness	fMRI BOLD
Abstinence effects						
Cohen et al. (2004) USA[61]	*Experimental group:* 6 smokers. Mean cig/day, gender mix, and age not reported. *Comparison group:* Within-subjects comparison	2×2 repeated-measures ANOVA Drug (nicotine, placebo) Task (2-Back, control)	*Experimental group:* Nicotine (2 cigarettes). *Comparison group:* None, 12 h abstinence	N-back	No self-reported behavioral data described	fMRI BOLD
David et al. (2007) UK[26]	*Experimental group:* 8 smokers. Mean 18 cig/day. 0% male. Mean age 55 years. *Comparison group:* Within-subjects comparison	2×2×4 repeated-measures ANOVA Cue (smoking, neutral) Smoking (satiated, abstinent) Session (1st or 2nd satiated, 1st or 2nd abstinent)	*Experimental group:* Ad libitum smoking. Mean CO 14.6 ppm. *Comparison group:* Overnight abstinence prescan. Mean CO 4.6 ppm	Pictorial cues Photos Smoking-related Neutral Gender discrimination task Key press	Self-reported craving & withdrawal Reaction times	fMRI BOLD

Study	Sample	Design	Group	Task	Measures	Imaging
Domino et al. (2000) USA[71]	*Experimental group:* 11 smokers, Mean 23 cig/day, 100% male, Mean age 34 years. *Comparison group:* Within-subjects comparison	2×2 repeated-measures ANOVA, Drug (nicotine, placebo), Hemisphere (right, left)	*Experimental group:* Nicotine nasal spray, Mean CO pre/post 7.2/5.4 ppm. *Comparison group:* Oleoresin of pepper placebo nasal spray, Mean CO pre/post 7.5/5.9 ppm	Nicotine nasal spray, No behavioral task	No self-reported or observed behavioral measures	FDG PET (regional glucose metabolism)
Jacobsen et al. (2006a) USA[63]	*Experimental group:* 35 smokers with prenatal nicotine exposure, Mean 14 cig/day, 17% male, Mean age 17 years. *Comparison group:* 26 smokers without prenatal nicotine exposure, Mean 9 cig/day, 42% male, Mean age 17 years	2×2×2×2 repeated-measures ANOVA, Prenatal exposure (yes, no), Drug (satiated, abstinent), Verbal working memory load (high, low), Nonverbal working memory load (high, low)	*Experimental group:* 24 h abstinence pre-scan or ad libitum smoking in counterbalanced sessions. *Comparison group:* Same	Visuospatial encoding & recognition task, Keypress	Cognitive & memory testing, Self-reported nicotine dependence, withdrawal, craving, depression, anxiety, ADHD symptoms, smoking quantity, Accuracy, Reaction times	fMRI BOLD
[a]Jacobsen et al. (2006b) USA[13]	*Experimental group:* 15 smokers with *DRD2* 957T/T or T/C genotypes, Mean 27 cig/day, 67% male, Mean age 37 years. *Comparison group:* 21 smokers with DRD2 957 C/C genotypes, Mean 24 cig/day, 57% male	2×2×2×2 repeated-measures ANOVA *DRD2* genotype (957 T/T or T/C, CC), Working memory (high load, low load), Attention (high load, low load), Drug (nicotine, placebo)	*Experimental group:* Nicotine patch (weight-based dose: 28 mg or 35 mg) or 15 h abstinence prescan in counterbalanced sessions, 2 levels working memory (1-back, 2-back), 2 levels selective attention load (binaural & dichotic stimuli), Mean CO not reported but plasma nicotine levels reported. *Comparison group:* Same paradigm	N-back, Keypress	Cognitive testingSelf-reported nicotine dependence, mood, withdrawal, craving, smoking quantity, Accuracy, Reaction times	fMRI BOLD

(continued)

Table 9.2 (continued)

Study	Subjects	Design	Experimental conditions	Paradigm	Measures	Modality
Jacobsen et al. (2007b) USA[41]	*Experimental group:* 20 tobacco and cannabis smokers. Mean 13 cig/day. 25% male. Mean age 17 years. *Comparison group:* 25 tobacco smokers with minimal cannabis smokers. Mean 17 cig/day. 28% male. Mean age 17 years	2 × 2 × 2 repeated-measures ANOVA. Cannabis use status (cannabis user, non-cannabis user). Drug (satiated, abstinent). Verbal working memory load (high, low)	24 h abstinence prescan & ad libitum smoking in counterbalanced sessions. *Experimental group:* Mean CO not reported. *Comparison group:* Mean CO not reported	Verbal working memory task	Verbal learning & memory, IQ, self-reported nicotine dependence, withdrawal, craving, depression, anxiety, PTSD symptoms	fMRI BOLD and functional connectivity
Lim et al. (2005) South Korea[29]	*Experimental group:* 1 smoker. 50 cig/day. Male. Age 56 years. *Comparison group:* 1 non-smoker. Male. Age 55 years	Case series. Within subjects comparison of Cue (smoking, neutral) and Smoking (satiated, abstinent)	*Experimental group:* 24 h abstinence prescan, Smoking, and sham smoking scanning sessions. Mean CO not reported for either participant. *Comparison group:* Smoking, and sham smoking	Pictorial cues Photos Smoking-related Neutral	None	fMRI BOLD
Mamede et al. (2007) Japan[72]	*Experimental group:* 10 smokers. Mean 16 cig/day. 100% male. Mean age 28 years. *Comparison group:* 6 non-smokers. 100% male. Mean age 23 years	2 × 3 × 8 repeated-measures ANOVA. Smoking status (smoker, non-smoker). Cessation duration (4 h, 10 days, 21 days). Brain region (frontal, parietal, temporal, occipital, basal ganglia, thalamus, brain stem, cerebellum)	*Experimental group:* Smokers who had abstained for 4 h, 10 days, or 21 days prescan. Mean CO not reported. No intervention other than radiotracer infusion. *Comparison group:* No intervention other than radiotracer infusion	No behavioral task	No self-reported or observed behavioral measures	5IA SPECT (temporal change in nicotinic acetylcholine receptor BP)
McClernon et al. (2005) USA[31]	*Experimental group:* 13 smokers. Mean 25 cig/day. 38% male. Mean age 30 years. *Comparison group:* Within-subjects comparison	2 × 2 × 4 repeated-measures ANOVA. Cue (smoking, neutral). Smoking (satiated, abstinent). Time (4, 6, 8, 10 s)	*Experimental group:* Ad libitum smoking. Mean CO 26.5 ppm. *Comparison group:* 10 h abstinence prescan. Mean CO 9.4 ppm	Pictorial cues Photos Smoking-related Neutral Target (animals) Keypress	Self-reported craving & mood	fMRI BOLD

McClernon et al. (2007a) USA[32]	*Experimental group:* 16 smokers Mean 23 cig/day 13% male Mean age 39 years *Comparison group:* Within-subjects comparison	$2 \times 3 \times 12$ repeated-measures ANOVA Cue (smoking, neutral, target) Smoking (baseline, nicotine patch + reduced-nicotine cigarettes, smoking cessation) Region (ventral & dorsal anterior cingulate gyrus, inferior frontal gyrus, middle frontal gyrus, superior frontal gyrus, amygdala, hippocampus, caudate, putamen, thalamus, ventral striatum, insula)	*Experimental group:* Three scanning sessions: Session 1: baseline following ad libitum smoking, mean CO 22.3 ppm Session 2: following 2 reduced nicotine cigarettes + nicotine 21 mg patch, mean CO 15.1 ppm Session 3: following 2–4 weeks of smoking cessation *Comparison group:* None	Pictorial cues Photos Smoking-related Neutral Target Keypress	Self-reported nicotine dependence, craving, withdrawal, mood, smoking quantity	fMRI BOLD
[a]McClernon et al. (2007b) USA[14]	DRD4 exon III genotype short (S)/long (L) alleles *Experimental group:* 7 smokers L/L or L/S genotypes Mean 23 cig/day 14% male Mean age 36 years *Comparison group:* 8 smokers with DRD4 gene S/S genotype Mean 23 cig/day 12% male Mean age 43 years	2×2 repeated-measures ANOVA Cue (smoking, neutral) Genotype (L/L or L/S, S/S)	*Experimental group:* Mean CO 18.0 ppm *Comparison group:* Mean CO 21.4 ppm Both genotype groups underwent same stimulus paradigm	Pictorial cues Photos Smoking-related Neutral Target Keypress	Self-reported nicotine dependence, craving, withdrawal, affect, appetite, arousal, arousal, somatic symptoms, smoking quantity	fMRI BOLD
McClernon et al. (2008) USA[33]	*Experimental group:* 30 smokers, subgroup of previously reported data from McClernon et al. (2005 "study 1"; 2007a "study 2") Pooled data: Mean 24 cig/day 23% male Mean age 36 years *Comparison group:* Within-subjects comparison	$2 \times 3 \times 12$ repeated-measures ANOVA Cue (smoking, neutral, target) Smoking (baseline, nicotine patch + reduced-nicotine cigarettes, smoking cessation) Sex (male, female) Region (ventral & dorsal anterior cingulate gyrus, inferior frontal gyrus, middle frontal gyrus, superior frontal gyrus, amygdala, hippocampus, caudate, putamen, thalamus, ventral striatum, insula) Post-hoc analyses Multiple regression with 4 covariates (nicotine dependence, craving, negative affect, sex)	See experimental conditions for studies 1 and 2 above Pooled prescan Mean CO 22.3 ppm	Pictorial cues Photos Smoking-related Neutral Target Keypress	Self-reported nicotine dependence, craving, withdrawal, affect, arousal, & smoking quantity	fMRI BOLD

(continued)

Table 9.2 (continued)

Study	Subjects		Design	Experimental conditions	Paradigm	Measures	Modality
McClernon et al. (2009) USA[37]	*Experimental group:* 18 smokers Mean 18 cig/day 39% male Mean age 29 years	*Comparison group:* Within-subjects comparison	2×2 repeated-measures ANOVA Cue (smoking, neutral) Smoking (satiated, abstinent)	*Experimental group:* Ad libitum smoking Mean CO not reported No nicotine *Comparison group:* 24 h abstinence prescan Mean CO not reported	Nicotine Pictorial cues Photos Smoking-related Neutral	Self-reported craving & withdrawal	fMRI BOLD
Montgomery et al. (2007) UK[73]	*Experimental group:* 10 smokers Mean 11 cig/day 70% male Mean age 30 years	*Comparison group:* Within-subjects comparison	2×2×3 repeated-measures ANOVA Drug (nicotine, no nicotine)	*Experimental group:* 12 h abstinence prescan Nicotine nasal spray 2 mg 50 min into scan *Comparison group:* Nicotine administration first 50 min of scan	Nicotine No behavioral task	Self-reported nicotine dependence, visual analog ratings of affect, hedonic, and physiological symptoms	[11C]raclopride PET (D2 receptor BP)
Mulligan et al. (2009) USA	*Experimental group:* 18 smokers Mean 17 cig/day 44% male Mean age 39 years	*Comparison group:* Within-subjects comparison	One way ANOVA Smoking (satiated, abstinent) Post-hoc Correlation of BOLD signal with number of reported early life stress (ELS) events	*Experimental group:* Overnight (15 hr) abstinence prescan. Two counterbalanced sessions. Nicotine patch Administration in one session. Placebo patch administration in the other session Mean CO not reported *Comparison group:* None	Go/No-Go task	Self-reported craving, smoking quantity, dependence, number of ELS events Accuracy	fMRI BOLD
Rose et al. (2007) USA[59]	*Experimental group:* 15 smokers Mean 23 cig/day 40% male Mean age 37 years	*Comparison group:* Within-subjects comparison	3×2×13 repeated-measures ANOVA Drug (baseline, 2 weeks nicotine patch+denicotinized cigarettes, 2 weeks after return to usual cigarettes) Hemisphere (right, left) Region (anterior cingulate cortex, prefrontal cortex, orbitofrontal cortex, temporal cortex, amygdala, thalamus, caudate, putamen, midbrain, superior & inferior colliculi, ventral striatum, pons) Post-hoc correlational analyses with behavioral & performance measures	*Experimental group:* Overnight abstinence prescan Session 1: baseline Session 2: following 2 weeks nicotine 21 mg patch+denicotinized cigarettes Session 3: following 2 weeks of returning to usual smoking Mean CO 12 ppm sessions 1 & 2; & 9 ppm session 3	Nicotine Continuous performance task Keypress	Self-reported nicotine dependence, withdrawal, craving, anxiety, somatic symptoms, dysphoria, stimulation, appetite, hedonic & physiological effects of smoking, smoking quantity Accuracy	[18F]-FDG PET (regional glucose metabolism)

Scott et al. (2007) USA[74]	*Experimental group:* 6 smokers Mean 17 cig/day 100% male Mean age 25 years *Comparison group:* Within-subjects comparison	3× ANOVA Within-subjects variable Drug (abstinent, low nicotine , high nicotine) Brain region Between-subject variables (D2 & μ-opioid receptor BPs)	*Experimental group:* Overnight abstinent prescan, smoked 2 denicotinized cigarettes, followed by 2 regular cigarettes 45 min later Mean CO not reported	Nicotine No behavioral task	Self-reported nicotine dependence, craving, affect ("relaxed", "nervous", "alert"), smoking quantity Plasma nicotine at each session	[¹¹C]carfentanil & [¹¹C] raclopride PET (μ-opioid & D2 receptor BPs)
Staley et al. (2006) USA[75]	*Experimental group:* 16 smokers Mean 20 cig/day 50% male Mean age 37 years *Comparison group:* 16 non-smokers 50% male Mean age 35 years	MANOVA Within-subjects (nicotine) Between-subjects (smoking status)	*Experimental group:* Mean 7 days prescan abstinence Mean CO 3.5 ppm *Comparison group:* Mean CO 1.0 ppm	No behavioral task	Self-reported nicotine dependence, withdrawal, smoking urges, smoking quantity, days to last cigarette	[¹²³I]5-IA SPECT
Stapleton et al. (2003) USA[76]	*Experimental group:* 6 smokers Mean cig/day not reported 100% male Mean age not reported *Comparison group:* Within-subjects comparison	2×2×2×30 repeated-measures ANOVA Drug (nicotine, placebo) Time (preinjection, postinjection) Hemisphere (right, left) Region (30 regions)	*Experimental group:* 1×1 mg nicotine infusion *Comparison group:* 1× saline infusion All participants overnight prescan abstinent, randomized to receive nicotine or placebo in counterbalanced sessions	Nicotine No behavioral task	Self-reported mood, fatigue & vigor, drug "feelings"	[¹⁸F]-FDG PET (regional glucose metabolism)
Tanabe et al. (2006) Japan[77]	*Experimental group:* 16 schizophrenics 50% smokers 75% male Mean age 38 years *Comparison group:* 16 controls 38% smokers 50% male Mean age 33 years Mean cig/day not reported for smokers.	2×2×4 repeated-measures ANOVA Drug (nicotine, placebo) Smooth pursuit eye movement (active, rest) Region (hippocampus, cingulate cortex, frontal eye fields, area MT)	*Experimental group:* Smokers 6 h prescan abstinence Nicotine 6 mg gum, placebo gum in counterbalanced sessions Mean CO not reported *Comparison group:* Non-smokers Nicotine 4 mg gum and placebo gum same protocol	Nicotine Smooth pursuit eye movement task	Self-reported nicotine dependence, positive & negative affect	fMRI BOLD

(continued)

Table 9.2 (continued)

Study	Subjects	Design	Experimental conditions	Paradigm	Measures	Modality
Tanabe et al. (2008) Japan[78]	*Experimental group:* 12 smokers Mean cig/day not reported 42% male Mean age 28 years *Comparison group:* Within-subjects comparison	2 × 3 repeated-measures ANOVA Drug (nicotine, placebo) Region (ventral striatum, thalamus, medial frontal cortex) Post-hoc correlational analyses with behavioral measures	*Experimental group:* Nicotine 6 mg gum Mean CO 23.0 ppm *Comparison group:* 16 h abstinence prescan Mean CO 6.3 ppm	Nicotine No behavioral task	Self-reported nicotine dependence, craving, withdrawal, & smoking quantity	MR dynamic susceptibility contrast (regional cerebral blood flow)
Wang et al. (2007) USA[38]	*Experimental group:* 14 smokers Mean 17 cig/day 43% male Mean age 39 years *Comparison group:* Within-subjects comparison	Repeated-measures ANOVA Smoking (satiety, abstinence) Cue (smoking, neutral) Post-hoc correlations of global & regional perfusion with craving	*Experimental group:* Smoking *Comparison group:* 12 h abstinence prescan Counterbalanced sessions	No behavioral task	Self-reported nicotine dependence, craving, smoking urges, smoking quantity	fMRI ASL (regional cerebral perfusion)
[a]Wang et al. (2008) USA[15]	*Experimental group:* 13 smokers Mean 17 cig/day 46% male Mean age 38 years *Comparison group:* Within-subjects comparison	2 × 2 × 2 repeated-measures ANOVA Smoking (satiated, abstinent) Genotype (wildtype allele, minor allele)	*Experimental group:* 24 h abstinence, then ad libitum smoking morning of scan Mean CO Not reported No nicotine *Comparison group:* 24 h prescan abstinence only Mean CO Not reported	Pictorial cues Photos Smoking-related Neutral	Genotype: *DRD2, COMT, OPRM* variants	fMRI ASL (regional cerebral perfusion)
Xu et al. (2005) USA[60]	*Experimental group:* 8 smokers Mean 19 cig/day 63% male Mean age 35 years *Comparison group:* Within-subjects comparison	2 × 2 repeated-measures ANOVA Task load (high, low) Smoking (abstinence, near-satiety)	*Experimental group:* ≤1.5 h abstinence Mean CO 22.5 ppm *Comparison group:* ≥14 h abstinence Mean CO 3.3 ppm	N-back	Self-reported nicotine dependence, craving, & withdrawal symptoms Key press Error rates Reaction times	fMRI BOLD

Xu et al. (2006) USA[62]	*Experimental group:* 6 smokers Mean cig/day not reported 50% male Mean age not reported *Comparison group:* Within-subjects comparison	2 × 2 repeated-measures ANOVA Task load (high, low) Smoking (abstinence, satiety)	*Experimental group:* Ad libitum smoking prior to scan Mean CO not reported *Comparison group:* ~13 h abstinence Mean CO not reported	*N*-back	Self-reported nicotine dependence, craving, & withdrawal symptoms Key press Error rates Reaction times	fMRI BOLD
Zubieta et al. (2005) USA[79]	*Experimental group:* 19 smokers Mean 16 cig/day 42% male Mean age 27 years *Comparison group:* Within-subjects comparison	MANOVA Smoking (low-nicotine cigarette, average nicotine cigarette) Session Region	*Experimental group:* 12 h abstinence prescan 6 scans counterbalanced Scan 1: baseline Scan 2: after 1st cigarette (nicotine-containing) Scan 3: baseline Scan 4: after 2nd cigarette (nicotine-containing) Scan 5: baseline Scan 6: after 3rd cigarette (denicotinized)	No behavioral tasks	Self-reported nicotine dependence, craving, somatic symptoms Pharmacokinetic & cardiovascular data	[^{15}O]H$_2$O PET (regional cerebral blood flow)
Task-free approaches						
Brody et al. (2004) USA[65]	*Experimental group:* 19 smokers Mean 26.2 cig/day 58% male Mean age 40 years *Comparison group:* 17 non-smokers 59% male Mean age 38 years	2 × 2 × 6 MANCOVA Smoking status (smoker, non-smoker) Hemisphere: (right, left) Brain region (dorsolateral prefrontal cortex, ventrolateral prefrontal cortex, dorsal anterior cingulate cortex ventral anterior cingulate cortex, thalamus)	*Experimental group:* Mean CO 18.3 ppm *Comparison group:* Mean CO 1.9 ppm	Task free	Self-reported nicotine dependence, depression, anxiety, smoking quantity	Structural MRI (gray matter volume)
Gallinat et al. (2006) Germany[66]	*Experimental group:* 22 smokers Mean 15 cig/day 55% male Mean age 30 years *Comparison group:* 23 never-smokers Mean age 31 years 52% male	2 × 2 MANCOVA Smoking status (smoker, never-smoker) Hemisphere: (right, left)	*Experimental group:* Mean CO not reported *Comparison group:* Mean CO not reported	Task free	Self-reported nicotine dependence & smoking quantity	Structural MRI (voxel-based morphometry)

(continued)

Table 9.2 (continued)

Study	Subjects	Design	Experimental conditions	Paradigm	Measures	Modality
Gallinat et al. (2007a) Germany[69]	*Experimental group:* 13 smokers Mean 15 cig/day 46% male Mean age 36 years *Comparison group:* 13 non-smokers 46% male Mean age 36 years	2 × 2 ANOVA Smoking status (smoker, non-smoker) Region (hippocampus, anterior cingulate cortex)	*Experimental group:* Mean CO not reported *Comparison group:* Mean CO not reported	Task free	Self-reported nicotine dependence & smoking quantity	Magnetic resonance spectroscopy (*N*-acety-laspartate, choline, creatine)
Gallinat et al. (2007b) Germany[70]	*Experimental group:* 13 smokers Mean 17 cig/day 38% male Mean age 35 years *Comparison groups:* 9 ex-smokers 56% male Mean age 42 years 16 never-smokers 50% male Mean age 33 years	2 × 2 ANOVA Smoking status (smokers, ex-smokers, never-smokers) Region (hippocampus, anterior cingulate cortex)	*Experimental group:* Mean CO not reported *Comparison groups:* Mean CO not reported	Task free	Self-reported nicotine dependence & smoking quantity	Magnetic resonance spectroscopy (glutamate)
Jacobsen et al. (2007c) USA[67]	*Experimental group:* 25 smokers with prenatal nicotine exposure Mean 16 cig/day 28% male Mean age 16 years 14 smokers without prenatal nicotine exposure Mean 14 cig/day 50% male Mean age 17 years *Comparison group:* 8 non-smokers with prenatal nicotine exposure	Mixed-model repeated-measures ANOVA Smoking status (smoker, non-smoker) Prenatal nicotine exposure (exposed, nonexposed) Region	*Experimental group:* Mean CO not reported *Comparison groups:* Mean CO not reported	Task free	Self-reported nicotine dependence, depression, cognitive testing, PTSD symptoms, smoking quantity	fMRI DTI (FA) Structural MRI (white matter volumetry)

50% male Mean age 16 years 20 non-smokers without prenatal nicotine exposure 40% male Mean age 16 years					fMRI DTI (FA, trace) Structural MRI (white matter volumetry)
Paul et al. (2008) USA[68] *Experimental group:* 10 smokers 60% male Mean age 39 years Mean cig/day not reported *Comparison group:* 10 non-smokers 40% male Mean age 39 years Post-hoc analysis: High vs. low nicotine dependence	2×3 MANOVA Separate models for FA, trace, & volumetry Smoking status (smoker, non-smoker) or nicotine dependence (high, low) Brain region (corpus collosum: body, genu, splenium)	*Experimental group:* Mean CO not reported *Comparison group:* Mean CO not reported	Task free	Self-reported nicotine dependence, depression, smoking quantity, stress	
Tregellas et al. (2007) USA[64] *Experimental group:* 32 schizophrenics (14 smokers, 18 non-smokers) Mean cig/day not reported 66% male Mean age 40 years *Comparison group:* 32 healthy controls (2 smokers, 30 non-smokers) 44% male Mean age 35 years	ANCOVA Regional gray matter volume Smoking status covariate	*Experimental group:* Mean CO not reported *Comparison group:* Mean CO not reported	Task free	No behavioral measures reported	Structural MRI (gray matter volume)

[a]Imaging genomic studies are not listed separately because genetic studies of neuroimaging phenotypes span most experimental approaches and functional neuroimaging modalities

[b]"DAT" refers to dopamine transporter gene. Radioligand abbreviations and acronyms defined in Table 9.1

as faces,[19] or a range of scenes intended to provoke specific emotional response (i.e., International Affective Picture Series, IAPS) to assess interpretation of the emotional valence of the cues and the emotional and behavioral response of the participants. Working memory tasks, such as the *N*-back discussed below, are useful in examining abstinence-induced or nicotine-induced effects on behavioral performance and neural activation. Indeed, as the behavioral phenomenon of tobacco craving is complex and encompasses interdependent hedonic, affective, and cognitive processes, smoking-related cues, emotional cues, and cognitive/working memory tasks can be used in concert to better understand the neural pathways involved in nicotine dependence.

Cue reactivity paradigms: Smoking-related cues exposure paradigms have been widely studied using fMRI and PET, with and without examination of abstinence effects, or nicotine effects in non-abstinent smokers. Visual, olfactory, and other sensory cues associated with smoking reliably evoke cigarette craving and are associated with smoking cessation relapse – a process known as "cue reactivity".[20–23] The introduction of functional neuroimaging approaches to cue reactivity research has made it possible to better elucidate the neurocircuitry of nicotine and tobacco reward and correlate behavioral measures with brain structure and function by providing a more direct window into neural activity than what was previously possible with electromyelographic and electroencephalographic methods and cognitive testing – which is also the case for examination of affective, attention, and working memory studies of nicotine dependence.

A germinal cue reactivity fMRI study by Due and colleagues, of 12 smokers and 6 never-smokers, examined the effect of smoking-related pictorial cues on fMRI BOLD signal activation in reward and visual spatial pathways.[24] Smokers who were abstinent overnight were exposed to a pseudorandom, event-related sequence of smoking images, neutral nonsmoking images, and rare target images. In smokers, the fMRI signal was greater after exposure to smoking-related images than after exposure to neutral images in seven regions of interest (ROI) right posterior amygdala, posterior hippocampus, ventral tegmental area, and medial thalamus (mesolimbic reward circuit), as well as in bilateral prefrontal and parietal cortex and right fusiform gyrus (visual spatial attention centers). The authors concluded that mesolimbic and extrastriate visual brain regions work in concert to process reward signaling to visual smoking-related stimuli that are more salient to smokers than nonsmoking related stimuli. No significant activation was seen in non-smokers. Within the ROI studied, there was greater activation following target images than neutral images in smokers. Subsequent to the study by Due and colleagues, there have been at least 17 additional smoking cue reactivity published fMRI studies[12,14,15,24–37] – of which, eight studies have examined abstinence effects[14,26,29,31–33,37,38] (Sect. 4.3).

FMRI studies using similar paradigms to and images from the International Smoking Image Series[39] have generated robust results for activation reward pathway brain regions (particularly the ventral striatum and orbitofrontal cortex),[27] visuospatial attention, and visuospatial and/or extrastriate/ventral visual processing regions (anterior cingulate gyrus, cuneus, fusiform gyrus, inferior temporal gyrus, parietal, & parahippocampal gyrus).[24,27,31] Many of the ROIs demonstrating activation in fMRI studies of smoking cues have been correlated with severity of tobacco craving or severity of nicotine dependence.[24,26,31,35] In general, non-smokers (often including ex-smokers and/or never-smokers) demonstrate either no significant activation with smoking cue exposure (vs. neutral cues) or significantly less activation when compared to smokers.[24,27]

A recent study conducted in our lab by Sweet and colleagues involved 15 dependent smokers using a smoking cue exposure paradigm.[36] Consistent with our pilot work, smoking cues elicited increased activity (t > ±4.63, $p < .05$, corrected) in visual cortices and left inferior frontal gyrus (IFG), and deactivation in the bilateral cuneus. Replication of the findings of other groups observing ventral striatum (inclusive of nucleus accumbens/NA) activation in association with smoking-related cue exposure was suggested in the present study. The left NA exhibited significantly (t = 2.336, $p = .035$) greater activity and the left insula tended to exhibit less activity (t = −2.029, $p = .062$) during the smoking cues. Activity in the left NA ($r = .572$, $p = .026$) and left insula exhibited relationships with cigarettes/day ($r = .611$, $p = .016$). There was a trend for this in the right insula ($r = .495$, $p = .060$). The left NA also exhibited a positive relationship with FTND ($r = .550$, $p = .034$). Figure 9.1 below illustrates the activation pattern observed in these smokers associated with smoking cue presentation. These data suggest, consistent with other cue reactivity findings by our group, a lateralization of neural activation such that in right-handed smokers, and correlation between indicants of nicotine dependence or craving severity and NA activation.[12,26–28,31]

Cognitive/working memory/affective processing paradigms: It is well established that nicotine withdrawal is associated with cognitive impairment, both in terms of working memory and attention deficits. Thus, working memory tasks such as the *N*-back and attention tasks provide a means for correlating abstinence-induced or nicotine-induced effects on cognitive function, and most studies employing these paradigms utilize abstinence-satiation or baseline-nicotine delivery repeated-measures designs (Sects. 4.2 and 4.3). However, there may only be two published studies have utilized working memory and attention paradigms without the additional pharmacodynamic evaluation of abstinence or nicotine administration.[40,41]

For example, in an fMRI study, Jacobsen and colleagues compared 33 adolescent smokers and non-smokers with history of prenatal nicotine exposure to 30 adolescent smokers and non-smoker without history of prenatal nicotine exposure utilizing auditory and visual selective and divided attention tasks.[42] Combined prenatal and adolescent nicotine exposure was associated with reductions in visual and auditory attention in females that were greatest in female smokers with prenatal exposure (combined exposure) relative to female smokers and non-smokers without prenatal exposure, but in males, there were marked deficits in auditory attention which suggested a greater vulnerability to neurological insult during development with combined exposure. Brain regions activated in association with simple vs. selective attention tasks included Brodman Areas (BA) 41/42 (anterior & posterior transverse temporal lobe area, respectively), inferior temporal gyrus, and lingual gyrus.

In an fMRI study by Finnerty and colleagues, nine abstinent smokers were presented with neutral, negatively, and positively valent images from the IAPS during FMRI.[40] While participants were in an abstinence/withdrawal state, there was not an abstinence/satiation contrast. The paradigm elicited changes in brain activity in 14 regions associated with visual processing, attention, and emotion. These regions were further examined for specific effects of negative emotion and relationships between this response and smoking severity as measured by cigarettes smoked per day. Two

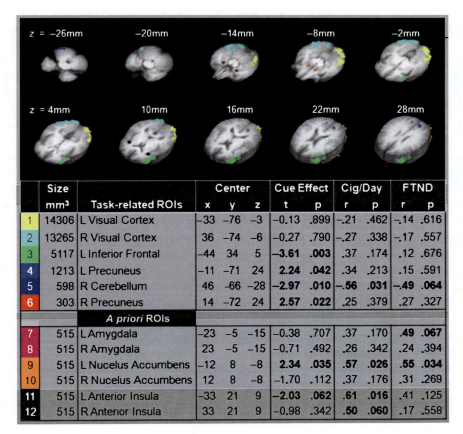

Fig. 9.1 Response to the cue reactivity paradigm, effects of cues, and relationship to the severity of nicotine dependence.[36] Statistical map of voxelwise analyses within six task-related regions of interest (ROIs) and six cue-related ROIs. T-scores for blood-oxygene-dependent-contrast are color-coded according to ROI and hemisphere, as indicated in first column of table. Data presented at the 37th Annual Meeting of the International Neuropsychological Society

of these regions demonstrated a significant positive correlation between the response to negative emotional stimuli and smoking severity. These included regions comprising a large cortical frontoparietal attentional network ($r=.73$, $p<.05$), including subcortical nuclei ($r=.68$, $p<.05$; caudate and thalamus). Findings suggest that in smokers experiencing withdrawal, greater smoking severity is associated with a greater brain response to negatively valenced stimuli. The largest region of increased activity was located in left frontoparietal regions previously associated with attention. These observations may reflect enhanced attention to negative stimuli in smokers experiencing withdrawal.

Cue exposure and cognitive/working memory studies using other modalities such as arterial spin labeling fMRI,[12,28] or for example, [18F]-fluorodeoxyglucose PET, have demonstrated similar activation patterns.[25,43] Whether the cues are pictorial photographs, video, or virtual environments, brain regions associated with reward processing, visuospatial and auditory attention, and working memory have been associated with cue reactivity and cognitive and affective task-related performance.[2]

Nicotine and/or Tobacco Effects

While most of the published functional neuroimaging studies of nicotine dependence incorporate nicotine delivery in some form (e.g., intravenously administered nicotine, ad libitum smoking, nicotine patch), it is important to make the distinction between studies examining abstinence effects (i.e., participants generally abstinent for 10 h or more and likely to be experiencing nicotine withdrawal symptoms) with effects of nicotine and/or tobacco smoking. Thus, studies examining abstinence effects are discussed separately.

Intravenous nicotine infusion: Very few of these studies administered nicotine via a controlled, intravenous (i.v.) route, and most, but not all, of such work has not utilized cue reactivity or cognitive /working memory or affective processing tasks.[33,44–47]

For example, Stein and colleagues[47] conducted a study of 16 active cigarette smokers using fMRI to identify sites of action of nicotine. Nicotine was administered in three, successive, i.v. dosages (0.75, 1.50, 2.25 mg/70 kg) following i.v. saline injection in separate, 20-min trials. Echo planar imaging (EPI) scans of the whole brain (volumes) were obtained every 6 s.

Dose-dependent increases in activation were observed in the nucleus accumbens, amygdala, cingulate, and frontal lobes. Dose-dependent relationships were also seen for several behavioral parameters including "drug liking", "rush", and "high". Of note, the Stein study did not include nonpharmacological stimuli (e.g., smoking-related visual cues, cognitive tasks, etc.). The same group followed up with a pharmacokinetic fMRI study of ten smokers administered an i.v. infusion of 1.5 mg nicotine in a saline vehicle using a waveform analysis protocol method.[44] Significant differences in activated voxels were demonstrated (contrasting pre/postnicotine infusion) in the cingulate cortex, insular cortex, angular gyrus, cuneus, putamen, hypothalamus, and amygdala.

We are aware of only two task-related nicotine infusion studies of nicotine dependence. In an fMRI study by Kumari and colleagues examining nicotine effects on N-back performance, nicotine infusion produced an increased BOLD response in anterior cingulate gyrus, superior frontal gyrus, and parietal cortex.[46] However, in a study of nicotine effects on photic stimulation by Jacobsen and colleagues, there was no effect of nicotine on photic-stimulation BOLD contrast in whole-brain voxelwise analyses.[45] It is not clear why nicotine would be expected to affect photic stimulation in a task-free paradigm. The latter study by Jacobsen and colleagues may suggest that nicotine effects are task-specific and, although not systematically evaluated, tasks that assess cognitive, emotional, and hedonic neural processes would, if this notion holds, be more sensitive to detection of nicotine effects on fMRI BOLD.

Noninvasive nicotine and/or tobacco administration: Noninvasive nicotine administration studies have utilized a wider array of behavioral and nonbehavioral (resting) paradigms.

At least two studies, using radioligands for dopamine D2 receptors have been published by Brody and colleagues[48] and Takahashi and colleagues.[49] Both studies finding that smoking decreases D2 receptor binding potential (BP), which indicates increased endogenous dopamine release.

Other studies have examined fMRI BOLD contract in association with attention cues,[50–56] or in relation to N-back performance on nicotine replacement therapies using examining cerebral perfusion with in a $H_2^{15}O$ PET study by Ernst and colleagues,[57] demonstrating nicotine effects increased regional cerebral perfusion in the anterior cingulate gyrus, prefrontal cortex and BA 44 (inferior temporal gyrus); and interregional connectivity in an fMRI study by Jacobsen and colleagues[58] demonstrating nicotine effects on connectivity of anterior cingulate gyrus to thalamus and thalamus to cortex, with the most marked effects in schizophrenic smokers.

Abstinence Effects on Task Performance

Neuroimaging studies on nicotine abstinence effects on task performance compose the largest subgroup of published studies discussed in this chapter and vary widely with regard to behavioral paradigms employed.

Cue reactivity paradigms: Studies of abstinence-induced effects on cue reactivity in smokers have demonstrated robust results with regard to activation of ROIs but some mixed results with regard to abstinence effects on correlations with behavioral measures such as tobacco craving. For example, McClernon and colleagues, using a within-subjects comparison of overnight abstinence to smoking satiation, reported greater cue reactivity associated with greater activation in the satiated state than the abstinent state in superior frontal gyrus, ventral anterior cingulate gyrus and the ventral striatum.[31] McClernon and colleagues did observe correlations between effects of abstinence on BOLD signal and craving in the middle frontal gyri.[31] David and colleagues demonstrated a significantly greater ventral striatum activation in the satiated vs. abstinent state in a study of female smokers, and there was a significant correlation between BOLD signal in the ventral striatum and tobacco craving in the abstinent prescan state, but there was no correlation observed in the ventral striatum in the study by McClernon and colleagues. Other studies by McClernon and other investigators have demonstrated greater activation in some, but not all visuospatial ROIs in the abstinent state compared to the satiated state.[32,33,59] Depending on the ROI, study design, and characteristics of the participants, some differences in activation patterns and behavioral correlation findings would be expected between studies. Each of these studies used different presentation formats (block vs. event-related) and differed in sample size and gender mix, differences which could explain some of the differences in findings.[33] This observation raises the issue of whether or not more efforts should be made in the field of nicotine dependence neuroimaging research to establish standardized cue exposure and other paradigms, which would lend itself to generaliz-

able findings, demonstration of replication, and also potentially to meta-analytic techniques. Without some degree of methodological harmonization, nonreplication of findings can be uninterpretable with regard to whether and which findings are spurious and which findings represent valid observations.

Cognitive/working memory/affective processing paradigms: In addition to studies of abstinence-effects on cue reactivity, there are a growing number of studies that have examined effects on working memory and other cognitive functions. In general, nicotine abstinence in dependent smokers results in impaired cognitive task performance using multiple paradigms. For example, in an fMRI study by Xu and colleagues, eight smokers were administered the N-back during a repeated-measures abstinence/satiation protocol.[60] Task-related activation was observed in the dorsolateral prefrontal cortex (DLFPC) and a significant interaction between task load (1-back, 2-back, & 3-back) and abstinence (abstinence, satiation) such that task-related activity was relatively low in the lower load (i.e., 1-back) condition during satiety and diminished with higher loads, but the opposite phenomenon was observed in the abstinence condition whereby task-related activity increased in this brain region at higher loads (i.e., 2-back & 3-back). These results are generally consistent with other fMRI studies of abstinence effects on N-back-related brain activation not only in DLPFC but other brain regions implicated in working memory and visuospatial attention (e.g., hippocampus & parahippocampal gyrus, inferior parietal and superior temporal gyri).[41,61,62]

In addition to abstinence-effect studies using the N-back, Jacobsen and colleagues have examined abstinence effects on task-related activation using visuospatial encoding[63] using fMRI; and Rose and colleagues[59] have examined abstinence-effects on task-related continuous performance using FDG PET (regional glucose metabolism). In the study by Jacobsen and colleagues, task-related activation was observed in the hippocampus and parahippocampal gyrus as well as medial temporal lobe. In the PET study by Rose and colleagues, demonstrated that task-induced neural activation increased in the ventral striatum, orbitofrontal cortex and pons when switching from denicotinized cigarettes to regular smoking. In the case of both of these studies, working memory task-related neural activation was enhanced in reward and visuospatial brain regions with nicotine compared to non-nicotine abstinence states.

Task-Free Approaches

In addition to fMRI studies examining reactivity to a behavioral task or pharmacological challenge, structural MRI for measurement of gray and white matter volumes, DTI, ASL, and connectivity analysis are informative approaches to examining specific neurobiological hypotheses.

For example, there have been at least three published MRI volumetric studies, by Brody and colleagues, Gallinat and colleagues, and Tregellas and colleagues that compared regional gray matter volumes between current smokers and ex-smokers and/or never-smokers,[64-66] with replication across studies for the observation that current smokers demonstrate diminished gray matter volumes in anterior brain reward regions including the anterior cingulate gyrus, DLPFC, and orbitofrontal cortex. In addition, there are only two published structural, and DTI studies of white matter volume and function, by Jacobsen and colleagues, and Paul and colleagues, and each study addressed very different clinical questions and examined different brain regions.[67,68] Finally, Gallinat and colleagues have used MRS to examine differences between smokers and non-smokers in N-acetylaspartate, choline, creatine, and glutamate levels.[69,70] These studies demonstrated differences between smokers and non-smokers only for N-acetylaspartate, for which there was reduced concentration in one region only (left hippocampus) in smokers compared to non-smokers. No differences were observed between smokers and non-smokers for regional choline, creatine, or glutamate levels.

Other task-free approaches have been used in nicotine-administration studies, particularly using PET to examine effects of nicotine replacement or infusion on receptor binding, which are discussed briefly above (Sects. 3.2 and 3.3) and described in Table 9.1.

Imaging Genomic Studies

Although only a small number of genetic neuroimaging studies have been conducted, two of the most promising findings come from studies using cue reactivity studies. McClernon and colleagues,[14] for example, found that smokers with a long version of the variable number of tandem repeats (VNTR) polymorphism in

exon III of the dopamine D4 receptor (*DRD4*) gene exhibited greater cue reactivity in the right superior frontal gyrus and right insula compared to individuals who were homozygous for the short version. Similarly, Franklin and colleagues[12] found that smokers with a 9-repeat versions of a VNTR polymorphism in the dopamine transporter gene *SLC6A3* exhibited augmented reactions to tobacco cues in the ventral striatum and orbitofrontal cortex, among multiple regions. Although these are only two studies, these findings indicate the promise of an imaging genetics approach to unraveling the variability in the motivational antecedents of smoking. Establishing these polymorphisms as robust predictors of tobacco cue reactivity and clarifying the role of differential reactivity to other aspects of smoking motivation will be high priorities in future studies.

Summary and Implications for Advancing the State of the Science of Nicotine Dependence Treatment

This chapter provides an introduction and overview into the rapidly growing field of functional neuroimaging for nicotine dependence research. It is evident that there has been wide variation in the specific behavioral paradigms, behavioral measures, study designs, and imaging approaches used in nicotine and tobacco studies. While this may be one of the strengths of functional neuroimaging in terms of the versatility of neuroimaging for addressing a range of neurobiological questions, it may also be a weakness in terms of the ability to demonstrate external validity of findings and to demonstrate replicable observations for cue reactivity, cognitive/working memory, attention, and many other types of behavioral tasks. Despite this wide variation in approaches and study designs, emerging trends have provided investigators with many consistent observations mapping brain regions of interest in humans, which until recently had only been demonstrated in animal studies. As the field advances, the use of imaging genomics and a new line of research, using functional neuroimaging in treatment studies, promises to contribute to important advances in the science of nicotine and tobacco treatment. Identification of genomic loci associated with nicotine dependence and smoking cessation drug efficacy points to specific brain regions and neurotransmitter pathways as logical targets for the development and testing of novel compounds and drug development. In addition, the treatment of diseases other than nicotine dependence, such as Parkinson's disease and Alzheimer's disease, may likewise be informed by the enhanced understanding of nicotine's effects on cholinergic function, movement disorders, and dementia. Challenges to the field will include more concerted efforts to harmonize paradigms across studies and process data in ways amenable to systematic review and meta-analysis, and finally to the translation of these preclinical findings to more efficacious treatments at the clinical bedside.

References

1. McClernon FJ, Gilbert DG (2004) Human functional neuroimaging in nicotine and tobacco research: basics, background, and beyond. Nicotine Tob Res 6(6):941–959
2. Ray R, Loughead J, Wang Z, Detre J, Yang E, Gur R et al (2008) Neuroimaging, genetics and the treatment of nicotine addiction. Behav Brain Res 193(2):159–169
3. Hukkanen J, Jacob P 3rd, Benowitz NL (2005) Metabolism and disposition kinetics of nicotine. Pharmacol Rev 57(1):79–115
4. Nestler EJ, Aghajanian GK (1997) Molecular and cellular basis of addiction. Science 278(5335):58–63
5. Di Chiara G (2000) Role of dopamine in the behavioural actions of nicotine related to addiction. Eur J Pharmacol 393(1–3): 295–314
6. Laviolette SR, van der Kooy D (2004) The neurobiology of nicotine addiction: bridging the gap from molecules to behaviour. Nat Rev Neurosci 5(1):55–65
7. Balfour DJ (2002) Neuroplasticity within the mesoaccumbens dopamine system and its role in tobacco dependence. Curr Drug Target CNS Neurol Disord 1(4):413–421
8. Robinson TE, Berridge KC (2001) Incentive-sensitization and addiction. Addiction 96(1):103–114
9. Robinson TE, Berridge KC (1993) The neural basis of drug craving: an incentive-sensitization theory of addiction. Brain Res Brain Res Rev 18(3):247–291
10. Tsukada H, Miyasato K, Kakiuchi T, Nishiyama S, Harada N, Domino EF (2002) Comparative effects of methamphetamine and nicotine on the striatal [(11)C]raclopride binding in unanesthetized monkeys. Synapse 45(4):207–212
11. Porjesz B, Begleiter H (2003) Alcoholism and human electrophysiology. Alcohol Res Health 27(2):153–160
12. Franklin TR, Lohoff FW, Wang Z, Sciortino N, Harper D, Li Y et al (2009) DAT genotype modulates brain and behavioral responses elicited by cigarette cues. Neuropsychopharmacology 34(3):717–728
13. Jacobsen LK, Pugh KR, Mencl WE, Gelernter J (2006) C957T polymorphism of the dopamine D2 receptor gene modulates the effect of nicotine on working memory performance and cortical processing efficiency. Psychopharmacology (Berl) 188(4):530–540

14. McClernon FJ, Hutchison KE, Rose JE, Kozink RV (2007) DRD4 VNTR polymorphism is associated with transient fMRI-BOLD responses to smoking cues. Psychopharmacology (Berl) 194(4):433–441
15. Wang Z, Ray R, Faith M, Tang K, Wileyto EP, Detre JA et al (2008) Nicotine abstinence-induced cerebral blood flow changes by genotype. Neurosci Lett 438(3):275–280
16. Jonsson EG, Nothen MM, Grunhage F, Farde L, Nakashima Y, Propping P et al (1999) Polymorphisms in the dopamine D2 receptor gene and their relationships to striatal dopamine receptor density of healthy volunteers. Mol Psychiatry 4(3): 290–296
17. Talbot PS, Laruelle M (2002) The role of in vivo molecular imaging with PET and SPECT in the elucidation of psychiatric drug action and new drug development. Eur Neuropsychopharmacol 12(6):503–511
18. Volkow ND, Rosen B, Farde L (1997) Imaging the living human brain: magnetic resonance imaging and positron emission tomography. Proc Natl Acad Sci U S A 94(7):2787–2788
19. Ekman P, Friesen W (1975) Unmasking the Face: A Guide to Recognizing Emotions from Facial Clues. Prentice Hall, Inc., Englewood Cliffs, NJ
20. Niaura R, Shadel WG, Abrams DB, Monti PM, Rohsenow DJ, Sirota A (1998) Individual differences in cue reactivity among smokers trying to quit: effects of gender and cue type. Addict Behav 23(2):209–224
21. Rohsenow DJ, Monti PM, Rubonis AV, Sirota AD, Niaura RS, Colby SM et al (1994) Cue reactivity as a predictor of drinking among male alcoholics. J Consult Clin Psychol 62(3):620–626
22. Rohsenow DJ, Niaura RS, Childress AR, Abrams DB, Monti PM (1990) Cue reactivity in addictive behaviors: theoretical and treatment implications. Int J Addict 25(7A-8A):957–993
23. Shadel WG, Niaura R, Abrams DB, Goldstein MG, Rohsenow DJ, Sirota AD et al (1998) Scripted imagery manipulations and smoking cue reactivity in a clinical sample of self-quitters. Exp Clin Psychopharmacol 6(2):179–186
24. Due DL, Huettel SA, Hall WG, Rubin DC (2002) Activation in mesolimbic and visuospatial neural circuits elicited by smoking cues: evidence from functional magnetic resonance imaging. Am J Psychiatry 159(6):954–960
25. Brody AL, Mandelkern MA, London ED, Childress AR, Lee GS, Bota RG et al (2002) Brain metabolic changes during cigarette craving. Arch Gen Psychiatry 59(12):1162–1172
26. David SP, Munafo MR, Johansen-Berg H, Mackillop J, Sweet LH, Cohen RA et al (2007) Effects of acute nicotine abstinence on cue-elicited ventral striatum/nucleus accumbens activation in female cigarette smokers: a functional magnetic resonance imaging study. Brain Imaging Behav 1(3–4):43–57
27. David SP, Munafo MR, Johansen-Berg H, Smith SM, Rogers RD, Matthews PM et al (2005) Ventral striatum/nucleus accumbens activation to smoking-related pictorial cues in smokers and nonsmokers: a functional magnetic resonance imaging study. Biol Psychiatry 58(6):488–494
28. Franklin TR, Wang Z, Wang J, Sciortino N, Harper D, Li Y et al (2007) Limbic activation to cigarette smoking cues independent of nicotine withdrawal: a perfusion fMRI study. Neuropsychopharmacology 32(11):2301–2309
29. Lim HK, Pae CU, Joo RH, Yoo SS, Choi BG, Kim DJ et al (2005) fMRI investigation on cue-induced smoking craving. J Psychiatr Res 39(3):333–335

30. McBride D, Barrett SP, Kelly JT, Aw A, Dagher A (2006) Effects of expectancy and abstinence on the neural response to smoking cues in cigarette smokers: an fMRI study. Neuropsychopharmacology 31(12):2728–2738

31. McClernon FJ, Hiott FB, Huettel SA, Rose JE (2005) Abstinence-induced changes in self-report craving correlate with event-related FMRI responses to smoking cues. Neuropsychopharmacology 30(10):1940–1947

32. McClernon FJ, Hiott FB, Liu J, Salley AN, Behm FM, Rose JE (2007) Selectively reduced responses to smoking cues in amygdala following extinction-based smoking cessation: results of a preliminary functional magnetic resonance imaging study. Addict Biol 12(3–4):503–512

33. McClernon FJ, Kozink RV, Rose JE (2008) Individual differences in nicotine dependence, withdrawal symptoms, and sex predict transient fMRI-BOLD responses to smoking cues. Neuropsychopharmacology 33(9):2148–2157

34. Okuyemi KS, Powell JN, Savage CR, Hall SB, Nollen N, Holsen LM et al (2006) Enhanced cue-elicited brain activation in African American compared with Caucasian smokers: an fMRI study. Addict Biol 11(1):97–106

35. Smolka MN, Buhler M, Klein S, Zimmermann U, Mann K, Heinz A et al (2006) Severity of nicotine dependence modulates cue-induced brain activity in regions involved in motor preparation and imagery. Psychopharmacology (Berl) 184(3–4):577–588

36. Sweet LH, Mackillop J, Weir L, et al. Brain response to smoking cues and relationships to severity of nicotine dependence. In: *Thirty-Seventh Annual Meeting International Neuropsychological Society*; February 11–14, 2009.

37. McClernon FJ, Kozink RV, Lutz AM, Rose JE (2009) 24-h smoking abstinence potentiates fMRI-BOLD activation to smoking cues in cerebral cortex and dorsal striatum. Psychopharmacology (Berl) 204(1):25–35

38. Wang Z, Faith M, Patterson F, Tang K, Kerrin K, Wileyto EP et al (2007) Neural substrates of abstinence-induced cigarette cravings in chronic smokers. J Neurosci 27(51):14035–14040

39. Gilbert DG, Rabinovitch NE (1998) International Smoking Image Series with Neutral Counterparts, 12th edn. Southern Illinois University, Carbondale, IL

40. Finnerty CE, FMRI response to negative emotional images among smokers in withdrawal. In: *2009 Joint Conference of SRNT and SRNT-Europe*. Saggart, Co. Dublin, Ireland: Society for Research on Nicotine & Tobacco; April 27–30, 2009.

41. Jacobsen LK, Pugh KR, Constable RT, Westerveld M, Mencl WE (2007) Functional correlates of verbal memory deficits emerging during nicotine withdrawal in abstinent adolescent cannabis users. Biol Psychiatry 61(1):31–40

42. Jacobsen LK, Slotkin TA, Mencl WE, Frost SJ, Pugh KR (2007) Gender-specific effects of prenatal and adolescent exposure to tobacco smoke on auditory and visual attention. Neuropsychopharmacology 32(12):2453–2464

43. Brody AL, Mandelkern MA, Lee G, Smith E, Sadeghi M, Saxena S et al (2004) Attenuation of cue-induced cigarette craving and anterior cingulate cortex activation in bupropion-treated smokers: a preliminary study. Psychiatry Res 130(3): 269–281

44. Bloom AS, Hoffmann RG, Fuller SA, Pankiewicz J, Harsch HH, Stein EA (1999) Determination of drug-induced changes in functional MRI signal using a pharmacokinetic model. Hum Brain Mapp 8(4):235–244

45. Jacobsen LK, Gore JC, Skudlarski P, Lacadie CM, Jatlow P, Krystal JH (2002) Impact of intravenous nicotine on BOLD signal response to photic stimulation. Magn Reson Imaging 20(2):141–145

46. Kumari V, Gray JA, ffytche DH, Mitterschiffthaler MT, Das M, Zachariah E et al (2003) Cognitive effects of nicotine in humans: an fMRI study. Neuroimage 19(3):1002–1013

47. Stein EA, Pankiewicz J, Harsch HH, Cho JK, Fuller SA, Hoffmann RG et al (1998) Nicotine-induced limbic cortical activation in the human brain: a functional MRI study. Am J Psychiatry 155(8):1009–1015

48. Brody AL, Mandelkern MA, Olmstead RE, Allen-Martinez Z, Scheibal D, Abrams AL et al (2009) Ventral striatal dopamine release in response to smoking a regular vs a denicotinized cigarette. Neuropsychopharmacology 34(2):282–289

49. Takahashi H, Fujimura Y, Hayashi M, Takano H, Kato M, Okubo Y et al (2008) Enhanced dopamine release by nicotine in cigarette smokers: a double-blind, randomized, placebo-controlled pilot study. Int J Neuropsychopharmacol 11(3):413–417

50. Giessing C, Fink GR, Rosler F, Thiel CM (2007) fMRI data predict individual differences of behavioral effects of nicotine: a partial least square analysis. J Cogn Neurosci 19(4): 658–670

51. Lawrence NS, Ross TJ, Stein EA (2002) Cognitive mechanisms of nicotine on visual attention. Neuron 36(3):539–548

52. Thiel CM, Fink GR (2007) Visual and auditory alertness: modality-specific and supramodal neural mechanisms and their modulation by nicotine. J Neurophysiol 97(4):2758–2768

53. Thiel CM, Fink GR (2008) Effects of the cholinergic agonist nicotine on reorienting of visual spatial attention and top-down attentional control. Neuroscience 152(2):381–390

54. Thiel CM, Zilles K, Fink GR (2005) Nicotine modulates reorienting of visuospatial attention and neural activity in human parietal cortex. Neuropsychopharmacology 30(4):810–820

55. Tregellas JR, Tanabe JL, Martin LF, Freedman R (2005) FMRI of response to nicotine during a smooth pursuit eye movement task in schizophrenia. Am J Psychiatry 162(2):391–393

56. Vossel S, Thiel CM, Fink GR (2008) Behavioral and neural effects of nicotine on visuospatial attentional reorienting in non-smoking subjects. Neuropsychopharmacology 33(4): 731–738

57. Ernst M, Matochik JA, Heishman SJ, Van Horn JD, Jons PH, Henningfield JE et al (2001) Effect of nicotine on brain activation during performance of a working memory task. Proc Natl Acad Sci U S A 98(8):4728–4733

58. Jacobsen LK, D'Souza DC, Mencl WE, Pugh KR, Skudlarski P, Krystal JH (2004) Nicotine effects on brain function and functional connectivity in schizophrenia. Biol Psychiatry 55(8):850–858

59. Rose JE, Behm FM, Salley AN, Bates JE, Coleman RE, Hawk TC et al (2007) Regional brain activity correlates of nicotine dependence. Neuropsychopharmacology 32(12):2441–2452

60. Xu J, Mendrek A, Cohen MS, Monterosso J, Rodriguez P, Simon SL et al (2005) Brain activity in cigarette smokers performing a working memory task: effect of smoking abstinence. Biol Psychiatry 58(2):143–150

61. Tobacco SfRoNa, ed. Nicotine satiation and abstinence effects on fMRI brain activation during verbal working memory. In: *10th Annual Society for Research on Nicotine and Tobacco Meeting*. Scotsdale, AZ: SRNT; February 18–21, 2004.

62. Xu J, Mendrek A, Cohen MS, Monterosso J, Simon S, Brody AL et al (2006) Effects of acute smoking on brain activity vary with abstinence in smokers performing the N-Back task: a preliminary study. Psychiatry Res 148(2–3):103–109

63. Jacobsen LK, Slotkin TA, Westerveld M, Mencl WE, Pugh KR (2006) Visuospatial memory deficits emerging during nicotine withdrawal in adolescents with prenatal exposure to active maternal smoking. Neuropsychopharmacology 31(7): 1550–1561

64. Tregellas JR, Shatti S, Tanabe JL, Martin LF, Gibson L, Wylie K et al (2007) Gray matter volume differences and the effects of smoking on gray matter in schizophrenia. Schizophr Res 97(1–3):242–249

65. Brody AL, Mandelkern MA, Jarvik ME, Lee GS, Smith EC, Huang JC et al (2004) Differences between smokers and nonsmokers in regional gray matter volumes and densities. Biol Psychiatry 55(1):77–84

66. Gallinat J, Meisenzahl E, Jacobsen LK, Kalus P, Bierbrauer J, Kienast T et al (2006) Smoking and structural brain deficits: a volumetric MR investigation. Eur J Neurosci 24(6):1744–1750

67. Jacobsen LK, Picciotto MR, Heath CJ, Frost SJ, Tsou KA, Dwan RA et al (2007) Prenatal and adolescent exposure to tobacco smoke modulates the development of white matter microstructure. J Neurosci 27(49):13491–13498

68. Paul RH, Grieve SM, Niaura R, David SP, Laidlaw DH, Cohen R et al (2008) Chronic cigarette smoking and the microstructural integrity of white matter in healthy adults: a diffusion tensor imaging study. Nicotine Tob Res 10(1):137–147

69. Gallinat J, Lang UE, Jacobsen LK, Bajbouj M, Kalus P, von Haebler D et al (2007) Abnormal hippocampal neurochemistry in smokers: evidence from proton magnetic resonance spectroscopy at 3 T. J Clin Psychopharmacol 27(1):80–84

70. Gallinat J, Schubert F (2007) Regional cerebral glutamate concentrations and chronic tobacco consumption. Pharmacopsychiatry 40(2):64–67

71. Domino EF, Minoshima S, Guthrie S, Ohl L, Ni L, Koeppe RA et al (2000) Nicotine effects on regional cerebral blood flow in awake, resting tobacco smokers. Synapse 38(3):313–321

72. Mamede M, Ishizu K, Ueda M, Mukai T, Iida Y, Kawashima H et al (2007) Temporal change in human nicotinic acetylcholine receptor after smoking cessation: 5IA SPECT study. J Nucl Med 48(11):1829–1835

73. Montgomery AJ, Lingford-Hughes AR, Egerton A, Nutt DJ, Grasby PM (2007) The effect of nicotine on striatal dopamine release in man: a [11C]raclopride PET study. Synapse 61(8):637–645

74. Scott DJ, Domino EF, Heitzeg MM, Koeppe RA, Ni L, Guthrie S et al (2007) Smoking modulation of mu-opioid and dopamine D2 receptor-mediated neurotransmission in humans. Neuropsychopharmacology 32(2):450–457

75. Staley JK, Krishnan-Sarin S, Cosgrove KP, Krantzler E, Frohlich E, Perry E et al (2006) Human tobacco smokers in early abstinence have higher levels of beta2* nicotinic acetylcholine receptors than nonsmokers. J Neurosci 26(34): 8707–8714

76. Stapleton JM, Gilson SF, Wong DF, Villemagne VL, Dannals RF, Grayson RF et al (2003) Intravenous nicotine reduces cerebral glucose metabolism: a preliminary study. Neuropsychopharmacology 28(4):765–772

77. Tanabe J, Tregellas JR, Martin LF, Freedman R (2006) Effects of nicotine on hippocampal and cingulate activity during smooth pursuit eye movement in schizophrenia. Biol Psychiatry 59(8):754–761

78. Tanabe J, Crowley T, Hutchison K, Miller D, Johnson G, Du YP et al (2008) Ventral striatal blood flow is altered by acute nicotine but not withdrawal from nicotine. Neuropsychopharmacology 33(3):627–633

79. Zubieta JK, Heitzeg MM, Xu Y, Koeppe RA, Ni L, Guthrie S et al (2005) Regional cerebral blood flow responses to smoking in tobacco smokers after overnight abstinence. Am J Psychiatry 162(3):567–577

Chapter 10
The Relationship Between Mood, Stress, and Tobacco Smoking

Espen Walderhaug, Kelly P. Cosgrove, Zubin Bhagwagar, and Alexander Neumeister

The primary addictive substance in tobacco is nicotine,[1] although other chemicals also contribute to the reinforcing properties of tobacco smoke.[2–12] Nicotine shares the reinforcing and dopamine-stimulating properties with other psychostimulants.[13] Nicotine exerts its effect on all humans; however, the abuse potential of tobacco smoking is probably exacerbated in individuals with depression, during high stress, and in people exhibiting negative emotions.[14] It is therefore of great interest to understand the neurobiological and behavioral effects of nicotine in healthy people and individuals with mood and anxiety disorders, all of which occur to be associated with high rates of nicotine dependence. Molecular imaging using single-photon emission computed tomography (SPECT) and positron emission tomography (PET) is currently the most powerful tool to better understand the relationship between nicotine addiction, mood, stress, and cognition; however, we have to acknowledge that this research is still in its infancy.

The Nicotinic Acetylcholine Receptors

Nicotine, the main addictive chemical in tobacco smoke, exerts its effects by binding to, activating, and desensitizing the nicotinic acetylcholine receptors (nAChRs) in the central nervous system and autonomic

ganglia.[15] All nAChRs are desensitized by nicotine. Neuronal nAChRs belong to a receptor family of ligand gated ion channel receptors[16] composed of a combination of α and non-α subunits. There are at least eight neuronal α subunits ($\alpha2$–$\alpha9$[17]) and at least three non-α subunits ($\beta2$–$\beta4$) that are 40–55% homologous to nAChR subunits found at the neuromuscular junction (reviewed in ref.[18]). Twelve genes for subunits associated with neuronal nAChRs have been identified in the mammalian genome, including $\alpha2$–$\alpha7$, $\alpha9$, $\alpha10$, $\beta2$–$\beta4$,[19,20]. nAChRs comprised of $\alpha7$ and $\alpha9$ are functional as monomeric receptors, characterized by low affinity for nicotinic agonists and high affinity for α-bungarotoxin. All other α subunits (i.e., 2–6) need coexpression of α and β pairs and are distinguished by high affinity for nicotinic agonists and low affinity for α-bungarotoxin.[20,21] These subunits can be divided into subfamilies based on sequence homology and phylogeny,[22,23] as well as on their pharmacological and physiological properties. $\alpha4$ and $\beta2$, combined with $\alpha5$, $\alpha6$, or $\beta3$, would comprise one family with widespread expression in the brain and high affinity for nicotine; $\alpha3$ and $\beta4$, along with $\alpha5$ and other third subunits, comprise a second family responsible for direct ganglionic neurotransmission with a more limited expression in brain and a somewhat lower sensitivity to nicotine; the $\alpha7$ subunit, which is able to form active homopentamers in vitro, comprises a third family of nAChRs with wide brain expression, a high permeability to calcium, and a low affinity for nicotine in vitro, although high affinity $\alpha7$-like responses have been seen in slices.[24] Animals that lack the $\beta2$ subunit of the nAChR ($\beta2^*$ nAChRs) have normal expression and function of receptors containing the $\beta4$ subunit ($\beta4^*$ nAChRs) and the homopentameric receptors of the $\alpha7$ class ($\alpha7^*$ nAChRs[24]). Similarly, the other lines of mutant mice isolate individual nAChR families that

A. Neumeister (✉)
Molecular Imaging Program of the National Center for PTSD, Clinical Neuroscience Division, VA Connecticut Healthcare System, (116-A) 950 Campbell Avenue, Bldg. 1, Room 9-174 (MSC 151E), West Haven, CT, 06516, USA
and
Mount Sinai School of Medicine, New York, NY, 10029, USA
e-mail: alexander.neumeister@mssm.edu

R.A. Cohen and L.H. Sweet (eds.), *Brain Imaging in Behavioral Medicine and Clinical Neuroscience*,
DOI 10.1007/978-1-4419-6373-4_10, © Springer Science+Business Media, LLC 2011

can then be targeted with more specific antagonists. Thus, these three nAChR subunit families appear to be relatively independent in their expression in brain.

Anatomical Localization

NAChRs are most prevalent in the thalamus, followed by the substantia nigra, striatum, hippocampus, entorhinal cortex, with the lowest densities in the cerebellar, parietal, and frontal cortices.[21,25-27] Regional differences in nAChR subunit combinations are likely determined by the relative ratio or type of subunits expressed by that region. The most common subunits expressed in human brain are $\alpha4$, $\alpha7$, and $\beta2$. In vitro immunological studies have demonstrated that $\alpha4$ is highest in cortical areas, $\alpha7$ is highest in lateral and medial geniculate, and the $\beta2$ is most dense in the striatum. The regional expression of $\alpha7$ differs between rodents and humans and illustrates the likelihood of species differences in nAChR expression and the importance of studies in living humans. $\alpha4\beta2$ and $\alpha3\beta2$ are the most common nAChR subtype in the striatal reward areas that are relevant to the neurobiology of addiction disorders.

In Vivo Imaging of the nAChR

Nicotinic agonist binding is higher in the gyrus rectus, thalamus, hippocampus, midbrain,[28,29] striatum, entorhinal, prefrontal, and temporal cortices, and cerebellum in postmortem brain from human smokers.[30,31] This increase in high-affinity nAChR is dose-dependent, based on the number of cigarettes smoked at death, and was reversible with binding levels returning to control values in subjects who had quit smoking for at least 2 months prior to death.[29] The upregulation is directly due to the regulatory effects of nicotine since chronic nicotine treatment in mice[32-37] and rats[38-42] results in a dose-dependent increase in high-affinity nicotinic agonist binding to $\beta2$-nAChR. After chronic nicotine administration to male baboons and male rhesus macaques using SPECT and [123I]5-IA,[43,44] it was noted that nicotinic agonist binding to $\beta2$-nAChR was decreased at 1–2 days abstinence from nicotine and increased only after 7 days of abstinence. Since urinary

cotinine levels were still very high at 1–2 days of abstinence, it is likely that the lower number of receptors at 1–2 days of abstinence reflects the interference of residual nicotine that was blocking radiotracer binding and not a true reflection of $\beta2$-nAChR number.

Until recently, it was impossible to image $\beta2$ nAChR in humans. First attempts with [11C]-nicotine and radiolabeled derivatives of epibatidine failed in vivo because of high nonspecific uptake, fast washout from brain, and neurotoxicity.[45] Recently [123I]5-I-A-85380 ([123I]5-IA[46]) and 2-[18F]fluoro-A-85380 have been labeled for SPECT and PET imaging, respectively.[46,47] 5-IA has high affinity (KD = 11 pM) for nAChR. In brain, the greatest uptake is thalamic, with moderate to low levels in the striatum, hippocampus, and cortex.[46,48] [123I]5-IA uptake in vivo is displaced by the agonists (−)-nicotine and cytisine, but not by noncompetitive antagonists mecamylamine, bupropion, cotinine, or the muscarinic antagonist (−)-scopolamine,[49,50] showing that [123I]5-IA binds to the nicotine binding site on $\beta2$ nAChR. The selectivity of [123I] 5-IA for $\beta2$-nAChR was confirmed autoradiographically in wild-type (+/+) mice, but not in mice lacking the nAChR $\beta2$ subunit (−/−).[50]

Staley et al recently examined nicotinic agonist binding to $\beta2$-nAChR in living smokers using [123I]5-IA SPECT.[51] All smokers were asked to abstain from smoking for 4–9 days prior to $\beta2$-nAChR. A 26–36% increase was noted throughout the cerebral cortical mantle, including the parietal, frontal, occipital, anterior cingulate, temporal, and cerebellar cortices, and striatum (26.9%), with less notable elevation in the thalamus (8.7%). A recent study by Brody et al[52] found that after smoking one puff, three puffs, one cigarette, or to satiety, the nAChRs occupied 33, 75, 88, and 95%, respectively, 3.1 h after smoking the cigarette, and they proposed that the occupancy would be even greater sooner postchallenge. The latest study by Staley et al[53] (see Fig. 10.1) examined changes in $\beta2$-nAChR availability during acute and prolonged abstinence from tobacco smoking. They found significantly higher $\beta2$-nAChR availability in smokers at 1 week of abstinence in the cortex, striatum, and cerebellum compared with the age-matched nonsmokers. The higher $\beta2$-nAChR availability persisted up to 1 month, and normalized to nonsmoker levels by 6–12 weeks of abstinence from tobacco smoking, which is consistent with the prolonged craving, withdrawal, and risk for relapse typical for cigarette addiction.[53]

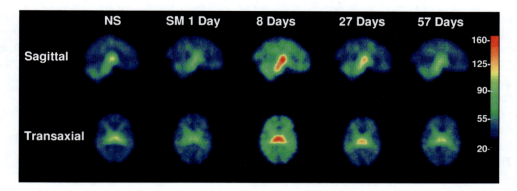

Fig. 10.1 Illustrates sagittal and tranasxial views of parametric images (VT/fP) of a representative nonsmoker (NS) compared to an age- and sex-matched smoker (SM) over the course of abstinence from cigarette smoking at 1 day, 8 days, 27 days, and 57 days. The subject was scanned with [^{123}I]5-IA-85380 and SPECT brain imaging. Note the increased β2*-nicotinic acetylcholine receptor availability at 8 days of abstinence marking tobacco smoking-induced upregulation of the receptor, which declines over the course of abstinence. At 1 day of abstinence, nicotine is still present in the brain interfering with radiotracer binding, thus it is critical to wait ~1 week for nicotine to clear from brain prior to imaging this receptor site in tobacco smokers

In Vivo Imaging of Monoamine Oxidase

Over 4,000 chemicals are contained in tobacco smoke, most of which have not been identified. Harman and norharman are centrally active, well-established monoamine oxidase (MAO) inhibitors[54] present in cigarettes. MAO-A and MAO-B are decreased by 28 and 40% respectively in brain[55–57] and platelets[58–60] of smokers. A recent study using a selective radioligand of MAO-A isoenzyme ([^{11}C]befloxatone) found that the binding potential in smokers, as compared to nonsmokers, was reduced by as much as 60% in cortical areas and around 40% in the caudate and thalamus.[61] These numbers are close to the expected effect on cerebral MAO-A levels obtained by the MAO inhibitors tranylcypromine[55] and moclobemide.[62] Smoking-associated MAO-A inhibition could have a mood-modulating effect in smokers, which counteracts the elevated cerebral MAO-A density found in untreated depressed patients.[63] This supports the theory that tobacco smoking is a "self-medication"[64,65] and could partly explain the high comorbidity between smoking and depression.[66] Prior to smoking cessation, smoking behavior is negatively correlated with platelet MAO activity, which normalizes by 4 weeks of smoking cessation.[67] Thus, MAO inhibition likely plays an important role in smoking cessation. Plasma norharman levels are negatively correlated with severity of craving in low dependence smokers.[68] While the cognitive effects of harman and norharman have not yet been directly studied, there are numerous studies on other MAO-A (moclobemide) and MAO-B (l-deprenyl) inhibitors that demonstrate cognitive effects in animals and humans.[69–77] MAO-A also plays a crucial role in the catabolism of amine neurotransmitters, such as dopamine, norepinephrine, and serotonin, and could therefore contribute to the addictive properties of tobacco smoking, in addition to mood, stress, and cognition in several different ways.

Nicotine Dependence and Major Depressive Disorder

Nicotine dependence is the most frequent comorbid lifetime disorder and the second most frequent *current* comorbid disorder among patients with major depressive disorder (MDD).[66] A lifetime history of MDD is a significant predictor of smoking onset[78–81] and failure to quit smoking.[82–86] MDD has also been shown to significantly contribute to the severity of nicotine dependence in adolescents.[78] Other research has shown that as depressive symptoms increase, smoking rates increase, and quit rates decrease.[83,87] A history of nicotine dependence increases the risk of first incidence of MDD.[79–81,88,89] Age of onset of smoking was found to be predictive of MDD, with the younger the age of nicotine use increasing the risk of eventual MDD.[81] Prenatal exposure increases risk of MDD, ADHD, substance-use disorders.[90] Patients with the melancholic depressive subtype have been shown to have higher rates of nicotine dependence compared with patients with undifferentiated depression.[91] Nicotine deprivation studies have shown reexposure to nicotine to reduce negative affect[92–94] and increase positive affect,[95,96] though these effects may be attributable to reversing the withdrawal. Nicotine has been shown to worsen induced negative mood in people with current or past history of MDD as well as in controls, to increase the effect of positive mood induction in dispelling negative mood induction in people with a past and current history of MDD, and to enhance induced positive mood induction in MDD.[97] Previous studies have also shown an increase in withdrawal and depressive symptoms during smoking cessation in people with a history of depression.[86,98–100]

The relationship between bipolar disorder and nicotine dependence is bidirectional as the odds ratios for nicotine dependence is estimated to be 3.9 and 3.5 for bipolar I and II disorders, respectively, in comparison with the general population.[88] Epidemiologic data from 2000 indicated that the lifetime prevalence of daily smoking among adults with bipolar disorder (BP) was 82.5%, more than twice as high compared to that of adults with no mental illness (39.1%), and higher than that of adults with lifetime major depression (59%).[101] Interestingly, Hughes et al (1986) reported that seven of ten patients experiencing a current episode of mania were smokers.[102]In a population-based study examining the prevalence of smoking for adults with psychiatric disorders ($N=4,411$), the current and lifetime prevalence of smoking was higher for persons with bipolar disorder, 60.6 and 81.8%, respectively, than persons with other psychiatric illnesses or persons with no psychiatric illness.[103] Finally, Morris et al found that 50.7% of 14,759 bipolar patients receiving treatment in community mental health centers were smokers.[104]

Nicotine administration normalizes sensory deficits, which are seen in both schizophrenia and bipolar disorder, suggesting that the high incidence of tobacco use in these patients may be an attempt of self-medication.[64,65] Consistent with this hypothesis, clinically significant symptoms of mania and depression have been reported following smoking cessation in some individuals.[105–107] In a recent study, smoking has been found to be associated with worse treatment outcomes in mania which emphasize the strong relationship between nicotinic receptor modulation and mood control.[108] Conflicting evidence regarding the relationship between nicotine and mood control might be explained by considering nicotine's complex neuropharmacology and the distribution of nicotinic receptors in neural circuits regulating responses to stress, the circadian rhythm, and behavioral reinforcement.

nAChRs Are Important Modulators of Serotonin

It seems likely that nAChRs play a primarily neuromodulatory role in the CNS rather than mediating direct synaptic transmission. A large proportion of nicotine binding sites are found on nerve terminals rather than in the postsynaptic membrane.[109] Accordingly, nicotine is known to modulate release of acetylcholine, dopamine, GABA, glutamate, norepinephrine, and serotonin from presynaptic terminals in several brain areas.[110–112] nAChRs on the cell bodies of neurons play a large role in calcium mobilization in the cell,[113] and this may be part of the mechanism underlying the increase in transmitter release caused by nicotine. Nicotinic antagonists can stimulate the serotonergic system,[114,115] although antagonists can also block the ability of nicotine to stimulate serotonin release,[114,116] suggesting that a balance of nicotinic activation and inhibition is important for regulation of the serotonin system. It is possible that the ability of mecamylamine to increase serotonin release is due to blockade of nAChRs on GABA terminals, as has been seen previously in the ventral tegmental area.[117] Thus, one potential mechanism underlying the antidepressant-like effects of nicotinic antagonists could be stimulation of transient serotonin release in selected brain areas such as the hippocampus and/or frontal cortex.

Cholinergic Hypothesis of Depression

A growing body of evidence suggests that the cholinergic system may be a potential target for the development of novel antidepressant compounds. Cholinergic hyperactivity has long been postulated to play a role in the pathophysiology of depression.[118,119] Stimulation of cholinergic systems with agents such as the cholinesterase inhibitor physostigmine can induce depression-like symptoms in individuals with affective disorders, as well as in normal subjects.[120,121] These findings are supported by animal studies demonstrating that the Flinders Sensitive Line of rats, selectively bred for increased sensitivity to cholinergic agents, show behavior that resembles symptoms of depression in humans.[122] Furthermore, inescapable footshock and swim stress, which are used to induce "depressive-like" states in rodents, can both induce a supersensitivity of the cholinergic system.[119,123] Scopolamine, an antimuscarinic agent, showed rapid and robust antidepressant responses in depressed patients who predominantly had poor prognoses.[124] Genetic studies also support a role for the acetylcholinergic system in the pathophysiology of depression. It has been shown that some polymorphisms of the muscarinic receptor gene are associated with an elevated incidence of depression.[125,126] In another recent study, the distribution of the two-base-pair deletion of the partially duplicated α7 nAChR genotype and alleles suggested a modest difference between depressive patients and control.[127] Together, these studies suggest that excessive activation of cholinergic systems may contribute to the pathophysiology of depression.

The Cholinergic System as a Therapeutic Target in Depression

As described above, there is growing evidence to suggest that the cholinergic system may be a potential target for the development of novel molecular approaches to the treatment of depression. Early studies found that antimuscarinic agents produce antidepressant-like effects. However, these findings were considered "false-positives" as there was a belief that these agents did not have an inherent antidepressant effect.[128] Moreover, rats bred selectively for increased sensitivity of muscarinic receptors showed putative behavioral analogs of depression, such as lethargy, reductions in self-stimulation, and increased behavioral despair, in the forced swim test (FST) in response to cholinomimetic drugs.[122,129] Recently, it has been shown that antagonism of central, but not peripheral, nAChRs has an antidepressant-like effect in mice in the tail suspension test and FST.[130] Both the β2 and α7-nAChR subunits are necessary for the antidepressant-like effect of

mecamylamine because mice lacking these subunits are insensitive to the effects of mecamylamine in the FST. Anticholinesterase inhibitors are drugs that inhibit the catabolism of acetylcholine,[131] increasing both the level and duration of action of acetylcholine. An increase of acetylcholinergic activity has been shown to be depressogenic, and physostigmine (an anticholinesterase inhibitor) exacerbated depressive symptoms in depressed patients with MDD and induced depressive symptoms in currently manic patients with bipolar disorder.[118,120,121,132,133] Further evidence comes from studies that show that neuroendocrine and pupillary responses to cholinomimetics[119,134] and polysomnographic responses to muscarinic receptor agonists[135] are exaggerated in depressed patients. An interesting side note is the issue of antidepressant induced side effects and specifically anticholinergic side effects. It has long been known that tricyclic antidepressant (TCA) agents exert potent antimuscarinic actions,[136,137] but these effects are thought to produce adverse effects without contributing to therapeutic efficacy.[138]

Classical Antidepressants Are nAChR Antagonists

If depression is associated with a hyperactive cholinergic system, then inhibition of cholinergic receptors might be expected to be antidepressant. Although it is clear that modulation of serotonergic and/or noradrenergic function is important for antidepressant efficacy, studies at the cellular, physiological, and behavioral levels have shown that a wide range of antidepressants also act as nAChR antagonists at clinically relevant doses. In cellular studies, TCAs, monoamine oxidase inhibitors, selective serototonin reuptake inhibitors (SSRIs), and atypical antidepressants have been shown to inhibit the function of nAChRs.[139–142] In physiological studies, TCAs, SSRIs, and bupropion inhibited nicotine-induced norepinephrine (NE) release from hippocampal and striatal slices.[143,144] In behavioral studies, bupropion inhibited the analgesic, motor, hypothermic, and convulsive effects of nicotine,[145] and the SSRI citalopram blocked the anxiolytic effects of chronic nicotine in the elevated plus maze.[146] Together, these studies provide strong evidence that different classes of antidepressants can inhibit nAChRs. Furthermore, both nicotine and mecamylamine potentiate the antidepressant-like effect of the TCA imipramine and the SSRI citalopram in the tail suspension test in mice,[147] providing evidence that nAChRs and antidepressants interact to affect behavior. Thus, nicotinic antagonism may be another important component for antidepressant efficacy.

Mood Stabilizers for Bipolar Disorder and the Cholinergic System

As described above, there is growing evidence to suggest that the cholinergic system may be a potential target for the development of novel molecular approaches to the treatment of depression. The anergic–anhedonic syndrome following a cholinergic agonist was found to be dose-dependent,[148] suggesting that the percent change (and perhaps the speed of change) in intrasynaptic acetylcholinergic concentration is critical. Administration of mood stabilizers such as repeated lithium treatment, divalproex, and atypical antipsychotic drugs (e.g., olanzapine, quetiapine, risperidone, aripiprazole) were reported to increase acetylcholinergic efflux in rat hippocampus and medial prefrontal cortex. The neuroendocrine and pupillary responses to cholinergic activity are increased in depressed subjects,[119] whereas manic subjects are hyporesponsive to cholinergic agents with respect to pupillary responses,[149] and improvement in mania with lithium and valproate is associated with normalization of pupillary responses,[150,151] consistent with the hypotheses that depression is associated with cholinergic overreactivity, whereas mania is associated with a hypocholinergic state.

Reduction in Acetylcholine Concentration Has Antidepressant Effect

Animal studies have also shown that chronic nicotine administration can elicit antidepressant-like effects in rats both in the learned helplessness[152] and the forced swim[153,154] paradigms. Furthermore, the nicotinic partial

agonist cytisine results in antidepressant-like effects in several behavioral paradigms in mice.[15] Because nicotine is a nicotinic receptor agonist, it may seem paradoxical that nicotine administration is antidepressant. If nicotine can relieve depressive symptoms, it might seem counterintuitive that physostigmine, which increases acetylcholine concentration, increases depressive symptoms. Further, several classes of nicotinic agonists have antidepressant actions in both human studies and animal models,[155,156] but several nicotinic antagonists have also shown to have potent antidepressant effects.[155,157] These data can be reconciled if the ability of nicotine to desensitize nAChRs is primarily responsible for its ability to alleviate depressive symptoms. Thus, nicotine and other nicotinic agonists and partial agonists may be antidepressant as they limit the ability of endogenous acetylcholine to signal through nAChRs. Similarly, nicotinic antagonists would exert the same effect on depressive symptoms by decreasing cholinergic tone on nAChRs. Data in human subjects support the idea that blockade rather than activation of nAChRs results in antidepressant-like effects. For example, the noncompetitive, nonselective nAChR antagonist mecamylamine as well as the nicotine patch, a mode of nicotine delivery biased toward desensitization of nAChRs, decrease symptoms of depression in depressed nonsmoking patients and patients with Tourette's syndrome.[158-160] Mecamylamine and the competitive nicotinic antagonist DhbE also have antidepressant-like properties in mice.[15,130] A number of studies have shown that chronic administration of nicotinic agonists (including nicotine through regular smoking or as delivered through the nicotine patch) can desensitize rather than activate nAChRs,[161] leading to functional antagonism.[162] Such an effect would be expected to be antidepressant [153,154]. Indeed, this hypothesis suggests that the increased depressive symptoms observed in some patients following acute cessation from smoking might be explained by the fact that the clearance of nicotine following smoking cessation coupled with persistent nAChR upregulation[51] results in increased ability of ACh to activate these upregulated nAChRs. Increased depressive symptoms following smoking cessation, in addition to other withdrawal symptoms, further consolidate the addiction and suggest that the high prevalence of tobacco use in MDD patients may be an attempt of self-medication.

Nicotine Dependence and Posttraumatic Stress Disorder

Post-traumatic Stress Disorder (PTSD) symptom severity, including depression, is positively correlated with increased smoking, and smokers report an increased urge of smoking in response to trauma. It can be suspected that this high rate of comorbidity between PTSD and smoking[163] is partially explained by the symptomatology of PTSD which includes anxiety, depression, cognitive deficits – all linked to dysfunctional brain acetylcholinergic systems and possible influence by nicotine, which binds to nAChRs (which are found in the thalamus, and less so in the striatum, hippocampus, and cortex). This raises the possibility that in a subpopulation of PTSD patients, nicotine may be exerting anxiolytic and antidepressant effects. Additionally, nicotinic agonists improve performance on tests of working memory, spatial and fear-associated learning, and noncompetitive nAChR antagonists such as mecamylamine impair working memory function in rodents and nonhuman primates.[164–180] Interestingly, unlike most other agonists, postmortem studies have shown that nicotine exposure appears to cause an upregulation of agonist binding to the receptor which may be related to the inactivation of receptor function which occurs with prolonged exposure. Thus, its anti-anxiety/ antidepressant action may be attributable to its paradoxical ability to reduce cholinergic activity. As an example, nicotine treatment diminishes symptoms in a learned helplessness[152] animal model and improves performance on a FST[153,154] measure in FSL rats, an animal model for depression selectively bred for cholinergic sensitivity.

Role of Nicotinic Acetylcholinergic System in Cognition and Behavior in PTSD

Nicotinic cholinergic systems are involved with several aspects of cognitive function including attention, learning, and memory. Nicotinic agonists improve performance on tests of working memory, spatial and fear-associated learning, and noncompetitive nAChR antagonists, such as mecamylamine, impair working memory function in rodents and nonhuman

primates.[164–180] Nicotine also acts upon nAChRs to release GABA, among other neurotransmitters, which is involved in control of mood. Lower GABA levels are seen in individuals with certain anxiety and depressive disorders.[181,182] It can therefore be assumed that the higher the number of nAChRs occupied, the more GABA and other neurotransmitters may be released, and the lower chances for mood and behavioral disorders. This can also be seen in the high prevalence of smoking in mental illness, especially schizophrenia and bipolar disorders. Abstinence from smoking has been shown to relate to enhanced number of psychotic symptoms as well as attentional and executive difficulties in subjects with schizophrenia.[183] Animal studies have shown that exposure to immobilization stress alters the levels of brain nAChR expression.[184] However, immobilization stress may not constitute a relevant model for PTSD in humans. PTSD patients typically show an enhanced inhibition of the hypothalamo-pituitary-adrenal (HPA) axis, which has been reliably reproduced by a single-prolonged stress (SPS) model in rats.[185] nAChR expression has not yet been studied in this model, but self-administration of nicotine in rats has been shown to modulate the sensitization of the HPA axis to stressors.[186]

Brain and Cognition

Some cognitive processes have been localized to specific areas in the brain (e.g., receptive language in Brodmann's areas 44 and 45), whereas others, such as vocabulary, are located throughout the brain. Highest density of nAChRs is in the thalamus, followed by the striatum, hippocampus, and the cortex. The thalamus plays an important role in overall cognitive abilities and has recently been implicated in semantic memory (e.g., in an fMRI study, Assaf et al[187] found more brain activation in the left thalamus during the processing of correct recall versus no recall trials). Most recent knowledge on striatal involvement in cognition comes from better understanding of Parkinson's disease and shows that it plays an important role in cognitive flexibility (ability to switch between tasks[188]). The hippocampus has been implicated in amnestic disorders and commonly associated with declarative memory. Studies of damage localized to the brain stem reveal surprising association with markedly impaired executive functioning, attention, and some memory processes.[189] In terms of the cortical regions, it is well established that the frontal lobes are associated with executive abilities, attention/concentration, among other processes; the temporal cortex is important in receptive and expressive language; the parietal lobes are involved in visuospatial abilities, the occipital cortex is deemed the "visual" cortex, and the cerebellum is involved in motor abilities and some forms of learning. The anterior cingulate is involved in many top-down and bottom-up processes, including learning and problem solving,[190] as well as in emotional processes. All of the described brain areas contain at least a detectable number of nAChRs, and future research should look at these regions of interest and compare the receptor occupancy with the results from cognitive task.

β₂-nAChR Availability in PTSD

To assess β₂-nAChR availability in PTSD, ten patients with PTSD (seven female, mean ± SD age = 41.8 ± 13.0 years) and ten age- and gender-matched healthy controls (seven female, mean ± SD age = 39.4 ± 14.5 years) were imaged using [^{123}I]5-IA SPECT Imaging.[191] Multivariate ANOVA considering all primary regions of interest showed a significant difference in [^{123}I]5-IA binding between controls and PTSD patients ($F=4.29$, $p=0.038$). Between-group differences were most pronounced in the mesiotemporal cortex where PTSD patients relative to controls showed significantly higher [^{123}I]5-IA binding ($F=6.20$, $p=0.030$, see Fig. 10.2). A nonsignificant trend was detected toward higher [^{123}I]5-IA binding when comparing the total group of PTSD patients (including four PTSD patients and three healthy control subjects with smoking history) versus controls ($F=2.91$, $p=0.057$). In PTSD patients, [^{123}I]5-IA binding did not correlate with CAPS-D scores or HDRS scores in any region of interest. [^{123}I]5-IA binding in PTSD patients was independent of a diagnosis of current or lifetime Major Depression or diagnosis of past alcohol abuse. This is the first study to support an involvement of β2-nAChRs in PTSD, showing a significant difference between PTSD patients and controls in [^{123}I]5-IA binding with most prominence in never-smoking individuals.

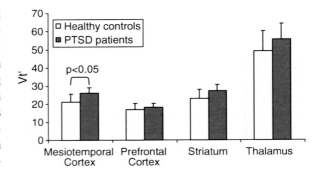

Fig. 10.2 Never-smoking PTSD patients compared to never-smoking healthy controls showed significant higher [^{123}I]5-IA binding in the mesiotemporal cortex (ANOVA: $F=6.21$, $p=0.030$; MANOVA: $F=4.29$, $p=0.038$). Shown are mean and standard deviation of regional [^{123}I]5-IA binding, as determined by V_T' (regional activity/total plasma parent)

The study by Czermak et al[191] found a difference in β2-nAChR availability between never-smoking healthy controls and never-smoking patients with PTSD. This difference was prominent in the mesiotemporal cortex, which includes two regions that have been consistently implicated in the neurocircuitry of PTSD: the amygdala und hippocampus.[192] Both regions have been shown to play a critical role in memory and may be involved in memory deficits shown by PTSD patients.[193] Decreases in hippocampal volume in PTSD patients have been shown to be inversely associated with verbal memory deficits,[192] and infusion of α4β2 nAChR antagonists in the amygdala and hippocampus both produced working memory impairments in rats.[194] The mesiotemporal cortex is anatomically and functionally closely connected to the thalamus, which also has been implicated in PTSD.[195] nAChRs modulate the vividness of dreams[196] and play an important role in learning and memory.[197] This raise the possibility that β2-nAChRs contribute to reexperiencing symptoms in PTSD by modulating the sensory input to the cortex and by modulating cortical neuroplasticity associated with learning and stress response. Furthermore, studies of Golf War veterans showed that these individuals exhibit deficits in working memory, sustained attention, initial learning (e.g., verbal), and retroactive interference. Some of these domains are serviced by the frontal lobes, which contain some nAChRs. Thalamus, which contains the largest amount of nicotinic receptors, also plays an important role in memory.

PTSD is associated with cognitive dysfunction, including memory impairment. Hippocampus (moderate levels of nAChRs) plays an important role in memory – especially in process of converting short-term memory into long-term stores, and the thalamus (high levels of nAChRs) has been implicated in semantic memory. Hippocampal volume decrease in PTSD has been detected by MRI scans, and decreased activation is detected by PET. Therefore, it is evident that areas containing nicotinic receptors are highly involved in cognitive processes, and their role in experiences and deficits associated with PTSD needs to be better understood.

Conclusion

There is an emerging body of evidence derived from imaging studies on nAChR and tobacco smoking, which provide data to better understand the clinical course of smoking in relation to mood, stress, and cognition. Tobacco smokers were found to have higher $\beta2$-nAChR availability at 1 week of abstinence before it returned to nonsmoker levels at 6–12 weeks of abstinence,[53,198] signifying the prolonged symptoms of craving and withdrawal observed in tobacco smokers. Exploring the cerebral MAO-A in vivo in smokers, Fowler et al[55] and Leroy et al[61] reported a widespread reduction of MAO-A activity clinically relevant to understand the high prevalence of smoking in MDD and PTSD patients. Never-smoking PTSD patients had higher β_2-nAChR binding in the mesiotemporal cortex when compared to never-smoking healthy controls.[191] Apart from documenting an involvement of β_2-nAChR in PTSD, this could have implications for future studies on tobacco smoking and cognition as the mesiotemporal cortex includes the amygdala and hippocampus,[192] both regions known to play a crucial role in memory and emotional regulation. Therefore, this receptor subtype may be directly involved in the neurobiology of mood and anxiety disorders or could be a modulator of other neurobiological systems which are involved in its etiology. Further studies should aim to further clarify the potential role of β_2-nAChRs in the comorbidity of smoking, MDD, and PTSD, as this represents important clinical problems. The findings discussed here also raise the possibility that the β_2-nAChR may be an interesting candidate for drug development.

References

1. Le Foll B, Goldberg SR. Effects of nicotine in experimental animals and humans: an update on addictive properties. *Handb Exp Pharmacol.* 2009;192:335–367.
2. Rose J, Tashkin D, Ertle A, Zinser M, Lafer R. Sensory blockade of smoking satisfaction. *Pharmacol Biochem Behav.* 1985;23L:289–293.
3. Rose J, Behm F. Refined cigarette smoke as a method for reducing nicotine intake. *Pharmacol Biochem Behav.* 1987;28:305–310.
4. Rose J, Levin E. Inter-relationships between conditioned and primary reinforcement in the maintenance of cigarette smoking. *Br J Addict.* 1991;86:605–609.
5. Rose J, Behm F, Levine E. The role of nicotine dose and sensory cues in the regulation of smoke intake. *Pharmacol Biochem Behav.* 1993;44:891–900.
6. Butschky M, Bailer D, Henningfield J, Pickworth W. Smoking without nicotine delivery decreases withdrawal in 12-hour abstinent smokers. *Pharmacol Biochem Behav.* 1995;50:91–96.
7. Gross J, Lee J, Stitzer M. Nicotine-containing versus de-nicotinized cigarettes: effects on craving and withdrawal. *Pharmacol Biochem Behav.* 1997;57:159–165.
8. Pickworth W, Fant R, Nelson R, Rohrer M, Henningfield J. Pharmacodynamic effects of new denicotinized cigarettes. *Nicotine Tob Res.* 1999;1:357–364.
9. Rose J, Westman E, Behm F, Johnson M, Goldberg J. Blockade of smoking satisfaction uisng the peripheral nicotinic antagonist trimethaphan. *Pharmacol Biochem Behav.* 1999;62:165–172.
10. Shahan T, Bickel W, Madden G, Badger G. Comparing the reinforcing efficacy of nicotine containing and de-nicotinized cigarettes: a behavioral economic analysis. *Psychopharmacology (Berl).* 1999;147:210–216.
11. Dallery J, Houtsmuller E, Pickworth W, Stitzer M. Effects of cigarette nicotine content and smoking pace on subsequent craving and smoking. *Psychopharmacology (Berl).* 2003;165: 172–180.
12. Rose J, Behm F, Westman E, Bates J, Salley A. Pharmacologic and sensorimotor components of satiation in cigarette smoking. *Pharmacol Biochem Behav.* 2003;76:243–250.
13. Picciotto MR. Common aspects of the action of nicotine and other drugs of abuse. *Drug Alcohol Depend.* 1998;51(1–2): 165–172.
14. Picciotto MR, Brunzell DH, Caldarone BJ. Effect of nicotine and nicotinic receptors on anxiety and depression. *Neuroreport.* 2002;13(9):1097–1106.
15. Mineur YS, Somenzi O, Picciotto MR. Cytisine, a partial agonist of high-affinity nicotinic acetylcholine receptors, has antidepressant-like properties in male C57BL/6J mice. *Neuropharmacology.* 2007;52(5):1256–1262.
16. Bertrand D, Changeux J. Nicotinic receptor: an allosteric protein specialized for intracellular communication. *Semin Neurosci.* 1992;7:75–90.
17. Elgoyhen AB, Johnson DS, Boulter J, Vetter DE, Heinemann S. Alpha 9: an acetylcholine receptor with novel pharmacological properties expressed in rat cochlear hair cells. *Cell.* 1994;79:705–715.

18. Sargent PB. The diversity of neuronal nicotinic acetylcholine receptors. *Annu Rev Neurosci.* 1993;16:403–443.

19. Gotti C, Fornasari D, Clementi F. Human neuronal nicotinic receptors. *Prog Neurobiol.* 1997;53:199–237.

20. Coplan JD, Smith ELP, Altemus M, et al. Variable foraging demand rearing: sustained elevations in cisternal cerebrospinal fluid corticotropin-releasing factor concentrations in adult primates. *Biol Psychiatry.* 2001;50(3):200–204.

21. Preisig M, Bellivier F, Fenton BT, et al. Association between bipolar disorder and monoamine oxidase A gene polymorphisms: results of a multicenter study. *Am J Psychiatry.* 2000;157:948–955.

22. Le Novere N, Corringer PJ, Changeux JP. The diversity of subunit composition in nAChRs: evolutionary origins, physiologic and pharmacologic consequences. *J Neurobiol.* 2002;53(4):447–456.

23. Le Novère N, Changeux J-P. Molecular evolution of the nicotinic acetylcholine receptor: an example of multigene family in excitable cells. *J Mol Evol.* 1995;40:155–172.

24. Zoli M, Léna C, Picciotto MR, Changeux J-P. Identification of four classes of brain nicotinic receptors using b2-mutant mice. *J Neurosci.* 1998;18:4461–4472.

25. Buss AH, Perry M. The aggression questionnaire. *J Pers Soc Psychol.* 1992;63(3):452–459.

26. Court J, Clementi F. Distribution of nicotinic subtypes in human brain. *Alzheimer Dis Assoc Disord.* 1995;9(suppl 2):6–14.

27. Perry A, Tarrier N, Morriss R, McCarthy E, Limb K. Randomised controlled trial of efficacy of teaching patients with bipolar disorder to identify early symptoms of relapse and obtain treatment. *Br Med J.* 1999;318: 149–153.

28. Benwell M, Balfour D, Anderson J. Evidence that tobacco smoking increases the density of (–)-[^{3}H]nicotine binding site in human brain. *J Neurochem.* 1988;50:1243–1247.

29. Breese C, Marks M, Logel J, et al. Effect of smoking history on [^{3}H]nicotine binding in human postmortem brain. *J Pharmacol Exp Ther.* 1997;282:7–13.

30. Court J, Lloyd S, Thomas N, et al. Dopamine and nicotinic receptor binding and the levels of dopamine and homovanillic acid in human brain related to tobacco use. *Neuroscience.* 1998;87:63–78.

31. Perry D, Dávila-García M, Stockmeier C, Kellar K. Increased nicotinic receptors in brains from smokers: membrane binding and autoradiography studies. *J Pharmacol Exp Ther.* 1999; 289:1545–1552.

32. Bhat R, Turner S, Selvaag S, Marks M, Collins A. Regulation of brain nicotinic receptors by chronic agonist infusion. *J Neurochem.* 1991;56:1932–1939.

33. Collins A, Marks M. Chronic nicotine exposure and brain nicotinic receptors – influence of genetic factors. *Prog Brain Res.* 1989;79:137–146.

34. Marks M, Stitzel J, Collins A. Time course study of the effects of chronic nicotine infusion on drug response and brain receptors. *J Pharmacol Exp Ther.* 1985;235:619–628.

35. Marks M, Romm E, Gaffney D, Collins A. Nicotine-induced tolerance and receptor changes in four mouse strains. *J Pharmacol Exp Ther.* 1986;237:809–819.

36. Marks M, Pauly J, Gross S, et al. Nicotine binding and nicotinic receptor subunit RNA after chronic nicotine treatment. *J Neurosci.* 1992;12:2765–2784.

37. Wonnacott S. The paradox of nicotinic acetylcholine receptor upregulation by nicotine. *Trends Pharmacol Sci.* 1990;11: 216–219.

38. Flores C, Rogers S, Pabreza L, Wolfe B, Kellar K. A subtype of nicotinic cholinergic receptor in rat brain is composed of alpha 4 and beta 2 subunits and is up-regulated by chronic nicotine treatment. *Mol Pharmacol.* 1992;41:31–37.

39. Ksir C, Hakan R, Kellar K. Chronic nicotine and locomoter activity: influences of exposure dose and test dose. *Psychopharmacology (Berl).* 1987;92:25–29.

40. Nordberg A, Romanelli L, Sundwall A, Bianchi C, Beani L. Effect of acute and subchronic nicotine treatment on cortical acetylchoine release and on nicotinic receptors in rats and guinea-pigs. *Br J Pharmacol.* 1989;98:71–78.

41. Schwartz R, Kellar K. Nicotinic cholinergic receptor binding sites in the brain: regulation in vivo. *Science.* 1983;220: 214–216.

42. Schwartz R, Kellar K. In vivo regulation of [^{3}H]acetylcholine recognition sites in brain by nicotinic cholinergic drugs. *J Neurochem.* 1985;45:427–433.

43. Kassiou M, Eberl S, Meikle S, et al. In vivo imaging of nicotinic receptor upregulation following chronic (–)-nicotine treatment in baboon using SPECT. *Nucl Med Biol.* 2001;28: 165–175.

44. Baldwin R, Zoghbi S, Staley J, et al. Chemical fate of the nicotinic acetylcholinergic radiotracer [^{123}I]5-IA-85380 in baboon brain and plasma. *Nucl Med Biol.* 2006;33:549–554.

45. Sedvall G, Farde L, Nyback H, et al. Recent advances in psychiatric brain imaging. *Acta Radiol Suppl.* 1990;374:113–115.

46. Horti AG, Koren AO, Lee KS, et al. Radiosynthesis and preliminary evaluation of 5-[$^{123/125}$I]iodo-3-(2(S)-azetidinylmethoxy)pyridine: a radioligand for nicotinic acetylcholine receptors. *Nucl Med Biol.* 1999;26(2):175–182.

47. Fan H, Scheffel UA, Rauseo P, et al. [$^{125/123}$I] 5-Iodo-3-pyridyl ethers: syntheses and binding to neuronal nicotinic acetylcholine receptors. *Nucl Med Biol.* 2001;28(8):911–921.

48. Chefer SI, Horti AG, Lee KS, et al. In vivo imaging of brain nicotinic acetylcholine receptors with 5-[^{123}I]iodo-A-85380 using single photon emission computed tomography. *Life Sci.* 1998;63(25):PL355-PL360.

49. Fujita M, Charney DS, Innis RB. Imaging serotonergic neurotransmission in depression: hippocampal pathophysiology may mirror global brain alterations. *Biol Psychiatry.* 2000;48(8):801–812.

50. Horti AG, Chefer SI, Mukhin AG, et al. 6-[^{18}F]fluoro-A-85380, a novel radioligand for in vivo imaging of central nicotinic acetylcholine receptors. *Life Sci.* 2000;67(4):463–469.

51. Staley J, Krishnan-Sarin S, Cosgrove K, et al. Human tobacco smokers in early abstinence have higher levels of beta2-nicotinic acetylcholine receptors than nonsmokers. *J Neurosci.* 2006;26(34):8707–8714.

52. Brody A, Mandelkern M, London E, et al. Cigarette smoking saturates brain alpha 4 beta 2 nicotinic acetylcholine receptors. *Arch Gen Psychiatry.* 2006;63:907–915.

53. Cosgrove KP, Batis J, Bois F, et al. Beta2-nicotinic acetylcholine receptor availability during acute and prolonged abstinence from tobacco smoking. *Arch Gen Psychiatry.* 2009;66(6):666–676.

54. Kahlil A, Steyn S, Castagnoli N. Isolation and characterization of monoamine oxidase inhibitor from tobacco leaves. *Chem Res Toxicol.* 2000;13:31–35.

55. Fowler JS, Volkow ND, Wang GJ, et al. Brain monoamine oxidase A inhibition in cigarette smokers. *Proc Natl Acad Sci U S A*. 1996;93(24):14065–14069.

56. Fowler JS, Volkow ND, Wang GJ, et al. Neuropharmacological actions of cigarette smoke: brain monoamine oxidase B (MAO B) inhibition. *J Addict Dis*. 1998;17(1):23–34.

57. Fowler JS, Volkow ND, Wang GJ, et al. Inhibition of monoamine oxidase B in the brains of smokers. *Nature*. 1996; 379(6567):733–736.

58. Berlin I, Said S, Spreux-Varoquaux O, Olivares R, Launay J-M, Peuch A. Monoamine oxidase A and B activities in heavy smokers. *Biol Psychol*. 1995;38:756–761.

59. Norman T, Chamberlain K, French M. Platelet monoamine oxidase: low activity in cigarette smokers. *Psychiatry Res*. 1987;20:199–205.

60. Norman T, Chamberlain K, French M. Platelet monoamine oxidase and cigarette smoking. *J Affect Disord*. 1987;4:73–77.

61. Leroy C, Bragulat V, Berlin I, et al. Cerebral monoamine oxidase A inhibition in tobacco smokers confirmed with PET and [^{11}C]befloxatone. *J Clin Psychopharmacol*. 2009;29(1): 86–88.

62. Ginovart N, Meyer JH, Boovariwala A, et al. Positron emission tomography quantification of [^{11}C]-harmine binding to monoamine oxidase-A in the human brain. *J Cereb Blood Flow Metab*. 2006;26(3):330–344.

63. Meyer JH, Ginovart N, Boovariwala A, et al. Elevated monoamine oxidase a levels in the brain: an explanation for the monoamine imbalance of major depression. *Arch Gen Psychiatry*. 2006;63(11):1209–1216.

64. Leonard S, Adler LE, Benhammou K, et al. Smoking and mental illness. *Pharmacol Biochem Behav*. 2001;70(4): 561–570.

65. Thaker G. Psychosis endophenotypes in schizophrenia and bipolar disorder. *Schizophr Bull*. 2008;34(4):720–721.

66. Zimmerman M, Chelminski I, McDermut W. Major depressive disorder and axis I diagnostic comorbidity. *J Clin Psychiatry*. 2002;63(3):187–193.

67. Rose J, Behm F, Ramsey C, Ritchie J. Platelet monoamine oxidase, smoking cessation and tobacco withdrawal symptoms. *Nicotine Tob Res*. 2001;3:383–390.

68. VanDenEijnden R, Spijkerman R, Fekkes D. Craving for cigarettes among low and high dependent smokers: impact of norharman. *Addict Biol*. 2003;8:463–472.

69. Wesnes K, Simpson P, Christmas L, Anand R, McClelland G. The effects of moclobemide on cognition. *J Neural Transm*. 1989;28:91–102.

70. Allain H, Lieury A, Brunet-Bourgin F, et al. Antidepressants and cognition: comparative effects of moclobemide, viloxazine and maprotiline. *Psychopharmacology (Berl)*. 1991; 106(suppl):S56–S61.

71. Fairweather D, Kerr J, Hindmarch I. The effects of moclobemide on psychomotor performance and cognitive function. *Int Clin Psychopharmacol*. 1993;8:43–47.

72. Dignemanse J, Berlin I, Payan C, Tede H, Puech A. Comparative investigation of the effect of moclobemide and toloxatone on monoamine oxidase activity and psychometric performance in healthy subjects. *Psychopharmacology (Berl)*. 1992;106:S68–S70.

73. Frank M, Braszko J. Moclobemide enhances aversively motivated learning and memory in rats. *Pol J Pharmacol*. 1999;1999:497–503.

74. Getova D, Dimitrova D, Roukounakis I. Effects of the antidepressant drug moclobemide on learning and memory in rats. *Methods Find Exp Clin Pharmacol*. 2003;25:811–815.

75. Knoll J. The pharmacology of selegiline ((−)deprenyl). New aspects. *Acta Neurol Scand*. 1988;80(suppl 126):83–91.

76. Brandeis R, Sapir M, Kapon Y, Borelli G, Cadel S, Valsecchi B. Improvement of cognitive function by MAO-B inhibitor l-deprenyl in aged rats. *Pharmacol Biochem Behav*. 1991;39: 297–304.

77. Gelowitz D, Richardson J, Wishart T, Yu P, Lai C-T. Chronic l-deprenyl or l-amphetamine: equal cognitive enhancement, unequal MAO inhibition. *Pharmacol Biochem Behav*. 1994;47:41–45.

78. Riggs PD, Mikulich SK, Whitmore EA, Crowley TJ. Relationship of ADHD, depression, and non-tobacco substance use disorders to nicotine dependence in substance-dependent delinquents. *Drug Alcohol Depend*. 1999;54(3): 195–205.

79. Breslau N, Kilbey MM, Andreski P. Nicotine dependence and major depression: new evidence from a prospective investigation. *Arch Gen Psychiatry*. 1993;50(1):31–35.

80. Brown RA, Lewinsohn PM, Seeley JR, Wagner EF. Cigarette smoking, major depression, and other psychiatric disorders among adolescents. *J Am Acad Child Adolesc Psychiatry*. 1996;35(12):1602–1610.

81. Scarinci IC, Thomas J, Brantley PJ, Jones GN. Examination of the temporal relationship between smoking and major depressive disorder among low-income women in public primary care clinics. *Am J Health Promot*. 2002;16(6):323–330.

82. Levine MD, Marcus MD, Perkins KA. A history of depression and smoking cessation outcomes among women concerned about post-cessation weight gain. *Nicotine Tob Res*. 2003;5(1):69–76.

83. Anda RF, Williamson DF, Escobedo LG, Mast EE, Giovino GA, Remington PL. Depression and the dynamics of smoking. A national perspective. *JAMA*. 1990;264(12):1541–1545.

84. Glassman AH, Helzer JE, Covey LS, et al. Smoking, smoking cessation, and major depression. *JAMA*. 1990;264(12): 1546–1549.

85. Glassman AH, Stetner F, Walsh BT, et al. Heavy smokers, smoking cessation, and clonidine. Results of a double-blind, randomized trial. *JAMA*. 1988;259(19):2863–2866.

86. Glassman AH, Covey LS, Dalack GW, et al. Smoking cessation, clonidine, and vulnerability to nicotine among dependent smokers. *Clin Pharmacol Ther*. 1993;54(6): 670–679.

87. Killen JD, Fortmann SP, Schatzberg A, Hayward C, Varady A. Onset of major depression during treatment for nicotine dependence. *Addict Behav*. 2003;28(3):461–470.

88. Grant BF, Hasin DS, Chou SP, Stinson FS, Dawson DA. Nicotine dependence and psychiatric disorders in the United States: results from the national epidemiologic survey on alcohol and related conditions. *Arch Gen Psychiatry*. 2004;61(11):1107–1115.

89. Quattrocki E, Baird A, Yurgelun-Todd D. Biological aspects of the link between smoking and depression. *Harv Rev Psychiatry*. 2000;8(3):99–110.

90. Paz R, Barsness B, Martenson T, Tanner D, Allan AM. Behavioral teratogenicity induced by nonforced maternal nicotine consumption. *Neuropsychopharmacology*. 2007;32(3): 693–699.

91. Leventhal AM, Francione Witt C, Zimmerman M. Associations between depression subtypes and substance use disorders. *Psychiatry Res.* 2008;161(1):43–50.

92. Gentry MV, Hammersley JJ, Hale CR, Nuwer PK, Meliska CJ. Nicotine patches improve mood and response speed in a lexical decision task. *Addict Behav.* 2000;25(4):549–557.

93. Masson CL, Gilbert DG. Cardiovascular and mood responses to quantified doses of cigarette smoke in oral contraceptive users and nonusers. *J Behav Med.* 1999;22(6):589–604.

94. Parrott AC. Nesbitt's paradox resolved? Stress and arousal modulation during cigarette smoking. *Addiction.* 1998;93(1): 27–39.

95. Pomerleau CS, Pomerleau OF. Euphoriant effects of nicotine in smokers. *Psychopharmacology (Berl).* 1992;108(4): 460–465.

96. Perkins KA, Doyle T, Ciccocioppo M, Conklin C, Sayette M, Caggiula A. Sex differences in the influence of nicotine dose instructions on the reinforcing and self-reported rewarding effects of smoking. *Psychopharmacology (Berl).* 2006;184(3–4):600–607.

97. Spring B, Cook JW, Appelhans B, et al. Nicotine effects on affective response in depression-prone smokers. *Psychopharmacology (Berl).* 2008;196(3):461–471.

98. Kalman D, Morissette SB, George TP. Co-morbidity of smoking in patients with psychiatric and substance use disorders. *Am J Addict.* 2005;14(2):106–123.

99. Pomerleau CS, Mehringer AM, Marks JL, Downey KK, Pomerleau OF. Effects of menstrual phase and smoking abstinence in smokers with and without a history of major depressive disorder. *Addict Behav.* 2000;25(4):483–497.

100. Williams JM, Ziedonis D. Addressing tobacco among individuals with a mental illness or an addiction. *Addict Behav.* 2004;29(6):1067–1083.

101. Lasser K, Boyd JW, Woolhandler S, Himmelstein DU, McCormick D, Bor DH. Smoking and mental illness: a population-based prevalence study. *JAMA.* 2000;284(20): 2606–2610.

102. Hughes JR, Hatsukami DK, Mitchell JE, Dahlgren LA. Prevalence of smoking among psychiatric outpatients. *Am J Psychiatry.* 1986;143(8):993–997.

103. Hennessy S, Bilker WB, Knauss JS, et al. Cardiac arrest and ventricular arrhythmia in patients taking antipsychotic drugs: cohort study using administrative data. *BMJ.* 2002;325(7372):1070.

104. Morris CD, Giese AA, Turnbull JJ, Dickinson M, Johnson-Nagel N. Predictors of tobacco use among persons with mental illnesses in a statewide population. *Psychiatr Serv.* 2006;57(7):1035–1038.

105. Labbate LA. Nicotine cessation, mania, and depression. *Am J Psychiatry.* 1992;149(5):708.

106. Benazzi F. Severe mania following abrupt nicotine withdrawal. *Am J Psychiatry.* 1989;146(12):1641.

107. Cohen SB. Mania after nicotine withdrawal. *Am J Psychiatry.* 1990;147(9):1254–1255.

108. Berk M, Ng F, Wang WV, et al. Going up in smoke: tobacco smoking is associated with worse treatment outcomes in mania. *J Affect Disord.* 2008;110(1–2):126–134.

109. Clarke PBS, Pert A. Autoradiographic evidence for nicotine receptors in nigrostriatal and mesolimbic dopaminergic neurons. *Brain Res.* 1985;348:355–358.

110. Giorguieff-Chesselet MF, Kemel ML, Wandscheer D, Glowinski J. Regulation of dopamine release by presynaptic nicotinic receptors in rat striatal slices: effect of nicotine in a low concentration. *Life Sci.* 1979;25:1257–1262.

111. Yoshida K, Kato Y, Imura H. Nicotine induced release of noradrenaline from hypothalamic synaptosomes. *Brain Res.* 1980;182:361–368.

112. Wonnacott S, Drasdo A, Sanderson E, Rowell P. Presynaptic nicotinic receptors and the modulation of transmission release. In: Block G, Marsh J, eds. *The Biology of Nicotine Dependence.* Chichester, UK: Wiley; 1990:87–105.

113. Muller-Oerlinghausen B, Muser-Causemann B, Volk J. Suicides and parasuicides in a high-risk patient group on and off lithium long-term medication. *J Affect Disord.* 1992;25:261–270.

114. Mihailescu S, Palomerorivero M, Meadehuerta P, Mazaflores A, Druckercolin R. Effects of nicotine and mecamylamine on rat dorsal raphe neurons. *Eur J Pharmacol.* 1998;360(1): 31–36.

115. File SE, Kenny PJ, Cheeta S. The role of the dorsal hippocampal serotonergic and cholinergic systems in the modulation of anxiety. *Pharmacol Biochem Behav.* 2000;66(1): 65–72.

116. Toth E, Sershen H, Hashim A, Vizi ES, Lajtha A. Effect of nicotine on extracellular levels of neurotransmitters assessed by microdialysis in various brain regions: role of glutamic acid. *Neurochem Res.* 1992;17(3):265–271.

117. Mansvelder HD, Keath JR, McGehee DS. Synaptic mechanisms underlie nicotine-induced excitability of brain reward areas. *Neuron.* 2002;33:905–919.

118. Janowsky DS, El-Yousef MK, Davis JM, Sekerke HJ. A cholinergic-adrenergic hypothesis of mania and depression. *Lancet.* 1972;2(7778):632–635.

119. Dilsaver SC. Pathophysiology of "cholinoceptor supersensitivity" in affective disorders. *Biol Psychiatry.* 1986;21(8–9): 813–829.

120. Risch SC, Cohen RM, Janowsky DS, Kalin NH, Murphy DL. Mood and behavioral effects of physostigmine on humans are accompanied by elevations in plasma beta-endorphin and cortisol. *Science.* 1980;209(4464):1545–1546.

121. Janowsky DS, Overstreet DH. Cholinergic dysfunction in depression. *Pharmacol Toxicol.* 1990;3:100–111.

122. Overstreet DH. The flinders sensitive line rats: a genetic animal model of depression. *Neurosci Biobehav Rev.* 1993;17(1):51–68.

123. Dilsaver SC, Greden JF, Snider RM. Antidepressant withdrawal syndromes: phenomenology and physiopathology. *Int Clin Psychopharmacol.* 1987;2:1–19.

124. Furey ML, Drevets WC. Antidepressant efficacy of the antimuscarinic drug Scopolamine: a randomized, placebo-controlled clinical trial. *Arch Gen Psychiatry.* 2006;63(10): 1121–1129.

125. Wang JC, Hinrichs AL, Stock H, et al. Evidence of common and specific genetic effects: association of the muscarinic acetylcholine receptor M2 (CHRM2) gene with alcohol dependence and major depressive syndrome. *Hum Mol Genet.* 2004;13(17):1903–1911.

126. Comings D, Wu S, Rostamkhani M, McGue M, Iacono WG, MacMurray JP. Association of the muscarinic cholinergic 2 receptor (*CHRM2*) gene with major depression in women. *Am J Med Genet.* 2002;114(5):527–529.

127. Lai IC, Hong C-J, Tsai S-J. Association study of nicotinic-receptor variants and major depressive disorder. *J Affect Disord*. 2001;66(1):79–82.

128. Browne RG. Effects of antidepressants and anticholinergics in a mouse "behavioral despair" test. *Eur J Pharmacol*. 1979;58(3):331–334.

129. Overstreet DH, Russell RW, Hay DA, Crocker AD. Selective breeding for increased cholinergic function – biometrical genetic-analysis of muscarinic responses. *Neuropsychopharmacology*. 1992;7(3):197–204.

130. Rabenstein RL, Caldarone BJ, Picciotto MR. The nicotinic antagonist mecamylamine has antidepressant-like effects in wild-type but not β2- or α7-nicotinic acetylcholine receptor subunit knockout mice. *Psychopharmacology (Berl)*. 2006;189(3):395–401.

131. Booij L, Swenne CA, Brosschot JF, Haffmans PMJ, Thayer JF, Van der Does AJW. Tryptophan depletion affects heart rate variability and impulsivity in remitted depressed patients with a history of suicidal ideation. *Biol Psychiatry*. 2006;60(5):507–514.

132. Risch SC, Kalin NH, Janowsky DS. Cholinergic challenges in affective-illness – behavioral and neuroendocrine correlates. *J Clin Psychopharmacol*. 1981;1(4):186–192.

133. Janowsky DS, El-Yousef MK, Davis JM. Acetylcholine and depression. *Psychosom Med*. 1974;36(3):248–257.

134. Rubin RT, O'Toole SM, Rhodes ME, Sekula LK, Czambel RK. Hypothalamo-pituitary-adrenal cortical responses to low-dose physostigmine and arginine vasopressin administration: sex differences between major depressives and matched control subjects. *Psychiatry Res*. 1999;89(1):1–20.

135. Berger M, Riemann D, Hochli D, Spiegel R. The cholinergic rapid eye movement sleep induction test with RS-86. State or trait marker of depression? *Arch Gen Psychiatry*. 1989;46(5):421–428.

136. Raisman R, Briley M, Langer SZ. Specific tricyclic antidepressant binding sites in rat brain. *Nature*. 1979;281(5727): 148–150.

137. Stanton T, Bolden-Watson C, Cusack B, Richelson E. Antagonism of the five cloned human muscarinic cholinergic receptors expressed in CHO-K1 cells by antidepressants and antihistaminics. *Biochem Pharmacol*. 1993;45(11): 2352–2354.

138. Schatzberg AF. Employing pharmacologic treatment of bipolar disorder to greatest effect. *J Clin Psychiatry*. 2004;65:15–20.

139. Dalley JW, Fryer TD, Brichard L, et al. Nucleus accumbens D2/3 receptors predict trait impulsivity and cocaine reinforcement. *Science*. 2007;315(5816):1267–1270.

140. Segurado R, Detera-Wadleigh SD, Levinson DF, et al. Genome scan meta-analysis of schizophrenia and bipolar disorder, part III: bipolar disorder. *Am J Hum Genet*. 2003;73(1):49–62.

141. Lopez-Valdes HE, Garcia-Colunga J. Antagonism of nicotinic acetylcholine receptors by inhibitors of monoamine uptake. *Mol Psychiatry*. 2001;6(5):511–519.

142. Garcia-Colunga J, Awad JN, Miledi R. Blockage of muscle and neuronal nicotinic acetylcholine receptors by fluoxetine (Prozac). *Proc Natl Acad Sci U S A*. 1997;94(5):2041–2044.

143. Miller DK, Sumithran SP, Dwoskin LP. Bupropion inhibits nicotine-evoked [$^{(3)}$H]overflow from rat striatal slices preloaded with [$^{(3)}$H]dopamine and from rat hippocampal slices preloaded with [$^{(3)}$H]norepinephrine. *J Pharmacol Exp Ther*. 2002;302(3):1113–1122.

144. Hennings EC, Kiss JP, De Oliveira K, Toth PT, Vizi ES. Nicotinic acetylcholine receptor antagonistic activity of monoamine uptake blockers in rat hippocampal slices. *J Neurochem*. 1999;73(3):1043–1050.

145. Slemmer JE, Martin BR, Damaj MI. Bupropion is a nicotinic antagonist. *J Pharmacol Exp Ther*. 2000;295:321–327.

146. Olausson P, Engel JA, Soderpalm B. Behavioral sensitization to nicotine is associated with behavioral disinhibition; counteraction by citalopram. *Psychopharmacologia*. 1999;142(2): 111–119.

147. Popik P, Kozela E, Krawczyk M. Nicotine and nicotinic receptor antagonists potentiate the antidepressant-like effects of imipramine and citalopram. *Br J Pharmacol*. 2003;139(6): 1196–1202.

148. Lesch KP, Rupprecht R, Poten B, et al. Endocrine responses to 5-hydroxytryptamine-1A receptor activation by ipsapirone in humans. *Biol Psychiatry*. 1989;26(2):203–205.

149. Sokolski KN, DeMet EM. Cholinergic sensitivity predicts severity of mania. *Psychiatry Res*. 2000;95(3):195–200.

150. Hrdina PD, Demeter E, Vu TB, Sotonyi P, Palkovits M. 5-HT uptake sites and 5-HT2 receptors in brain of antidepressant-free suicide victims/depressives: increase in 5-HT2 sites in cortex and amygdala. *Brain Res*. 1993;614(1–2): 37–44.

151. Sokolski KN, DeMet EM. Pupillary cholinergic sensitivity to pilocarpine increases in manic lithium responders. *Biol Psychiatry*. 1999;45(12):1580–1584.

152. Semba J, Mataki C, Yamada S, Nankai M, Toru M. Antidepressant-like effects of chronic nicotine on learned helplessness paradigm in rats. *Biol Psychiatry*. 1998;43(5): 389–391.

153. Djuric VJ, Dunn E, Overstreet DH, Dragomir A, Steiner M. Antidepressant effect of ingested nicotine in female rats of Flinders resistant and sensitive lines. *Physiol Behav*. 1999;67(4):533–537.

154. Tizabi Y, Overstreet DH, Rezvani AH, et al. Antidepressant effects of nicotine in an animal model of depression. *Psychopharmacology (Berl)*. 1999;142(2):193–199.

155. Ferguson SM, Brodkin JD, Lloyd GK, Menzaghi F. Antidepressant-like effects of the subtype-selective nicotinic acetylcholine receptor agonist, SIB-1508Y, in the learned helplessness rat model of depression. *Psychopharmacology (Berl)*. 2000;152(3):295–303.

156. Gatto GJ, Bohme GA, Caldwell WS, et al. TC-1734: an orally active neuronal nicotinic acetylcholine receptor modulator with antidepressant, neuroprotective and long-lasting cognitive effects. *CNS Drug Rev*. 2004;10(2): 147–166.

157. Shytle RD, Silver AA, Sheehan KH, Sheehan DV, Sanberg PR. Neuronal nicotinic receptor inhibition for treating mood disorders: preliminary controlled evidence with mecamylamine. *Depress Anxiety*. 2002;16(3):89–92.

158. George TP, Sacco KA, Vessicchio JC, Weinberger AH, Shytle RD. Nicotinic antagonist augmentation of selective serotonin reuptake inhibitor-refractory major depressive disorder: a preliminary study. *J Clin Psychopharmacol*. 2008;28(3):340–344.

159. Mihailescu S, Drucker-Colin R. Nicotine, brain nicotinic receptors, and neuropsychiatric disorders. *Arch Med Res.* 2000;31(2):131–144.

160. Dursun SM, Kutcher S. Smoking, nicotine and psychiatric disorders: evidence for therapeutic role, controversies and implications for future research. *Med Hypotheses.* 1999;52(2):101–109.

161. Reitstetter R, Lukas RJ, Gruener R. Dependence of nicotinic acetylcholine receptor recovery from desensitization on the duration of agonist exposure. *J Pharmacol Exp Ther.* 1999;289(2):656–660.

162. Gentry CL, Lukas RJ. Regulation of nicotinic acetylcholine receptor numbers and function by chronic nicotine exposure. *Curr Drug Targets CNS Neurol Disord.* 2002;1(4):359–385.

163. Breslau N, Davis GC, Schultz LR. Posttraumatic stress disorder and the incidence of nicotine, alcohol, and other drug disorders in persons who have experienced trauma. *Arch Gen Psychiatry.* 2003;60(3):289–294.

164. Bovet D, Bovet-Nitti F, Oliverio A. Effects of nicotine on avoidance conditioning of inbred strains of mice. *Psychopharmacologia.* 1966;10:1–5.

165. Levin E, Rose J. Nicotinic and muscarinic interactions and choice accuracy in the radial arm maze. *Brain Res Bull.* 1991;27:125–128.

166. Levin E. Nicotinic systems and cognitive function. *Psychopharmacology (Berl).* 1992;108:417–431.

167. Levin E, Briggs S, Christopher N, Rose J. Chronic nicotinic stimulation and blockade effects on working memory. *Behav Pharmacol.* 1993;4:179–182.

168. Brioni J, Arneric S. Nicotinic receptor agonists facilitate retention of avoidance training: participation in dopaminergic mechanisms. *Behav Neural Biol.* 1993;59:57–62.

169. Levin E, Briggs S, Christopher NC, Auman JT. Working memory performance and cholinergic effects in the ventral tegmental area and substantia nigra. *Brain Res.* 1994;657: 165–170.

170. Rusted J, Graupner L, O'Connell N, Nicholls C. Does nicotine improve cognitive performance? *Psychopharmacology (Berl).* 1994;115:547–549.

171. Sansone M, Battaglia M, Castellano C. Effect of caffeine and nicotine on avoidance learning in mice: lack of interaction. *J Pharm Pharmacol.* 1994;46:765–767.

172. Levin E, Kim P, Meray R. Chronic nicotine effects on working and reference memory in the 16-arm radial maze: interactions with D1 agonist and antagonist drugs. *Psychopharmacology (Berl).* 1996;127:25–30.

173. Levin E, Christopher N, Briggs S, Auman J. Chronic nicotinic and dopaminergic effects on spatial working memory performance in rats. *Drug Dev Res.* 1996;39:29–35.

174. Levin E, Torry D. Acute and chronic nicotine effects on working memory in aged rats. *Psychopharmacology (Berl).* 1996;123:88–97.

175. Zarrindast M, Sadegh M, Shafaghi B. Effects of nicotine on memory retrieval in mice. *Eur J Pharmacol.* 1996;295: 1–6.

176. Newhouse P, Potter A, Levin E. Nicotinic system involvement in Alzheimer's and Parkinson's diseases: implications for therapeutics. *Drugs Aging.* 1997;11:206–228.

177. Levin E, Simon B. Nicotinic acetylcholine involvement in cognitive function in animals. *Psychopharmacology (Berl).* 1998;138:217–230.

178. Gould T, Wehner J. Nicotine enhancement of contextual fear conditioning. *Behav Brain Res.* 1999;102:31–39.

179. Picciotto M, Calderone B, King S, Zachariou V. Nicotinic receptors in the brain: links between molecular biology and behavior. *Neuropsychopharmacology.* 2000;22:451–465.

180. Stolerman I, Mirza N, Hahn B, Shoaib M. Nicotine in an animal model of attention. *Eur J Pharmacol.* 2000;393: 147–154.

181. Sanacora G, Gueorguieva R, Epperson C, et al. Subtype-specific alterations of gamma-aminobutyric acid and glutamate in patients with major depression. *Arch Gen Psychiatry.* 2004;61:705–713.

182. Lydiard R. The role of GABA in anxiety disorders. *J Clin Psychol.* 2003;64:21–27.

183. Sacco K, Bannon K, George T. Effects of cigarette smoking on spatial working memory and attentional deficits in schizophrenia: involvement of nicotinic receptor mechanisms. *Arch Gen Psychiatry.* 2005;62:649–659.

184. Takita M. Alteration of brain nicotinic receptors induced by immobilization stress and nicotine in rats. *Brain Res.* 1995;681:190–192.

185. Kohda K, Harada K, Kato K, et al. Glucocorticoid receptor activation is involved in producing abnormal phenotypes of single-prolonged stress rats: a putative post-traumatic stress disorder model. *Neuroscience.* 2007;148:22–33.

186. Chen H, Fu Y, Sharp BM. Chronic nicotine self-administration augments hypothalamic-pituitary-adrenal responses to mild acute stress. *Neuropsychopharmacology.* 2008;33(4): 721–730.

187. Assaf M, Calhoun V, Kuzu C, et al. Neural correlates of the object-recall process in semantic memory. *Psychiatry Res.* 2006;147:115–126.

188. Cools R, Ivry RB, D'Esposito M. The human striatum is necessary for responding to changes in stimulus relevance. *J Cogn Neurosci.* 2006;18(12):1973–1983.

189. Garrard P, Bradshaw D, Jäger HR, Thompson AJ, Losseff N, Playford D. Cognitive dysfunction after isolated brain stem insult. An underdiagnosed cause of long term morbidity. *J Neurol Neurosurg Psychiatry.* 2002;73:191–194.

190. Allman JM, Hakeem A, Erwin JM, Nimchinsk E, Hof P. The anterior cingulate cortex: the evolution of an interface between emotion and cognition. *Ann N Y Acad Sci.* 2001;935: 107–117.

191. Czermak C, Staley JK, Kasserman S, et al. Beta2 nicotinic acetylcholine receptor availability in post-traumatic stress disorder. *Int J Neuropsychopharmacol.* 2008;11(3):419–424.

192. Shin L, Rauch S, Pitman RK. Amygdala, medial prefrontal cortex, and hippocampal function in PTSD. *Ann N Y Acad Sci.* 2006;1071:67–79.

193. Ehlers A, Hackmann A, Michael T. Intrusive re-experiencing in post-traumatic stress disorder: phenomenology, theory, and therapy. *Memory.* 2004;12:403–415.

194. Levin E, McClernon F, Rezvani A. Nicotinic effects on cognitive function: behavioral characterization, pharmacological specification, and anatomic localization. *Psychopharmacology (Berl).* 2006;184:523–539.

195. Lanius R, Williamson P, Densmore M, et al. The nature of traumatic memories: a 4-T FMRI functional connectivity analysis. *Am J Psychiatry*. 2004;161:36–44.

196. Page F, Coleman G, Conduit R. The effect of transdermal nicotine patches on sleep and dreams. *Physiol Behav*. 2006;88:425–432.

197. Gotti C, Clementi F. Neuronal nicotinic receptors: from structure to pathology. *Prog Neurobiol*. 2004;74:363–396.

198. Mamede M, Ishizu K, Ueda M, et al. Temporal change in human nicotinic acetylcholine receptor after smoking cessation: 5IA SPECT study. *J Nucl Med*. 2007;48(11): 1829–1835.

Chapter 11
Imaging Substance Use and Misuse: Psychostimulants

Tara L. White

Introduction

Neuroimaging provides a dynamic window on the effects of psychoactive substances on the structure and function of human brain. As a field, neuroimaging of substance abuse is broad and includes investigation of processes involved in chronic drug effects and addiction such as craving, compulsive drug seeking, and compulsive drug use; initial drug effects that include sedative, stimulant, cognitive, and behavioral effects; and potential between-person factors relevant to substance use and misuse such as gender, family history, age, and other factors. Given this scope, this chapter has been restricted to three main topical areas: (1) *overarching research questions* in neuroimaging of substance use and misuse, (2) *methodological issues* typically encountered in the field, and (3) *between-person factors that may confer a vulnerability to, or protection from, the development and maintenance of substance use and misuse*. Many substances have been studied using neuroimaging methods, including alcohol, nicotine, opiates, cannabinoids, cocaine, and amphetamine. The present chapter focuses on the classic psychostimulants cocaine and amphetamine which serve as archetypal drugs of abuse because of their impact on dopamine, which is processed by the brain as highly salient and which motivates the approach and acquisition of the drug.[105]

T.L. White (✉)
Center for Alcohol and Addiction Studies,
Department of Community Health, Brown University,
Box G-S121-4, Providence, RI 02912, USA
e-mail: Tara_White@Brown.edu

Public Health Impact

Substance use and misuse carries enormous personal and societal costs, with monetary costs estimated at over half a trillion dollars annually in the United States due to medical-related, crime-related, and productivity-related losses related to illicit and licit drug use.[67,74,104] This figure, while compelling, does not take into account the human costs of substance abuse and addiction, which are virtually inestimable and include family, employment and educational problems, domestic violence, and child abuse.[67] Substance use and misuse thus represents a significant public health problem. Neuroimaging can provide information about the neural mechanisms involved in the sequelae of drug addiction, where and how brain systems of potentially vulnerable individuals are sensitive to drugs of abuse, and functional evidence that can be used to guide the development of high-impact prevention and treatment efforts.

Methodological Issues

Methodological issues in addiction transcend specific imaging techniques, and involve issues of study design and interpretation, research ethics, sample heterogeneity, and sample size. *Study design and interpretation*: Neuroimaging studies typically compare separate groups of participants, such as individuals with and without drug dependence. Fewer studies follow the same participants over time to determine time-dependent changes in brain structure or function. Reliance on cross-sectional designs can make determination of causality difficult. Prospective designs and longitudinal approaches help delineate whether differences

R.A. Cohen and L.H. Sweet (eds.), *Brain Imaging in Behavioral Medicine and Clinical Neuroscience*,
DOI 10.1007/978-1-4419-6373-4_11, © Springer Science+Business Media, LLC 2011

between groups exist due to preexisting factors or as a consequence of drug exposure. *Research ethics*: Neuroimaging of acute and chronic drug effects need to be attuned to whether participants are seeking treatment for their substance use; for ethical reasons, any substance or cue related to a substance should not be administered to an individual currently seeking treatment for his/her substance use. Certificates of confidentiality are often required to protect participant confidentiality with regard to drug status and security of participant identity. *Sample heterogeneity*: Substance use and misuse can involve a wide range of drugs, consumption patterns, and history of prior drug exposure, and there is inherent heterogeneity in most study samples. To address this issue, researchers can prospectively collect data to quantify potential sources of variation in their sample, to distinguish the between-subject and within-subject factors that may impact outcomes under study. *Sample size*: Use of large sample sizes increases statistical power, which reduces but does not eliminate the impact of heterogeneity within and between samples.

Overarching Research Questions of Interest

Pressing research questions in this area include the *immediate impact* of psychoactive drugs on function in addiction-relevant circuits; the *chronic impact* of drugs on the structure and function of the human brain; and the neural mechanisms involved in *craving*, *withdrawal*, and *relapse* to drugs of abuse. Each of these questions has spawned a large literature, which is reviewed in brief below.

Acute Drug Effects

Substantive issue: Substances that produce dependence and abuse typically cause a reversible, time-bound state of intoxication after initial drug consumption. When this state is accompanied by significant maladaptive behavioral or psychological changes, as well as by clinically relevant negative impact on the individual's behavioral, social, or occupational functioning,

substance intoxication can reach the status of a diagnosable (though reversible) Axis I condition.[3] Neuroimaging of acute drug effects provides information about the specific neural systems activated by drugs during periods of intoxication. This information assists in understanding the brain mechanisms that mediate the subjective and behavioral impact of drugs immediately after drug consumption.

Empirical approaches: *Populations and study drugs*: Neuroimaging of acute drug effects has been conducted to date for a fairly wide range of drugs, which include but are not limited to alcohol, nicotine, cocaine, amphetamine, and MDMA (ecstacy). *Methods*: Neuroimaging of acute drug effects can be accomplished using positron emission tomography (PET) and functional magnetic resonance imaging (fMRI) methods. PET when used with the specific D_2 dopamine radioligand [^{11}C]raclopride provides evidence of a drug's acute impact on dopamine, due to competitive displacement of the radioligand from D_2 receptors after drug-induced dopamine release. PET data can be correlated with other outcomes, such as participant ratings of subjective effects experienced after drug administration (e.g., elation, rush, drug liking, drug wanting), to determine the association between drug-induced DA release and the subjective or behavioral impact of the drug.[105] fMRI is used during the peak period of drug effects and compared to placebo responses either within or between subjects, during performance of a cognitive or behavioral task, to assess the acute impact of the drug on functiones in emotional, cognitive, and attentional circuits.

Findings: Amphetamine. PET data indicate that amphetamine causes increased dopamine release in incentive motivational circuits, the magnitude of which is positively associated with subjects' reports of drug-induced euphoria.[26] Existing fMRI data suggest that amphetamine may amplify ongoing brain activation. d-amphetamine increased fMRI signal strength in right prefrontal regions during working memory tasks[65] and increased the number of activated voxels in primary auditory and sensorimotor cortices during auditory vigilance tasks and motor tasks, respectively.[103] In PET studies, d-amphetamine specifically increases task-dependent regional cerebral blood flow[64] and increases the glucose metabolism observed during performance of continuous attention tasks.[28] While it is widely appreciated that performing a motor task, auditory vigilance task, or working memory task increases the neural activity in brain regions that mediate these activities, it is less well known that in each case amphetamine causes further increases in the activity in each region. These data indicate that across techniques, d-amphetamine appears capable of acting as a general amplifier of brain activation, modulating activity depending on ongoing stimulus and task demands. *Methamphetamine* (METH): There have been two fMRI studies of the acute impact of METH consumption on brain processing. These include work by Kleinschmidt and colleagues[50], who demonstrated in seven healthy young volunteers that i.v. METH (15 mg) produced BOLD signal increases in subcortical gray, cerebellum, and frontotemporal regions compared to predrug and placebo conditions, and Völlm and colleagues[110] who demonstrated in seven psychostimulant-naïve volunteers that i.v. METH (0.15 mg/kg dose i.v.) activated medial orbitrofrontal cortex, rostral ACC, and ventral striatum, with ratings of "mind-racing" correlating with activation in the last two regions. These studies relied on the time course of the drug effect[50] and button-press ratings of subjective effects[110] to delineate the effects of METH on brain function.

Overall findings: Imaging using PET methods indicates that drugs of abuse achieve their subjective rewarding effects through the speed at which they increase dopamine in limbic regions such as nucleus accumbens.[26,105] Drugs that produce a rapid but short-acting effect on brain dopamine have high potential for abuse due to the association between rapid DA increases and positive subjective impact of the drug and the association between rapid drug clearance and readministration of the drug (for discussion, see ref. [105]).

Chronic Drug Effects

Substantive issue: One of the challenges of understanding substance abuse is the fact that while many individuals may use psychoactive drugs, not all users go on to develop addiction. The repeated use of drugs creates the opportunity for neural systems activated by temporary exposure to the substance to undergo substantial structural and functional remodeling. Neuroimaging can provide insight as to the nature and chronicity of the structural impact of psychoactive

drugs, when consumed repeatedly over long periods of time. This provides important information about the substrates altered in addiction which may assist in the development of novel therapeutics for addiction.

Empirical approaches: *Populations and study drugs*: The impact of chronic drug exposure is well studied and typically investigates effects in active or abstinent substance abusers, compared to healthy controls. *Methods*: The impact of chronic drug use can be investigated using a wide variety of methods, including PET, structural MRI, and MR spectroscopy, which provide information about receptor and transporter densities, gray and white matter volumes, and metabolite concentrations, respectively (see ref. [37] for review).

Findings: Cocaine: Chronic cocaine use has been associated with volumetric and structural changes in human brain. Cocaine abusers display reduced gray matter in frontal cortex, despite abstinence from cocaine for the prior 3-week period.[63] Cocaine-dependent samples also display enlarged basal ganglia compared to healthy controls[47], which may relate to psychoses associated with psychostimulant abuse.[37] PET studies indicate multiple changes in dopamine targets, including reduction in D_2 dopamine receptor density in striatum in detoxified cocaine abusers,[106,109] which may relate to reductions in salience of nondrug compared to drug stimuli in cocaine abusers, and reduced interest in, and involvement with, natural (nondrug) sources of reward in the environment.[105] *Methamphetamine*: METH use and misuse has significant impact on brain structure. There are regional changes in interhemispheric white matter tracts,[69] reduced frontal white-matter integrity,[19] and gray-matter deficits in hippocampus, cingulate, limbic, and paralimbic cortices[101] in abstinent METH abusers which may reflect neurotoxicity and neuroinflammation involving activated microglial proceses.[16,89] Chronic methamphetamine abusers also display enlarged striatum (caudate, globus pallidus, and putamen[16,17]) during the first 4 months of abstinence which may be due to neuroinflammation, a direct trophic effect of dopamine or a side effect of high occupancy of D1-receptors in this region with chronic drug-induced DA (for review, see ref. [16]). PET studies indicate reductions in dopamine transporter, serotonin transporter, vesicular monoamine transporter, and D_2 receptor densities in striatum in methamphetamine abusers[16] which tend to be associated with amount and duration of methamphetamine use and may reflect neuroadaptive changes during drug exposure and abstinence.[16]

Craving

Substantive issue: Stimuli (cues) in the environment previously associated with drug use are able to trigger motivational circuits and elicit a high motivation to use these drugs. The craving state that results contributes to both the continuation of drug use and relapse. Neuroimaging of craving is important because craving has been found to predict posttreatment substance use outcomes for smoking[92,93] and cocaine dependence[78] and is thus an important target for intervention. Analysis of situations in which substance-dependent patients relapse finds that many involve craving,[62,80] and cocaine-dependent patients who use more urge-specific coping skills after treatment have less cocaine relapse.[79] Developing additional ways by which substance-dependent patients can reduce their craving urges is an important target for treatment research. Neuroimaging techniques provide a noninvasive method for understanding the neurobiological basis of craving states and their potential alleviation in humans.

Empirical approaches: Populations and study drugs: Drug-cue-related craving states have been most widely studied with fMRI for two drugs, cocaine and alcohol. For ethical reasons, study participants are most often current users who are not seeking treatment for their substance use. Individuals are studied during a period of abstinence from their drug of choice. *Methods*: In order to permit neuroimaging during craving, study participants are presented with drug cues through visual, auditory, or sensory modalities (e.g., pictures, scripts read aloud, scents, or holding a cigarette) in a blocked- or event-related design while lying prone within an MR scanner. Craving ratings are assessed by key-press on an MRI compatible keypad.

Specific findings: For cocaine, cue-related activity has been most widely documented in the anterior cingulate.[38] This activity temporally precedes[113] and positively correlates with the self-reported craving for cocaine (e.g., r's > 0.8[60]). Neural correlates of cocaine-cue-induced craving are not restricted to this region and involve a wide network of emotional, reward-related, and attentional circuits activated by these stimuli in cocaine users (e.g., left dorsolateral prefrontal cortex[60]; nucleus accumbens, parahippocampal gyrus, lateral prefrontal cortex, amygdala[12]; right inferior parietal, caudate/lateral dorsal nucleus[38]). These fMRI findings are similar to findings with PET, which indicate increased metabolic activity in dorsolateral prefrontal cortex, amygdala, medial temporal cortex, anterior cingulate, cerebellum, and insula during cue-induced cocaine craving.[18,45,111]

Overall findings: Exposure to drug cues is associated with increased activity in a number of common brain regions in adult addicts, which include the anterior cingulate, nucleus accumbens, dorsolateral prefrontal cortex, and amygdala. Craving occurs within the context of chronic reductions in dopamine activity and changes in structural components of dopamine systems, including reduced dopamine D_2 receptor density in the striatum and orbitofrontal cortex.[105] These reductions are thought to relate to a state of anhedonia, or inability to experience pleasure, against which drug-cue stimuli achieve relative salience and attentional and motivational capture (for discussion, see ref. [105]).

Withdrawal

Substantive issue: Withdrawal is the development of a substance-specific syndrome after the cessation of or reduction in substance use, particularly when individual has used the drug heavily or over a long period of time.[3] Specific symptoms experienced during withdrawal vary and are typically the opposite of symptoms experienced during acute drug intoxication.[3] For psychostimulants, withdrawal begins from 12 h to 4 days after initial cessation of use and involves symptoms of anhedonia, depressed mood, increased appetite, increased sleep, fatigue, concentration problems, mental confusion, suicidality, drug craving, irritability, and restlessness, with symptoms of anhedonia lasting 2–12 weeks during protracted abstinence (for review, see refs. [5,21,39]). Neuroimaging during withdrawal is important because the negative emotional effects and lack of motivational drive coincide with initial efforts at detoxification or reduction in use, making the first week of abstinence from psychostimulants a period in which individuals are at heightened risk for craving, relapse, and treatment failure. Insights provided by neuroimaging during the first week of abstinence may help inform the development of behavioral, psychological, or pharmacologic interventions to assist quit attempts during this difficult period.[59]

Empirical approaches: Populations and study drugs: Withdrawal has been relatively well studied for alcohol, nicotine, and cocaine. *Populations*: Study participants are typically individuals seeking treatment, who are enrolled in a neuroimaging study early in their treatment period, or who are not treatment-seeking but who are willing to abstain from drug consumption as a part of a research study. *Methods*: Individuals are studied during a period of drug abstinence, such as 4–7 days abstinence from methamphetamine[59] and 1–4 weeks' abstinence from cocaine.[108] Neuroimaging methods deployed to investigate acute effects of withdrawal on brain function include PET using [18F]fluorodeoxyglucose to investigate cerebral glucose metabolism and self-ratings of depression and anxiety,[59] and length of abstinence (1 week vs. 2–4 weeks[108]).

Findings: The first week of abstinence from cocaine has been found to be associated with higher levels of overall brain metabolism and higher metabolism in basal ganglia and orbital frontal cortex compared to controls,[108] an effect that decreases with length of abstinence when studied cross-sectionally (1 week vs. 2–4 weeks[108]). During the first 7 days of abstinence from methamphetamine, ratings of depression correlate with elevated glucose metabolism in amygdala and perigenual anterior cingulate gyrus, and state anxiety ratings during this period are correlated with low glucose metabolism in the left insula.[59] These data indicate that alterations in amygdala and insula function are related to negative mood during early abstinence.[59]

Relapse

Substantive issue: While treatment has many long-term successes, many patients relapse repeatedly on their path toward abstinence. Addiction has been described as a chronically relapsing condition that is highly treatment resistant.[91] While relapse is a persistent feature of addiction, it has also been construed as

contributing to learning processes and the path to long-term recovery ([102]; for discussion, see ref. [53]). Objective measures from a national sample indicate that approximately 33% of individuals treated for cocaine dependence remain abstinent 5 years after treatment.[36] It is essential to develop improved methods to decrease relapse and increase the number of patients who develop lasting abstinence. Neuroimaging methods are beginning to identify prospective predictors of relapse, which may, in the future, lead to methods with specificity and sensitivity to identify markers of recovery and vulnerability on a single-subject basis (for discussion, see ref. [75]).

Empirical approaches: Populations and study drugs: Prediction of relapse is most powerfully achieved using longitudinal studies of individuals with current addiction. Several prospective studies of relapse have been conducted using neuroimaging techniques. These studies have focused on participants with methamphetamine dependence[71] or cocaine dependence,[51,97] who are treatment-seeking for their substance use,[71,97] abstinent at fMRI assessment (3–4 weeks abstinence[71], 2-week inpatient detoxification[51], 2–4 week inpatient treatment[96,97]), and followed-up 10 weeks, 90 days, and 1 year after neuroimaging assessment for indications of relapse (10 weeks[51], 90 days[96], 370 days[71]).

Methods: Methods used to assess predictors of relapse include fMRI assessments during decision-making, exposure to drug cues, and emotional stress, with the aim of identifying differences between relapsers and nonrelapsers in future follow-up. Specific paradigms include investigation of fMRI responses during performance of a two-choice prediction task in methamphetamine-dependent subjects, to test decision-making processing and its relationship to relapse 1 year later[71]; fMRI responses during viewing of video images of cocaine smoking in cocaine-dependent subjects, to test brain responses to drug cues and relapse 10 weeks later[51]; and fMRI responses during exposure to subject-specific scripts of stressful vs. nonstressful life events, to test the association between stress reactivity and relapse 90 days later.[96,97]

Findings: fMRI protocols focusing on decision-making, drug-cue processing, and emotional distress have identified a number of predictors of relapse. For instance, decision-making on the two-choice prediction task typically activates prefrontal cortex, striatum, posterior parietal, and anterior insula[70]; in METH-dependent men who later relapsed ($n=18$), reduced or reversed activation patterns were observed in right insula, right middle temporal gyrus, and right posterior cingulate during performance of the task compared to participants who did not relapse during follow-up ($n=22$[71]; for discussion, see ref. [75]). These results suggest reduced activation in decision-making circuits in individuals who later relapse, particularly in regions that are involved in assessing potential negative outcomes (e.g., insula[71,75]). In response to the cocaine cue fMRI paradigm, individuals who later relapsed displayed increased activation in left posterior cingulate, sensory, and motor areas compared to those who did not relapse over the 10-week follow-up period.[51] The fMRI associations were more strongly predictive of relapse than were participants' self-reports of craving to the cocaine-cue stimuli used in the fMRI scan protocol,[51] demonstrating the power of the neuroimaging approach. In response to the emotional stress fMRI paradigm, greater stress-induced signal change in medial prefrontal cortex (Brodmann areas 9 and 10) was associated with shorter time to relapse during the initial 90-day follow-up.[97] These data collectively indicate that activation in decision-making circuits, cue-processing, and stress-response circuits can predict later relapse in individuals with psychostimulant addiction who have undergone treatment and are attempting to maintain long-term abstinence. Much additional work must be done, however, before these methods have diagnostic utility for predicting relapse on either a group- or case-by-case basis (for an excellent discussion of this issue, see ref. [75]).

Between-Person Factors

Substantive issue: It is estimated that 20.1 million Americans aged 12 years and older – 8% of the population – have used illicit drugs in the past month. Of these, 1.9 million Americans – 0.7% of the population – have used cocaine in the past month, and 6.2 million Americans – 2.5% of the population – have used prescription-type psychotherapeutic drugs for nonmedical purposes in the past month.[86] Despite these numbers, only a minority of individuals who consume a drug go on to develop problems of drug dependence and addiction.[105] Because of the disconnect between the numbers of individuals consuming illicit drugs and those

who go on to develop problems of drug dependence, identifying specific factors that pose an increased risk or protection from addiction will assist in preventing and intervening in the course of this chronic brain disease.

There is now considerable evidence that healthy individuals vary in their neurochemical and psychological responses to the same dose of a psychostimulant drug. For instance, interindividual variability exists in d-amphetamine's effects on subjective activation and positive mood,[11,26,31,94] and on anxiety and cortisol released by this drug.[22,48,68,84,85,94] Because of this variability, individual differences factors are likely to be very important for understanding and preventing drug addiction. Specific between-subject factors of potentially high impact include gender, family history, prior use, age, and temperament. These are described in turn below.

Gender: While there are greater numbers of male than female drug abusers in the human population, animal and human evidence indicates that females transition to addiction more quickly after initial drug and alcohol exposure (for review, see ref. [30]). In women, drinking problems often develop later but display a "telescoping" or accelerated course in which females progress quickly from onset of drinking to later stages of alcoholism.[54] This more rapid transition from initial drug use to dependence may involve females' more pronounced sensitization after repeated exposure to stimulant drugs compared to males.[99,121] For patients who develop alcoholism relatively early (i.e., before the age of 25), greater proportions of female than male patients go on to develop severe alcohol problems (for review, see ref. [54]). This finding is consistent with greater acquisition of stimulant self-administration, escalation of use, and priming-induced relapse (reinstatement) in females compared to males in animal studies (for review, see refs. [30,82]). Differences in sensitivity to stimulant drugs have also been observed across the menstrual cycle in humans.[116] Gender differences are thus an important factor to consider in the neuroimaging of drug effects and transitions to consider in in drug abuse.

Family and personal history: A family history of alcoholism and substance abuse is one of the strongest predictors of substance abuse risk in healthy populations and deserves significant attention as a between-subjects factor. *Prior use*: Because regular consumption is required for dependence to occur, investigation of prior use of addictive agents, in individuals without current dependence, provides insight regarding sequelae leading to addiction.

Age: Distinct age-related responses and developmental differences in drug use indicate that adolescence may constitute a critical period of vulnerability for addiction. The prefrontal cortex, amygdala, nucleus accumbens, and anterior cingulate and orbital-frontal cortices undergo significant refinement and maturation during adolescence, which include changes in gray and white matter volume that reflect age-dependent processes of synaptic pruning, cell death, and myelination (for review, see ref. [95]). An increased risk for addiction in adolescence is thought to relate to several mechanisms, including but not limited to early life stress and stress during adolescence, which impacts regions involved in addiction (hippocampus, nucleus accumbens, prefrontal cortex, see ref. [4]).

Temperament/personality: Emotional and behavioral responses to stimulants relate to normal personality traits in healthy volunteers. These include measures of sensation seeking which have been found to be positively associated with d-amphetamine effects on subjective stimulation, arousal, and elevated mood.[20,46,87] Because sensation seeking measures individuals' responses to external rewards as well as their tendency to fearlessly approach potentially harmful situations, this phenotype can be measured as two separable components, extraversion and fearlessness[100], which are involved in stimulant drug effects on mood and behavior (see refs. [115,117,118]). These between-subject difference factors – gender, family history, prior use, age, and temperament – can be studied using multiple imaging modalities, including PET and structural and functional MRI.

Empirical approaches: Populations and study drugs: Investigation of individual differences can be done using either between-subjects or between-groups designs, in which the study sample is separated on one or more factors of interest (e.g., gender; family history). This can be done prospectively, as two separate groups, or post hoc, as factors in the data analysis. Between-person factors that can be operationalized as continuous variables (for instance, age, prior use, temperament/personality) can be either studied using a two-group design (with cutoff values separating the groups) or treated analytically as regressors, the latter of which increases statistical power.

Methods: Between-person factors in addictive processes have been studied using the entire range of neuroimaging methods available, including fMRI, MRI, PET, SPECT, and MRS.

Findings: Gender. Neuroimaging studies have identified gender differences in acute dopamine released by drugs of abuse in humans and in functional brain responses to the drug cues and stress cues that can precipitate relapse, with a different pattern of risk factors emerging for males and females. For instance, PET studies using [11C] raclopride indicate greater dopamine release in ventral striatum after amphetamine, and greater self-reports of positive subjective effects of the drug, in male participants compared to female participants.[66] Studies using ^{1}H-MRS indicate decreases in frontal NAA concentrations in abstinent male, but not female, cocaine users, suggesting neuronal injury in men due to long-standing cocaine use (for review, see ref. [61]). Cocaine-dependent males have been found to display greater fMRI activation than cocaine-dependent females in paralimbic regions (left uncus, right claustrum, Brodmann's area 20) in response to drug cues compared to stress cues.[57] The above findings suggest that males are more sensitive to drug-induced dopamine release and drug cues than females, and suggest a neuroprotective effect of estrogen on long-term impact of stimulant drugs on brain structure (for discussion, see ref. [66]). In contrast, cocaine-dependent females have been found to display greater fMRI activation in frontal and limbic regions in response to stress imagery than do cocaine-dependent males, in regions such as anterior cingulate and insula which are involved in craving and relapse.[58] These data suggest the existence of different neural vulnerabilities to stress- and drug cue-related relapse in women and men.

Findings: Family history. Studies investigating *fMRI* responses in family history positive individuals have identified reduced amygdala responses to fear faces (mean age of 23.5 years[41]), decreased frontal responses during response inhibition tasks (ages 12–14[88]), and decreased anterior insula responses to loss of monetary reward[8] in adolescents and young adults whose families contain alcoholics, compared to age-matched controls who do not have a family history of alcoholism. These data implicate frontal and limbic circuit involvement in the genetic vulnerability to alcoholism and substance abuse. Youth with a family history of alcoholism have not been found to differ from controls on other outcomes, such as striatal response to monetary reward, in the same tasks.[8] This pattern of findings suggests that the reduced response to rewards, regularly observed in stimulant dependence, is likely a consequence rather than a cause of drug dependence and that the genetic vulnerability to substance abuse may specifically involve variation in negative affective and behavioral inhibition processes. *Structural MRI* and neurocognitive tests indicate a positive relationship between white matter volume, cognitive performance, and information processing speed in females without a family history of substance abuse.[95] This relationship has not been demonstrated in adolescents who have a family history of substance abuse.[95] These data suggest that structural brain maturational processes may confer some protection from substance abuse. Potential candidates include development-related increases in myelination, which may be causally related to maturational changes in cognition in girls without a family history of substance abuse,[95] which could be a protective factor in these low-risk individuals.

Findings: Prior use. Contributions of prior use can be difficult to disentangle in individuals with ongoing substance use problems. Contributions of this life history factor are most readily evaluated in individuals who have previously used a given substance, but are not currently dependent. When investigated in such individuals, it has been found that moderate to heavy drinkers display *decreased amygdala activation* during risk taking on the stop signal task,[119] and *elevated activation in mesocorticolimbic regions* (prefrontal cortex, striatum, ventral tegmental area) in response to alcohol taste cues[35] compared to lighter drinkers. These findings indicate that past alcohol use is associated with altered function in circuits relevant to emotion and behavioral control. In MRS investigations, subjects with high prior levels of alcohol consumption have been found to display increased choline signal in frontal white matter.[27] This indicates an increase in membrane turnover in individuals with high prior alcohol consumption, with possible implication for health of myelin sheaths in this area.[27] The above findings indicate that prior drug and alcohol use history is associated with functional and structural differences in brain regions involved in addiction. Current use is associated with striatal responses to drug-related cues, which is most likely due to cue-related conditioning processes.

Findings: Age. Investigations with [^{123}I]IBZM SPECT indicate that the positive subjective effects of amphetamine (i.e., happiness, energy) are positively correlated with the magnitude of dopamine released by the drug and are negatively correlated with subjects' age, such that younger participants report a stronger subjective impact of the drug.[1] In a pilot fMRI study of d-amphetamine using a behavioral risk task, men under age 21 showed increased intensity of activation in response to high rewards in anterior cingulate and insula and showed greater volumes recruited under amphetamine in anterior cingulate compared to older subjects. These data suggest that young men could be relatively sensitive to amphetamine and high-risk, high-value rewards compared to older individuals who experience the same stimuli.[114] Young age appears to confer increased subjective drug effects upon initial use[1] and may confer increased activational responses to environmental reward and the drug itself.[114] There are documented age-related differences in chronic drug impact on brain structure, such that individuals with cocaine dependence display age-related declines in gray matter volume in temporal cortex that are not observed in control subjects.[6] Age appears to be a potentially potent between-subjects factor mediating the short- and long-term impact of psychostimulants on brain structure and function.

Findings: Temperament/personality. Normal personality traits have been found to relate to between-subject differences in a number of neuroimaging outcomes. These include dopamine response to alcohol, dopamine response to amphetamine, and sensitization of dopamine response to amphetamine, assessed by [^{11}C] raclopride/PET methods[9,10,55,76]; glucose metabolism in orbital frontal cortex, assessed by FDG/PET[43]; and ventral striatal responses to incentive cues, assessed by fMRI.[8,52] While alcohol and stimulant drugs cause rises in dopamine in the ventral striatum which correlate with the subjective impact of the drug,[26,55] there are between-subject differences in the magnitude of this effect. Individuals who have higher trait scores on measures of novelty seeking display greater magnitude of change in [^{11}C] raclopride binding in ventral striatum after consumption of alcohol ($n = 6$ males[9]), and after consumption of d-amphetamine ($r = 0.79$, $n = 8$ males[55]). High scores on trait novelty seeking also relate to the magnitude of a long-term sensitization in DA response to psychostimulants, when stimulants are administered to healthy volunteers on three separate test days scheduled 2–3 days apart, with follow-up up to 1 year later ($n = 10$ males[10]). There is additional evidence that these effects differ by gender. Correlations between trait sensation seeking and ventral striatal dopamine release, as identified by [18F]fallypride PET scans, were found to be positive in men ($r = 0.8$, $n = 7$) but not women ($r = -0.7$, $n = 6$; see ref. [76]), underscoring the importance of investigating gender differences. For individuals without substance dependence, these findings indicate that personality traits related to novelty seeking are important in modulating the acute responses to stimulant drugs, and the drug-related escalation of brain responses after repeated drug exposure, particularly in young adult males. Replication and extension of these findings using larger sample sizes and attention to potential gender differences are important next steps in this area.

In individuals with stimulant dependence, the personality measure of trait fearlessness [low MPQ Harm Avoidance (HA)] has been found to relate to metabolism in orbitalfrontal gyrus. Methamphametamine-dependent individuals with high scores on trait fear (HA) had higher relative orbitofrontal gyrus metabolism at rest than those with low scores on this trait [$r = +0.57$, $n = 14$ (11 women)[43]]. This finding indicates a role of orbitofrontal gyrus in the failure to avoid physically dangerous situations and inhibit drug consumption in psychostimulant dependence,[43] and a role of trait fearlessness in modulating functional brain outcomes after the onset of drug dependence.

Overarching Models of Substance Use and Misuse

Neuroimaging findings such as those described above have been incorporated into several overarching models of substance use, dependence and addiction. These include the "Impaired Response Inhibition and Salience Attribution" model (I-RISA model[44]), which posits a special role for frontal dysregulation in altered drug reinforcement, craving, bingeing, and withdrawal, which are theorized to involve the nucleus accumbens, amygdala, and anterior cingulate and thalamo-orbital frontal cortex; the "incentive sensitization" model,[77] which proposes drug-induced increase in cue-elicited

motor approach of drug involves drug-induced changes in nucleus accumbens and prefrontal cortex; the "negative reinforcement/reward allostasis" model (see ref. [2]), which proposes that repeated drug use produces increased drug motivation, tolerance, and consumption through an accumulation of negative reinforcement-antagonized function in midbrain dopamine reward circuits, amygdala, and lateral hypothalamus[2]; *behavioral economic models*[33], which posit a special role for personality traits of impulsivity or present-centeredness in facilitating low risk: high benefit payoff judgments that encourage drug intake; and the "two factor dopamine model,"[56] which proposes that repeated use of psychostimulant drugs leads to systematic perturbation of DA transmission based on the presence (sensitization and increased DA transmission) and absence (decreased DA transmission) of drug-paired cues.[56] These models are not mutually exclusive, but describe overlapping processes involved in the acquisition and continuation of drug use despite negative consequences.

Summary: Regions involved in the various aspects and stages of addiction include areas involved in motivation, reward processing, decision-making, and behavioral control. These include the *orbitofrontal cortex*, located above the sinus which is involved in stimulus evaluation and valence; the *nucleus accumbens*, located in the ventral base of the human forebrain, which is a key structure for reward and incentive motivation; the *amygdala*, which responds to the intensity of rewarding and aversive stimuli and links motivationally relevant events with neutral stimuli; and the *anterior cingulate*, which has a high concentration of dopaminergic receptors and is interconnected with multiple regions involved in behavioral inhibition and emotional processing (e.g., OFC, amygdala[7]).

Unanswered Questions and Future Directions: Identifying Vulnerability and Protective Factors

As described above, there is a growing literature that indicates that there are individual differences in the direction and magnitude of stimulant effects on mood and behavior. The origin of these individual differences is not well understood but appears to involve several distinct risk factors – the personality trait of

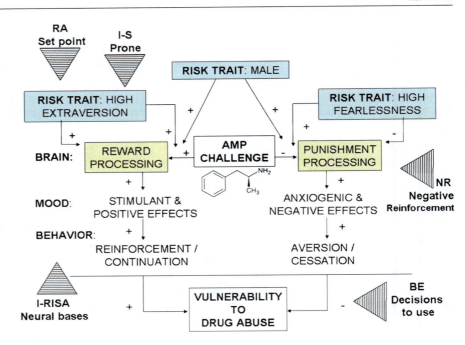

Fig. 11.1. Between-person differences in the vulnerability to amphetamine effects (VENTURE model), in relation to other theoretical models of addiction. Abbreviations: RA = reward allostasis (ref. 2); I-S = incentive sensitization (ref. 77); I-RISA = impaired response inhibition and salience attribution (ref. 44); NR = negative reinforcement (ref. 2) ; BE = behavioral economic (e.g., ref 33) models. AMP = amphetamine, a prototypic psychostimulant

extraversion, the personality trait of fearlessness (which constitutes a separate trait), and maleness. These are summarized in the VENTURE model of risk, which is outlined in Fig. 11.1.

To date, many investigations of personality differences in stimulant drug effects have used measures of sensation seeking in the assessment of potential risk traits, for instance, TPQ novelty seeking, SSS-V sensation seeking, and EPQ-Psychoticism. These measures have been found to be positively associated with d-amphetamine effects on number of outcomes, including subjective stimulation,[46] arousal,[20] and elevated mood.[87] Sensation seeking measures individuals' responses to external rewards as well as their tendency to fearlessly approach potentially harmful situations[13,42,122,123], which can be psychometrically separated into multiple separable components, such as the stable tendencies toward extraversion and fearlessness.[100,118] When dissociated, these two traits appear to be *separately* relevant to amphetamine effects on mood and behavior. For instance, the personality trait of fearlessness, measured by participants' MPQ Harm Avoidance (HA), has been found to predict the magnitude of subjective activation responses to d-amphetamine,[118] while related scales such as thrill and adventure seeking (TAS) and interpersonal aggressiveness (MPQ Aggression) predict the timing and magnitude of cortisol rise responses to d-amphetamine.[115] Thus, individuals who are predispositionally fearless (bold individuals) appear to experience larger subjective activational and larger and faster neuroendocrine responses to the same dose of a stimulant than do individuals who are predispositionally timid. These between-person differences suggest that high trait fearlessness could be a risk factor for drug abuse by decreasing the negative emotional processing of punishers in fearless individuals after drug consumption which would increase the risk of continued drug use despite negative consequences (Fig. 11.1). There is additional evidence that a separate trait, trait extraversion, modulates the acute *behavioral effects* of stimulant drugs. Amphetamine impacts behavioral impulsivity on a computerized gambling task [Balloon Analogue Risk Task (BART)], and there are individual differences in the magnitude and direction of this effect, such that drug-induced *increases* in risk behavior have been observed in males with high trait extraversion, whereas drug-induced decreases in risk behavior have been observed in males with low scores on this trait. This produces a correlation ($r=+0.6$) between drug-induced risk behavior and extraversion in males (for discussion, see ref. [117]). The personality trait of extraversion, thus, appears to modulate both the direction and magnitude of behavioral impulsivity after stimulant drug consumption. This could constitute a specific risk factor for continued drug use, a risk factor that is outlined in the left portion of the VENTURE model (Fig. 11.1).

The clarification of *the neural basis of specific sources of individual differences* in stimulant drug effects on brain, emotion, and behavior, using empirically derived personality measures with an orthogonal or quasi-orthogonal factor structure (such as those described above) is an emerging area of research. Future research in this area will assist in the delineation of the specific vulnerability and protective factors in individuals who have exposure to drugs, but who are not yet drug dependent.

Developing Effective Treatment Options

Addiction to psychostimulants follows a chronically relapsing course, for which there is currently no pharmacological treatment.[90] Available treatment options for psychostimulant dependence are currently limited to psychosocial interventions; of which community reinforcement, voucher reinforcement, and motivational interviewing programs appear to be most effective.[90] Other programs, such as detoxification, cue exposure, and 12-step programs, appear to be relatively less effective against stimulant dependence.[90]

Future pharmacological treatments with potential utility against psychostimulant addiction include the dopamine agonist bupropion, the mixed monoamine agonist/antagonist mirtazapine, GABA receptor agonists baclofen and topiramate,[81] disulfiram, which inhibits dopamine-β-hydroxylase to reduce synthesis of NE[98,112], lofexidine, an α-2 receptor antagonist, and atomoxetine, which blocks norepinephrine transporter (see ref. [98]). Other potential therapeutics include modafinil, a selective α-1 receptor agonist with stimulant-like properties,[91] and novel dopamine/serotonin releasers such as PAL-287[83] which are potential "agonist therapy" for psychostimulant addiction.[83,91]

Existing neuroimaging findings have suggested some novel targets for future treatment options, in light of the acute and chronic impacts of addictive drugs.[105] These include treatment options targeted at (1) reducing the reward associated with the drug while increasing the reward associated with nondrug stimuli in the individual's environment, to remediate the heightened incentive salience of the drug and its cues; (2) reducing learned (conditioned) behaviors associated with the drug, to reduce the drive to obtain and consume the drug; and (3) improving frontal functions of inhibitory control and executive function, to remediate drug-related deficits in these regions and improve volitional control over behavior.[105,107] These new ideas should help guide future treatment development for psychostimulant addiction, which remains, at present, highly resistant to treatment.

Novel Applications of Real-Time fMRI for Substance Abuse Research and Treatment

Real-time fMRI is a nascent technology with potential long-term applications for substance abuse. To date, most real-time fMRI studies have focused on cortical regions, such as somatomotor cortex,[24] auditory cortex,[120] insular cortex,[14] medial frontal cortex,[72] and anterior cingulate cortex (ACC[24,25]). Fewer real-time fMRI investigations focus on subject-driven modulation of signal in subcortical structures, such as amygdala[73] or nucleus accumbens.[15]

Several real-time studies have focused on regions with known involvement in addiction. For instance, deCharms and colleagues have developed procedures for real-time imaging and feedback of BOLD fMRI signal to participants based on activity in anterior cingulate; using a 60-s visualization paradigm, and feedback of BOLD signal through a brain–computer interface of scrolling timeseries fMRI signal and a real-time fire intensity graphic.[23,25] The majority of real-time fMRI protocols have involved healthy subjects who are typically between 18 and 45 years of age (e.g., range of 20–45 years with a mean age of 30.4 years[34], range of 18–37 years with a mean age of 23.5 years[25], range of 25–40 years[29], range of 20–35 years[40]). A minority of studies have used clinical populations such as brain tumor patients intraoperatively,[32] epileptic patients,[34,49] or chronic pain patients.[23,25]

Because addiction can be construed as a disorder involving the supranormal stimulation of reward circuits which results in altered learning in those circuits, real-time fMRI methods could have utility for the treatment of addiction, by producing patient-initiated modulation of reward responses to either drug-related or nondrug stimuli. The extremely high public health cost of addiction, combined with our current lack of efficacious treatments, suggests that real-time fMRI could have a place in our future therapeutic arsenal against this refractory brain disease.

Acknowledgements This work was supported by the National Institute on Drug Abuse (NIDA) grants DA020725 and DA017178 to TL White.

References

1. Abi-Dargham A, Kegeles LS, Martinez D, Innis RB, Laruelle M. Dopamine mediation of positive reinforcing effects of amphetamine in stimulant naïve healthy volunteers: results from a large cohort. *Eur Neuropsychopharmacol.* 2003;13(6): 459–468.
2. Ahmed SH, Koob GF. Transition to drug addiction: a negative reinforcement model based on an allostatic decrease in reward function. *Psychopharmacology (Berl).* 2005;180: 473–490.
3. American Psychiatric Association. *Diagnostic and Statistical Manual of Mental Disorders.* 4th ed. Washington, DC: American Psychiatric Press; 1994.
4. Andersen SL, Teicher MH. Desperately driven and no brakes: developmental stress exposure and subsequent risk for substance abuse. *Neurosci Biobehav Rev.* 2009;33(4):516–524.
5. Barr AM, Markou A. Psychostimulant withdrawal as an inducing condition in animal models of depression. *Neurosci Biobehav Rev.* 2005;29(4–5):675–706.
6. Bartzokis G, Beckson M, Lu PH, Nuechterlein KH, Edwards N, Mintz J. Age-related changes in frontal and temporal lobe volumes in men: a magnetic resonance imaging study. *Arch Gen Psychiatry.* 2001;58(5):461–465.
7. Baskin-Sommers A, White TL, Sommers I. Neurobiology of addiction. In: Fisher GL, Roget NA, Fisher GL, Roget NA, eds. *Encyclopedia of Substance Abuse, Prevention, Treatment, and Recovery.* Newbury Park, CA: SAGE Publications; 2008. ISBN # 9781412950848.
8. Bjork JM, Knutson B, Hommer DW. Incentive-elicited striatal activation in adolescent children of alcoholics. *Addiction.* 2008;103(8):1308–1319.
9. Boileau I, Assaad JM, Pihl RO, et al. Alcohol promotes dopamine release in the human nucleus accumbens. *Synapse.* 2003;49(4):226–231.
10. Boileau I, Dagher A, Leyton M, et al. Modeling sensitization to stimulants in humans: an [^{11}C]raclopride/positron emission tomography study in healthy men. *Arch Gen Psychiatry.* 2006;63(12):1386–1395.
11. Brauer LH, de Wit H. Role of dopamine in d-amphetamine-induced euphoria in normal, healthy volunteers. *Exp Clin Psychopharmacol.* 1995;3:371–381.
12. Breiter HC, Gollub RL, Weisskoff RM, et al. Acute effects of cocaine on human brain activity and emotion. *Neuron.* 1997;19:591–611.
13. Campbell JB, Heller JF. Correlations of extraversion, impulsivity and sociability with sensation seeking and MBTI-introversion. *Pers Individ Dif.* 1987;8:133–136.
14. Caria A, Veit R, Sitaram R, et al. Regulation of anterior insular cortex activity using real-time fMRI. *Neuroimage.* 2007;35(3):1238–1246.
15. Carelli RM, Wightman RM. Functional microcircuitry in the accumbens underlying drug addiction: insights from real-time signaling during behavior. *Curr Opin Neurobiol.* 2004; 14(6):763–768.

16. Chang L, Alicata D, Ernst T, Volkow N. Structural and metabolic brain changes in the striatum associated with methamphetamine abuse. *Addiction.* 2007;102(suppl 1):16–32.
17. Chang L, Cloak C, Patterson K, Grob C, Miller EN, Ernst T. Enlarged striatum in abstinent methamphetamine abusers: a possible compensatory response. *Biol Psychiatry.* 2005;57(9):967–974.
18. Childress AR, Mozley PD, McElgin W, Fitzgerald J, Reivich M, O'Brien CP. Limbic activation during cue-induced cocaine craving. *Am J Psychiatry.* 1999;156:11–18.
19. Chung A, Lyoo IK, Kim SJ, et al. Decreased frontal white-matter integrity in abstinent methamphetamine abusers. *Int J Neuropsychopharmacol.* 2007;10(6):765–775.
20. Corr PJ, Kumari V. Individual differences in mood reactions to d-amphetamine: a test of three personality factors. *J Psychopharmacol.* 2000;14:371–377.
21. Covington HE 3rd, Miczek KA. Vocalizations during withdrawal from opiates and cocaine: possible expressions of affective distress. *Eur J Pharmacol.* 2003;467(1–3):1–13.
22. de Wit H, Uhlenhuth EH, Johanson CE. Individual differences in the reinforcing and subjective effects of amphetamine and diazepam. *Drug Alcohol Depend.* 1986;16:341–360.
23. deCharms RC. Reading and controlling human brain activation using real-time functional magnetic resonance imaging. *Trends Cogn Sci.* 2007;11(11):473–481 [review].
24. deCharms RC, Christoff K, Glover GH, Pauly JM, Whitfield S, Gabrieli JD. Learned regulation of spatially localized brain activation using real-time fMRI. *Neuroimage.* 2004;21(1): 436–443.
25. deCharms RC, Maeda F, Glover GH, et al. Control over brain activation and pain learned by using real-time functional MRI. *Proc Natl Acad Sci U S A.* 2005;102(51): 18626–18631.
26. Drevets WC, Gautier C, Price JC, et al. Amphetamine-induced dopamine release in human ventral striatum correlates with euphoria. *Biol Psychiatry.* 2001;49(2):81–96.
27. Ende G, Walter S, Welzel H, et al. Alcohol consumption significantly influences the MR signal of frontal choline-containing compounds. *Neuroimage.* 2006;32(2):740–746.
28. Ernst M, Zametkin AJ, Matochik J, et al. Intravenous dextroamphetamine and brain glucose metabolism. *Neuropsychopharmacology.* 1997;6:391–401.
29. Esposito F, Seifritz E, Formisano E, et al. Real-time independent component analysis of fMRI time-series. *Neuroimage.* 2003;20(4):2209–2224.
30. Fattore L, Altea S, Fratta W. Sex differences in drug addiction: a review of animal and human studies. *Womens Health (Lond Engl).* 2008;4:51–65.
31. Feeney S, Goodall E, Silverstone T. The effect of d- and l-fenfluramine (and their interactions with d-amphetamine) on psychomotor function and mood. *Int Clin Psychopharmacol.* 1996;11:89–99.
32. Feigl GC, Safavi-Abbasi S, Gharabaghi A, et al. Real-time 3T fMRI data of brain tumour patients for intra-operative localization of primary motor areas. *Eur J Surg Oncol.* 2008;34(6):708–715.
33. Ferguson BS. Economic modeling of the rational consumption of addictive substances. *Subst Use Misuse.* 2006;41:573–603.
34. Fernández G, de Greiff A, von Oertzen J, et al. Language mapping in less than 15 minutes: real-time functional MRI during routine clinical investigation. *Neuroimage.* 2001; 14(3):585–594.

35. Filbey FM, Claus E, Audette AR, et al. Exposure to the taste of alcohol elicits activation of the mesocorticolimbic neurocircuitry. *Neuropsychopharmacology*. 2008;33(6):1391–1401.
36. Flynn PM, Joe GW, Broome KM, Simpson DD, Brown BS. Looking back on cocaine dependence: reasons for recovery. *Am J Addict*. 2003;12(5):398–411.
37. Fowler JS, Volkow ND, Kassed CA, Chang L. Imaging the addicted human brain. *Sci Pract Perspect*. 2007;3(2):4–16.
38. Garavan H, Pankiewicz J, Bloom A, et al. Cue-induced cocaine craving: neuroanatomical specificity for drug users and drug stimuli. *Am J Psychiatry*. 2000;157(11):1789–1798.
39. Gawin FH. Cocaine addiction: psychology and neurophysiology. *Science*. 1991;251(5001):1580–1586.
40. Gembris D, Taylor JG, Schor S, Frings W, Suter D, Posse S. Functional magnetic resonance imaging in real time (FIRE): sliding-window correlation analysis and reference-vector optimization. *Magn Reson Med*. 2000;43(2):259–268.
41. Glahn DC, Lovallo WR, Fox PT. Reduced amygdala activation in young adults at high risk of alcoholism: studies from the Oklahoma family health patterns project. *Biol Psychiatry*. 2007;61(11):1306–1309.
42. Glicksohn J, Abulafia J. Embedding sensation seeking within the big three. *Pers Individ Dif*. 1998;25:1085–1099.
43. Goldstein RZ, Volkow ND, Chang L, et al. The orbitofrontal cortex in methamphetamine addiction: involvement in fear. *Neuroreport*. 2002;13(17):2253–2257.
44. Goldstein RZ, Volkow ND. Drug addiction and its underlying neurobiological basis: neuroimaging evidence for the involvement of the frontal cortex. *Am J Psychiatry*. 2002;159(10):1642–1652.
45. Grant S, London ED, Newlin DB, et al. Activation of memory circuits during cue-elicited cocaine craving. *Proc Natl Acad Sci U S A*. 1996;93:12040–12045.
46. Hutchison KE, Wood MD, Swift R. Personality factors moderate subjective and psychophysiological responses to d-amphetamine in humans. *Exp Clin Psychopharmacol*. 1999;7:493–501.
47. Jacobsen LK, Giedd JN, Gottschalk C, Kosten TR, Krystal JH. Quantitative morphology of the caudate and putamen in patients with cocaine dependence. *Am J Psychiatry*. 2001; 158(3): 486–489.
48. Kavoussi RJ, Coccaro EF. The amphetamine challenge test correlates with affective lability in healthy volunteers. *Psychiatry Res*. 1993;48:219–228.
49. Kesavadas C, Thomas B, Sujesh S, et al. Real-time functional MR imaging (fMRI) for presurgical evaluation of paediatric epilepsy. *Pediatr Radiol*. 2007;37(10):964–974.
50. Kleinschmidt A, Bruhn H, Krüger G, Merboldt KD, Stoppe G, Frahm J. Effects of sedation, stimulation, and placebo on cerebral blood oxygenation: a magnetic resonance neuroimaging study of psychotropic drug action. *NMR Biomed*. 1999;12(5):286–292.
51. Kosten TR, Scanley BE, Tucker KA, et al. Cue-induced brain activity changes and relapse in cocaine-dependent patients. *Neuropsychopharmacology*. 2006;31(3):644–650.
52. Leland DS, Arce E, Feinstein JS, Paulus MP. Young adult stimulant users' increased striatal activation during uncertainty is related to impulsivity. *Neuroimage*. 2006;33(2):725–731.
53. Leukefeld CG, Tims FM. Relapse and recovery in drug abuse: research and practice. *Subst Use Misuse*. 1989;24(3):189–201.
54. Lex BW. Some gender differences in alcohol and polysubstance users. *Health Psychol*. 1991;10(2):121–132.
55. Leyton M, Boileau I, Benkelfat C, Diksic M, Baker G, Dagher A. Amphetamine-induced increases in extracellular dopamine, drug wanting, and novelty seeking: a PET/[^{11}C] raclopride study in healthy men. *Neuropsychopharmacology*. 2002;27(6):1027–1035.
56. Leyton M. Conditioned and sensitized responses to stimulant drugs in humans. *Prog Neuropsychopharmacol Biol Psychiatry*. 2007;31(8):1601–1613.
57. Li CS, Kemp K, Milivojevic V, Sinha R. Neuroimaging study of sex differences in the neuropathology of cocaine abuse. *Gend Med*. 2005;2(3):174–182.
58. Li CS, Kosten TR, Sinha R. Sex differences in brain activation during stress imagery in abstinent cocaine users: a functional magnetic resonance imaging study. *Biol Psychiatry*. 2005;57(5):487–494.
59. London ED, Simon SL, Berman SM, et al. Mood disturbances and regional cerebral metabolic abnormalities in recently abstinent methamphetamine abusers. *Arch Gen Psychiatry*. 2004;61(1):73–84.
60. Maas LC, Lukas SE, Kaufman JJ, et al. Functional magnetic resonance imaging of human brain activation during cui-induced cocaine craving. *Am J Psychiatry*. 1998;155:124–126.
61. Magalhaes AC. Functional magnetic resonance and spectroscopy in drug and substance abuse. *Top Magn Reson Imaging*. 2005;16(3):247–251.
62. Marlatt GA, Gordon JR. *Relapse Prevention*. New York, N.Y.: Guilford Press; 1985.
63. Matochik JA, London ED, Eldreth DA, Cadet JL, Bolla KI. Frontal cortical tissue composition in abstinent cocaine abusers: a magnetic resonance imaging study. *Neuroimage*. 2003;19(3):1095–1102.
64. Mattay VS, Berman KF, Ostrem JL, et al. Dextroamphetamine enhances "neural network-specific" physiological signals: a positron-emission tomography rCBF study. *J Neurosci*. 1996;16:4816–4822.
65. Mattay VS, Callicott JH, Bertolino A, et al. Effects of dextroamphetamine on cognitive performance and cortical activation. *Neuroimage*. 2000;12:268–275.
66. Munro CA, McCaul ME, Wong DF, et al. Sex differences in striatal dopamine release in healthy adults. *Biol Psychiatry*. 2006;59(10):966–974.
67. National Institute on Drug Abuse (NIDA). NIDA infofacts: understanding drug abuse and addiction. http://www.drugabuse.gov/infofacts/understand.html; 2009 Accessed 26.10.2009.
68. Nurnberger JI Jr, Gershon ES, Simmons S, et al. Behavioral, biochemical and neuroendocrine responses to amphetamine in normal twins and 'well-state' bipolar patients. *Psychoneuroendocrinology*. 1982;7:163–176.
69. Oh JS, Lyoo IK, Sung YH, et al. Shape changes of the corpus callosum in abstinent methamphetamine users. *Neurosci Lett*. 2005;384(1–2):76–81.
70. Paulus MP, Hozack N, Zauscher B, et al. Prefrontal, parietal, and temporal cortex networks underlie decision-making in the presence of uncertainty. *Neuroimage*. 2001;13(1):91–100.
71. Paulus MP, Tapert SF, Schuckit MA. Neural activation patterns of methamphetamine-dependent subjects during decision making predict relapse. *Arch Gen Psychiatry*. 2005; 62(7):761–768.
72. Phan KL, Fitzgerald DA, Gao K, Moore GJ, Tancer ME, Posse S. Real-time fMRI of cortico-limbic brain activity during emotional processing. *Neuroreport*. 2004; 15(3):527–532.

73. Posse S, Fitzgerald D, Gao K, et al. Real-time fMRI of temporolimbic regions detects amygdala activation during single-trial self-induced sadness. *Neuroimage*. 2003;18(3):760–768.

74. RAND Drug Policy Research Center. *Cocaine: The First Decade*, vol. 1. Santa Monica, CA: Drug Policy Research Center; 1992:1–4.

75. Reske M, Paulus MP. Predicting treatment outcome in stimulant dependence. *Ann N Y Acad Sci*. 2008;1141:270–283.

76. Riccardi P, Zald D, Li R, et al. Sex differences in amphetamine-induced displacement of [(18)F]fallypride in striatal and extrastriatal regions: a PET study. *Am J Psychiatry*. 2006;163(9):1639–1641.

77. Robinson TE, Berridge KC. Addiction. *Annu Rev Psychol*. 2003;54:25–53.

78. Rohsenow DJ, Martin RA, Eaton CA, Monti PM. Cocaine craving as a predictor of treatment attrition and outcomes after residential treatment for cocaine dependence. *J Stud Alcohol Drugs*. 2007;68(5):641–648.

79. Rohsenow DJ, Martin RA, Monti PM. Urge-specific and lifestyle coping strategies of cocaine abusers: relationships to treatment outcomes. *Drug Alcohol Depend*. 2005;78(2): 211–219.

80. Rohsenow DJ, Monti PM. Relapse among cocaine abusers: theoretical, methodological, and treatment considerations. In: Tims FM, Leukefeld CG, Platt JJ, eds. *Relapse and Recovery in Addictions*. New Haven, CT: Yale University Press; 2001:355–378.

81. Rose ME, Grant JE. Pharmacotherapy for methamphetamine dependence: a review of the pathophysiology of methamphetamine addiction and the theoretical basis and efficacy of pharmacotherapeutic interventions. *Ann Clin Psychiatry*. 2008;20(3):145–155.

82. Roth ME, Cosgrove KP, Carroll ME. Sex differences in the vulnerability to drug abuse: a review of preclinical studies. *Neurosci Biobehav Rev*. 2004;28(6):533–546.

83. Rothman RB, Blough BE, Baumann MH. Dual dopamine/serotonin releasers: potential treatment agents for stimulant addiction. *Exp Clin Psychopharmacol*. 2008;16(6):458–474.

84. Sachar EJ, Halbreich U, Asnis GM, Nathan RS, Halpern FS, Ostrow L. Paradoxical cortisol responses to dextroamphetamine in endogenous depression. *Arch Gen Psychiatry*. 1981;38:1113–1117.

85. Sachar EJ, Puig-Antich J, Ryan ND, et al. Three tests of cortisol secretion in adult endogenous depressives. *Acta Psychiatr Scand*. 1985;71:1–8.

86. Substance Abuse and Mental Health Services Administration (SAMHSA). *Results from the 2008 National Survey on Drug Use and Health: National Findings (Office of Applied Studies, NSDUH Series H-36, HHS Publication No. SMA 09–4434)*. Rockville, MD: SAMHSA; 2009.

87. Sax KW, Strakowski SM. Enhanced behavioral response to repeated d-amphetamine and personality traits in humans. *Biol Psychiatry*. 1998;44:1192–1195.

88. Schweinsburg AD, Paulus MP, Barlett VC, et al. An FMRI study of response inhibition in youths with a family history of alcoholism. *Ann N Y Acad Sci*. 2004;1021:391–394.

89. Sekine Y, Ouchi Y, Sugihara G, et al. Methamphetamine causes microglial activation in the brains of human abusers. *J Neurosci*. 2008;28(22):5756–5761.

90. Shearer J. Psychosocial approaches to psychostimulant dependence: a systematic review. *J Subst Abuse Treat*. 2007;32(1):41–52.

91. Shearer J. The principles of agonist pharmacotherapy for psychostimulant dependence. *Drug Alcohol Rev*. 2008; 27(3):301–308.

92. Shiffman S, Engberg J, Paty J, et al. A day at a time: predicting smoking lapse from daily urge. *J Abnorm Psychol*. 1997;106:133–152.

93. Shiffman S, Paty J, Gnys M, Kassel J, Hickox M. First lapses to smoking: within subject analysis of real time reports. *J Consult Clin Psychol*. 1996;64:366–379.

94. Silberman EK, Reus VI, Jimerson DC, Lynott AM, Post RM. Heterogeneity of amphetamine response in depressed patients. *Am J Psychiatry*. 1981;138:1302–1307.

95. Silveri MM, Tzilos GK, Yurgelun-Todd DA. Relationship between white matter volume and cognitive performance during adolescence: effects of age, sex and risk for drug use. *Addiction*. 2008;103(9):1509–1520.

96. Sinha R, Garcia M, Paliwal P, Kreek MJ, Rounsaville BJ. Stress-induced cocaine craving and hypothalamic-pituitary-adrenal responses are predictive of cocaine relapse outcomes. *Arch Gen Psychiatry*. 2006;63(3):324–331.

97. Sinha R, Li CS. Imaging stress- and cue-induced drug and alcohol craving: association with relapse and clinical implications. *Drug Alcohol Rev*. 2007;26(1):25–31.

98. Sofuoglu M, Sewell RA. Norepinephrine and stimulant addiction. *Addict Biol*. 2009;14(2):119–129.

99. Strakowski SM, Sax KW, Rosenberg HL, DelBello MP, Adler CM. Human response to repeated low-dose d-amphetamine: evidence for behavioral enhancement and tolerance. *Neuropsychopharmacology*. 2001;25(4):548–554.

100. Tellegen A. *Brief Manual for the Multidimensional Personality Questionnaire*. Unpublished manuscript, University of Minnesota, Minneapolis; 1982.

101. Thompson PM, Hayashi KM, Simon SL, et al. Structural abnormalities in the brains of human subjects who use methamphetamine. *J Neurosci*. 2004;24(26):6028–6036.

102. Tims FM, Leukefeld CG, Platt JJ, eds. *Relapse and Recovery in Addictions*. New Haven, CT: Yale University Press; 2001.

103. Uftring SJ, Wachtel SR, Chu D, McCandless C, Levin DN, de Wit H. An fMRI study of the effect of amphetamine on brain activity. *Neuropsychopharmacology*. 2001;25:925–935.

104. Volkow ND. Fiscal Year 2010 Budget request before the senate subcommittee on Labor-HHS-Education Appropriations – statement of Nora D. Volkow, M.D. http://www.nida.nih.gov/Testimony/5-21-09Testimony.html; 2009 Accessed 5.21.09.

105. Schuh LM, Schuh KJ, Hennigfield JE. Pharacologic determinants of tobacco dependence. Am. J. Ther. 1996;3:335–341.

106. Volkow ND, Fowler JS, Wang GJ, et al. Decreased dopamine D_2 receptor availability is associated with reduced frontal metabolism in cocaine abusers. *Synapse*. 1993;14(2):169–177.

107. Volkow ND, Fowler JS, Wang GJ, Swanson JM, Telang F. Dopamine in drug abuse and addiction: results of imaging studies and treatment implications. *Arch Neurol*. 2007;64(11):1575–1579.

108. Volkow ND, Fowler JS, Wolf AP, et al. Changes in brain glucose metabolism in cocaine dependence and withdrawal. *Am J Psychiatry*. 1991;148(5):621–626.

109. Volkow ND, Wang GJ, Fowler JS, et al. Cocaine uptake is decreased in the brain of detoxified cocaine abusers. *Neuropsychopharmacology*. 1996;14(3):159–168.

110. Völlm BA, de Araujo IE, Cowen PJ, et al. Methamphetamine activates reward circuitry in drug naïve human subjects. *Neuropsychopharmacology*. 2004;29(9):1715–1722.

111. Wang GJ, Volkow ND, Fowler JS, et al. Regional brain metabolic activation during craving elicited by recall of previous drug experiences. *Life Sci*. 1999;64:775–784.

112. Weinshenker D, Schroeder JP. There and back again: a tale of norepinephrine and drug addiction. *Neuropsychopharmacology*. 2007;32(7):1433–1451.

113. Wexler BE, Gottschalk CH, Fulbright RK, et al. Functional magnetic resonance imaging of cocaine craving. *Am J Psychiatry*. 2001;158(1):86–95.

114. White TL, Baskin-Sommers A, Cohen RA, Sweet LH. Age and brain responses to reward and d-amphetamine in healthy volunteers using a novel impulsivity/risk task (BART). Organization for Human Brain Mapping annual meeting. Chicago, IL. *Neuroimage*. 2007;36(suppl 1):S107.

115. White TL, Grover VK, de Wit H. Cortisol effects of d-amphetamine relate to traits of fearlessness and aggression but not anxiety in healthy humans. *Pharmacol Biochem Behav*. 2006;85:123–131.

116. White TL, Justice AJH, de Wit H. Differential subjective effects of d-amphetamine by gender, hormone levels and menstrual cycle phase. *Pharmacol Biochem Behav*. 2002;73:729–741.

117. White TL, Lejuez CW, de Wit H. Personality and gender differences in effects of d-amphetamine on risk-taking. *Exp Clin Psychopharmacol*. 2007;15(6):599–609.

118. White TL, Lott D, de Wit H. Personality and the subjective effects of acute amphetamine in healthy volunteers. *Neuropsychopharmacology*. 2006;31(5):1064–1074.

119. Yan P, Li CS. Decreased amygdala activation during risk taking in non-dependent habitual alcohol users: a preliminary fMRI study of the stop signal task. *Am J Drug Alcohol Abuse*. 2009;35(5):284–289.

120. Yoo SS, Lee JH, O'Leary H, Lee V, Choo SE, Jolesz FA. Functional magnetic resonance imaging-mediated learning of increased activity in auditory areas. *Neuroreport*. 2007;18(18):1915–1920.

121. Zilberman M, Tavares H, el-Guebaly N. Gender similarities and differences: the prevalence and course of alcohol- and other substance-related disorders. *J Addict Dis*. 2003;22:61–74.

122. Zuckerman M. P-impulsive sensation seeking and its behavioral, psychophysiological biochemical correlates. *Neuropsychobiology*. 1993;28:30–36.

123. Zuckerman M. Personality in the third dimension: a psychobiological approach. *Pers Individ Dif*. 1989;10:391–418.

Chapter 12
Eating Disorders

Angelo Del Parigi and Ellen Schur

As commonly defined, eating disorders are persistent abnormalities of eating behavior that affect physical or mental health. Traditionally, eating disorders identify psychiatric conditions characterized by compulsive eating or extreme avoidance of eating, epitomized by bulimia nervosa (BN) and anorexia nervosa (AN), respectively. Another rather well-characterized eating disorder is binge eating disorder (BED), which can lead to weight gain, obesity, and related comorbidities, but it is not specific to any metabolic condition or disease. Although not included among eating disorders, we submit that "garden variety" (i.e., nonspecific) chronic overeating that leads to weight gain and obesity meets the basic criterion for eating disorders. Overeaters challenge the homeostasis of energy balance by ingesting food in excess of their needs and clearly develop a pathological condition, overweight–obesity, that undermines their physical health, meeting our common definition of an eating disorder. In this chapter, therefore, we will take a comprehensive approach and illustrate the neuroimaging evidence accrued on nonspecific overeating, BED, bulimia nervosa, and anorexia nervosa.

Overeating

Overeating – that is, eating in excess of energy needs – is a behavioral outcome of various conditions that span several chapters of psychiatric and metabolic pathology. Despite this diversity of causes and triggers, the result of overeating sustained over time is weight gain and eventual obesity, unless overeating is counteracted by practices (e.g., purging) or conditions (malabsorption due to medical conditions or consequent to surgical interventions) that limit the intestinal absorption of nutrients. As such, overeating is the elective target of behavioral and biological studies aimed at identifying, on a different scale, the characteristics, phenotypes, and genotypes of weight gain and obesity.

Investigations of the biology of weight gain and obesity have targeted the central nervous system (CNS), based on decades of research in animal models of obesity.[1] With the same purpose, overeating has become the subject of intense investigation by neuroimaging scientists interested in discovering neural substrates of the propensity to weight gain and obesity.

The neuroimaging investigation of nonspecific overeating has mainly focused on overweight and obese individuals. This experimental choice is based on the observation that excessive energy intake is a common phenotype of overweight–obesity. However, linking overeating to actual weight gain has proved exceptionally difficult, most likely because it is inherently challenging to measure energy intake in free-living individuals.[2] In the last decade, functional neuroimaging has been instrumental in identifying neurofunctional differences between obese and normal-weight individuals in their response to food-related stimuli.

Functional neuroimaging offers the possibility of exploring the whole brain at once without *a priori* region-specific hypotheses, making this technology an appealing choice to probe differences in brain function between overeaters and normal eaters, and obese and normal-weight individuals. This option has opened a window for appreciating the complexity of the neural substrates of overeating in humans beyond the regions and circuits evidenced by research in animal models.

A.D. Parigi (✉)
Clinical Development Endocrine, Pfizer Inc., 235 East 42nd Street, MailStop 219/8/2, New York, NY 10017, USA
e-mail: Angelo.DelParigi@pfizer.com

R.A. Cohen and L.H. Sweet (eds.), *Brain Imaging in Behavioral Medicine and Clinical Neuroscience*, DOI 10.1007/978-1-4419-6373-4_12, © Springer Science+Business Media, LLC 2011

In fact, a number of brain regions involved in cognitive and emotional processing have been reported to be activated in response to food-related stimuli, supporting the notion that eating behavior in humans is an idiosyncratic behavior, driven not only by the need to compensate for acute and chronic energy imbalances, but also by emotional, cultural, and cognitive factors that often override energy homeostasis in the initiation and termination of an eating episode.

Sensory Cues

Sight, smell, taste, and "mouth feel" are the fundamental means of appreciating food and, as such, are screeners, gatekeepers, and primary reinforcers of eating choices. At the same time, the anticipation of a forthcoming meal is conducive to physiological and psychological phenomena (i.e., cephalic phase response and expectation of reward) that prepare the organism for ingesting food. In addition, for a number of technical and logistic reasons, sensory stimulation is experimentally suitable for functional neuroimaging.

Thus, it is no surprise that the first report of neurofunctional differences between obese and normalweight individuals by Karhunen et al focused on the brain's response to visual stimulation by pictures of food vs. control images (pictures of a landscape), using single photon emission computed tomography (SPECT) to measure changes in regional cerebral blood flow (rCBF) as a proxy for local neural activity.[3] This study found that obese women responded to visual stimulation by pictures of food with increased neural activity in the right parietal and temporal cortices, but it observed no changes in normal-weight women. The investigators also reported that changes in neural activity in the parietal cortex were associated with increased feelings of hunger, as elicited by viewing food pictures.[3]

More refined experimental designs and settings have used functional magnetic resonance imaging (fMRI) to assess brain responses by measuring blood oxygen level-dependent (BOLD) contrasts. This method has evaluated differential responses to visual stimulation by pictures of high-calorie food, low-calorie food, and nonfood stimuli in obese and normal-weight women. In nonhungry nor satiated (after at least 1.5 h of fasting) obese compared with normal-weight women,

the dorsal striatum showed a greater response to pictures of high-calorie food than to neutral stimuli.[4] The dorsal striatum is a region of special interest because it is rich in dopamine D2 receptors (DRD2), which are involved in reward processing. These receptors were reported to be abnormally scarce in morbidly obese individuals compared with controls in a positron emission tomography (PET) study using a specific radioligand (^{11}C-raclopride) for DRD2.[5] Furthermore, a direct relationship between body mass index (BMI), over a 20–45 kg/m^2 range, and brain activation in response to high-calorie food pictures was described in women in several regions involved in the control of energy intake, including the dorsal striatum, anterior insula, posterior cingulate, and lateral orbitofrontal cortex (OFC).[4]

In slightly different experimental conditions, a study of moderately hungry women (8–9 h fast, after skipping lunch) has recently reported a greater activation in response to high-calorie food pictures vs. neutral stimuli in a series of cortical and subcortical regions of interest, including the OFC, medial prefrontal cortex, insula, anterior cingulate cortex, amygdala, nucleus accumbens, ventral pallidum, caudate, putamen, and hippocampus. A widespread greater response in obese compared with normal-weight women was also observed in response to high-calorie vs. low-calorie food pictures, except for the putamen.[6]

The oral sensory experience of food, encompassing taste, smell, and mouth feel, has also been investigated in obese individuals. Using PET and ^{15}O-water to measure changes in rCBF, Del Parigi et al assessed the brain response to oral administration of 2 ml of a liquid meal after a 36-h fast, shortly before consuming the same meal to satiation.[7] Compared with lean individuals, obese subjects exhibited greater increases in neural activity in the middle-dorsal insula and midbrain, and greater decreases in the posterior cingulate and the temporal and orbitofrontal cortices. Furthermore, body fat percentage, glycemia, and disinhibition (i.e., the susceptibility of eating behavior to emotional factors and sensory cues) were independent correlates of the neural response in the middle-dorsal insular cortex,[7] an area implicated in many sensorial and appetitive functions, including craving for food[8] and oral appreciation of food texture.[9] The sensory experience of food, again stimulated by 2 ml of a liquid meal, has also been reported to elicit a middle insular response in formerly obese individuals,[10] who had achieved and maintained normal body weight through diet and physical exercise despite a past history of severe obesity. In these phenotypically lean individuals, who have a history of persistent dieting to fight their propensity to regain weight, an obese-like response points to the possible existence of neural risk factors for weight gain, pending validation in longitudinal studies.

Consumption of Food

Although the brain response to food sensory cues has provided a fertile field for investigating the central regulation of energy intake, the actual consumption of food is what defines human eating behavior, representing the outcome of various motivational, cognitive, and metabolic factors. The frequency and caloric content of meals are the two quantitative factors that determine the magnitude of energy intake. In particular, the caloric content of a meal is the natural target of dietary interventions for weight loss, while manipulations of meal volume and macronutrient composition are often used instrumentally to elicit satiety in response to a smaller energy intake. Despite this compelling evidence for meal consumption as the key behavioral phenomenon of interest, investigations of the brain response to ingesting a meal have been much less frequent than investigations of the response to food sensory cues. This bias hinges on the fact that consumption of food presents several experimental challenges in a functional neuroimaging setting.

PET studies using ^{15}O-water to measure changes in rCBF have made a substantial contribution to our understanding of the differences between obese and normal-weight individuals and their relevance to the pathophysiology of obesity. One study reported the brain response to consuming a satiating liquid meal (supplying 50% of resting energy expenditure) after a 36-h fast in obese, normal weight, and formerly obese individuals. Consuming a meal was found to elicit differential responses in obese and normal-weight individuals in cortical and subcortical regions, including the OFC, hypothalamus, insula, hippocampus, and prefrontal cortex, which is recognized as the pivotal area for top-down control of behavioral responses.[2,11–13]

These responses were also generally consistent in men and women, with the exception of the hypothalamus,[14] and were confirmed as areas involved in controlling eating behavior in a study of brain response to ingesting a solution of 75 g of glucose, which reported analogous differences between obese and normal-weight individuals.[15] Similar results were reported by a study of brain response to the consumption of a preferred food (chocolate).[16] Del Parigi et al also observed that formerly obese individuals had an obese-like response in the posterior hippocampus, which is involved in complex functions such as learning, memory, craving for food, and enteroception. As discussed before, these results raise the possibility that the posterior hippocampus may exhibit a functional marker of risk for weight gain.[2]

Taken together, the evidence collected in the investigation of the brain response to the consumption of a meal and its obesity-related abnormalities, while also encompassing regions of interest suggested by robust evidence from animal models of obesity, such as the hypothalamus, has clearly pointed to brain regions involved in emotional and cognitive processing which are natural correlates of the hedonic and cognitive dimensions of human eating behavior. As a reflection of its whole brain at once recording capability, functional neuroimaging has opened new avenues for investigating the central control of eating behavior and has drawn the attention to such brain regions as the dorsal prefrontal cortex (DPFC), which has undergone the greatest phylogenetic development in humans and is central to the cognitive control of human behaviors.

In fact, a group of successful dieters, characterized by a higher level of cognitive control over eating behavior than nondieters, showed a greater activation in the DPFC in response to consuming a satiating liquid meal.[17] This increase in activity was directly proportional to the degree of dietary restraint that they exhibited.[17] In addition, the response in the DPFC was inversely correlated with the response in the OFC, a multimodal associative area where sensory and visceral inputs elicited by food ingestion converge and are decoded for reward value.[17] This interplay between DPFC and OFC is of special interest, given that these frontal regions are reciprocally interconnected. Furthermore, the emergence of metabolic and sensorial information related to food ingestion (bottom-up processing) to the cognitive level is thought to take place in the OFC, raising the possibility that in response to meal ingestion, an inhibitory feedback circuit links the DPFC and the OFC in successful dieters, which could be instrumental in maintaining their restrained eating behavior.

Notably, prefrontal activity measured by[18] F-fluorodeoxyglucose (FDG, a marker of local brain metabolic activity) was also found to be directly correlated in morbidly obese subjects with striatal DRD2 receptor availability, as measured by[11] C-raclopride. This correlation suggests that prefrontal projections of striatal dopaminergic pathways may modulate the control of food intake.[18] On the other hand, greater prefrontal activation in response to food pictures was also observed using BOLD-fMRI in women with AN compared with women with BN, possibly confirming an inhibitory role of this brain region on the drive to eat.[19]

Binge Eating Disorder

BED is defined by recurrent episodes of eating large amounts of food, with a sense of lack of control over eating and without the inappropriate compensatory behaviors that characterize BN.[20] It was given a provisional eating disorder diagnosis in the Diagnostic and Statistic Manual, Version IV,[20] and there have been calls for its inclusion in subsequent versions.[21]

A handful of functional neuroimaging studies in individuals with BED have been published. Increases in neural activity in the left frontal and prefrontal regions were reported by Karhunen et al in obese binge eaters in response to a food cue by using SPECT and Tc-99m-HMPAO.[3] Similar relative increases in left brain activity are also present in BN, where a loss of normal right/left asymmetry in brain activity has been reported.[22–25] Furthermore, patients with fronto-temporal dementia who engage in compulsive binge eating demonstrate atrophy of the right ventral insula, OFC, and striatum,[26] all of which are involved in regulating taste perception and food intake. In particular, reduced OFC activity is associated with higher volumes of food intake despite satiation.[27] Thus, findings from diverse studies connect binge eating episodes to a loss or relative reduction in function in prefrontal and orbitofrontal cortical regions of the right brain.

This loss of function may reflect underlying alteration of neurotransmitter activity, although no data on cortical regions are available for individuals with BED. Nevertheless, midbrain serotonin activity may be reduced in obese binge eaters compared with obese controls,[28] while treatment with psychotherapy and fluoxetine (a selective serotonin-reuptake inhibitor also effective in treatment of symptoms in BN) leads to improvements in symptoms that correlate with improvements in 5-HT transporter binding.[29] Thus, preliminary evidence suggests that BED may have distinguishing neurobiological abnormalities similar to those observed in nonspecific overeating and BN.

Bulimia Nervosa

BN is defined by recurrent episodes of binge eating (on average, at least twice a week for 3 months) followed by inappropriate compensatory behaviors such as purging, fasting, or excessive physical exercise. The episodes occur in response to exaggerated concerns about weight and body appearance.[20] The lifetime prevalence rate for BN in the general population is about 1%,[30] but among younger women it is substantially higher, with 4.5% of women aged 18–24 years meeting diagnostic criteria for BN.[31] Without treatment, BN usually has a chronic course.[32] Both behavioral therapies[33] and pharmacologic treatment with antidepressant drugs[34] are effective in reducing symptoms, but relapse is common, given the absence of specific therapies targeting neurobiological defects.

Structural and Global Functional Deficits

Structural and functional abnormalities of the brain in BN have been investigated by neuroimaging. Enlarged ventricles and widening of cortical sulci were documented by computed tomography scans in approximately 40% of normal-weight patients with BN,[35] and reduced cerebral/cranial ratios have also been documented.[36] However, after long-term recovery, women with a history of BN showed no evidence of persistent brain abnormalities.[37] Thus, while a small proportion of people who are acutely ill with BN show neuroimaging signs consistent with cerebral atrophy, these changes appear to resolve with recovery. Because they are also present in normal-weight bulimic subjects, these changes may be neural correlates of disturbed endocrine or metabolic factors rather than to loss of body adiposity.[35]

Global brain function is also abnormal during the acute phase of BN. Using FDG and PET, women with

BN were found to have globally and regionally reduced glucose metabolism compared with controls,[38] but other studies found no differences.[22,39,40] In addition, normal brain glucose metabolism is characterized by an asymmetry with right greater than left brain activity, a feature which is absent in women with BN.[22–25] Nevertheless, after long-term (at least 1 year) recovery from BN, brain function assessed by measuring rCBF did not differ between controls and recovered women.[41] Thus, changes in brain structure and function are associated with symptomatic BN. These abnormalities appear to resolve following treatment and represent neither a predisposing trait nor long-lasting sequelae of the disorder. As noted above, a relative reduction in right-sided brain activity has been observed in obese persons with BED,[3] suggesting that these findings may be specific to binge eating behaviors.

Abnormal Processing of Food Reward and Taste

One hypothesis regarding both BN and nonspecific overeating is that neural signaling or neurotransmitter function is reduced in cortical and reward processing brain regions. Much of this research has focused on the role of serotonin, an approach that is further supported by the relief of bulimic symptoms associated with selective serotonin-reuptake inhibitors treatment. More importantly, it is possible to measure synaptic serotonin transporter binding by using specific radioligands and PET, thus assessing more directly the role of serotonin transmission in neuropsychiatric disorders such as BN.[42] For this purpose,[18] F-altanserin has been used to quantify serotonin 2A receptors (5-HT2A) and carbonyl-[11] C 100635 (^{11}C-WAY100635) to quantify serotonin 1A receptors (5-HT1A).[43] In fact, increased 5-HT1A receptor binding in cortical regions, including the prefrontal and cingulate cortex, has been documented using ^{11}C-WAY100635.[44] As these findings point to brain regions involved in cognitive control of behavior, the authors speculate that an abnormal serotonin tone in these regions might be a correlate of impaired impulse control in women with BN who are actively binge eating. Abnormalities in cingulate cortex activity may be persistent, as reduced activity was found in the right anterior cingulate cortex and left

cuneus in recovered bulimic women in response to a glucose solution on the tongue. This finding supports the hypothesis that an impaired response to rewarding gustatory stimulation, possibly related to an abnormal serotonergic tone, may play a role in BN.[45]

Other brain regions implicated by studies of the serotonergic system include the hypothalamus, thalamus,[46] and medial OFC.[47] Taken together, this cumulative evidence suggests that functional impairment in serotonin transmission is present at multiple levels of receptor and synaptic function[48] and that it affects brain regions involved in the regulation of food intake, executive control of behavior, and reward processing, although findings are not fully consistent across studies.[49] It is tempting to believe that BN is associated with varying degrees of abnormalities in the serotonergic system, similar to the ones found in binge eating individuals,[28] but direct comparisons have not yet been made.

In addition, a PET study using[11] C-carfentanil[50] reported that the mu-opioid system, which is involved in processing hedonic information about food, is altered in bulimic women, who showed decreased receptor binding in the insular cortex, a region involved in many functions, including taste[51] and enteroceptive cue processing.[52] However, this study could not resolve whether the downregulation of mu-opioid receptors was a consequence of pathological eating or a marker of susceptibility.[50] Longitudinal studies are warranted to address this question.

Abnormal Body Image Perception and Response to Food Cues

In a study comparing brain responses to food vs. nonfood visual stimuli, patients with BN were distinguished from controls by their response to food photographs, as shown by greater activation in the left ventromedial prefrontal cortex, left occipital cortex, and cerebellum, and smaller activation in the anterior and lateral regions of the prefrontal cortex.[19] The smaller prefrontal activation could signify reduced ability to control a behavioral response, either to visual food cues or to food intake itself,[19] but specific studies are warranted to test these hypotheses. Perception of body shape in BN has also been studied using BOLD-fMRI. Data suggest that patients with eating disorders have less activity in occipito-temporal and parietal regions known to be involved in the recognition of animate forms.[53] The findings in women with BN were intermediate to those in women with AN and healthy controls, suggesting that the abnormal brain response to body shape in BN is less extreme than that in AN.[53]

Considerations for Future Work

These results suggest several promising avenues for future research, including studies of brain response to food cues and/or food consumption, neurotransmitter function, and the use of neuroimaging to monitor response to treatment. Further studies of BN may also benefit from comparisons with other groups that exhibit binge eating behavior, in order to resolve specific correlates of impaired impulse control. Studies of BN patients are more feasible than those of AN patients, because it is easier to control for potential confounding by body weight by choosing weight-matched controls. On the other hand, factors such as recent restriction of food intake vs. bingeing and purging behavior also need to be accounted for as they could potentially introduce additional variability into the results, even in recovered patients.[54]

Anorexia Nervosa

The clinical criteria for a diagnosis of AN include: (1) refusal to maintain body weight at or above a minimal normal weight for age and height; (2) intense fear of gaining weight or becoming fat, even though underweight; (3) disturbance in the way in which one's body weight or shape is experienced; (4) in postmenarchal females, amenorrhea.[20] The mortality rate for AN is the highest of any psychiatric disorder, with about 15% of patients dying as a result of complications of the disease.[55] Acute intensive treatment aims at maintaining body weight within a medically safe range. Beyond acute management, however, therapeutic options remain limited. Pharmacological trials have been disappointing, and no standardized approach has been established for postintensive treatment.[34] Evidence for the efficacy of behavioral interventions is sparse, but some data indicate that cognitive-behavioral therapy

may reduce relapse in adults and that family therapy may be helpful in adolescents.[56]

Structural Abnormalities

Neuroimaging studies have documented striking structural abnormalities in the brain during AN.[57–61] Computed tomography studies were among the first to report a pathological enlargement of ventricles and/or sulci consistent with cerebral atrophy during paroxysms of the disease.[62–67] Because these changes were reported to be reversible upon body weight recovery,[61,65,68–75] the term "pseudoatrophy" was suggested as a more descriptive definition.[76] Nutritional deficiencies consequent to insufficient food intake have been proposed to cause the condition.[73] Pseudoatrophy has also been confirmed by MRI in adults[71,72,77] and adolescents.[73,78,79] Cerebral matter loss appears to occur diffusely in the brain, in both gray and white matter.[75,79]

As noted above, several studies documented at least partial reversibility of this condition after weight recovery, but other evidence indicates that normalization in some brain regions may be incomplete.[71,72,80] For example, after weight recovery, AN patients have been reported to have persistently reduced volume in the hippocampus–amygdala,[81] anterior cingulate,[82] and total gray matter.[80] Even after at least 1 year of normalized body weight, AN patients showed reduced gray matter volume, suggesting that the effects on the brain are long-lasting.[83] In summary, while brain atrophy and increased ventricular volume substantially improve with weight regain, it is possible that specific brain matter losses persist after recovery. Predisposing or contributing factors to such deficits are not defined, but possibilities include a persistently altered metabolic state, severe structural damage, or unknown preexisting factors. Longitudinal studies are warranted to shed light on the natural history of these brain matter losses in the context of the disease course.

Despite the imaging evidence for marked brain abnormalities, pseudoatrophy has not been associated with changes in cognitive performance,[71] nor were hippocampal reductions correlated with hippocampal-dependent memory function.[84] On the contrary, a shrunken anterior cingulate was, in fact, associated with lower performance intelligence quotient (IQ) in another study.[85]

In conclusion, abnormalities in brain structure have been consistently documented in patients with AN. These changes are compatible with cerebral atrophy, are associated with extreme weight loss and very low BMI,[86] and are thought to be consequent to starvation.[87] It has been estimated that pseudoatrophy is present in 26–75% of AN patients.[59] While many studies have documented partial or complete resolution with weight regain, others suggest that a global deficit may persist long after weight normalization. Some structural defects have been associated with cognitive impairment. Because patients with AN present striking structural abnormalities, functional neuroimaging studies performed during the acute phase of the disorder should not apply normal anatomical parameters, whether in morphology or in hemodynamics, to functional mapping.

Deficits in Global and Regional Brain Function

Consistent with the structural changes discussed above, deficits in global and regional brain function are found during acute AN. Underweight young women with AN have significantly lower global cerebral glucose metabolism by FDG-PET.[88,89] Findings of similarities between women with AN and women with depression have led to suppositions that the observed differences may be related to weight loss, nutritional deficiency, and/or depressed mood.[90] Global deficits in brain function appear to resolve with weight regain[89,91] and after long-term recovery.[92]

Abnormalities in function across cortical regions have been consistently identified. While a relative hypermetabolism has been demonstrated in the inferior frontal cortex[40,89] and in limbic regions, including the thalamus and amygdala–hippocampus complex,[93] most studies reported hypofunction. Affected regions include the posterior and anterior cingulate cortices,[93–96] prefrontal cortex,[93,94] middle temporal gyrus,[94] superior temporal gyrus,[94] superior frontal cortex,[88,89] parietal lobe,[88–90,96] occipital lobes,[96] and insula.[96] Anterior cingulate hypoperfusion may be specific to restrictor-type AN.[97]

However, one would expect increased activity in regions involved in executive control of behavior as a neural correlate of the cognitive control over eating exercised by anorexic women. One possible explanation is that malnutrition and metabolic disturbances result in combinations of global and regional functional deficits that may mask increases in brain activity associated with rigid control over eating. These global and regional abnormalities during acute AN improve with refeeding in most cortical regions, including the parietal and occipital lobes, insula,[96] and cingulate cortex.[95] However, according to other reports, some of these brain regions may not recover, including the anterior cingulate,[96] temporoparietal, and OFC regions.[98] In addition, provision of testosterone significantly increases regional cerebral glucose metabolism in the posterior cingulate cortex.[94] On the whole, it appears that reduced activity during acute AN reflects the physiologic state of starvation and is not a causal factor leading to the presentation of disordered eating.

These functional deficits have been linked to cognitive impairment. In AN patients, impaired cognitive function is associated with reduced cerebral metabolism in the prefrontal cortex.[99] Cerebral hypoperfusion in the temporal lobe has also been implicated in impaired visual-spatial ability, impaired complex visual memory, and enhanced information processing.[100]

In sum, regional and global brain metabolism and perfusion abnormalities have been identified in AN, with potential implications for cognitive function during the acute illness. These abnormalities have not been conclusively linked to the pathophysiology of the disorder, and may, in fact, mask causal or correlative neuroimaging findings.

Serotonin and Dopamine Transmission

Theories regarding a role for serotonin transmission in the etiology of eating disorders are based on serotonin's documented role in mood and compulsivity disorders, as well as on evidence of low cerebrospinal fluid serotonin during acute AN that rebounds to elevated levels after recovery.[101,102]

As in some studies of BN,[47] reduced 5-HT2A binding in the parietal, frontal, and occipital lobes has been shown in women with AN.[103] Not all studies concur,[104] however, perhaps because of differences in serotonergic tone between the subtypes (bulimic vs. restricting) of AN.[105] Changes in serotonergic tone may be persistent. For example, in women recovered for more than 1 year, the presence of reduced 5-HT2A receptor binding compared with controls supports theories that excess serotonin transmission may contribute to the development of the disorder and may be detected even after recovery.[106] The amygdala, hippocampus, and cingulate cortex have been implicated.[106,107]

During the acute phase of AN, 5-HT1A receptor activity appears to be elevated in regions including the prefrontal cortex and lateral OFC, temporal lobe, parietal cortex, and dorsal raphe nuclei, as measured by PET.[104] After recovery, 5-HT1A receptor binding increased in women with prior binge eating/purging-type AN but not in women recovered from restricting-type AN.[108] Again, these findings emphasize the need for precise categorization of AN subtypes in order to reach firm conclusions regarding the interpretation of neuroimaging findings. A study of the serotonin transporter (5-HTT) also found that subtypes of AN were distinguished after recovery by differences in 5-HTT binding patterns in the dorsal raphe nucleus and anteroventral striatum.[54] These results suggest that reduced serotonergic activity in fronto-temporal regions in both lean and recovered AN patients may be correlates of the typical personality profile of eating disorder patients in terms of perfectionism and compulsivity.[109]

These data point to dysregulation in serotonergic pathways in cortical and limbic centers in AN that may contribute to traits of anxiety, perfectionism, and compulsivity.[48] The persistence of abnormalities after recovery suggests that altered serotonin transmission may be either a characteristic of eating disorders or a risk factor predisposing to their development.[110] Relative imbalances of 5-HT1A vs. 5-HT2A activity could also contribute to the rigid behavioral control exhibited in AN.[104] Yet despite a growing body of evidence for altered serotonin transmission in AN and after recovery from AN, causal interpretations must be made with caution, given the lack of prospective data or evidence that manipulations of serotonin activity can alter the course of the illness.[111]

As known, dopamine signaling plays a major role in regulating normal eating behavior,[112] but neuroimaging data on its role in eating disorders are scarce. An abnormality in the dopaminergic system in the ventral striatum (either decreased intrasynaptic dopamine availability or increased density of D2/D3 receptors) was documented by a study using PET and ^{11}C-raclopride to compare a group of formerly AN patients with controls.[113] Abnormalities in neurotransmitter systems implicated in eating behavior, including serotonin, dopamine, and histamine,[114] clearly represent a promising field of research into the pathophysiology of AN and may yield new targets for drug development.[115]

Disturbed Relationships to Food

AN is characterized by an abnormal relationship with food intake, and investigations into the neural correlates of this relationship have generated interesting but sometimes inconsistent results. In an fMRI study assessing brain response to visual food cues, AN patients showed less activation than controls in the inferior parietal lobe while satiated[116] and in the right visual occipital cortex while fasting,[116] suggesting a reduced salience of food cues regardless of the state of energy balance. Increased response to visual food cues in the lingual gyrus and left medial prefrontal cortex also have been reported.[19,117] Findings of greater activation in response to visual food cues in medial prefrontal cortical regions may reflect rigid control of food intake and, along with anterior cingulate activation, have been found to persist after recovery.[117] In contrast, greater responses to visual food stimuli in the lateral and apical prefrontal cortices are associated with recovery, while reduced responses characterize individuals with persistent symptoms.[117]

Women who recovered from restricting-type AN exhibited a reduced response to a sucrose and water solution in the insular cortex and striatum,[118] regions involved in central processing of taste and food reward. However, in patients with active AN, viewing pictures of high-calorie beverages was associated with an increased response in the insula, as well as in the anterior cingulate gyrus and amygdala–hippocampal region.[119] In the context of the more extensive structural and functional deficits observed in AN, differences in central processing of food stimuli might reflect an altered interplay between different brain regions and pathways.[120] Such changes may be especially pronounced in the management of potentially conflicting information, where the anterior cingulate is thought to play a fundamental role in the cognitive control of hunger.

Abnormal Body Image Perception

fMRI investigations have used a variety of experimental designs to identify a neural basis for the distorted body image and self-perception found in patients with AN. The left middle frontal gyrus and right posterior cingulate gyrus neural activities were correlated with reported body dissatisfaction in one study,[121] whereas activity in the right medial prefrontal cortex was associated with the degree of aversion produced by body figure drawings in another study.[53] Studies using self-images to trigger brain responses reported less activity in attentional and perceptual regions (including the cuneus, lingual gyrus, medial frontal gyrus, and insula) in AN patients than in controls,[122] possibly as a correlate of altered self-perceptions.

In response to visual stimulation by distorted self-images, an increased activation in AN patients compared with controls has been reported in the right amygdala, right fusiform gyrus, and brainstem,[123] as well as in the inferior parietal lobule.[124] The amygdala and parahippocampal gyrus were also stimulated by reading unpleasant words concerning body image.[125] Taken together, these findings may indicate potential fearful or aversive responses to body image cues, particularly in the case of the amygdalar response. However, conclusions are limited by the wide array of experimental approaches and the variability of results across studies, while the fundamental question of whether perceptual abnormalities in assessing body shape precede or follow the onset of the disorder remains open.

Conclusions and Considerations for Future Work

The acute underweight phase of AN is associated with structural changes in the brain that are evocative of cerebral atrophy. These changes generally reverse with weight regain. Parallel functional changes also occur, potentially affecting cognitive processing. Although these functional abnormalities appear to resolve with weight regain, they may limit the ability of some neuroimaging techniques to examine differences in brain function between acutely ill anorexic patients and controls.

One promising area, both for neuroimaging research and for potential pharmacological targets, is the role of neurotransmitters in AN, including serotonin and dopamine. Hypothesis-testing studies should now proceed with focused experimental designs aimed at defining the role of several regions of interest in the pathophysiology of the disorder and the manifestation

of specific symptoms. Such regions include the anterior cingulate cortex, striatum, and amygdala. Finally, longitudinal studies are needed to discern the neurological bases of AN, and of other eating disorders, starting with high-risk groups that may show signatures of functional aberrations before the onset of the disorder.

References

1. Morton GJ, Cummings DE, Baskin DG, Barsh GS, Schwartz MW. Central nervous system control of food intake and body weight. *Nature*. 2006;443(7109):289–295.
2. DelParigi A, Pannacciulli N, Le DN, Tataranni PA. In pursuit of neural risk factors for weight gain in humans. *Neurobiol Aging*. 2005;26(suppl 1):50–55.
3. Karhunen LJ, Vanninen EJ, Kuikka JT, Lappalainen RI, Tiihonen J, Uusitupa MI. Regional cerebral blood flow during exposure to food in obese binge eating women. *Psychiatry Res*. 2000;99(1):29–42.
4. Rothemund Y, Preuschhof C, Bohner G, et al. Differential activation of the dorsal striatum by high-calorie visual food stimuli in obese individuals. *Neuroimage*. 2007;37(2):410–421.
5. Wang GJ, Volkow ND, Logan J, et al. Brain dopamine and obesity. *Lancet*. 2001;357(9253):354–357.
6. Stoeckel LE, Weller RE, Cook EW, Twieg DB, Knowlton RC, Cox JE. Widespread reward-system activation in obese women in response to pictures of high-calorie foods. *Neuroimage*. 2008;41(2):636–647.
7. DelParigi A, Chen K, Salbe AD, Reiman EM, Tataranni PA. Sensory experience of food and obesity: a positron emission tomography study of the brain regions affected by tasting a liquid meal after a prolonged fast. *Neuroimage*. 2005;24(2):436–443.
8. Pelchat ML, Johnson A, Chan R, Valdez J, Ragland JD. Images of desire: food-craving activation during fMRI. *Neuroimage*. 2004;23(4):1486–1493.
9. de Araujo IE, Rolls ET, Kringelbach ML, McGlone F, Phillips N. Taste-olfactory convergence, and the representation of the pleasantness of flavour, in the human brain. *Eur J Neurosci*. 2003;18(7):2059–2068.
10. DelParigi A, Chen K, Salbe AD, et al. Persistence of abnormal neural responses to a meal in postobese individuals. *Int J Obes Relat Metab Disord*. 2004;28(3):370–377.
11. Del Parigi A, Gautier JF, Chen K, et al. Neuroimaging and obesity: mapping the brain responses to hunger and satiation in humans using positron emission tomography. *Ann N Y Acad Sci*. 2002;967:389–397.
12. Gautier JF, Del Parigi A, Chen K, et al. Effect of satiation on brain activity in obese and lean women. *Obes Res*. 2001;9(11):676–684.
13. Tataranni PA, DelParigi A. Functional neuroimaging: a new generation of human brain studies in obesity research. *Obes Rev*. 2003;4(4):229–238.
14. Del Parigi A, Chen K, Gautier JF, et al. Sex differences in the human brain's response to hunger and satiation. *Am J Clin Nutr*. 2002;75(6):1017–1022.

15. Matsuda M, Liu Y, Mahankali S, et al. Altered hypothalamic function in response to glucose ingestion in obese humans. *Diabetes*. 1999;48(9):1801–1806.

16. Small DM, Zatorre RJ, Dagher A, Evans AC, Jones-Gotman M. Changes in brain activity related to eating chocolate: from pleasure to aversion. *Brain*. 2001;124(Pt 9):1720–1733.

17. DelParigi A, Chen K, Salbe AD, et al. Successful dieters have increased neural activity in cortical areas involved in the control of behavior. *Int J Obes (Lond)*. 2007;31(3):440–448.

18. Volkow ND, Wang GJ, Telang F, et al. Low dopamine striatal D2 receptors are associated with prefrontal metabolism in obese subjects: possible contributing factors. *Neuroimage*. 2008;42(4):1537–1543.

19. Uher R, Murphy T, Brammer MJ, et al. Medial prefrontal cortex activity associated with symptom provocation in eating disorders. *Am J Psychiatry*. 2004;161(7):1238–1246.

20. American Psychiatric Association. *Diagnostic and Statistical Manual of Mental Disorders, Version IV*. Washington, DC: American Psychiatric Association; 1994.

21. Striegel-Moore RH, Franko DL. Should binge eating disorder be included in the DSM-V? A critical review of the state of the evidence. *Annu Rev Clin Psychol*. 2008;4:305–324.

22. Andreason PJ, Altemus M, Zametkin AJ, King AC, Lucinio J, Cohen RM. Regional cerebral glucose metabolism in bulimia nervosa. *Am J Psychiatry*. 1992;149(11):1506–1513.

23. Wu JC, Hagman J, Buchsbaum MS, et al. Greater left cerebral hemispheric metabolism in bulimia assessed by positron emission tomography. *Am J Psychiatry*. 1990;147(3):309–312.

24. Hagman JO, Buchsbaum MS, Wu JC, Rao SJ, Reynolds CA, Blinder BJ. Comparison of regional brain metabolism in bulimia nervosa and affective disorder assessed with positron emission tomography. *J Affect Disord*. 1990;19(3):153–162.

25. Nozoe S, Naruo T, Yonekura R, et al. Comparison of regional cerebral blood flow in patients with eating disorders. *Brain Res Bull*. 1995;36(3):251–255.

26. Woolley JD, Gorno-Tempini ML, Seeley WW, et al. Binge eating is associated with right orbitofrontal-insular-striatal atrophy in frontotemporal dementia. *Neurology*. 2007;69 (14):1424–1433.

27. Batterham RL, ffytche DH, Rosenthal JM, et al. PYY modulation of cortical and hypothalamic brain areas predicts feeding behaviour in humans. *Nature*. 2007;450(7166): 106–109.

28. Kuikka JT, Tammela L, Karhunen L, et al. Reduced serotonin transporter binding in binge eating women. *Psychopharmacology (Berl)*. 2001;155(3):310–314.

29. Tammela LI, Rissanen A, Kuikka JT, et al. Treatment improves serotonin transporter binding and reduces binge eating. *Psychopharmacology (Berl)*. 2003;170(1):89–93.

30. Garfinkel PE, Lin E, Goering P, et al. Bulimia nervosa in a Canadian community sample: prevalence and comparison of subgroups. *Am J Psychiatry*. 1995;152(7):1052–1058.

31. Bushnell JA, Wells JE, Hornblow AR, Oakley-Browne MA, Joyce P. Prevalence of three bulimia syndromes in the general population. *Psychol Med*. 1990;20(3):671–680.

32. Fairburn CG, Cooper Z, Doll HA, Norman P, O'Connor M. The natural course of bulimia nervosa and binge eating disorder in young women. *Arch Gen Psychiatry*. 2000; 57(7):659–665.

33. Wilson GT, Fairburn CC, Agras WS, Walsh BT, Kraemer H. Cognitive-behavioral therapy for bulimia nervosa: time course and mechanisms of change. *J Consult Clin Psychol*. 2002;70(2):267–274.

34. Walsh BT. Pharmacologic treatment of anorexia nervosa and bulimia nervosa. In: Fairburn CG, Brownell KD, eds. *Eating Disorders and Obesity: A Comprehensive Handbook*. New York, NY: Guilford Press; 2002:325–329.

35. Krieg JC, Lauer C, Pirke KM. Structural brain abnormalities in patients with bulimia nervosa. *Psychiatry Res*. 1989;27(1):39–48.

36. Hoffman GW, Ellinwood EH Jr, Rockwell WJ, Herfkens RJ, Nishita JK, Guthrie LF. Cerebral atrophy in bulimia. *Biol Psychiatry*. 1989;25(7):894–902.

37. Wagner A, Greer P, Bailer UF, et al. Normal brain tissue volumes after long-term recovery in anorexia and bulimia nervosa. *Biol Psychiatry*. 2006;59(3):291–293.

38. Delvenne V, Goldman S, Simon Y, De Maertelaer V, Lotstra F. Brain hypometabolism of glucose in bulimia nervosa. *Int J Eat Disord*. 1997;21(4):313–320.

39. Krieg JC, Holthoff V, Schreiber W, Pirke KM, Herholz K. Glucose metabolism in the caudate nuclei of patients with eating disorders, measured by PET. *Eur Arch Psychiatry Clin Neurosci*. 1991;240(6):331–333.

40. Delvenne V, Goldman S, De Maertelaer V, Lotstra F. Brain glucose metabolism in eating disorders assessed by positron emission tomography. *Int J Eat Disord*. 1999;25(1):29–37.

41. Frank GK, Kaye WH, Greer P, Meltzer CC, Price JC. Regional cerebral blood flow after recovery from bulimia nervosa. *Psychiatry Res*. 2000;100(1):31–39.

42. Hesse S, Barthel H, Schwarz J, Sabri O, Muller U. Advances in in vivo imaging of serotonergic neurons in neuropsychiatric disorders. *Neurosci Biobehav Rev*. 2004;28(6):547–563.

43. Barbarich NC, Kaye WH, Jimerson D. Neurotransmitter and imaging studies in anorexia nervosa: new targets for treatment. *Curr Drug Targets CNS Neurol Disord*. 2003;2 (1):61–72.

44. Tiihonen J, Keski-Rahkonen A, Lopponen M, et al. Brain serotonin 1A receptor binding in bulimia nervosa. *Biol Psychiatry*. 2004;55(8):871–873.

45. Frank GK, Wagner A, Achenbach S, et al. Altered brain activity in women recovered from bulimic-type eating disorders after a glucose challenge: a pilot study. *Int J Eat Disord*. 2006;39(1):76–79.

46. Tauscher J, Pirker W, Willeit M, et al. [123I] beta-CIT and single photon emission computed tomography reveal reduced brain serotonin transporter availability in bulimia nervosa. *Biol Psychiatry*. 2001;49(4):326–332.

47. Kaye WH, Frank GK, Meltzer CC, et al. Altered serotonin 2A receptor activity in women who have recovered from bulimia nervosa. *Am J Psychiatry*. 2001;158(7):1152–1155.

48. Kaye WH, Frank GK, Bailer UF, et al. Serotonin alterations in anorexia and bulimia nervosa: new insights from imaging studies. *Physiol Behav*. 2005;85(1):73–81.

49. Goethals I, Vervaet M, Audenaert K, et al. Comparison of cortical 5-HT2A receptor binding in bulimia nervosa patients and healthy volunteers. *Am J Psychiatry*. 2004; 161(10):1916–1918.

50. Bencherif B, Guarda AS, Colantuoni C, Ravert HT, Dannals RF, Frost JJ. Regional mu-opioid receptor binding in insular cortex is decreased in bulimia nervosa and correlates inversely with fasting behavior. *J Nucl Med*. 2005; 46(8):1349–1351.

51. Rolls ET. Taste, olfactory, and food texture processing in the brain, and the control of food intake. *Physiol Behav.* 2005;85(1):45–56.
52. Critchley HD, Wiens S, Rotshtein P, Ohman A, Dolan RJ. Neural systems supporting interoceptive awareness. *Nat Neurosci.* 2004;7(2):189–195.
53. Uher R, Murphy T, Friederich HC, et al. Functional neuro-anatomy of body shape perception in healthy and eating-disordered women. *Biol Psychiatry.* 2005;58(12):990–997.
54. Bailer UF, Frank GK, Henry SE, et al. Serotonin transporter binding after recovery from eating disorders. *Psychopharmacology (Berl).* 2007;195(3):315–324.
55. Zipfel S, Lowe B, Reas DL, Deter HC, Herzog W. Long-term prognosis in anorexia nervosa: lessons from a 21-year follow-up study. *Lancet.* 2000;355(9205):721–722.
56. Bulik CM, Berkman ND, Brownley KA, Sedway JA, Lohr KN. Anorexia nervosa treatment: a systematic review of randomized controlled trials. *Int J Eat Disord.* 2007; 40(4):310–320.
57. Hendren RL, De Backer I, Pandina GJ. Review of neuroimaging studies of child and adolescent psychiatric disorders from the past 10 years. *J Am Acad Child Adolesc Psychiatry.* 2000;39(7):815–828.
58. Kerem NC, Katzman DK. Brain structure and function in adolescents with anorexia nervosa. *Adolesc Med.* 2003; 14(1):109–118.
59. Mazzetti di Pietralata G. Imaging techniques in the management of anorexia and bulimia nervosa. *Eat Weight Disord.* 2002;7(2):146–151.
60. Herholz K. Neuroimaging in anorexia nervosa. *Psychiatry Res.* 1996;62(1):105–110.
61. Krieg JC. Eating disorders as assessed by cranial computerized tomography (CCT, dSPECT, PET). *Adv Exp Med Biol.* 1991;291:223–229.
62. Enzmann DR, Lane B. Cranial computed tomography findings in anorexia nervosa. *J Comput Assist Tomogr.* 1977;1(4):410–414.
63. Krieg JC, Pirke KM, Lauer C, Backmund H. Endocrine, metabolic, and cranial computed tomographic findings in anorexia nervosa. *Biol Psychiatry.* 1988;23(4):377–387.
64. Datlof S, Coleman PD, Forbes GB, Kreipe RE. Ventricular dilation on CAT scans of patients with anorexia nervosa. *Am J Psychiatry.* 1986;143(1):96–98.
65. Dolan RJ, Mitchell J, Wakeling A. Structural brain changes in patients with anorexia nervosa. *Psychol Med.* 1988; 18(2):349–353.
66. Lankenau H, Swigar ME, Bhimani S, Luchins D, Quinlan DM. Cranial CT scans in eating disorder patients and controls. *Compr Psychiatry.* 1985;26(2):136–147.
67. Palazidou E, Robinson P, Lishman WA. Neuroradiological and neuropsychological assessment in anorexia nervosa. *Psychol Med.* 1990;20(3):521–527.
68. Heinz ER, Martinez J, Haenggeli A. Reversibility of cerebral atrophy in anorexia nervosa and Cushing's syndrome. *J Comput Assist Tomogr.* 1977;1(4):415–418.
69. Kohlmeyer K, Lehmkuhl G, Poutska F. Computed tomography of anorexia nervosa. *AJNR Am J Neuroradiol.* 1983;4(3):437–438.
70. Artmann H, Grau H, Adelmann M, Schleiffer R. Reversible and non-reversible enlargement of cerebrospinal fluid spaces in anorexia nervosa. *Neuroradiology.* 1985;27(4):304–312.
71. Kingston K, Szmukler G, Andrewes D, Tress B, Desmond P. Neuropsychological and structural brain changes in anorexia nervosa before and after refeeding. *Psychol Med.* 1996;26(1):15–28.
72. Neumarker KJ, Bzufka WM, Dudeck U, Hein J, Neumarker U. Are there specific disabilities of number processing in adolescent patients with Anorexia nervosa? Evidence from clinical and neuropsychological data when compared to morphometric measures from magnetic resonance imaging. *Eur Child Adolesc Psychiatry.* 2000;9(suppl 2):II111–II121.
73. Golden NH, Ashtari M, Kohn MR, et al. Reversibility of cerebral ventricular enlargement in anorexia nervosa, demonstrated by quantitative magnetic resonance imaging. *J Pediatr.* 1996;128(2):296–301.
74. Swayze VW 2nd, Andersen A, Arndt S, et al. Reversibility of brain tissue loss in anorexia nervosa assessed with a computerized Talairach 3-D proportional grid. *Psychol Med.* 1996;26(2):381–390.
75. Swayze VW 2nd, Andersen AE, Andreasen NC, Arndt S, Sato Y, Ziebell S. Brain tissue volume segmentation in patients with anorexia nervosa before and after weight normalization. *Int J Eat Disord.* 2003;33(1):33–44.
76. Sein P, Searson S, Nicol AR, Hall K. Anorexia nervosa and pseudo-atrophy of the brain. *Br J Psychiatry.* 1981;139: 257–258.
77. Hoffman GW Jr, Ellinwood EH Jr, Rockwell WJ, Herfkens RJ, Nishita JK, Guthrie LF. Cerebral atrophy in anorexia nervosa: a pilot study. *Biol Psychiatry.* 1989;26(3):321–324.
78. Kornreich L, Shapira A, Horev G, Danziger Y, Tyano S, Mimouni M. CT and MR evaluation of the brain in patients with anorexia nervosa. *AJNR Am J Neuroradiol.* 1991; 12(6):1213–1216.
79. Katzman DK, Lambe EK, Mikulis DJ, Ridgley JN, Goldbloom DS, Zipursky RB. Cerebral gray matter and white matter volume deficits in adolescent girls with anorexia nervosa. *J Pediatr.* 1996;129(6):794–803.
80. Katzman DK, Zipursky RB, Lambe EK, Mikulis DJ. A longitudinal magnetic resonance imaging study of brain changes in adolescents with anorexia nervosa. *Arch Pediatr Adolesc Med.* 1997;151(8):793–797.
81. Giordano GD, Renzetti P, Parodi RC, et al. Volume measurement with magnetic resonance imaging of hippocampus-amygdala formation in patients with anorexia nervosa. *J Endocrinol Invest.* 2001;24(7):510–514.
82. Muhlau M, Gaser C, Ilg R, et al. Gray matter decrease of the anterior cingulate cortex in anorexia nervosa. *Am J Psychiatry.* 2007;164(12):1850–1857.
83. Lambe EK, Katzman DK, Mikulis DJ, Kennedy SH, Zipursky RB. Cerebral gray matter volume deficits after weight recovery from anorexia nervosa. *Arch Gen Psychiatry.* 1997;54(6):537–542.
84. Connan F, Murphy F, Connor SE, et al. Hippocampal volume and cognitive function in anorexia nervosa. *Psychiatry Res.* 2006;146(2):117–125.
85. McCormick LM, Keel PK, Brumm MC, et al. Implications of starvation-induced change in right dorsal anterior cingulate volume in anorexia nervosa. *Int J Eat Disord.* 2008;41(7):602–610.
86. Kohn MR, Ashtari M, Golden NH, et al. Structural brain changes and malnutrition in anorexia nervosa. *Ann N Y Acad Sci.* 1997;817:398–399.

87. Katzman DK, Christensen B, Young AR, Zipursky RB. Starving the brain: structural abnormalities and cognitive impairment in adolescents with anorexia nervosa. *Semin Clin Neuropsychiatry.* 2001;6(2):146–152.

88. Delvenne V, Lotstra F, Goldman S, et al. Brain hypometabolism of glucose in anorexia nervosa: a PET scan study. *Biol Psychiatry.* 1995;37(3):161–169.

89. Delvenne V, Goldman S, De Maertelaer V, Simon Y, Luxen A, Lotstra F. Brain hypometabolism of glucose in anorexia nervosa: normalization after weight gain. *Biol Psychiatry.* 1996;40(8):761–768.

90. Delvenne V, Goldman S, Biver F, et al. Brain hypometabolism of glucose in low-weight depressed patients and in anorectic patients: a consequence of starvation? *J Affect Disord.* 1997;44(1):69–77.

91. Kuruoglu AC, Kapucu O, Atasever T, Arikan Z, Isik E, Unlu M. Technetium-99 m-HMPAO brain SPECT in anorexia nervosa. *J Nucl Med.* 1998;39(2):304–306.

92. Frank GK, Bailer UF, Meltzer CC, et al. Regional cerebral blood flow after recovery from anorexia or bulimia nervosa. *Int J Eat Disord.* 2007;40(6):488–492.

93. Takano A, Shiga T, Kitagawa N, et al. Abnormal neuronal network in anorexia nervosa studied with I-123-IMP SPECT. *Psychiatry Res.* 2001;107(1):45–50.

94. Miller KK, Deckersbach T, Rauch SL, et al. Testosterone administration attenuates regional brain hypometabolism in women with anorexia nervosa. *Psychiatry Res.* 2004; 132(3):197–207.

95. Matsumoto R, Kitabayashi Y, Narumoto J, et al. Regional cerebral blood flow changes associated with interoceptive awareness in the recovery process of anorexia nervosa. *Prog Neuropsychopharmacol Biol Psychiatry.* 2006;30(7): 1265–1270.

96. Kojima S, Nagai N, Nakabeppu Y, et al. Comparison of regional cerebral blood flow in patients with anorexia nervosa before and after weight gain. *Psychiatry Res.* 2005;140(3):251–258.

97. Naruo T, Nakabeppu Y, Deguchi D, et al. Decreases in blood perfusion of the anterior cingulate gyri in Anorexia Nervosa Restricters assessed by SPECT image analysis. *BMC Psychiatry.* 2001;1:2.

98. Rastam M, Bjure J, Vestergren E, et al. Regional cerebral blood flow in weight-restored anorexia nervosa: a preliminary study. *Dev Med Child Neurol.* 2001;43(4):239–242.

99. Ohrmann P, Kersting A, Suslow T, et al. Proton magnetic resonance spectroscopy in anorexia nervosa: correlations with cognition. *Neuroreport.* 2004;15(3):549–553.

100. Lask B, Gordon I, Christie D, Frampton I, Chowdhury U, Watkins B. Functional neuroimaging in early-onset anorexia nervosa. *Int J Eat Disord.* 2005;37(Suppl):S49–S51; discussion S87–S49.

101. Kaye WH, Gwirtsman HE, George DT, Jimerson DC, Ebert MH. CSF 5-HIAA concentrations in anorexia nervosa: reduced values in underweight subjects normalize after weight gain. *Biol Psychiatry.* 1988;23(1):102–105.

102. Wolfe BE, Metzger E, Jimerson DC. Research update on serotonin function in bulimia nervosa and anorexia nervosa. *Psychopharmacol Bull.* 1997;33(3):345–354.

103. Audenaert K, Van Laere K, Dumont F, et al. Decreased 5-HT2a receptor binding in patients with anorexia nervosa. *J Nucl Med.* 2003;44(2):163–169.

104. Bailer UF, Frank GK, Henry SE, et al. Exaggerated 5-HT1A but normal 5-HT2A receptor activity in individuals ill with anorexia nervosa. *Biol Psychiatry.* 2007;61(9):1090–1099.

105. Goethals I, Vervaet M, Audenaert K, et al. Differences of cortical 5-HT2A receptor binding index with SPECT in subtypes of anorexia nervosa: relationship with personality traits? *J Psychiatr Res.* 2007;41(5):455–458.

106. Frank GK, Kaye WH, Meltzer CC, et al. Reduced 5-HT2A receptor binding after recovery from anorexia nervosa. *Biol Psychiatry.* 2002;52(9):896–906.

107. Bailer UF, Price JC, Meltzer CC, et al. Altered 5-HT(2A) receptor binding after recovery from bulimia-type anorexia nervosa: relationships to harm avoidance and drive for thinness. *Neuropsychopharmacology.* 2004;29(6):1143–1155.

108. Bailer UF, Frank GK, Henry SE, et al. Altered brain serotonin 5-HT1A receptor binding after recovery from anorexia nervosa measured by positron emission tomography and [carbonyl11C]WAY-100635. *Arch Gen Psychiatry.* 2005;62(9):1032–1041.

109. Galusca B, Costes N, Zito NG, et al. Organic background of restrictive-type anorexia nervosa suggested by increased serotonin(1A) receptor binding in right frontotemporal cortex of both lean and recovered patients: [(18)F]MPPF PET scan study. *Biol Psychiatry.* 2008;64(11):1009–1013.

110. Kaye WH, Bailer UF, Frank GK, Wagner A, Henry SE. Brain imaging of serotonin after recovery from anorexia and bulimia nervosa. *Physiol Behav.* 2005;86(1–2):15–17.

111. Walsh BT, Devlin MJ. Eating disorders: progress and problems. *Science.* 1998;280(5368):1387–1390.

112. Kelley AE, Baldo BA, Pratt WE, Will MJ. Corticostriatal-hypothalamic circuitry and food motivation: integration of energy, action and reward. *Physiol Behav.* 2005;86(5): 773–795.

113. Frank GK, Bailer UF, Henry SE, et al. Increased dopamine D2/D3 receptor binding after recovery from anorexia nervosa measured by positron emission tomography and [11c]raclopride. *Biol Psychiatry.* 2005;58(11):908–912.

114. Yoshizawa M, Tashiro M, Fukudo S, et al. Increased brain histamine H1 receptor binding in patients with anorexia nervosa. *Biol Psychiatry.* 2009;65(4):329–335.

115. Frank GK, Kaye WH. Positron emission tomography studies in eating disorders: multireceptor brain imaging, correlates with behavior and implications for pharmacotherapy. *Nucl Med Biol.* 2005;32(7):755–761.

116. Santel S, Baving L, Krauel K, Munte TF, Rotte M. Hunger and satiety in anorexia nervosa: fMRI during cognitive processing of food pictures. *Brain Res.* 2006;1114:138–148.

117. Uher R, Brammer MJ, Murphy T, et al. Recovery and chronicity in anorexia nervosa: brain activity associated with differential outcomes. *Biol Psychiatry.* 2003;54(9): 934–942.

118. Wagner A, Aizenstein H, Mazurkewicz L, et al. Altered insula response to taste stimuli in individuals recovered from restricting-type anorexia nervosa. *Neuropsychopharmacology.* 2008;33(3):513–523.

119. Ellison Z, Foong J, Howard R, Bullmore E, Williams S, Treasure J. Functional anatomy of calorie fear in anorexia nervosa. *Lancet.* 1998;352(9135):1192.

120. Wagner A, Aizenstein H, Venkatraman VK, et al. Altered reward processing in women recovered from anorexia nervosa. *Am J Psychiatry.* 2007;164(12):1842–1849.

121. Goethals I, Vervaet M, Audenaert K, Jacobs F, Ham H, Van Heeringen C. Does regional brain perfusion correlate with eating disorder symptoms in anorexia and bulimia nervosa patients? *J Psychiatr Res.* 2007;41(12):1005–1011.
122. Sachdev P, Mondraty N, Wen W, Gulliford K. Brains of anorexia nervosa patients process self-images differently from non-self-images: an fMRI study. *Neuropsychologia.* 2008;46(8):2161–2168.
123. Seeger G, Braus DF, Ruf M, Goldberger U, Schmidt MH. Body image distortion reveals amygdala activation in patients with anorexia nervosa – a functional magnetic resonance imaging study. *Neurosci Lett.* 2002;326(1): 25–28.
124. Wagner A, Ruf M, Braus DF, Schmidt MH. Neuronal activity changes and body image distortion in anorexia nervosa. *Neuroreport.* 2003;14(17):2193–2197.
125. Shirao N, Okamoto Y, Okada G, Okamoto Y, Yamawaki S. Temporomesial activation in young females associated with unpleasant words concerning body image. *Neuropsychobiology.* 2003;48(3):136–142.

Chapter 13
Structural and Functional Neuroimaging in Obesity

Kelly Stanek, Joseph Smith, and John Gunstad

Introduction

An estimated one-third of American adults are obese[1], and the proportion of obese adults has been shown to increase with age through midlife [2]. Obesity throughout the lifespan is associated with greater cardiovascular risk[2,3] and increased mortality,[3,4] as well as negative psychosocial sequelae[5] and psychiatric comorbidity[6,7], including a variety of maladaptive eating/dieting patterns (e.g., binge eating, emotional eating, weight cycling).[8,9]

Growing evidence also suggests that cognitive impairment is common in both younger and older obese adults.[7,10–14] Obesity has been associated with increased risk for Alzheimer's and vascular dementia,[15–18] even independent of cardiovascular risk factors and other medical comorbidities.[19,20] While the neuropathological mechanisms for these cognitive changes are not yet fully understood, elevated body mass and adiposity have been linked to alterations in brain structure, function, and chemistry prior to the onset of dementia.

Recent advances in neuroimaging allow for identification and analysis of these morphological and functional brain changes in obese individuals, demonstrated by a growing body of literature that employs diverse methods, including computerized tomography, magnetic resonance, and spectroscopic imaging techniques, to examine global and regional abnormalities. The goals of this chapter are to summarize neuroimaging findings of morphological and functional brain alterations in obesity, to identify possible limitations of the existing literature, and to highlight directions for continued research.

Morphological Brain Alterations

Evidence for structural brain alterations in obesity have been demonstrated using a variety of imaging modalities.

Computed Tomography

Morphological changes in gray and white matter, including global and regional atrophy, have been widely examined using Computed Tomography (CT). For example, Gustafson and colleagues[21,22] followed body mass index (BMI) and obesity-related health problems in 290 women for up to 24 years. Using CT, they demonstrated that increased BMI throughout midlife was independently associated with latelife brain alterations, including greater temporal atrophy[21] and white matter lesions.[22]

Longitudinal research also suggests that some regional abnormalities may improve following bariatric surgery. Using CT scans, Berginer and colleagues[23] found larger cortical sulci and a trend toward smaller ventricles in obese bariatric surgery candidates when compared to nonobese control subjects. Interestingly, analyses showed postsurgical increases in cerebral spinal fluid spaces, particularly the frontal interhemispheric fissure. The authors compare these findings to the brain involution found in anorexia nervosa and malnutrition and attribute possible, and potentially reversible, postoperative fluid shifts to nutritional deprivation coinciding with rapid weight loss.

J. Gunstad (✉)
Kent State University, Kent, OH, USA
and
Summa Health System, Kent State University,
221 Kent Hall Addition, Kent, OH, USA
e-mail: jgunstad@kent.edu

R.A. Cohen and L.H. Sweet (eds.), *Brain Imaging in Behavioral Medicine and Clinical Neuroscience*,
DOI 10.1007/978-1-4419-6373-4_13, © Springer Science+Business Media, LLC 2011

Magnetic Resonance Imaging

Magnetic Resonance Imaging (MRI) has been employed in similar studies to produce more detailed images of brain tissue than possible with CT. Volumetric analyses are widely used to relate alterations in brain volume to increased adiposity and body mass across the lifespan, and voxel-based morphometry (VBM) is increasingly employed to measure associations between body weight and regional brain alterations.[24-29]

For instance, Gunstad and colleagues[24] used MRI to examine brain volume and BMI in a sample of 201 men and women across the lifespan (age range 17–79) free from medical and psychiatric disorders. Results indicated that otherwise healthy obese individuals had significantly smaller whole brain volumes and total gray matter volumes than healthy nonobese individuals, even after controlling for age. While they found no significant differences in total white matter volume or regional gray matter volumes, trends towards smaller parietal and temporal region volumes in obese individuals were reported.[24]

Similarly, Taki and colleagues[26] used MRI and volumetric analysis to demonstrate an inverse association between BMI and global gray matter ratio in a large sample of Japanese men (average age 45 years) after adjusting for relevant clinical and demographic variables, although no significant correlations occurred in female participants. Using VBM, the authors found both negative and positive associations between BMI and regional gray matter volume in men, including negative associations with midbrain and bilateral temporal, frontal, and anterior cerebellar area volume, and positive associations with volume of the bilateral thalami, caudate head, posterior cerebellar, and additional frontal and temporal areas. These results suggest a range of regional alterations in obesity, with an overall decrease in global gray matter volume.[26]

Ward and colleagues[27] demonstrated an association between BMI and reduced global brain volume in a sample of 114 middle-aged adults. In older adults, Jagust and colleagues examined the relationship between central adiposity, measured by waist–hip ratio, and hippocampal volume and white matter hyperintensities (WMH) on MRI. They found evidence for an inverse association between waist–hip ratio and hippocampal volume and a positive association between waist–hip ratio and WMH, after adjusting for elevated body mass and other relevant clinical variables, in their sample of 112 Latino men and women.

Pannacciulli and colleagues[25] applied VBM to examine regional gray and white matter densities in 24 obese and 36 lean younger adults. Significant differences included reduced gray matter density in several prefrontal, cerebellar, and basal regions, as well as in several regions implicated in taste processing, in obese individuals. Greater gray matter density was also found in several, primarily occipital, regions in obese individuals.

While several studies highlighted above reported independent positive associations between obesity and white matter lesions in older adults,[22,28] Pannacciuli and colleagues[25] found that white matter density was greater in the putamen of obese versus lean individuals, although no other differences in white matter density emerged. Haltia and colleagues[29] also reported greater white matter volume in several basal brain regions of obese versus lean individuals, which was reduced following postdieting weight loss.[29] The exact reason for these inconsistent findings is unknown and requires further investigation.

Diffusion-Weighted Imaging

Diffusion techniques provide information about brain alterations by examining local movement of water molecules. Alkan and colleagues[30] employed Diffusion-Weighted Imaging (DWI) in a sample of 81 obese younger adults and 29 nonobese counterparts. The obese group showed alterations in fluid distribution in several brain regions involved in hunger and satiety, including the hypothalamus, hippocampal gyrus, amygdala, insula, cerebellum, and midbrain.[30]

Positron Emission Tomography and Magnetic Resonance Spectroscopy

Resting state Magnetic Resonance Spectroscopy (MRS) and Positron Emission Tomography (PET) data can be used to provide evidence for alterations of regional cerebral metabolism and markers of neuronal and glial integrity. Gazdzinski and colleagues[31] employed MRS to demonstrate reduced concentrations of N-acetylaspartate in frontal gray matter and frontal, parietal, and temporal white matter of obese individuals. Reduced concentrations of choline-containing metabolite were also demonstrated in the frontal white matter of the same obese individuals.[31] The authors interpret these metabolic alterations as indications of cell loss and membrane breakdown, respectively, in the associated brain regions.[31]

PET research has demonstrated an inverse association between BMI and resting metabolism in prefrontal regions which was also positively associated with performance on tests of memory and executive function.[32] PET also revealed higher resting metabolic activity in brain regions involved in oral sensation in obese subjects.[33]

Summary of Morphological Brain Alterations in Obesity

Multiple neuroimaging modalities have been employed to explore morphological brain alterations involved in the cognitive impairment and increased risk for dementia found in obese adults. Cross-sectional and longitudinal research indicates a variety of structural alterations related to elevated body mass and adiposity in men and women across the lifespan. Prominent findings include reduced global brain volume, regional alterations of predominately frontal and temporal brain areas, and increased occurrence of WMH.[21,22,24–28] These structural findings are consistent with cognitive findings of impairments in executive function, memory, working memory, and psychomotor speed in obese individuals.[7,10–14,16–19] Though additional work is needed, these structural abnormalities on neuroimaging may also provide insight into the elevated dementia risk in obese older adults. Further support for neuropathological changes in obesity prior to dementia onset comes from autopsy studies, which demonstrate positive associations between adiposity and markers of AD, including the expression of tau and amyloid precursor proteins[34] as well as the accumulation of amyloid-β peptide, even in healthy individuals.[35] Additional structural findings provide evidence for obesity-related fluid alterations, white matter expansion, and increased resting metabolism in several brain regions that may be implicated in eating processes.[25,29,30,33] In summary, various types of neuroimaging have been employed to explore a range of structural brain alterations associated with weight gain and obesity. Further understanding of the role of brain alterations in pathological eating processes can be explored using functional imaging techniques, which are reviewed in the following section.

Functional Brain Alterations

After early fMRI studies demonstrated that the neural activity following food ingestion could be visualized,[36] researchers began mapping the complicated neural aspects of eating behavior. A complete review of this rapidly advancing field is beyond the scope of this chapter, but several studies with implications for understanding functional neuroimaging in obese individuals are briefly presented.

Functional Imaging of Eating Behavior

Studies using functional neuroimaging to examine eating behavior typically employ variations on several research paradigms. A common approach asks study participants to view images of food that have been categorized into low- and high-calorie foods, with greater neural activation typically found for the more desirable, high-calorie foods. More recent studies have involved manipulation of actual food intake during scanning. These innovative studies employ sophisticated delivery systems to introduce small quantities of liquid substances into participants' mouths in a standardized manner (e.g., standardized quantity of substance, timing of administration). A third common approach involves scanning individuals after a period of fasting and then immediately following ingestion of food.

This body of research suggests that neural activation to presentation of food cues and/or food ingestion is influenced by a number of factors, including:

- Time elapsed since last meal/food ingestion[37,38]
- Trait reward sensitivity[39]
- Degree of hunger/satiety, including length of fasting[40,41]
- Nature of taste stimulus (e.g., sweet vs. other tastes)[40]
- Cravings for specific foods (i.e., chocolate)[42]
- Evidence for the neural pattern of satiety sensations from gastric distention[43] 2008)

Research in this area has begun to reveal the complex pattern of neural processes involved in eating behavior and find that even minor changes can produce large effects. Consistent with this, it is perhaps not surprising that persons with eating disorders exhibit altered patterns of neural activation in brain regions important for eating behaviors. The few studies in this area have demonstrated that individuals with anorexia nervosa, bulimia nervosa, and binge eating disorder differ from controls in numerous ways.[44-47] Similarly, persons with Prader–Willi syndrome, a genetic disorder at chromosome 15 that produces hyperphagia, exhibit abnormal activation patterns on functional neuroimaging.[48-51]

Just as studies have begun to examine the association between altered neural patterns in response to food and eating pathology, researchers have started to identify compelling interactions between circulating biomarkers important for appetite/satiety and findings on neuroimaging. For example, persons with a genetic-resistance to leptin viewed food pictures during fMRI before and following leptin replacement.[52] Leptin replacement reduced reported hunger and altered neural response to food cues, including greater activation in frontal gyri, cingulate gyrus, and midbrain. These brain regions have considerable importance for behavioral control and thus may contribute to the improved eating behavior in these individuals above and beyond that expected by circulating leptin levels. Other studies in leptin-deficit persons show similar effects.[53] Similarly, a recent study has revealed that levels of a biomarker linked to satiety (glucagons-like peptide-1) correlated with activation in multiple brain regions important for eating behavior, including the dorsolateral prefrontal cortex and hypothalamus.[54]

Taken in sum, neuroimaging studies in both healthy and patient samples have begun to clarify many aspects of eating and food-related processing by the brain. Such findings lay the groundwork for a better understanding of neural activity in obese individuals.

Functional Imaging in Obesity

Functional imaging studies in obese individuals have typically been patterned after the food cue/ingestion studies introduced above and compare the neural response of obese individuals to lean controls. For example, a recent study revealed a greater neural response to pictures of high-calorie foods in obese women relative to normal-weight controls.[55] These differences emerged in a number of regions linked to emotion and eating/feeding behavior, including the orbitofrontal cortex, amygdale, nucleus accumbens, insula, and anterior cingulate. Perhaps more interestingly, obese individuals showed greater neural activation in these brain regions to pictures of high-calorie foods (e.g., desserts, pancakes with syrup, ribs) than low-calorie foods (e.g., vegetables, fish). In another study using visually presented food cues, obese persons with binge-eating behavior showed greater activation in the premotor cortex to depictions of desserts and high fat salty snacks[56] Patterns of activation did not differ in obese persons without binge-eating tendencies or in lean binge-eaters, suggesting a possible interaction between excess weight and eating pathology.

In an elegantly designed study, DelParigi and colleagues[57] examined regional cerebral blood flow (rCBF) changes in obese and lean participants to a small amount (i.e. 2 ml) of a liquid meal after a 36-h fast. Obese individuals differed from lean participants in multiple brain regions, including the midbrain, middle-dorsal insular cortex, temporal cortex, and cingulate cortex. Interestingly, the intensity of insular response was proportional to body composition, with greater obesity being associated with greater activation. The authors note that this pattern of activation indicates that obese individuals show differences in sensory, associative, and paralimbic areas relative to lean controls.

In addition to examining response to visual food cues or actual food ingestion, a recent study has explored possible differences in the anticipation of food intake in obese and lean adolescent girls.[58] Obese participants showed greater activation in regions important for gustatory and somatosensory functions when anticipating chocolate milkshake rather than a saliva-like control substance. Obese individuals also showed medium effect sized differences from controls when tasting the milkshake, including increased activation in regions important for food reward such as the cingulate gyrus, Rolandic operculum, and posterior insula. Greater activation patterns in some regions corresponded with BMI during both anticipation (e.g., temporal operculum) and consummatory conditions (e.g., insula/frontoparietal operculum). This study also revealed a large, inverse association between BMI and activation in the caudate nucleus during food consumption. The authors interpret this finding as potential further support for reduced dopamine receptor availability or a complex pattern of hypo-/hyperfrontality in the food response of obese individuals.

Other studies have also found evidence for an important role of dopamine availability in obese individuals. Regional brain glucose metabolism was measured in a sample of healthy adults at rest and during completion of a numerical computations task.[59] Higher BMI was associated with lower metabolism in frontal brain regions on imaging and reduced performance on standard neuropsychological tests. These findings again implicate the possibility of dopamine dysregulation in obese individuals, perhaps accounting for the observed difficulties in executive function and eating/feeding behavior. Further evidence for the role of dopamine receptors in the dysregulation of prefrontal activity in obese individuals also comes from that research team.[60] PET imaging revealed that obese individuals had lower striatal D2 receptor availability, which correlated with measures of metabolism in multiple frontal and somatosensory regions. The authors discuss the interesting possibility that the reduced activation in frontal brain regions may be a cause (rather than an effect) of obesity. Impulsive behavior or reduced self-monitoring could easily lead to weight gain and eventual excess weight. Prospective studies are much needed to examine this possibility.

In addition to this growing collection of studies delineating differences in neural activation between obese individuals and their lean-weight counterparts, researchers have also begun to determine possible mechanisms for these differences. Using a single-blind crossover design, obese individuals were scanned after 10% loss of initial body weight with either injected leptin or placebo.[61] Neural activation to visual depictions of food and nonfood cues was compared across time points. A complicated pattern of increased and decreased activation emerged following weight loss, including a number of frontal and limbic regions. Interestingly, leptin replacement reversed many of these changes in the sample, implicating leptin in a broad range of cognitive abilities, including emotion regulation, higher order cognitive abilities like executive functioning, in addition to eating/feeding behaviors.

Limitations of Current Research

Although studies to date have provided important information regarding both structural and functional brain correlates of body parameters, improvements in research design will likely clarify the nature and meaning of these findings, as well as further elucidate mechanisms for observed alterations. For example, prospective studies in the neuroimaging of obesity are much needed. As described above, obesity is associated with risk for Alzheimer's disease and cognitive decline.[7,10–14,16–19] Such studies suggest that obesity produces adverse brain changes that are best documented by prospective studies. Similarly, there is the exciting possibility that substantial weight loss may alter neural response to food cues/ingestion. Using PET imaging, DelParigi and colleagues[57] examined response to a liquid meal in Normal weight, Obese, and Postobese (i.e., normal weight persons who were formerly obese) individuals. As in past studies, obese individuals differed from Normal weight persons. However, Postobese individuals showed mixed patterns. Although activation patterns were generally similar to normal weight individuals, postobese participants showed continued abnormal activation in several regions, including the cingulate, insula, and hippocampus. This study and others using similar samples (e.g., Le et al.[62,63]) identify several important hypotheses for continued work, including: (1) neural response to food may change following weight loss, (2) a sustained period of obesity may produce permanent dysregulation in response to food cues or food ingestion, and (3) specific patterns of neural activation may predispose individuals to eventually become obese.

In addition to answering these and other important questions, prospective studies can determine the possible impact of comorbid conditions on the observed findings. For example, obese individuals are at elevated risk for hypertension.[64] However, even subtle changes in blood pressure can produce changes in the BOLD signal used for fMRI studies.[65] Prospective studies will clarify the actual differences in neural activation between obese and normal weight individuals.

Future Directions

Neuroimaging studies in obese participants holds great promise for better understanding feeding behavior, eating pathology, and neurocognitive decline. Advanced neuroimaging techniques will help clarify mechanisms for pathology and the possible obesity by aging interaction. For example, researchers interested in the cognitive impact of obesity are strongly encouraged to employ diffusion tensor imaging (DTI) to determine the integrity of white matter pathways in this population. Reduced functional connectivity as measured by DTI is associated with the cognitive deficits commonly found in obese individuals (e.g., executive dysfunction) and may provide key insight into these processes.[10,66]

Similarly, mechanistic studies are much needed to better understand the association between obesity and neural activity and the possibility of common pathways for vulnerability. One such example is the association among obesity, neural activity, and leptin. As noted above,[52,53] leptin appears to moderate the neural response to food cues. Recent work also demonstrates that leptin is independently associated with cognitive test performance and the volume of gray matter regions.[67,68] A better understanding of this complex interaction may advance understanding of a wide range of phenomena.

A final area for future study involves a better understanding of the impact of obesity in older adults. The prevalence of obesity and proportion of older adults are both increasing, highlighting a need to better understand the effects of obesity on the aging brain. In addition to further work clarifying the mechanisms by which obesity appears to accelerate cognitive aging, novel uses of neuroimaging may reveal new connections. For example, older adults often exhibit a period of appetite and/or weight loss prior to diagnosis of dementia.[69,70] A recent study has found that appetite loss in persons with Alzheimer's disease is associated with altered perfusion on SPECT in frontal and temporal regions.[71] Determining whether functional abnormalities to food cues/ingestion can be found in persons with mild cognitive impairment may help identify those persons most likely to convert.

Summary and Conclusion

Recent advances in neuroimaging have allowed for the development of a growing literature regarding morphological and functional brain alterations in obesity. Structural neuroimaging has proved useful in clarifying the nature and mechanisms for cognitive impairment and increased risk of dementia in this population. Likewise, functional neuroimaging has identified important differences in food-related neural activation in obese versus lean individuals that may clarify mechanisms for maladaptive eating behavior and weight gain.

Although much work is still needed, neuroimaging has proven to be an invaluable tool for examining the complex relationships between structure, function, and chemistry of the human brain and eating behavior and overweight – information that may ultimately aid the development of preventative and treatment strategies and reduce the individual and societal impact of obesity and associated cognitive and functional decline.

References

1. Ogden CL, Carroll MD, McDowell MA, Flegal KM. *Obesity among adults in the United States – no change since 2003–2004. NCHS data brief no 1.* Hyattsville, MD: National Center for Health Statistics; 2007.
2. de Lusignan S, Hague N, van Vlymen J, et al. A study of cardiovascular risk in overweight and obese people in England. *Eur J Gen Pract.* 2006;12(1):19–29.
3. Ogden CL, Yanovski SZ, Carroll MD, Flegal KM. The epidemiology of obesity. *Gastroenterology.* 2007;132:2087–2102.
4. Adams KF, Schatzkin A, Harris TB, et al. Overweight, obesity, and mortality in a large prospective cohort of persons 50 to 71 years old. *N Engl J Med.* 2006;355(8):763–778.
5. Mond JM, Rodgers B, Hay PJ, et al. Obesity and impairment in psychosocial functioning in women: the mediating role of eating disorder features. *Obesity (Silver Spring).* 2007;15(11):2769–2779.
6. Simon GE, Von Korff M, Saunders K, et al. Association between obesity and psychiatric disorders in the US adult population. *Arch Gen Psychiatry.* 2006;63(7):824–830.
7. Cserjési R, Luminet O, Poncelet AS, László L. Altered executive function in obesity. Exploration of the role of affective states on cognitive abilities. *Appetite.* 2009;52:535–539.
8. Ricca V, Castellini G, Lo Sauro C, et al. Correlations between binge eating and emotional eating in a sample of overweight subjects. *Appetite.* 2009;53(3):418–421.
9. Petroni ML, Villanova N, Avagnina S, et al. Psychological distress in morbid obesity in relation to weight history. *Obes Surg.* 2007;17(3):391–399.
10. Gunstad J, Paul RH, Cohen RA, Tate DF, Spitznagel MB, Gordon E. Elevated body mass index is associated with executive dysfunction in otherwise healthy adults. *Compr Psychiatry.* 2007;48:57–61.
11. Gunstad J, Paul RH, Cohen RA, Tate DF, Gordon E. Obesity is associated with memory deficits in young and middle-aged adults. *Eat Weight Disord.* 2006;11:15–19.
12. Cournot M, Marquié JC, Ansiau D, et al. Relation between body mass index and cognitive function in healthy middle-aged men and women. *Neurology.* 2006;67:1208–1214.
13. Waldstein SR, Katzel LI. Interactive relations of central versus total obesity and blood pressure to cognitive function. *Int J Obes.* 2006;30:201–207.
14. Sabia S, Kivimaki M, Shipley MJ, Marmot MG, Singh-Manoux A. Body mass index over the adult life course and cognition in late midlife: the Whitehall II Cohort Study. *Am J Clin Nutr.* 2009;89(2):601–607.

15. Beydoun MA, Beydoun HA, Wang Y. Obesity and central obesity as risk factors for incident dementia and its subtypes: a systematic review and meta-analysis. *Obes Rev.* 2008; 9(3):204–218.

16. Razay G, Vreugdenhil A, Wilcock G. Obesity, abdominal obesity and Alzheimer disease. *Dement Geriatr Cogn Disord.* 2006;22:173–176.

17. Whitmer RA, Gunderson EP, Barrett-Connor E, Quesenberry CP Jr, Yaffe K. Obesity in middle age and future risk of dementia: a 27 year longitudinal population based study. *BMJ.* 2005;330(7504):1360.

18. Fitzpatrick AL, Kuller LH, Lopez OL, et al. Midlife and late-life obesity and the risk of dementia: Cardiovascular Health Study. *Arch Neurol.* 2009;66(3):336–342.

19. Whitmer RA, Gunderson EP, Quesenberry CP, Zhou J, Yaffe K. Body mass index in midlife and risk of Alzheimer disease and vascular dementia. *Curr Alzheimer Res.* 2007;4:103–109.

20. Fergenbaum JH, Bruce S, Lou W, Hanley AJ, Greenwood C, Young TK. Obesity and lowered cognitive performance in a Canadian first nations population. *Obesity.* 2009;17(10): 1957–1963.

21. Gustafson D, Lissner L, Bengtsson C, Bjorkelund C, Skoog I. A 24-year follow-up of body mass index and cerebral atrophy. *Neurology.* 2004;63(10):1990–1991.

22. Gustafson DR, Steen B, Skoog I. Body mass index and white matter lesions in elderly women. An 18-year longitudinal study. *Int Psychogeriatr.* 2004;16:327–336.

23. Berginer VM, Solomon H, Hirsch M, et al. Brain computed tomography in morbid obesity before and after gastric restriction surgery: a prospective quantitative study. *Neuroradiology.* 1987;29:540–543.

24. Gunstad J, Paul R, Cohen R, et al. Relationship between body mass index and brain volume in healthy adults. *Int J Neurosci.* 2008;118:1582–1593.

25. Pannacciulli N, Del Parigi A, Chen K, Le DNT, Reiman EM, Tataranni PA. Brain abnormalities in human obesity: a voxel-based morphometric study. *Neuroimage.* 2006;31:1419–1425.

26. Taki Y, Kinomura S, Sato K, et al. Relationship between body mass index and gray matter volume in 1, 428 healthy individuals. *Obesity.* 2008;16(1):119–124.

27. Ward MA, Carlsson CM, Trivedi MA, Sager MA, Johnson SC. The effect of body mass index on global brain volume in middle-aged adults: a cross sectional study. *BMC Neurol.* 2005;5:23.

28. Jagust W, Harvey D, Mungas D, Haan M. Central obesity and the aging brain. *Arch Neurol.* 2005;62(10):1545–1548.

29. Haltia LT, Viljanen A, Parkkola R, et al. Brain white matter expansion in human obesity and the recovering effect of dieting. *J Clin Endocrinol Metab.* 2007;92(8):3278–3284.

30. Alkan A, Sahin I, Keskin L, et al. Diffusion-weighted imaging features of brain in obesity. *Magn Reson Imaging.* 2008;26:446–450.

31. Gazdzinski S, Kornak J, Weiner MW, Meyerhoff DJ. Body mass index and magnetic resonance markers of brain integrity in adults. *Ann Neurol.* 2008;63(5):652–657.

32. Volkow ND, Wang GJ, Telang F, et al. Inverse association between BMI and prefrontal metabolic activity in healthy adults. *Obesity.* 2009;17(1):60–65.

33. Wang GJ, Volkow ND, Felder C, et al. Enhanced resting activity of the oral somatosensory cortex in obese subjects. *Neuroreport.* 2002;13(9):1151–1155.

34. Mrak RE. Alzheimer-type neuropathological changes in morbidly obese individuals. *Clin Neuropathol.* 2009;28:40–45.

35. Balakrishnan K, Verdile G, Mehta PD, et al. Plasma Abeta42 correlates positively with increased body fat in healthy individuals. *J Alzheimers Dis.* 2005;8(3):269–282.

36. Liu Y, Gao J, Liu H, Fox P. The temporal response of the brain after eating revealed by functional MRI. *Nature.* 2000;405:1058–1062.

37. Cornier M, von Kaenel S, Bessesen D, Tregellas J. Effects of overfeeding on the neuronal response to visual food cues. *Am J Clin Nutr.* 2007;86:965–971.

38. Holsen L, Zarcone J, Thomposon T, et al. Neural mechanism underlying food motivation in children and adolescents. *Neuroimage.* 2005;27:669–676.

39. Beaver J, Lawrence A, van Ditzhuijzen J, Davis M, Woods A, Calder A. Individual differences in reward drive predict neural responses to images of food. *J Neurosci.* 2006;26: 5160–5166.

40. Haase L, Cerf-Ducastel B, Murphy C. Cortical activation in response to pure taste stimuli during the physiological states of hunger and satiety. *Neuroimage.* 2008;44:1008–1021.

41. Porubska K, Veit R, Preissl H, Fritsche A, Birbaumer N. Subjective feeling of appetite modulates brain activity: an fMRI study. *Neuroimage.* 2006;32:1273–1280.

42. Rolls ET, McCabe C. Enhanced affective brain representations of chocolate in cravers vs. non-cravers. *Eur J Neurosci.* 2007;26:1067–1076.

43. Wang GJ, Tomasi D, Backus W, et al. Gastric distention activates satiety circuitry in the human brain. *Neuroimage.* 2008;39:1824–1831.

44. Penas-Lledo EM, Loeb KL, Martin L, Fan J. Anterior cingulated activity in bulimia nervosa: a fMRI case study. *Eat Weight Disord.* 2007;12:78–82.

45. Marsh R, Steinglass JE, Gerber AJ, et al. Deficient activity in the neural systems that mediate self-regulatory control in bulimia nervosa. *Arch Gen Psychiatry.* 2009;66(1):51–63.

46. Castro-Fornieles J, Bargallo N, La'zaro L, et al. Adolescent anorexia nervosa: cross-sectional and follow-up frontal gray matter disturbances detected with proton magnetic resonance spectroscopy. *J Psychiatr Res.* 2007;41:952–958.

47. Schienle A, Schafer A, Hermann A, Vaitl D. Binge-eating disorder: reward sensitivity and brain activation to images of food. *Biol Psychiatry.* 2009;65:654–661.

48. Dimitropoulos A, Schultz RT. Food-related neural circuitry in Prader–Willi syndrome: response to high- versus low-calorie foods. *J Autism Dev Disord.* 2008;38:1642–1653.

49. Holsen LM, Zarcone JR, Brooks WM, et al. Neural mechanisms underlying hyperphagia in Prader–Willi syndrome. *Obesity.* 2006;14(6):1028–1037.

50. Miller JL, James GA, Goldstone AP, et al. Enhanced activation of reward mediating prefrontal regions in response to food stimuli in Prader–Willi syndrome. *J Neurol Neurosurg Psychiatry.* 2007;78:615–619.

51. Shapira NA, Lessig MC, He AG, James GA, Driscoll DJ, Liu Y. Satiety dysfunction in Prader–Willi syndrome demonstrated by fMRI. *J Neurol Neurosurg Psychiatry.* 2005;76:260–262.

52. Baicy K, London E, Monterosso J, et al. Leptin replacement alters brain response to food cues in genetically leptin-deficient adults. *Proc Natl Acad Sci U S A.* 2007;104: 18276–18279.

53. Farooqi S, Bullmore E, Keogh J, Gillard J, O'Rahilly S, Fletcher P. Leptin regulates striatal regions and human eating behavior. *Science*. 2007;317:1355.

54. Pannacciulli N, Le D, Salbe A, et al. Postprandial glucagons-like peptide-1 (GLP-1) response is positively associated with changes in neuronal activity of brain areas implicated in satiety and food intake regulation in humans. *Nueroimage*. 2007;25:511–517.

55. Stoeckel L, Weller R, Cook E, Twieg D, Knowlton R, Cox J. Widespread reward-system activation in obese women in response to pictures of high-calorie foods. *Neuroimage*. 2008;41:636–647.

56. Geliebter A, Ladell T, Logan M, Schweider T, Sharafi M, Hirsch J. Responsivity to food stimuli in obese and lean binge eaters using functional MRI. *Appetite*. 2006;46:31–35.

57. DelParigi A, Chen K, Salbe A, Reiman E, Tataranni PA. Sensory experience of food and obesity: a positron emission tomography study of brain regions affected by tasting a liquid meal after a prolonged fast. *Neuroimage*. 2005; 24:436–443.

58. Stice E, Spoor S, Bohon C, Veldhuizen M, Small D. Relation of reward from food intake and anticipated food intake to obesity: a functional magnetic resonance imaging study. *J Abnorm Psychol*. 2008;117:924–935.

59. Volkow N, Wang G, Telang F, et al. Inverse association between BMI and prefrontal metabolic activity in healthy adults. *Obesity*. 2008;17:60–65.

60. Volkow N, Wang G, Telang F, et al. Low dopamine striatal D2 receptors are associated with prefrontal metabolism in obese subjects: possible contributing factors. *Neuroimage*. 2008;42:1537–1543.

61. Rosenbaum M, Sy M, Pavlovich K, Leibel R, Hirsch J. Leptin reverses weight loss-induced changes in regional neural activity response to visual food stimuli. *J Clin Invest*. 2008;118:2583–2591.

62. DelParigi A, Chen K, Salbe A, et al. Persistence of abnormal neural responses to a meal in postobese individuals. *Int J Obes*. 2004;28:370–377.

63. Le DS, Pannacciulli N, Chen K, et al. Less activation in the left dorsolateral prefrontal cortex in the reanalysis of the response to a meal in obese than in lean women and its association with successful weight loss. *Am J Clin Nutr*. 2007;86(3):573–579.

64. Diaz ME. Hypertension and obesity. *J Hum Hypertens*. 2002;16(1):18–22.

65. Wang R, Foniok T, Wamsteeker JI, et al. Transient blood pressure changes affect the functional magnetic resonance imaging detection of cerebral activation. *Neuroimage*. 2006;31(1):1–11.

66. Chen TF, Chen YF, Cheng TW, Hua MS, Liu HM, Chiu MJ. Executive dysfunction and periventricular diffusion tensor changes in amnesic mild cognitive impairment and early Alzheimer's disease. *Hum Brain Mapp*. 2009;30(11): 3826–3836.

67. Gunstad J, Spitznagel MB, Keary TA, et al. Serum leptin levels are associated with cognitive function in older adults. *Brain Res*. 2008;1230:233–236.

68. Pannacciulli N, Le DS, Chen K, Reiman EM, Krakoff J. Relationships between plasma leptin concentrations and human brain structure: a voxel-based morphometric study. *Neurosci Lett*. 2007;412(3):248–253.

69. Knopman DS, Edland SD, Cha RH, Petersen RC, Rocca WA. Incident dementia in women is preceded by weight loss by at least a decade. *Neurology*. 2007;69(8):739–746.

70. Stewart R, Masaki K, Xue QL, et al. A 32-year prospective study of change in body weight and incident dementia: the Honolulu–Asia Aging Study. *Arch Neurol*. 2005;62(1):55–60.

71. Ismail Z, Hermann N, Rothenburg L, et al. A functional neuroimaging study of appetite loss in Alzheimer's disease. *J Neurol Sci*. 2008;271:97–100.

Chapter 14
Neuropsychology and Neuroimaging in Metabolic Dysfunction

Jason J. Hassenstab

Metabolic Dysfunction: from Obesity to Insulin Resistance to Insulin Dependence

Within the last 20 years, the worldwide prevalence of obesity in industrialized nations has reached epidemic proportions. Nowhere is this more evident than in the USA. According to the Centers for Disease Control, in 1991, there were only four states with adult obesity prevalence rates above 15%. By 2007, however, there was only one state with *less* than 20% and 30 states had prevalence rates higher than 25%.[12] The health consequences of obesity are many, and nearly all individuals with sustained obesity will develop metabolic dysfunction. In fact, the spectrum of health conditions that comprises metabolic dysfunction is most often etiologically linked to obesity and includes disruptions in the body's response to and production of insulin and resulting damage from hyperglycemia and hypoglycemia, hypertension, systemic inflammatory processes, and dyslipidemia – among others.[37] These metabolic abnormalities tend to cluster together in the obese individual, and are often referred to as *metabolic syndrome.*[25] With a current prevalence of approximately 40% among individuals over 50 years of age,[28] the costs associated with metabolic syndrome are significant. Analyses of Medicare expenditures indicate that individuals with metabolic syndrome incur 20–40% more health care costs over a 10-year period, representing a significant drain on the public health system in the USA.[18]

Metabolic syndrome is considered to be a "prediabetic" state associated with the development of type 2 diabetes as well as more significant cardiovascular and cerebrovascular disease.[1] When metabolic dysfunction becomes more severe, decreasing insulin sensitivity and decreasing insulin generation cause serum glucose levels to elevate even further, eventually reaching threshold for a diagnosis of type 2 diabetes, which has been criticized as an evolving and somewhat arbitrary cutoff.[85] Several studies have found that type 2 diabetes is related to cognitive impairment and structural brain abnormalities,[32] and some have speculated on an association with dementia.[8] At less extreme levels of metabolic dysfunction, there is accumulating evidence that the cluster of risk factors that comprise the metabolic syndrome may be related to subtle cognitive deficits and macroscopic brain insult.[42,57,99,100]

The role of metabolic dysfunction in neuropsychology and neuroimaging is extraordinarily complex, and until recently has been studied part and parcel with little regard for the highly correlated components of metabolic disorder that typically "travel together." As such, this chapter will outline the major findings in neurocognitive and neuroimaging studies of metabolic dysfunction, with a concentration on disorders of abnormal insulin functioning followed by concise coverage of hypertension and the emerging literature on obesity. It is important to note that while this chapter attempts to provide a comprehensive outline of these issues, it should not be considered an exhaustive resource due to the vast scope of the literature. Further, etiological determinants of human brain abnormalities in metabolic disorders represent a relatively undeveloped area of clinical research and are based largely on theoretical assumptions derived from nonhuman research.

J.J. Hassenstab (✉)
Departments of Neurology and Psychology,
Washington University Medical School in St. Louis,
St. Louis, MO 63108, USA
e-mail: jasonhassenstab@yahoo.com

R.A. Cohen and L.H. Sweet (eds.), *Brain Imaging in Behavioral Medicine and Clinical Neuroscience*,
DOI 10.1007/978-1-4419-6373-4_14, © Springer Science+Business Media, LLC 2011

Insulin Resistance

For several years, it was widely assumed that the brain was an insulin insensitive organ, based on the perception that insulin was simply too large a molecule to effectively transport across the blood–brain barrier.[81] Several lines of evidence suggest that this notion is erroneous, although insulin does not appear to have as prominent a role in regulating glucose uptake in the brain as it does in peripheral tissues.[82] However, chronic disruptions in systemic insulin levels, often seen in individuals with *insulin resistance*, can have multiple deleterious effects on brain functioning. Insulin resistance can be described as a pathological condition in which muscle, liver, and adipose tissue become resistant to normal circulating levels of insulin, resulting in an increase in insulin secretion and elevated serum glucose concentration.[76] Insulin resistance is an early phenomenon in the course of developing type 2 diabetes.[83] The precise causative pathway of insulin resistance is only partially understood, however, there are clearly inheritable contributions and the role of obesity appears to be of significance.

In direct association with insulin resistance, serum glucose levels become more variable and generally increase in peripheral tissues and in the central nervous system. Even subtle dysregulation of glucose can have profound effects on brain functioning, perhaps because the human brain constitutes only 2% of body mass, but uses 25% of the body's available glucose.[60] Terms such as impaired glucose tolerance, hyperglycemia, and glucose dysregulation have subtle distinctions, but typically are referring to disruptions in glucose utilization that are intricately tied to insulin functioning and can be considered part of the larger syndrome of insulin resistance. For purposes of clarity, the term insulin resistance will be used as much as possible throughout this chapter.

Insulin Resistance and Cognitive Functioning

The effects of chronic and acute insulin resistance on cognitive functioning have been well documented in adults across the lifespan. Several studies in healthy young adults have shown direct relationships between insulin resistance and cognitive functioning. For example Awad and colleagues,[5] administered glucose tolerance tests to undergraduate students and divided them into better and poorer glucoregulatory groups on the basis of glucose challenge tests. The subjects were tested on various measures of declarative verbal memory including list learning tests and paragraph recall from the Wechsler Memory Scale Third Edition (WMS-III[97]). Subjects with poorer glucoregulatory control performed more poorly than subjects with better glucoregulatory control across all measures, regardless of condition (placebo solution versus glucose solution). These results suggest that the relationship between insulin resistance and cognitive functioning cannot be accounted for solely by aging or other metabolic dysfunction associated with advanced age.

Insulin resistance can impact cognition in adults in mid-life as well. Using data from the NHANES III study, Pavlik, Hyman, and Doody[72] analyzed cognitive and metabolic variables in 3,270 subjects who ranged in age from 30 to 59 years. After controlling for age, gender, education, and poverty/income ratio, poorer cognitive performance was seen in subjects with hyperglycemia on measures of processing speed and memory. Similarly, middle-aged subjects with carefully diagnosed type 2 diabetes have lower scores on tests of memory, abstract reasoning, and verbal fluency.[54] Cognitive impairments associated with insulin resistance appear to increase with age, even among individuals without type 2 diabetes. Studies of healthy, nondiabetic, middle-aged, and elderly participants have found that after controlling for differences in levels of education, older subjects with poorer glucoregulation as determined by oral glucose tolerance tests, had worse performance on tests of working memory, immediate and delayed verbal memory, and executive functioning.[65] Similarly, in a larger study of middle-aged and elderly subjects with metabolic syndrome, insulin resistance explained more variance in performance on a comprehensive battery of declarative memory than other metabolic syndrome components even after controlling for a strictly defined diagnosis of type 2 diabetes.[42] Collectively, these studies establish that cognitive impairments are readily detectable in nondiabetic and type 2 diabetic populations with insulin resistance, which suggests that cognitive functions may become impaired prior to the level of glucoregulatory dysfunction seen in type 2 diabetes. Studies that evaluate cognitive functioning in diabetic individuals before and after successful treatment show that some of the cognitive deficits observed in type 2 diabetes may be directly attributed to the impact of insulin resistance and are attenuated by improvement of glucose control.[64] However, emerging evidence suggests that cognitive deficits associated with insulin resistance may become irreversible in subjects with moderate-to-severe type 2 diabetes and continue to increase with advancing age.[36]

In sum, it appears that there is a relationship between insulin resistance and cognitive functioning and that this relationship can be seen throughout the lifespan. The most commonly observed cognitive deficits associated with insulin resistance are verbal memory deficits, followed by processing speed deficits, and executive functioning deficits. Visuospatial abilities, attention and concentration, and language and verbal functioning are largely preserved.[5]

Neuropathology and Neuroimaging in Insulin Resistance

There is compelling evidence that insulin resistance and resultant hyperglycemia have direct and indirect relationships with structural changes throughout the brain, including gray matter and white matter. The hippocampus is most consistently linked to insulin resistance, and the frontal lobes appear to have some associations as well. Glucose is metabolized at different rates throughout the cerebrum, and certain areas, including the hippocampal formation, exhibit differential utilization depending upon age.[5] McNay et al[63] compared extracellular glucose levels in the hippocampus of rats and performance on a simple or complex maze-learning task. Completion of the complex maze resulted in a 32% decrease in extracellular glucose levels, and the simple maze resulted in an 11% reduction in extracellular glucose. Exogenous administration of glucose resulted in improved overall performance on the complex maze with no reduction in extracellular glucose, indicating that an increase in proximally available glucose contributed to improved performance. In subsequent studies using the same paradigm, it was observed that decreased extracellular glucose levels in the hippocampus were much more pronounced in aged rats than in younger rats,[62] suggesting that glucose supply fluctuates in relation to neuronal demand and that variable glucose levels associated with normal aging

and insulin resistance may have more impact on brain areas with higher glucose demand.

Declarative memory has well-established links with the medial temporal lobe including the hippocampal areas, and structural MRI studies have found direct associations between hippocampal volumes, performance on declarative memory tests, and glucose regulation. For example, nondiabetic middle-aged and older adults with poorer glucose regulation tend to have smaller hippocampal volumes and worse memory performance on paragraph learning and recall when compared with age and education-matched controls with normal glucose regulation.[16] In this sample, memory performance and glucose regulation were not associated with overall brain volume reductions, or specific reductions in other brain regions including proximal temporal lobe structures such as the parahippocampal gyrus and the superior temporal gyrus. This suggests that the memory deficits observed in individuals with insulin resistance and resultant glucose dysregulation appear to be associated specifically with hippocampal function. Convit et al[16] speculate that activation-induced attenuation in hippocampal glucose levels may lead to a state of functional hypoglycemia, which may limit hippocampal encoding. Convit[15] subsequently proposed a theoretical mechanism by which this process may occur. Since glucose cannot penetrate the blood–brain barrier, its transport must be actively facilitated by glucose transporters of the GLUT family, specifically the GLUT1 glucose transporter located in the endothelial cells of blood vessels.[35] Convit proposed that in order to compensate for acute reductions in cellular glucose levels that occur during activation of the hippocampus, capillary dilation must be increased so that more GLUT1 transporters are in contact with the blood, a process known as capillary recruitment.[29] Dysfunction in capillary recruitment is associated with insulin resistance and type 2 diabetes, and therefore a breakdown in the ability to compensate for acute drops in hippocampal glucose following hippocampal activation may lead to a functional hypoglycemic state and contribute to the cognitive deficits that have been associated with diabetes and insulin resistance. It is likely that this functional hypoglycemia is not limited to hippocampal activation and may be more widespread. However, the hippocampus has been shown to be differentially sensitive to damage from hypoglycemia.[14,61] Over time, a syndrome of chronic functional hypoglycemia may lead to hippocampal damage and volume loss.

Brownlee[11] has proposed an additional model for damage to hippocampal neurons that focuses on the role of hyperglycemia in type 2 diabetes rather than hypoglycemia at lower levels of insulin resistance. Brownlee proposes that microvascular endothelial cells are damaged by hyperglycemia in individuals with diabetes, which impairs transport of glucose across the blood–brain barrier. In addition, the metabolism of excess glucose in individuals with hyperglycemia may produce superoxides that damage hippocampal neurons directly. This model is somewhat limited by the lack of a mechanism for understanding hippocampal damage at lower levels of insulin resistance. Hyperglycemia itself may pose a direct threat to general brain integrity. Emerging evidence from neurobiological studies in rodents, primates, and humans have focused on the role of advanced glycation end products (AGEs). AGEs are sugar-derived toxic substances that form at a slow but constant rate in the normal body. In hyperglycemic individuals, as in diabetes, their formation is markedly accelerated because of the increased availability of glucose.[74] AGEs cause damage by altering proteins, which can interfere with cell structure and function throughout the body and brain. AGEs also negatively interact with a variety of cell receptors, causing endocytosis and oxidative and inflammatory states, which directly cause damage to the brain.[24]

Aside from its role in the regulation of glucose uptake, insulin may have unique contributions to brain dysfunction. In rodent models of insulin resistance, insulin signaling pathways are impaired throughout the cerebral cortex and in particular the hippocampus, where insulin-binding sites are concentrated.[21,66] These lines of evidence suggest that insulin and insulin receptors may be involved in learning and memory consolidation.[102] This has not been thoroughly examined outside of the rodent literature, although it suggests that some declarative memory deficits seen in individuals with insulin resistance may be related to impaired insulin receptor signaling in the hippocampus. Insulin also appears to be intricately tied to vascular function. Contraction and dilation of blood vessels is correlated with circulating insulin levels.[92] Insulin regulates nitric oxide production in vascular endothelial cells, which at normal levels of insulin is thought to help regulate metabolic and hemodynamic homeostasis. In pathologic states, however, these insulin signaling pathways become disrupted by hyperglycemia and inflammation, resulting in endothelial dysfunction.[67] Accordingly,

it has been well documented that endothelial function is impaired in peripheral tissues of individuals with insulin resistance, even at the early stages of disease onset.[45,89,92,101] Evidence that cerebral vasculature emulates findings from studies in peripheral vasculature in humans is not yet confirmed, however, the parallels between peripheral and cerebral blood vessels suggests that insulin resistance may cause abnormalities of the cerebral microvasculature.[34] To that end, middle-aged adults with insulin resistance exhibit reduced arteriolar-to-venular ratio, an index of retinal vessel health.[88]

In addition to endothelial dysfunction, insulin resistance is associated with increased cerebral vascular reactivity and decreased cerebral blood flow.[69,98] Vascular reactivity plays a critical role in the regulation of cerebral blood flow and during periods of high glucose demand (i.e. during taxing cognitive tasks), increased cerebral vascular reactivity may lead to decreased glucose availability. Accordingly, decreases in cerebral blood flow have been imaged at the level of the hippocampus in individuals with type 2 diabetes and were correlated with reduced performance on declarative memory tests sensitive to hippocampal function.[98] These findings appear to complement the model of Convit[15] discussed above. In each case, insulin resistance contributes to a state of functional hypoglycemia, but via different processes.

The literature on insulin resistance and type 2 diabetes often makes reference to an increased risk of Alzheimer's disease in this population. Indeed, some large-scale epidemiological population studies have found an increased risk for AD among individuals with type 2 diabetes.[59,71] However, these studies have to be interpreted carefully when inferring causal relationships. A systematic review of these large-scale studies found that the incidence of "any dementia", including vascular dementia and AD was higher in individuals with diabetes than among those without diabetes.[8] Also, detailed data on glycemic control, insulin levels, and antidiabetic medication use are largely unreported in these studies. Ronnemma et al[78] followed a large sample for over 30 years and found a relative risk of 1.3 for developing AD among those with insulin resistance at mid-life. While this is a statistically significant finding, a relative risk of 1.3 for developing AD is rather small and seems especially weak in comparison to studies where low education (after adjustments for age and gender) conferred a relative risk of 4.0.[70] There are some possible physiological links between insulin resistance and the regulation of beta-amyloid peptide,[17,96] one of the markers of AD. It is possible that there is an etiological link between diabetes and AD in humans, however, aside from epidemiological studies, there is currently very little supportive evidence. Perhaps the most compelling argument against the link can be found in autopsy neuropathology studies. A study of 233 older Catholic clergy in the Religious Orders Study found that diabetes was related to cerebral infarction, but was not related to global AD pathology score, or to specific measures of neuritic plaques, diffuse plaques or tangles, or to amyloid burden.[4] Other autopsy studies found no difference in the amount of AD pathology in patients with diabetes[44,73], and another study found that persons with diabetes actually had fewer neuritic plaques and neurofibrillary tangles compared with persons without diabetes.[6,7]

Neuroimaging in Diabetes

Collectively, imaging findings from diabetes populations reinforce the vulnerability theories of the medial temporal regions and susceptibility for subcortical ischemic vascular abnormalities. For example, in older males with longstanding type 2 diabetes, odds ratios for hippocampal atrophy and subcortical infarction are two to three times that of age-matched controls (Fig. 14.1).[50,51,91] Several studies using ordinal rating scales of white matter lesions (WMLs) detected on structural MRI have found associations between diabetes and WMLs (e.g.[20,58]), although these results appear to be less consistent. In addition, metaanalyses show that lacunar infarcts are more common in diabetic populations.[91] As mentioned above, several studies have found a direct link between diabetes and medial temporal lobe atrophy using structural MRI.[9,32,43] There is clearly a more general pattern of cerebral atrophy in diabetic populations, and results from studies using automated volumetric techniques on structural MRI have found smaller overall gray matter volumes and smaller gray matter volumes in prefrontal regions in subjects with insulin resistance and type 2 diabetes.[42,53] There are a few magnetic resonance spectroscopy (MRS) studies that have examined cerebral metabolism in diabetes. MRS is typically used to detect neurochemical interactions that are correlated with cognitive

processes. The most widely used methods are ^{1}H-MRS and ^{31}P-MRS, which detect absolute concentrations or ratios of compounds that contain hydrogen and phosphorus. Studies have shown that *N*-acetyl aspartate (NAA), which is associated with neuronal viability, reliably correlates with cognitive functioning in normal subjects.[79] In studies of diabetes, results have been somewhat hetergeneous, but most have found decreased NAA ratios and increased *myo*-inositol-to-creatine ratios, suggesting decreased viability of neurons.[47,52] SPECT and PET studies in diabetes have generally found decreased cerebral blood flow in diabetic populations, particularly in patients with longstanding diabetes and multiple hypoglycemic episodes.[68,91] Interestingly, induced hyperglycemia in otherwise healthy older subjects without diabetes has been found to alter cerebral blood flow patterns as measured by FDG-PET. During periods of mild hyperglycemia, FDG uptake was decreased in gray matter across nearly all regions, mainly in the frontal and temporal lobes, and the posterior regions of the cingulate cortex.[48]

In summary, there are several possible mechanisms through which the brain can sustain damage via insulin resistance and diabetes. Generalized damage from hyperglycemia can occur due to increased oxidative and inflammatory states, and via AGEs interference in protein synthesis. Hyperglycemia can impair capillary recruitment leading to decreased glucose transport across the blood–brain barrier, leaving less glucose available during periods of high demand. Disrupted insulin signaling is associated with endothelial dysfunction and may contribute directly to brain dysfunction by impairing glucose uptake, especially in brain areas with high concentrations of insulin receptors and high glucose demand. Accordingly, the hippocampus has a disproportionate concentration of insulin receptors and high glucose demand and is highly sensitive to damage from complications of insulin resistance. Decreased vascular reactivity related to disrupted insulin signaling may lead to decreased cerebral blood flow, further attenuating glucose availability during periods of high glucose demand, and exacerbating a syndrome of functional hypoglycemia and resultant tissue damage in sensitive brain areas such as the hippocampus. Neuroimaging studies in insulin resistance and diabetes reinforce the structural vulnerability theories of the hippocampal regions and also suggest that brain activity may be altered in key areas related to cognitive performance.

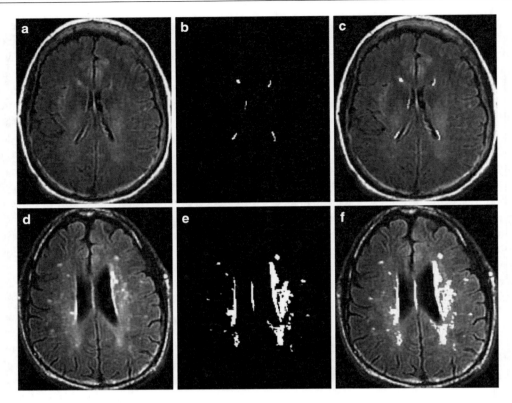

Fig. 14.1 Axial slices at the level of the ventricles for a control (**a**–**c**) and a diabetic (**d**–**f**) subject. The three columns represent the FLAIR image (**a** and **d**), the WMHs segmentation (**b** and **e**), and the overlay of the segmentation on the FLAIR image (**c** and **f**), respectively. From Novak et al.[69] Reprinted with permission from The American Diabetes Association

Hypertension and Cognitive Functioning

Similar to studies of insulin resistance and cognition, there is a substantial literature on the impact of hypertension on cognition. Early studies of hypertension found gross impairments in cognition among subjects with hypertension, yet were flawed by poor experimental control, limited sample sizes, and the inclusion of subjects with extreme cases of hypertension as well as subjects with hypertension-related complications. By the 1960s and 1970s, researchers were beginning to better understand the effect of aging on cognition and designed studies examining hypertension and cognition with better methodology. From approximately 1970–1990, a number of large-scale population-based prospective studies brought forth even more convincing evidence of an association between hypertension and cognition, but mostly relied upon global measures of cognition and did not include measures sensitive to specific patterns of cognitive decline. In addition, these studies tended to evaluate only elderly subjects and were inconsistent in applying adjustments for potentially confounding variables such as antihypertensive medication use, ethnicity, depression, and other factors present in metabolic syndrome such as impaired glucose tolerance glucose tolerance, obesity, and dyslipidemia.[94] More recent investigations have used more stringently controlled designs that adjusted for several confounding variables, but results have been inconsistent depending upon the population and the cognitive measures used. Overall, results suggest a link between hypertension and reduced cognitive abilities across the lifespan.

Data from the original Framingham Study[26] indicate that after controlling for age, gender, occupation, antihypertensive medication usage, alcohol consumption, and smoking status, chronic hypertension was associated with poor overall memory performance, as indicated by an education adjusted composite score derived from several tests of learning and memory. Similarly, Cerhan et al[13] using data from the Atherosclerosis Risk in Communities Study examined the effect of several atherosclerosis risk factors including hypertension on cognition in 14,000 middle-aged adults. Among 3,700 participants with hypertension (58% female), there were small but significant differences from controls on measures of verbal memory, processing speed, and verbal fluency. It should be noted, however, that these were extremely small effects, mostly on the order of 10–20% of one standard deviation.

More recent studies have made progress in the application of more stringently controlled experimental designs. In several studies of elderly subjects, the associations between hypertension and cognitive performance have been confounded by changes in blood pressure associated with the onset of dementia and the inclusion of subjects on antihypertensive medications and with end-organ damage such as stroke. Harrington et al[41] designed a study that attempted to circumvent these methodological issues. A computerized cognitive assessment was administered to 107 untreated hypertensives and 116 normotensives, both of which were free from dementia or end-organ damage. The cognitive assessment was based on existing neuropsychological tests of memory and attention. Results revealed that the hypertensives were slower on reaction time tests, had lower scores on recall and recognition memory, and made more accuracy errors across all measures. Using data from the Swedish study of Men born in 1914, a prospective study of cardiovascular disease, Andre-Petersson et al[86] found that subjects with hypertension, after controlling for cardiovascular risk factors, antihypertensive medication use, depression, and stroke history, scored significantly lower on tests of psychomotor speed and visuospatial ability. However, when the hypertensives were divided by severity levels, the results were limited to the highest levels of hypertension (systolic >179 mmHg or diastolic > 110 mmHg). Interestingly, the lowest levels of hypertension were associated with slightly better performance on cognitive tasks than normotensives. In addition, this study is unique in that all participants were of extremely similar age, education, and ethnicity. Overall, the findings from this study indicate an inverse relationship between blood pressure and cognitive abilities in elderly males. In a recent study by Kuo et al,[56] 70 elderly subjects had resting blood pressure readings on three different occasions before completing the Trail Making Test part B

(Trails B),[77] a verbal fluency test, and the Logical Memory I&II and Visual Reproduction I&II tests from the WMS-III.[97] After controlling for differences in ethnicity, gender, age, education, alcohol use, medication use, and BMI, there was a significant association between levels of blood pressure and cognitive impairment risk. Each 10 mmHg increase in systolic blood pressure was associated with a 2.31-fold increase in risk for impairment in overall Trails B completion time and total number of sequencing errors. The authors conclude that increases in blood pressure increase risk of frontal-executive impairments in otherwise healthy elders. Interestingly, van Boxtel et al[90] conducted a very similar study on a similar population and found no clear associations between blood pressure and cognitive functioning regardless of age.

The role of age in studies of cognition and blood pressure has received considerable attention as a potential confounder that must be controlled for in data analyses; however, the literature on hypertension and cognition in younger adults is limited. Elias et al[22] attempted to elucidate the impact of hypertension on cognition by comparing two age groups in a well-controlled longitudinal study of 529 community-dwelling adults. The first group ranged in age from 18 to 46 and the second group ranged in age from 47 to 83. All subjects were tested on two to four occasions approximately 4 years apart using selected subtests from the original Wechsler intelligence scale. A significant main effect of blood pressure was found on the Picture Completion, Block Design, and Object Assembly subtests, regardless of age. The authors concluded that hypertension negatively impacted upon cognition at all age levels. However, age of hypertension onset and other metabolic syndrome components were not included in the analysis and a large number of subjects were lost to follow up, especially in the younger age group.

Neuroimaging and Hypertension

There is a growing literature on the impact of hypertension in mid-life and late-life cognitive decline and associated reductions in brain integrity. Swan et al[87] investigated this association using the original data from the National Heart, Lung, and Blood Institute Twin Study for the mid-life time points and data from follow-up studies that included MRI for the late-life time points. Data from structural MRI and a comprehensive battery of cognitive tests were analyzed. Subjects with high mid-life blood pressure experienced a greater decline in cognitive performance and had larger white matter hyperintensity (WMHI) volumes and greater overall brain atrophy at follow up than did those with lower mid-life blood pressure. Swan et al[87] conclude that the long-term impact of hypertension on decline in late-life cognitive functioning is likely to be mediated by structural damage to the brain.

Further studies of the relationship between mid-life blood pressure and structural brain changes in late-life have exhibited intriguing results. In an MRI study of 513 subjects whose blood pressure was routinely monitored over an approximately 20-year period, den Heijer et al[43] found associations between blood pressure levels over time and overall brain tissue volume. Both high ($\geq$ 90 mmHg) and low ($\leq$ 65 mmHg) diastolic blood pressure were positively associated with degree of cortical atrophy. Similarly, DeCarli et al[19] found associations between mid-life blood pressure and late-life brain tissue volume in 414 men involved in the NHLBI Twin Study. In addition, blood pressure was directly related to WMHI volumes. The authors conclude that mid-life blood pressure is significantly associated with later-life brain and WMHI volumes, which may be a subclinical expression of cerebrovascular disease.

Cross-sectional analyses of brain integrity and hypertension have also revealed structural brain abnormalities. Sierra et al[84] used ambulatory blood pressure measurements, where blood pressure is repeatedly monitored over a 24 h period, in 66 middle-aged untreated hypertensives that were otherwise healthy. MRI scans revealed the presence of subtle WMLs in 40.9% of subjects. Subjects with WMLs had significantly higher ambulatory blood pressure than subjects without WMLs, after controlling for age. Similarly, Goldstein et al[33] investigated ambulatory blood pressure values and brain volumes in healthy elderly. A highly significant association was found between increases in blood pressure and reductions in overall brain volume. These studies confirm the results from previous, less stringent studies where the presence of WMLs has been reported to be associated with hypertension.[30]

There is some evidence that the frontal lobes may be differentially sensitive to damage from hypertension. Raz et al[75] compared 40 medication-controlled hypertensive subjects with 40 well-matched control subjects on measures of perseveration, working memory, fluid reasoning, and vocabulary knowledge. In addition, brain volumes and WMHI were measured via MRI. Relative to controls, hypertensive subjects had smaller prefrontal cortex and underlying white matter volumes as well as an overall increase in frontal lobe WMHI. Hypertensive subjects made significantly more perseverative errors on the Wisconsin Card Sorting Test. The authors conclude that prefrontal lobe damage and executive function are associated with hypertension, and this effect was evident despite antihypertensive medication use. However, this study did not account for other cardiovascular risk factors, which Gold et al[31] have found to have significant associations with frontal lobe integrity in studies of hypertension.

Gold et al[31] evaluated executive functioning, glucocorticoid feedback, and brain volumes in 27 hypertensive subjects and 27 well-matched control subjects. After adjusting for differences in age, gender, and BMI, hypertensives performed significantly worse than controls on the Stoop test and the Tower of London.[80] Moreover, hypertensives exhibited a trend toward smaller frontal lobe volumes, but impaired glucocorticoid feedback was significantly associated with frontal lobe atrophy. The authors conclude that impaired glucocorticoid feedback may partly account for the prefrontal volume reductions present in patients with hypertension.

In sum, elevation in blood pressure has adverse impacts on cognitive functioning and increases the likelihood of the development of structural brain abnormalities. Results from several studies of hypertension and cognition reveal that in general, hypertensives are found to perform more poorly on tests of processing speed, memory, and attention and less consistently on tests of mental flexibility and abstract reasoning. In addition, hypertension has been shown to increase the likelihood of structural brain abnormalities including overall brain tissue loss, white matter hyperintensities, and frontal lobe abnormalities.

Neuropsychology of Obesity

Despite the substantial increase in the prevalence of obesity in the USA and throughout the world, there is an extremely modest literature that directly examines the neurocognitive manifestations of obesity. In addition to obesity's direct impact on cognition, there is an emerging literature on the relationship between early and mid-life obesity and the development of dementia in later-life. However, studies of obesity and cognition in general have been subject to criticism for several reasons. The majority of studies have inconsistently controlled for confounding variables such as psychiatric comorbidity and other cardiovascular risk factors such as metabolic dysfunction. Studies investigating cognition and obesity have relied on global measures of cognition, and relatively few have used more sensitive cognitive measures. Of the population-based studies, only a few have included women and these had dramatically conflicting results. In addition, obesity has typically been measured using BMI, which can overlook the importance of the distribution of adipose tissue throughout the body and its relationship to cognitive functioning. Of the few existing studies directly examining cognition in obese subjects using sensitive measures of cognitive functioning, currently only one has attempted to distinguish between central obesity as measured by waist circumference and generalized obesity as measured by BMI.

In a population-based study of 467 South Korean elders, Jeong et al[46] found an association between lower mental status scores and increases in BMI. When different measures of obesity were applied, including ethnicity-corrected waist circumference values, subjects with waist circumference and BMI values in the obese range had the lowest mental status scores. This association was observed after adjusting for age, education, alcohol use, smoking status, marital status, and other metabolic syndrome components.

A population-based study of 504 elderly Swedish males investigated the relationship between several vascular risk factors and cognitive functioning.[49] This study utilized the MMSE and several standard neuropsychological measures adapted for a Swedish population. After controlling for age, education, stroke history, smoking status, and other components of metabolic syndrome, subjects with higher BMI performed more poorly on the digit span and the Trail Making Test B.[77] The authors concluded that obesity was related to decreased performance on tests of attention and executive functioning. However, the sample used for this study was exceptionally unhealthy and had very low levels of education. Approximately 30% of subjects had poorly controlled hypertension, and approximately 20% of subjects had verified cardiovascular disease. Only 44% had 5 or more years of education.

Elias et al[23] examined the independent effects of obesity and hypertension on cognitive functioning in subjects enrolled in the Framingham Heart Study. Using a prospective design, 1,423 White community-dwelling subjects (61% female) were administered selected subtests from the WAIS, the WMS, and customized language tests including verbal fluency. After adjusting for differences in age, education, occupation, alcohol use, smoking, cholesterol levels, and diabetes, results were different for men and women. Significant effects of hypertension and obesity were observed in men only on tests of mental status and tests of learning and memory. Obesity and hypertension were associated with lower cognitive functioning in middle-aged and elderly men, and the effects of obesity and hypertension were interdependent, wherein the presence of both risk factors resulted in lower levels of cognitive functioning and the presence of only one or the other was not significant. The authors conclude that obesity alone, or hypertension alone, could not account for the reductions in cognitive performance observed. Therefore, obesity and hypertension may share common mechanisms by which they affect cognition in males.

In contrast, Kuo et al[55] investigated the impact of obesity on cognition in 2,684 community-dwelling elderly (76% female, 26% African American) undergoing several different types of lifestyle interventions. Measures included the MMSE, two list learning tasks, a paragraph recall task, verbal reasoning tasks, a continuous performance measure, and digit-symbol coding. After controlling for intervention groupings, age, race, sex, education levels, and metabolic syndrome components including hypertension, overweight subjects had better overall cognitive performance in terms of verbal reasoning and processing speed. However, this study may have been flawed by sampling errors, including low mean scores on mental status examinations, and self-report of overall health status.

There has been some interest in the relationship between obesity and attention-deficit/hyperactivity disorder (ADHD). Altfas[2] investigated the prevalence of ADHD among 215 bariatric patients and found an overall sample prevalence of 27.4%, with substantial increases in ADHD prevalence in more extreme cases of obesity. However, patients were diagnosed with ADHD based on self-report and were not tested on established measures of attention. In addition, the sample was composed of over 91% females and several potential confounding factors including metabolic syndrome components were not accounted for. In a more well-balanced design using structured interviews and objective testing, Fleming et al[27] found that overweight and obese women had substantial increases in ADHD prevalence, yet this study did not account for potential metabolic confounders.

Waldstein and Katzel[93] conducted the only study to date that has directly examined central obesity and cognitive functioning using sensitive neuropsychological measures. In this study, 90 healthy white middle-aged and older adults (37% female) underwent comprehensive neuropsychological testing. Results indicated that after adjustment for age, education, gender, and other components of metabolic syndrome, significant interactions between waist circumference and blood pressure accounted for a significant amount of variance on the Grooved Pegboard Test and the Stroop interference score. The authors conclude that independent of other confounding variables, the combination of greater waist circumference and higher blood pressure was associated with reduced performance on tests of psychomotor speed and executive functioning. Similar to Elias et al,[23] there was a cumulative effect of obesity and blood pressure – neither obesity alone nor blood pressure alone was associated with reductions in cognitive functioning.

Obesity and Brain Function

Gustafson et al[40] investigated the relationship between BMI, blood pressure, and the presence of WMLs as measured by computerized tomography (CT) scans in a representative sample of 27 subjects. Subjects with increased BMI at ages 70, 75, and 79 were more likely to exhibit WMLs at 85 and 88 years of age, regardless of other cardiovascular factors including hypertension. In a third study using subjects from this same population, Gustafson et al[39] measured atrophy of the temporal, frontal, occipital, and parietal lobes based on CT scans collected in 1992. Increases in BMI were significantly associated with temporal lobe atrophy such that a one point increase in BMI increased the risk of temporal lobe atrophy by 13–16% of the base rate risk. These studies were limited by several factors, including possibly imprecise volumetric measurements obtained via CT scans and by not incorporating multiple measures of obesity including skinfold thickness and waist circumference.

At least two recent MRI studies have shown associations between obesity and total brain volumes. Ward et al[95] assessed the relationship between BMI and brain volumes in a sample of 114 white middle-aged adults (62% female). After controlling for other potentially confounding cardiovascular risk factors, a significant interaction was found between age and BMI, where increases in age and BMI predicted reductions in normalized brain volumes. This study is unique in that it examined the impact of BMI and brain volumes in an otherwise healthy middle-aged sample. Gunstad et al[38] used automated anatomical labeling and voxel-based morphometry to assess total brain volume and total gray matter volume in obese, overweight, and normal control subjects of a wide range of ages (17–79 years). The most obese individuals were found to have smaller whole brain and gray matter volumes, after correction for demographic differences.

The use of FMRI in neuropsychological studies of obesity is in a state of relative infancy. Based on findings from Gunstad et al,[38] Cohen (2009, personal communication) conducted a pilot FMRI study of 12 obese and 12 nonobese healthy adults comparing their FMRI response on the n-back task. Obese participants showed abnormal FMRI response with reduced signal intensity in ROIs on the 2-back ($p<0.01$), but increased response (volume of activated voxels) on the 1-back in areas outside the primary ROIs, suggesting compensatory brain response due to effortful task demands. Another study found that FMRI response during declarative memory tasks was greater in the posterior cingulate cortex and in regions of the frontal and temporal lobes among overweight and hypertensive elderly, indicating an abnormal response to cognitive processes in cognitively intact older adults with increased vascular risk.[10]

In sum, there is emerging evidence indicating that obesity may directly and negatively impact cognitive abilities; however, it is not clear whether the relationship between obesity and cognitive functioning can exist independent of hypertension. The most stringently controlled studies using the most comprehensive and sensitive measures of cognition have consistently found that obesity and hypertension appear to cluster together to produce a small, but cumulative effect on cognition mainly on tests of psychomotor speed and executive functioning.

Neuroimaging studies of neuropsychological functioning in obesity are few in number, but appear to support some relationship between obesity, hypertension, and decreased overall brain volumes and increased brain response to cognitive challenge relative to control subjects.

Conclusion

Imaging methodology will certainly continue to improve and should have the much needed impact of increasing our sensitivity to detect subtle changes in the brains of individuals with metabolic dysfunction across the lifespan. One cannot stress enough the importance of using the most sensitive techniques available when imaging metabolic disorders, especially in middle-aged or younger samples where accumulating evidence of structural and functional changes are still emerging and need to be distinguished reliably from normal aging or disease processes intricately tied to aging.

References

1. Alberti K, Zimmet PZ. Definition, diagnosis and classification of diabetes mellitus and its complications. Part 1: diagnosis and classification of diabetes mellitus. Provisional report of a WHO consultation. *Diabet Med*. 1998;15(7):539–553.
2. Altfas JR. Prevalence of attention deficit/hyperactivity disorder among adults in obesity treatment. *BMC Psychiatry*. 2002;2:1–8.
3. André-Petersson L, Hagberg B, Janzon L, Steen G. A comparison of cognitive ability in normotensive and hypertensive 68-yearold men: results from population study" men born in 1914," in Malmö, Sweden. *Exp Aging Res*. 2001;27(4): 319–340.
4. Arvanitakis Z, Schneider JA, Wilson RS, et al. Diabetes is related to cerebral infarction but not to AD pathology in older persons. *Neurology*. 2006;67(11):1960.
5. Awad N, Gagnon M, Messier C. The relationship between impaired glucose tolerance, type 2 diabetes, and cognitive function. *J Clin Exp Neuropsychol*. 2004;26(8):1044–1080.
6. Beeri MS, Schmeidler J, Silverman JM, et al. Insulin in combination with other diabetes medication is associated with less Alzheimer neuropathology. *Neurology*. 2008;71(10):750.
7. Beeri MS, Silverman JM, Davis KL, et al. Type 2 diabetes is negatively associated with Alzheimer's disease neuropathology. *J Geront A Biol Med Sci*. 2005;60(4):471–475.
8. Biessels GJ, Staekenborg S, Brunner E, Brayne C, Scheltens P. Risk of dementia in diabetes mellitus: a systematic review. *Lancet Neurol*. 2006;5(1):64–74.

9. Brands AMA, Biessels GJ, Kappelle LJ, et al. Cognitive functioning and brain MRI in patients with type 1 and type 2 diabetes mellitus: a comparative study. *Dement Geriatr Cogn Disord*. 2007;23(5):343–350.
10. Braskie, MN, Small, GW, Bookheimer, SY. Vascular health risks and fMRI activation during a memory task in older adults. *Neurobiol Aging*. 2008;31(9):1532–1542.
11. Brownlee M. Biochemistry and molecular cell biology of diabetic complications. *Nature*. 2001;414:813–818.
12. Centers for Disease Control and Prevention (CDC). *Behavioral Risk Factor Surveillance System Survey Data*. Atlanta, Georgia: US Department of Health and Human Services, Centers for Disease Control and Prevention; 2008.
13. Cerhan JR, Folsom AR, Mortimer JA, et al. Correlates of cognitive function in middle-aged adults. *Gerontology*. 1998;44:95–105.
14. Cervos-Navarro J, Diemer NH. Selective vulnerability in brain hypoxia. *Crit Rev Neurobiol*. 1991;6(3):149–182.
15. Convit A. Links between cognitive impairment in insulin resistance: An explanatory model. *Neurobiol Aging*. 2005; 26S:S31–35.
16. Convit A, Wolf OT, Tarshish C, de Leon MJ. Reduced glucose tolerance is associated with poor memory performance and hippocampal atrophy among normal elderly. *Proc Natl Acad Sci*. 2003;100(4):2019–2022.
17. Craft S, Watson GS. Insulin and neurodegenerative disease: shared and specific mechanisms. *Lancet Neurol*. 2004; 3(3):169–178.
18. Curtis LH, Hammill BG, Bethel MA, Anstrom KJ, Gottdiener JS, Schulman KA. Costs of the metabolic syndrome in elderly individuals: findings from the Cardiovascular Health Study. *Diabetes Care*. 2007;30(10):2553–2558.
19. DeCarli C, Miller BL, Swan GE, et al. Predictors of brain morphology for the men of the NHLBI twin study. *Stroke*. 1999;30:529–536.
20. Dejgaard A, Gade A, Larsson H, Balle V, Parving HH. Evidence for diabetic encephalopathy. *Diabet Med*. 1991;8(2): 162–167.
21. Dore S, Kar S, Rowe W, Quirion R. Distribution and levels of [125I] IGF-I,[125I] IGF-II and [125I] insulin receptor binding sites in the hippocampus of aged memory-unimpaired and-impaired rats. *Neuroscience*. 1997;80(4): 1033–1040.
22. Elias PK, Elias MF, Robbins MA, Budge MM. Blood pressure-related cognitive decline does age make a difference? *Hypertension*. 2004;44:631–636.
23. Elias MF, Elias PK, Sullivan LM, Wolf PA, D'Agostino RB. Lower cognitive function in the presence of obesity and hypertension: the Framingham heart study. *Int J Obes Relat Metab Disord*. 2003;27(2):260–268.
24. Evans JL, Goldfine ID, Maddux BA, Grodsky GM. Oxidative stress and stress-activated signaling pathways: A unifying hypothesis of type 2 diabetes. *Endocrinol Rev*. 2002; 23:599–622.
25. Executive Summary of The Third Report of The National Cholesterol Education Program (NCEP) Expert Panel on Detection, Evaluation, And Treatment of High Blood Cholesterol In Adults (Adult Treatment Panel III). Expert panel on detection, evaluation, and treatment of high blood cholesterol in adults. *JAMA*. 2001;285(19):2486–2497.

26. Farmer ME, Kittner SJ, Abbott RD, Wolz MM, Wolf PA, White LR. Longitudinally measured blood pressure, antihypertensive medication use, and cognitive performance: the Framingham Study. *J Clin Epidemiol*. 1990;43(5): 475.

27. Fleming JP, Levy LD, Levitan RD. Symptoms of attention deficit hyperactivity disorder in severely obese women. *Eat Weight Disord*. 2005;10(1):10–13.

28. Ford ES. Prevalence of the metabolic syndrome defined by the International Diabetes Federation among adults in the U.S. *Diabetes Care*. 2005;28(11):2745–2749.

29. Frankel HM, Garcia E, Malik F, Weiss JK, Weiss HR. Effect of acetazolamide on cerebral blood flow and capillary potency. *J Appl Physiol*. 1992;73(5):1756–1761.

30. Fukuda H, Kitani M. Differences between treated and untreated hypertensive subjects in the extent of periventricular hyperintensities observed on brain MRI. *Stroke*. 1995;26(9):1593–1597.

31. Gold SM, Dziobek I, Rogers K, Bayoumy A, McHugh PF, Convit A. Hypertension and hypothalamo-pituitary-adrenal axis hyperactivity affect frontal lobe integrity. *J Clin Endocrinol Metab*. 2005;90(6):3262–3267.

32. Gold SM, Dziobek I, Sweat V, et al. Hippocampal damage and memory impairments as possible early brain complications of type 2 diabetes. *Diabetologia*. 2007;50(4): 711–719.

33. Goldstein IB, Bartzokis G, Guthrie D, Shapiro D. Ambulatory blood pressure and brain atrophy in the healthy elderly. *Neurology*. 2002;59(5):713–719.

34. Goto I. Pathological studies on the intracerebral and retinal arteries in cerebrovascular and noncerebrovascular diseases. *Stroke*. 1975;6(3):263–269.

35. Gould GW, Bell GI. Facilitative glucose transporters: an expanding family. *Trends Biochem Sci*. 1990;15(1):18.

36. Greenwood CE. Dietary carbohydrate, glucose regulation, and cognitive performance in elderly persons. *Nutr Rev*. 2003;61(5):S68–S74.

37. Grundy SM, Cleeman JI, Daniels SR, et al. Diagnosis and management of the metabolic syndrome: an American Heart Association/National Heart, Lung, and Blood Institute Scientific Statement. *Circulation*. 2005;112(17): 2735–2752.

38. Gunstad J, Paul RH, Cohen RA, Tate DF, Spitznagel MB, Gordon E. Elevated body mass index is associated with executive dysfunction in otherwise healthy adults. *Compr Psychiatry*. 2007;48(1):57–61.

39. Gustafson D, Lissner L, Bengtsson C, Bjorkelund C, Skoog I. A 24-year follow-up of body mass index and cerebral atrophy. *Neurology*. 2004;63:1876–1881.

40. Gustafson D, Steen B, Skoog I. Body mass index and white matter lesions in elderly women. An 18-year longitudinal study. *Int Psychogeriatr*. 2004;16(3):327–336.

41. Harrington F, Saxby BK, McKeith IG, Wesnes K, Ford GA. Cognitive performance in hypertensive and normotensive older subjects. *Hypertension*. 2000;36(6):1079–1082.

42. Hassenstab, J. *A longitudinal study of the impact of the metabolic syndrome on cognition and brain volumes in normal aging*. Unpublished doctoral dissertation, Fordham University, New York; 2008.

43. den Heijer T, Vermeer SE, Dijk EJ, et al. Type 2 diabetes and atrophy of medial temporal lobe structures on brain MRI. *Diabetologia*. 2003;46(12):1604–1610.

44. Heitner J, Dickson D. Diabetics do not have increased Alzheimer-type pathology compared with age-matched control subjects. *A retrospective postmortem immunocytochemical and histofluorescent study Neurology*. 1997;49(5):1306–1311.

45. Hsueh WA, Lyon CJ, Quiñones MJ. Insulin resistance and the endothelium. *Am J Med*. 2004;117(2):109–117.

46. Jeong SK, Nam HS, Son MH, Son EJ, Cho KH. Interactive effect of obesity indexes on cognition. *Dement Geriatr Cogn Disord*. 2005;19:91–96.

47. Kario K, Ishikawa J, Hoshide S, et al. Diabetic brain damage in hypertension role of renin–angiotensin system. *Hypertension*. 2005;45:887–893.

48. Kawasaki K, Ishii K, Saito Y, Oda K, Kimura Y, Ishiwata K. Influence of mild hyperglycemia on cerebral FDG distribution patterns calculated by statistical parametric mapping. *Ann Nucl Med*. 2008;22(3):191–200.

49. Kilander L, Nyman H, Boberg M, Hansson L, Lithell H. Hypertension is related to cognitive impairment: A 20-year follow-up of 99 men. *Hypertension*. 1998;31:780–786.

50. Korf ESC, van Straaten ECW, de Leeuw FE, et al. Diabetes mellitus, hypertension and medial temporal lobe atrophy: the LADIS study. *Diabetic Med*. 2007;24(2):166.

51. Korf ESC, White LR, Scheltens P, Launer LJ. Brain aging in very old men with type 2 diabetes. *Diabetes Care*. 2006;29(10): 2268–2274.

52. Kreis R, Ross BD. Cerebral metabolic disturbances in patients with subacute and chronic diabetes mellitus: detection with proton MR spectroscopy. *Radiology*. 1992;184(1):123–130.

53. Kumar A, Haroon E, Darwin C, et al. Gray matter prefrontal changes in type 2 diabetes detected using MRI. *J Magn Reson Imaging*. 2008;27(1):14–19.

54. Kumari M, Marmot M. Diabetes and cognitive function in a middle-aged cohort Findings from the Whitehall II study. *Neurology*. 2005;65(10):1597–1603.

55. Kuo HK, Jones RN, Milberg WP, Tennstedt S, Talbot L, et al. Cognitive function in normal-weight, overweight, and obese older adults: An analysis of the advanced cognitive training for independent and vital elderly cohort. *J Am Geriatr Soc*. 2006;54:97–103.

56. Kuo HK, Sorond F, Iloputaife I, Gagnon M, Milberg W, Lipsitz LA. Effect of blood pressure on cognitive functions in elderly persons. *J Gerontol A Biol Med Sci*. 2004;59(11): 1191–1194.

57. Kwon HM, Kim BJ, Lee SH, Choi SH, Oh BH, Yoon BW. Metabolic syndrome as an independent risk factor of silent brain infarction in healthy people. *Stroke*. 2006;37:466–470.

58. Lazarus R, Prettyman R, Cherryman G. White matter lesions on magnetic resonance imaging and their relationship with vascular risk factors in memory clinic attenders. *Int J Geriatr Psychiatry*. 2005;20(3):274–279.

59. MacKnight C, Rockwood K, Awalt E, McDowell I. Diabetes mellitus and the risk of dementia, Alzheimer's disease and vascular cognitive impairment in the Canadian Study of Health and Aging. *Dement Geriatr Cogn Disord*. 2002;14:77–83.

60. Magistretti PJ, Pellerin L. Cellular mechanisms of brain energy metabolism. Relevance to functional brain imaging and to neurodegenerative disorders. *Ann N Y Acad Sci*. 1996;777:380–387.

61. McEwen BS. Possible mechanisms for atrophy of the human hippocampus. *Mol Psychiatry*. 1997;2(3):255–262.

62. McNay EC, Gold PE. Age-related differences in hippocampal extracellular fluid glucose concentration during behavioral testing and following systemic glucose administration. *J Gerontol A Biol Sci Med Sci.* 2001;56A(2):B66–B71.

63. McNay EC, Fries TM, Gold PE. Decreases in rat extracellular hippocampal glucose concentration associated with cognitive demand during a spatial task. *Proc Natl Acad Sci USA.* 2000;97(6):2881–2885.

64. Messier C. Glucose improvement of memory: a review. *Eur J Pharmacol.* 2004;490(1–3):33.

65. Messier C, Tsiakas M, Gagnon M, Desrochers A, Awad N. Effect of age and glucoregulation on cognitive performance. *Neurobiol Aging.* 2004;24(7):985–1003.

66. Mielke JG, Taghibiglou C, Liu L, et al. A biochemical and functional characterization of diet-induced brain insulin resistance. *J Neurochem.* 2005;93(6):1568.

67. Muniyappa R, Iantorno M, Quon MJ. An Integrated View of Insulin Resistance and Endothelial Dysfunction. *Endocrinol Metab Clin North Am.* 2008;37(3):685–711.

68. Nagamachi S, Nishikawa T, Ono S, et al. Regional cerebral blood flow in diabetic patients: evaluation by N-isopropyl-123I-IMP with SPECT. *Nucl Med Commun.* 1994;15(6):455.

69. Novak V, Last D, Alsop DC, et al. Cerebral blood flow velocity and periventricular white matter hyperintensities in type 2 diabetes. *Diabetes Care.* 2006;29(7):1529–1534.

70. Ott A, Breteler MMB, van Harskamp F, et al. Prevalence of Alzheimer's disease and vascular dementia: association with education. The Rotterdam study. *Br Med J.* 1995;310(6985): 970–973.

71. Ott A, Stolk RP, Van Harskamp F, Pols HAP, Hofman A, Breteler MMB. Diabetes mellitus and the risk of dementia The Rotterdam Study. *Neurology.* 1999;53(9):1937–1937.

72. Pavlik VN, Hyman DJ, Doody R. Cardiovascular risk factors and cognitive function in adults 30–59 years of age (NHANES III). *Neuroepidemiology.* 2005;24:42–50.

73. Peila R, Rodriguez BL, Launer LJ. Type 2 diabetes, APOE gene, and the risk for dementia and related pathologies: The Honolulu-Asia Aging study. *Diabetes.* 2002;51(4):1256–1262.

74. Peppa M, Uribarri J, Vlassara H. Glucose, advanced glycation end products, and diabetes complications: What is new and what works. *Clinical Diabetes.* 2003;21(4):186–187.

75. Raz N, Rodrigue KM, Acker JD. Hypertension and the brain: Vulnerability of the prefrontal regions and executive functions. *Behav Neurosci.* 2003;117(6):1169–1180.

76. Reaven GM. Role of insulin resistance in human disease (syndrome X): an expanded definition. *Annu Rev Med.* 1993;44(1): 121–131.

77. Reitan RM. The relation of the Trail Making Test to organic brain damage. *J Consult Psychol.* 1955;19(5):393–394.

78. Ronnema E, Zethelius B, Sundelof J, et al. Impaired insulin secretion increases the risk of Alzheimer disease. *Neurology.* 2008;71(14):1065.

79. Ross AJ, Sachdev PS. Magnetic resonance spectroscopy in cognitive research. *Brain Res Rev.* 2004;44(2–3):83–102.

80. Shallice T. Specific impairments of planning. *Philos Trans R Soc Lond Biol.* 1982;298:199–209.

81. Schwartz MW, Porte D. Diabetes, obesity, and the brain. *Science.* 2005;307:375–379.

82. Seaquist ER, Damberg GS, Tkac I, Gruetter R. The effect of insulin on in vivo cerebral glucose concentrations and rates of glucose transport/metabolism in humans. *Diabetes.* 2001;50(10):2203.

83. Sesti G. Pathophysiology of insulin resistance. *Best Pract Res Clin Endocrinol Metab.* 2006;20(4):665–679.

84. Sierra C, de la Sierra A, Mercader J, Gomez-Angelats E, Urbano-Marquea A, Coca A. Silent cerebral white matter lesions in middle-aged essential hypertensive patients. *J Hypertens.* 2001;20:519–524.

85. Starr VL, Convit A. Diabetes, sugar-coated but harmful to the brain. *Curr Opin Pharmacol.* 2007;7(6):638–642.

86. Steen G, Hagberg B, Johnson G, Steen B. Cognitive function, cognitive style and life satisfaction in a 68-year-old male population. *Compr Gerontol B.* 1987;1(2):54.

87. Swan GE, DeCarli C, Miller BL, et al. Association of midlife blood pressure to late-life cognitive decline and brain morphology. *Neurology.* 1998;51(4):986–993.

88. Tirsi A, Bruehl H, Sweat V, et al. Retinal vessel abnormalities are associated with elevated fasting insulin levels and cerebral atrophy in nondiabetic individuals. *Ophthalmology.* 2009;116(6):1175–1181.

89. Tooke JE, Goh KL. Endotheliopathy precedes type 2 diabetes. *Diabetes Care.* 1998;21(12):2047–2049.

90. van Boxtel MPJ, Gaillard C, Houx PJ, Buntinx F, de Leeuw PW, Jolles J. Can the blood pressure predict cognitive task performance in a healthy population sample? *J Hypertens.* 1997;15(10):1069.

91. van Harten B, de Leeuw FE, Weinstein HC, Scheltens P, Biessels GJ. Brain imaging in patients with diabetes. *Diabetes Care.* 2006;29(11):2539–2548.

92. Vinik AI, Erbas T, Park TS, Stansberry KB, Scanelli JA, Pittenger GL. Dermal neurovascular dysfunction in type 2 diabetes. *Diabetes Care.* 2001;24(8):1468.

93. Waldstein SR, Katzel LI. Interactive relations of central versus total obesity and blood pressure to cognitive function. *Int J Obes (Lond).* 2006;30(1):201–207.

94. Waldstein SR, Manuck SB, Ryan CM, Muldoon MF. Neuropsychological correlates of hypertension: review and methodologic considerations. *Psychol Bull.* 1991;110(3): 451–468.

95. Ward MA, Carlsson CM, Trivedi MA, Sager MA, Johnson SC. The effect of body mass index on global brain volume in middle-aged adults: A cross sectional study. *BMC Neurology.* 2005;5:1–7.

96. Watson GS, Peskind ER, Asthana S, et al. Insulin increases CSF Aß42 levels in normal older adults. *Neurology.* 2003;60(12):1899–1903.

97. Wechsler D. *Wechsler Memory Scale-Third Edition.* New York: Psychological Corporation; 1997.

98. Wu W, Brickman AM, Luchsinger J, et al. The brain in the age of old: the hippocampal formation is targeted differentially by diseases of late life. *Ann Neurol.* 2008;64(6):698–706.

99. Yaffe K, Haan M, Blackwell T, Cherkasova E, Whitmer RA, West N. Metabolic syndrome and cognitive decline in elderly Latinos: findings from the Sacramento Area Latino Study of Aging study. *J Am Geriatr Soc.* 2007;55(5):758–762.

100. Yaffe K, Kanaya A, Lindquist K, et al. The metabolic syndrome, inflammation, and risk of cognitive decline. *JAMA.* 2004;292(18):2237–2242.

101. Yki-Järvinen H. Insulin resistance and endothelial dysfunction. *Best Pract Res Clin Endocrinol Metab.* 2003;17(3): 411–430.

102. Zhao WQ, Chen H, Quon MJ, Alkon DL. Insulin and the insulin receptor in experimental models of learning and memory. *Eur J Pharmacol.* 2004;490(1–3):71–81.

Chapter 15
Neuroimaging of Cardiovascular Disease

Ronald A. Cohen

Cardiovascular disease (CVD) remains the leading cause of death in this country, underlying over 700,000 deaths per year.[1] CVD prevalence increases dramatically with advanced age, hence significant CVD is present in over 70% of people 75 years of age or older, and is the leading cause of mortality and morbidity in Western society. 84.7% of people who die of CVD are 65 years of age or older[1,2] With improved survival from acute cardiac events, older adults are often faced with the prospect of living with chronic heart disease, including severe CVD. Besides its obvious effects on physical wellbeing, CVD causes significant psychological, social, and economic hardship[3–8] and contributes to depression and psychiatric problems.[4–6,9–16]

Severe CVD, such as heart failure (HF), also predisposes people to cerebrovascular disease, which eventually may lead to cognitive dysfunction.[17–24] Though brain dysfunction is most likely to occur among people with severe CVD, many people with milder forms of CVD experience cognitive impairments,[25–27] though these have historically received less attention than CVD-associated psychosocial problems. There is compelling evidence that cognitive functioning is an important determinant of health status, quality of life (QOL), and ultimately, functional ability.[10,28–30] These effects limit the ability of the elderly to age successfully. We have previously shown that even subtle cognitive problems among CVD patients affect their QOL, their ability to benefit from treatment (e.g., cardiac rehabilitation), and may also be a harbinger of more serious problems.[28] Resulting cerebrovascular disease may eventually lead

to functional impairments and even vascular dementia (VaD).[20,31–35] This scenario provides a compelling reason to study the neurobehavioral mechanisms underlying the development of brain vascular cognitive impairment (VCI) secondary to CVD in the elderly.

The relationship between CVD and brain dysfunction is not yet fully understood. While CVD and cerebrovascular disease share common pathophysiology and comorbidity,[31,36–43] the cause of CVD-associated cerebrovascular changes and brain dysfunction is often difficult to disentangle, except in cases where acute cardioembolic stroke has occurred,[44–47] though there is considerable evidence that such changes can develop when there is chronic cerebral hypoperfusion and/or microvascular disease associated with CVD. Yet, relatively large gaps exist in knowledge regarding the longitudinal course of the progression from systemic vascular risk factors to the clinical disorder of VCI and dementia among certain people as they reach advanced. CVD is a major health problem among the elderly.

Questions regarding that needed to be resolved include: (1) Which systemic vascular disturbances associated with CVD exert the greatest affect on the brain and cognitive function in the absence of comorbid stroke? (2) How do CVD-associated cognitive problems progress to VCI? (3) To what extent do systemic vascular disturbances affect cerebral perfusion and brain dysfunction? (4) How do cardiac function and systemic hemodynamic function (endothelial function, atherosclerotic burden, etc.) interact to affect cerebral perfusion and brain dysfunction in CVD patients? (5) To what extent is the brain disturbances secondary to CVD linked to hypoperfusion versus cerebral metabolic abnormalities occurring in association with the underlying vascular disease? and (6) Is multimodal neuroimaging conducted in conjunction with neurocognitive examination of patients with CVD useful in establishing the basis for brain dysfunction and prognosis?

R.A. Cohen (✉)
Department of Psychiatry and Human Behavior
and the Institute for Brain Science, Warren Alpert Medical
School of Brown University, Providence, RI 02912, USA
e-mail: RCohen@lifespan.org

R.A. Cohen and L.H. Sweet (eds.), *Brain Imaging in Behavioral Medicine and Clinical Neuroscience*,
DOI 10.1007/978-1-4419-6373-4_15, © Springer Science+Business Media, LLC 2011

Rationale for Neuroimaging in CVD

Research directed at the neuroimaging of CVD and efforts to develop these methods for clinical use are driven largely by the fact that neuroimaging has the potential to provide power biomarkers of the cerebral neuronal, vascular, and metabolic disturbances occurring secondary to CVD. Neuroimaging has revolutionized brain science, enabling investigators to examine brain–behavior relationships, as well as abnormalities in anatomic microstructure, physiology, and metabolism. Magnetic resonance imaging (MRI) methods are powerful as they are noninvasive with high temporal and spatial resolution, enabling detection of subtle brain abnormalities and brain changes over time. Functional magnetic resonance imaging (FMRI) enables measurement of physiological activation across a priori brain regions of interest (ROIs) on specific cognitive, emotional, or other behavioral tasks that challenge specific functional brain systems,[48–52] while other MR-based methods such as MRS and ASL provide measures of metabolic and physiological disturbance. To date, hundreds of MR-based studies have been conducted showing abnormalities of brain structure and function in patients with AD, MCI, cerebrovascular disease, and systemic disorders, such as CVD and diabetes.

The current chapter was written with two primary goals in mind: (1) To briefly summarize current clinical and research evidence on the effects of CVD on the brain and on neurocognitive function as derived from studies employing neuroimaging methods; (2) To illustrate how these methods help to resolve particular questions that are not easily accomplished through standard clinical approaches. With these goals in mind, it would be useful to first examine some of our reasons for initiating studies of the neuropsychological effects of CVD over a decade ago, and why neuroimaging methods were introduced into these efforts.

Vascular Influences on Neurodegenerative Brain Disease

Our focus on CVD-associated brain dysfunction was an outgrowth of earlier research on the pathophysiology of neurodegenerative brain disease, such as AD. In the late 1980s, there was a growing sense that Alzheimer's disease did not account for all of the cases of dementia that were seen in memory disorder clinics. While the diagnostic entity "Binswanger's disease" had existed for many years and provided an alternative basis for dementia secondary to chronic cerebrovascular disease, this disorder was not well understood. Dementia secondary to multiple cerebral infarctions was an alternative basis for dementia, though many patients seemed to develop dementia secondary to cerebrovascular disease without evidence of multiple large vessel infarctions. This eventually led to NIH-led workgroups aimed at achieving greater clinical and research consensus on the nature of VaD. VaD was subsequently recognized as a clinical entity when the Diagnostic Statistical Manual was revised (DSM-IV, 1993).

Evidence from Studies of VCI

These led our group and other to conduct studies aimed at the cerebrovascular basis of dementia and possible precursors of VaD in patients with cerebrovascular and/or cardiovascular disease.[32,53–64] One of the key findings from these studies was that counter to our expectations, VaD had considerable overlap with AD. Despite compelling evidence that cerebrovascular disease is responsible for the development of dementia in certain patients, efforts to differentiate pure cases of VaD from AD have proven to be extremely difficult. Our own research suggested that many of the clinical heuristics that were thought to distinguish the two types of dementia (e.g., stepwise course, patchy cognitive profile, correlation of cognitive decline with discrete vascular events) did not consistently differentiate VaD patients in large between-group comparison studies. Furthermore, while it was generally thought that patients with a VaD had a different cognitive profile than AD patients, our results suggested that the groups were more similar than different in their cognitive presentation. Complicating the issue even more, we found that white matter hyperintensities (WMH) on MRI, considered to be an indicator of cerebral microvascular disease underlying VaD, were strongly associated with reduced speed of processing and problems on attention and executive control tasks, but were not significantly correlated with dementia severity or global cognitive function.[32,65] It was clear that story underlying the development of VaD was much more complicated than we originally anticipated.

One of our primary conclusions from this initial research was that by the time patients with suspected VaD were demented their cognitive dysfunction was quite global and no longer showed the specificity that would be predicted based on knowledge of the brain systems affected by microvascular disease. Either the more selective areas of cognitive impairment seen among patients who were not fully demented were converging into more global brain disturbance as the disease progressed, or neuronal degeneration of the type seen in Alzheimer's disease was occurring either as a result of the cerebrovascular disturbance or in addition to it. A solution to this quandary seemed to require that longitudinal studies focus on patients at earlier stages of cerebrovascular disease severity to examine how more severe brain disturbance develops among patients who have not experienced large cerebral infarctions. For this reason, we began a series of studies aimed at patients with CVD who had not experienced clinical stroke to examine what factors contributed to the development of VCI. To accomplish this goal, we also realized that it would be important to examine the relationship between disturbances occurring at the cardiac and systemic vascular level and changes occurring in the brain. This chapter reviews efforts to use structural and functional brain imaging methods in conjunction with clinical methods for cardiac and systemic vascular assessment to address these clinical neuroscience questions.

Pathophysiological Considerations

An important question implicit to our research in this area was how CVD affects progressive cognitive decline and brain abnormalities in the elderly. Accordingly, it is useful to briefly review what is known about the pathogenesis of neurodegenerative brain disease and the potential role of vascular disease. The cognitive and functional deterioration associated with of AD is known to involve progressive neuronal and synaptic loss[66–68] linked to neuritic plaques containing β-amyloid (Aβ)[69–73] and neurofibrillary tangles containing phosphorylated tau within neurons.[74–81] Beyond these characteristics, a large research literature suggests that the pathophysiology of AD is extremely complex, influenced by multiple genetic and environmental factors.[82,83] Aβ[69–73] and its precursor protein[84–86] occur in senile plaques,[84] around blood vessels,[87] and some forms cross the BBB. Deposition of amyloid occurs in the walls of the cerebral vasculature resulting in cerebral amyloid angiopathy (CAA)[88] in both cognitively normal elderly and people with AD. While capillary deposits of Aβ have been long observed, their influence is not well understood.[89,90] Recent studies suggest that they may play an important role in AD,[89–91] with some types of CAA identified based on whether Aβ deposits were found in cortical capillaries.[89–91] The APOE4 allele was found four times more common in CAA cases in which amyloid was detectable in capillaries,[91] and capillary Aβ deposition correlates with AD neuropathology,[89,90] suggesting that APOE, microvascular and AD pathogenesis are linked.

Microvascular Disease in AD

Microvascular disease is a common autopsy finding in the brains of elderly patients, and significant microvascular pathology including reduced vascular density, atrophic and coiling vessels, glomerular loop formations, and vascular Aβ deposits has been described in AD.[92–94] Aging animals and humans have also been found to exhibit more subtle alterations of arteriolar and capillary morphology. Such alterations are characterized by changes in connective tissue and smooth muscle,[95] thickening of the basement membrane,[96,97] thinning and loss of the endothelial cells,[98] an increase in endothelial pinocytotic vesicles,[99] loss of endothelial mitochondria,[100] and an increase in pericytes.[101,102] The laminar and regional distribution of these microvascular alterations typically correlates with the presence of neuropathological lesions (neurofibrillary tangles and Aβ deposits) suggesting a role for microvascular damage in AD pathology.[94,103,104] Various elements of the vascular basement membrane have all been found within senile plaques.[95,105–111] As we will discuss subsequently, evidence of microvascular disease in AD is also supported by epidemiological data and neuroimaging findings of subcortical and WMH. Numerous neuroimaging studies have shown decreased cerebral blood flow (CBF) to brain areas known to be affected in AD[112–114] and also CBF abnormalities in AD itself.[115–117] Structural imaging studies have also shown an increase in small vessel disease in AD.[118–122]

Contribution of Blood–Brain Barrier Dysfunction

Neurogenic regions close to cerebrospinal fluid (CSF), dentate gyrus, and subventricular zone support

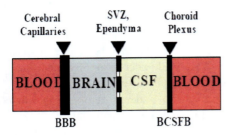

Fig. 15.1 Brain microvessels (BBB), a tight endothelial barrier, form interstitial fluid in the brain. Choroid plexus epithelium (BCSFB) also screens l0arge plasma solutes and secretes CSF. Macromolecules in CSF readily diffuse across the permeable ependyma into brain to exert trophic effects on neurons, and stem cells in SVZ. Regulated transport at all interfaces is disrupted in aging/disese

cognition but are vulnerable to oxidative/inflammatory damage, common late in life. Healthy synapses rely on regular vascular perfusion, sound microvascular function, and continuous bulk flow of interstitial fluid/CSF. Aging is accompanied by lower blood flow, breakdown of the blood–brain (BBB) and CSF barriers, and dwindling CSF circulation. Normal barrier interfaces in the CNS are depicted in Fig. 15.1. Sporadic AD is exacerbated by the failure of homeostatic transport interfaces in brain capillaries and choroid plexus epithelium. Preservation of cognition depends on stable brain fluid homeostasis. Given the presumed role of Aβ accumulation or clearance in AD pathogenesis, BBB disturbances may account for an association between vascular disease and AD. Clinical studies using the CSF/serum protein ratios have pointed to BBB disturbances in AD, with Aβ entering the brain passively via a leaky BBB,[84,123] and by active transport across the BBB.[124–133] The receptor for advanced glycation endproducts (RAGE) transports Aβ from the systemic circulation across the blood–brain barrier,[125] and it is transported out of the brain by low-density lipoprotein[126] and P-glycoprotein (P-gp).[132,133] Various neurotoxic responses occur during Aβ binding; nonenzymatic glycoxidation, proinflammatory cytokine-like mediators, and the DNA-binding protein, amphoterin.[134] Interactions between RAGE and glycation endproducts cause a major inflammatory response, and vascular injury, most notably in diabetes mellitus and renal failure.[106] RAGE expression is "upregulated" as Aβ concentrations increase,[106,107] and is found in AD brains in neurons, astrocytes, microglia, but most notably around Aβ plaques and neurofibrillary tangles. When Aβ binds to RAGE in extremely small concentrations, a cellular cascade occurs causing release of inflammatory cytokines.[106] RAGE is expressed in both endothelial and smooth muscle cells of blood vessels,[107] and Aβ in interaction with RAGE with suppresses CBF,[125] which can increase ischemia and cytotoxic damage in AD. Low-density lipoprotein receptors, involved in cholesterol and ApoE metabolism,[135] are also expressed in the endothelium of the cerebral microvasculature.[126] Taken as a whole, strong relationships exist among BBB, microvascular dysfunction, lipoprotein metabolism, proinflammatory responses, and neuropathology, providing a compelling rationale for this line of research.

Glucose- insulin metabolic and blood–brain-barrier disturbances in neurodegenerative disease are particularly interesting when examining the interface between vascular and neurodegenerative disease. Insulin and insulin-like growth factor expression impairments occur in AD and affect neural signaling mechanisms.[136–139] Reduced glucose utilization and deficient energy metabolism occur early in the course of disease, and suggest a role for impaired insulin signaling in the pathogenesis of AD.[140,141] These abnormalities are associated with reduced levels of insulin receptor substrate (IRS) mRNA, tau mRNA, IRS-associated phosphatidylinositol 3-kinase, and phospho-Akt (activated), and increased glycogen synthase kinase-3beta activity and amyloid precursor protein mRNA expression. The strikingly reduced CNS expression of genes encoding insulin, IGF-I, and IGF-II, and insulin and IGF receptors, suggests that AD may represent a neuroendocrine factor that resembles, yet is distinct from diabetes mellitus. This work is complemented by studies focusing intracellular accumulations of misfolded proteins with cytotoxicity to specialized cell types. These proteins create selective vulnerability of certain steps within key signaling, metabolic cycle control, and homeostatic pathways, and may contribute AD pathogenesis through amyloid toxicity within three essential homeostatic mechanisms: (1) the proteasome degradation machinery, (2) the insulin-PI3K/Akt responsive signaling pathway, and (3) mitochondrial function. The fact that diabetes, insulin, and lipid metabolism, and other related risk factors strongly underlie the development of both CVD and cerebrovascular disease provides another link between CVD and brain neurodegeneration.

Capillaries and Cerebral Arterioles Disruption in AD

We have found that thinning and discontinuities within the vascular basement membrane are associated with leakage of plasma protein across the BBB in AD.[142–144] Prothrombin was found in capillary walls, neuropil around microvessels in severe AD, with endothelial leakage of prothrombin greatest among patients with an APOE4 allele.[144] This work will be extended in future studies to lower molecular weight proteins to probe brain specimens from patients with prodromal AD. Other related ongoing research focuses on studying cortical arteriolar pathology at various Braak stages and APOE genotypes.[143] This study is revealing marked depletion of smooth muscle actin coincident with buildup of vascular Aβ with a strong association between progressively accumulating arteriolar amyloid and augmentations in both wall thickness and lumen width. Our working model is that progressing amyloid angiopathy harms the contractile apparatus and thus the CBF autoregulation.[379] This likely devastates downstream capillaries.[354] Our observations lend further support to the idea that microvascular damage has a role, perhaps relatively early, brain neurodegenerative pathology.

CVD-Associated Neurocognitive and Brain Dysfunction

There is now considerable evidence that many elderly people with CVD experience cognitive problems. While young people with minimal coronary artery disease are unlikely to experience significant cognitive problems, the elderly are vulnerable to impairments, particularly in the context of severe and chronic CVD. There is now a plethora of clinical evidence that many people with severe CVD experience cognitive problems and that various etiological factors affect brain function, including hypertension, reduced cardiac output, and heart failure.[7,9,12,15,16,23,25–28,36,40,145–177] Probably, the largest body of literature has focused on adverse neurocognitive outcome associated with cardiothoracic surgery, in particular coronary artery bypass graph (CABG), and valve replacement surgery.[178–184]

The most well-established and robust links between CVD and brain function occur among patients with heart failure.[185–190] Severe brain damage is common among people who survive cardiac arrest.[172,177,191] However, milder brain dysfunction also occurs among people with chronic severe CVD, who have not experienced complete cessation of CBF. Typically, attention-executive functioning and speed of processing are most affected in people with CVD,[192,193] though as discussed later memory and other cognitive functions decline as well.

In an effort to better understand the relationship between the vascular and metabolic disturbances associated with CVD and neurocognitive dysfunction, we have conducted several prospective studies different cohorts of CVD patients. Our initial studies focused on patients enrolled in cardiac rehabilitation (CR) who were attempting to modify maladaptive behaviors and their lifestyle in an effort to prevent worsening of their CVD. The CR patients had weaker cognitive performance compared to a healthy control group.[28,147] Over 20% of patients over age 70 had MMSE scores suggestive of possible dementia. CR patients exhibited weaker performance on attention/executive and learning indices (WRMT, Digit Symbol, verbal fluency (COWAT), with the COWAT being the best discriminator of CR from non-CR participants.[193] CR patients showed improvements on Trail Making and Digit Symbol Coding after completion of CR (Trail ($p = 0.02$) compared to patients not in CR. Both hypertension and impaired ventricular ejection fraction (EF) were associated with cognitive impairments in CR patients.[28,147] These findings suggested that some CVD patients without evidence of overt functional decline were still experiencing cognitive difficulties, perhaps due to subtle cerebrovascular pathology.

Studies by our group and others provide compelling evidence that poor functional outcome among elderly CVD patients is partly attributable to cognitive problems.[13–27] Accordingly, we examined the relationship between baseline cognitive performance and health satisfaction/QOL pre- and post-CR.[28] Prior to CR patients had poor overall rating on both physical (PCS) and mental health (MCS) indices of the SF-36, a measure of health status, compared people without CVD. Cognitive performance was strongly associated with both baseline health status and change. Patients with greater cognitive impairment (Digit Symbol, Verbal Fluency, Similarities, and RMT) showed less improvement from CR. There are various reasons that brain dysfunction and cognitive problems would affect QOL in people with CVD.[194–212] In modern society, intact cognition is increasingly important for mastery of various instrumental activities of daily living.[213–221] Cognitive ability also proves to be an important determinant of self-esteem related to mastery in one's environment, and ultimately emotional experience.[222–224] Furthermore, cognitive impairment is directly linked to overall health status, as brain disturbances often reflect broader physical problems. Neurocognitive dysfunction also limits ability for effective self-care,[28,222–224] interfering with people's ability to learn and modify behavior and lifestyle.

The results from this initial CR study motivated larger prospective longitudinal studies of CVD-associated brain dysfunction that have provided much of the neurocognitive and neuroimaging data that serve as the basis for our discussion in this chapter. In the first of these longitudinal studies, we followed 186 people with chronic CVD (mean age = 69.2 ± 7.6 years) for 36-months. Baseline analyses of data from the R01-AG179751 cohort have indicated mild deficits of psychomotor and information processing speed and efficiency (e.g., Grooved Pegboard, Digit Symbol Coding), and recall and learning efficiency.[192,193] The need for additional studies of systemic vascular influences on brain function was reinforced.

In a subsequent study, we focused of the effects of reduced systemic perfusion associated with heart failure.[225] People with heart failure performed worse than people with mild CVD and no heart failure on measures of executive functioning and psychomotor speed. Lower ejection fraction was associated with weaker global cognition, performance on measures of executive functioning, immediate memory, and to a lesser extent delayed memory, suggesting that reduced systemic perfusion is associated with cognitive deficits with severe CVD and failing heart function. As a follow-up to our investigation of heart failure, we examined the effects of ventricular stimulation aimed at increasing systemic perfusion.[226] Patients with heart failure exhibited improvements in quality of life and also cognitive function that were associated with improvements in cardiac function. These findings suggest that systemic perfusion is important to insure functional capacity and that enhancing perfusion improves functioning, illustrating the potential value of focusing on preserving and improving cardiac function in the elderly. To clarify the causal nature of the suggested mechanism, studies simultaneously examining cardiac function, cerebral perfusion, and cognition are necessary.

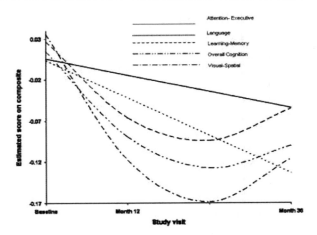

Fig. 15.2 Neurocognitive decline over 36 months among patients with chronic CVD[227]. Significant worsening of performance was evident particularly with respect to learning and memory, visuospatial, and overall cognitive functioning

Cognitive Change Over Time in CVD

We examined the degree to which people with severe CVD from this same cohort experienced cognitive decline over 36-months. CVD patients exhibited significant declines across cognitive domains, including overall cognitive function.[227] As shown in the figure, participants tended to improve between 12-months and 36-months of baseline, though this was attributable to improvements among some heart failure patients due to ventricular stimulation therapy (Fig. 15.2).

Vascular and Metabolic Contributions

A number of specific vascular and metabolic risk factors are known to be associated with the development of brain dysfunction and cognitive impairment among people without identified CVD, including *dislipidemia*[228–243] and hypertension,[244–252] with increasing prevalence with age occurring in greater than 85% of elderly CVD patients. Evidence of reduced cognitive function in community samples of people with chronic HTN has been described in a number of past studies of people without actual large vessel stroke.[253–255]

HTN prevalence increases among people over the age of 70 results occurring in greater than 85% of elderly CVD patients. Chronic HTN induces small vessel stiffening due to progressive replacement of media by collagen (hyalinization) and altered permeability to circulating proteins and fibrinoid changes,[40,146,153,159,256,257] which makes it an important systemic vascular factor. Spikes in systolic pressure and blood pressure variability can contribute to hypoperfusion, fluid exudation, and increased water content in subcortical regions, as seen as hyperintensities on T-2 weighted MRI. HTN causes cerebral microvascular damage and hypoperfusion and reflects cerebrovascular dysregulation.[258,259] As it is also among vascular factors associated with diminished neurocognitive performance in the elderly, HTN remains an important predictor of age-associated functional outcome in CVD.[15,145–148,151,154–158]

Diabetes/Insulin resistance,[148,260–284] which increases stroke risk,[148,260–270] and contributes to endothelial dysfunction, impaired vessel distensibility, and hemodynamic dysregulation,[271–284] and may affect cognition due to direct metabolic effects on neuronal function,[281,285–307] *as well as contribute to* neurodegenerative disease.[281,283,284,286,287,294,308–314] *Obesity*. Obesity increases risk of CVD and stroke.[315–317] Studies have linked obesity with reduced cognitive performance, even among people without other significant comorbidity.[318–326] These risk factors often coexist in certain people and in combination constitute "*metabolic syndrome*", *which involves* nonalcohol-related fatty liver. Approximately 25% of adults meets the clinical criteria for metabolic syndrome,[327–329] including about 44% of people over 55 years of age.[329] It has been strongly implicated as underlying the development of diabetes mellitus, heart disease, and stroke. There is growing consensus that metabolic syndrome is a major public health issue, reflected by the WHO and AHA (http://www.americanheart.org) and NHLBI (http://www.nhlbi.nih.gov) classification.[329–333] People with vascular-metabolic risk factors experience subtle cerebrovascular abnormalities that affect neurocognitive functioning even when there has been no history of prior stroke.[334–337] Neuroimaging approaches to the study of metabolic syndrome are reviewed elsewhere in the book (see Chap. 14).

Cerebral Hypoperfusion as a Basis for CVD-Associated Brain Dysfunction

The brain requires a constant supply of blood to sustain neural function with rapid cellular glucose metabolism changes to <10% within a minute of cessation, resulting in a cascade of metabolic events (e.g., entry of extracellular water, calcium and sodium into neurons).[338–340] Loss of hemodynamic autoregulation, ion channel failure and impaired neuronal response occur within seconds. Chronic cerebral hypoperfusion eventually affects brain functioning, particularly as people reach advanced age.[16,160,189,341–359] Maintaining normal cerebrovascular function requires relatively intact systemic hemodynamic function.[360] There is mounting evidence that metabolic factors including hyperlipidemia and insulin resistance contribute to endothelial dysfunction, atherosclerotic burden, and hemodynamic dysregulation, resulting in decreased regional CBF (rCBF) as people age.[288,361–373] This in turn causes cumulative subacute brain abnormalities, including microvascular disturbance resulting in brain lesions, even in the absence of acute stroke.[288,372,374,375] Cerebral hypoperfusion has been identified as an etiological factor in VaD,[341] though it remains not fully understood. Microvascular changes due to chronic hypoperfusion tend to go undetected, making this an important area of study among people "at risk". The ability to compensate for changes in CBF is a critical determinant of whether brain dysfunction occurs.[360] Cardiac disease was once thought to have little bearing on brain function because of cerebral hemodynamic autoregulation and the efficiency of collateral circulation.[376–378] This is largely true for young relative healthy adults, though with advanced age and the co-occurrence of systemic vascular disease, these autoregulatory processes breakdown, and the brain cannot compensate for hypoperfusion. Cerebral vessels lose their hemodynamic reactivity and autoregulation ability as endothelial function breaks down[360] due to aging and vascular disease.[14,37,379–384] Flow-mediated brachial artery response has been studied extensively as a measure of systemic endothelial and hemodynamic function.[385–389] Impaired systemic response has been found to relate to cerebrovascular dysfunction,[390,391] stroke risk and microvascular disease.[392–404] It has been shown by our group to be associated with cognitive function and WMH on MRI.[405,406] Vascular thickening and stiffening, results in a loss of distensibility (i.e., vessel elasticity), which reduces baroreceptor response and hemodynamic autoregulation, as vessels lose adaptability to change in blood pressure, flow and oxygen supply.[399,407–410]

Systemic Vascular Contributions

The effects of impaired cardiac output on brain function are not ubiquitous. Some patients with heart failure continue to function well despite reduced cardiac function, while others have major cognitive problems. This seems to depend on whether cerebral hypoperfusion results from reduced cardiac output in a particular patient, which in turn depends on the ability of the cerebrovascular system to compensate for perfusion changes.[360] Cardiac disease was once thought to have little bearing on brain function because of cerebral hemodynamic autoregulation and the efficiency of collateral circulation.[376–378] This is largely true for young relative healthy adults, though with advanced age and the co-occurrence of systemic vascular disease, these autoregulatory processes breakdown, and the brain cannot compensate for hypoperfusion.

Cardiac Output

Cerebral perfusion ultimately depends on the heart's pumping capacity much cardiac output and.[411–417] Left ventricular Ejection Fraction (EF) is the most widely used clinical measure of pumping efficiency, with EF <40% being clinically significant.[2,418–421] Cardiac output can also be measured and reflects the actual volume of blood expelled by the heart.[419,422] The Framingham Study data shows dramatic increases in heart failure in the elderly. Whereas only 1–2 new heart failure cases per 1,000 occur in adults under age 54 years, 13–14 cases per 100 occur among those 75–84 years, with a fourfold to sixfold increase in those over 85 years.[412–416,423] This has enormous implications, contributing to morbidity and mortality in the elderly. Exercise intolerance is compounded by the natural muscle atrophy (sarcopenia) and weakening with normal aging, resulting in a vicious cycle of infirmity exacerbating a cascade of deconditioning as measured by functional indices such as VO2 peak and 6 min walk distance and eventual mortality. Reduced EF and cardiac output both relate to cognitive impairment.[160,162] Our preliminary data points to the importance of reduced cardiac output in CVD-associated cognitive impairment, but additional research is needed to better understand this effect.

Cerebral Hemodynamic Autoregulatory Failure

The adverse effects reduced cardiac output do not occur in isolation in most CVD patients. Furthermore, not all people with heart failure experience cerebrovascular disturbance. Chronically reduced cardiac output is likely to have its greatest impact when in occurs in the context of impaired cerebral hemodynamic function. Impaired vascular reactivity and cerebral hemodynamic dysregulation has been related to cerebrovascular dysfunction.[390,391] Two factors appear to be particularly important in this regard: (1) endothelial function and (2) atherosclerotic burden. As endothelial function becomes impaired, cerebral vessels lose their ability to react to hemodynamic changes.[360] The biochemical bases of these effects are quite complex and beyond the scope of the current discussion. However, the critical issue is that many of the factors that contribute to CVD and HF also contribute to systemic endothelial dysfunction. Atherosclerotic burden appears to be very important in this regard, affecting both characteristics of vascular smooth muscle and also contributing to reduced luminal diameter.

Vascular Burden

Atherosclerosis causes narrowing of coronary, systemic, and cerebral blood vessels, including the cerebral arteries, leading to thrombosis and occlusion of large vessels, and structural changes of penetrating arteries and arterioles that branch from these large vessels (arteriosclerosis).[392–404] Atheromatous deposits in the subintima may affect the small vessels, with lipohyalinosis when both arterial and arteriolar processes occur in arteriosclerosis, with altered membrane permeability. A vicious cycle develops in the elderly, as hypertension caused in part by increased peripheral resistance causes damage to the arterial walls with an increase in quantities of collagen and a decrease in elastin, which in turn leads to vessel hypertrophy, with associated thickening and stiffening. Vascular stiffening contributes to altered baroreceptor response and impaired autoregulation in the elderly, making the cerebral vasculature less able to adapt to changes in blood pressure, blood flow, and oxygen supply.[399,407–410] Subcortical structures, such as the basal ganglia and deep subcortical and periventricular white matter, are very vulnerable to the effects of arteriolosclerosis due to poor collateral blood supply, whereas the subcortical U fibers, the corpus callosum, and cortical structures are usually spared. Small vessel narrowing can cause chronic hypoperfusion leading to demyelination, gliosis, and softening of the white matter. Advancing age, chronic hypertension, past cerebral ischemic events, and diabetes mellitus are major risk factors for these changes, which ultimately cause hypoperfusion and probably contribute to cognitive changes. Accordingly, in our studies of CVD effects on brain function, we have typically measured carotid intimal thickness and stiffness to provide indices of the degree of vascular burden associated with atherosclerosis and systemic vascular disease.[399,409,410]

Endothelial Disturbance

Vascular endothelial function become impaired with aging and CVD.[14,37,379-384] The ability of the endothelium to react to hemodynamic changes and reduced cardiac output is essential to the maintenance of CBF and brain functions.[37,383,384] Such reactivity is dependent of the integrity of autoregulatory mechanisms. Hemodynamic dysregulation increases with age[417,424-428] and with it the ability to compensate for perfusion variability. Cerebral vasoreactivity is difficult to directly measure in clinical situations, in large part because anatomic (e.g., skull) and physiological constraints. Flow-mediated brachial artery response has been studied extensively as measure of endothelial responsivity.[385-389] It is robust and relatively easy to measure reliably. It will be used in this project as a proxy of cerebrovascular vessel reactivity, and impairment of autoregulation (Fig. 15.3).

Systemic Vascular Measurement

Given these considerations, there are compelling reasons for assessing the degree of systemic vascular impairment when trying to determine the likelihood of associated brain dysfunction. We have focused our investigations on four vascular measures: (1) Cardiac output, (2) Blood pressure, (3) Vascular burden, and (4) Endothelial function when examining the systemic vascular precursors of cerebrovascular disease in CVD patients. Fortunately, reliable and valid noninvasive methods exist for assessing each of these factors, including (a) cardiac output for assessing heart function/perfusion, (b) Flow-mediated

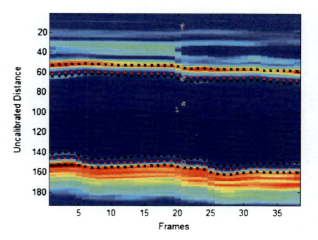

Fig. 15.3 Digitized carotid ultrasound of the type used to measure the thickness of the carotid intima media. (IMT). This method enables multiple measurements to be recorded from a small section of the carotid artery and is able to produce extremely reliable IMT measures

brachial artery reactivity (BAR) for measuring endothelial and smooth muscle functioning, (c) Carotid intima media thickness (IMT) and stiffness for assessing vascular atherosclerotic burden and also endothelial damage, and (d) blood pressure variability, which provides a measure of systolic and diastolic tone. An illustration of the method for IMT measurement is shown in the adjacent figure. These approaches are interest to our discussion of neuroimaging as they illustrate parallel methods for measuring systemic function that can be used to examine relationships of systemic and cerebrovascular abnormalities. They are not direct measures of cerebral perfusion or hemodynamic state, but rather serve as potential proxy measures. In the case of IMT, carotid ultrasound is used to characterize differences in the structural characteristics of the artery and to differentiate the intima media. Thickening of this vessel membrane is linked to atherosclerotic load and a breakdown of endothelial function, which in turn points to greater risk of hemodynamic failure. Our research has focused on examining the relationship between these measures of systemic vascular dysfunction and functional and structural brain imaging indices that provide more direct measures of evolving cerebrovascular disease, such as cerebral perfusion as measured by arterial spin labeling (ASL) with MRI and early structural brain changes, including WMH on FLAIR MRI imaging and diffusion tensor imaging (DTI), which are discussed later (Fig. 15.4).

Task	IMT (mm)	Systolic Variance	BAR (Δ)	CO (l/min)	Diastolic Variance
Executive Index	−0.34[***]	0.19[*]	0.19[*]	0.13[#]	0.07
COWAT	−0.20[*]	−0.06	0.28[**]	−0.19[**]	−0.06
Digit Span	−0.26[***]	−0.04	0.21[*]	0.04	0.05
GPB	0.23[**]	0.10	−0.12	0.06	0.09
Cancellation	0.33[***]	0.15[*]	−0.18[*]	−0.15[*]	0.02
Stroop Test	−0.29[**]	−0.16[*]	0.25[**]	−0.09	0.06
Coding	−0.31[***]	−0.12[#]	0.17[*]	−0.12[#]	−0.09
Trails A	0.14[#]	0.14[*]	0.04	0.07	0.07
Trails B	0.32[***]	0.16[*]	0.06	0.10	−0.03
Language Index	0.08	0.03	0.08	0.02	0.01
Memory Index	0.10	0.11	0.05	0.10	0.07
Total WMH	−0.63**	0.22	−0.22	0.01	−0.15
WMH/WBV	−0.49**	0.28#	.26[*]	0.01	−0.14
WBV	0.26	−0.29[*]	−0.35[**]	−0.32[*]	−0.23[#]

Fig. 15.4 Relationships between systemic vascular measures, neurocognitive, and MRI white matter hypertenstities (WMH) as found by Cohen et al. Strong associations between

Systemic Vascular and Neurocognitive Function

As part of R01-AG179751 we examined how four systemic vascular indices at baseline relate to baseline cognitive functioning and also change in functioning over 36 months. These results have been published in a series of papers published over the past 6 years.[59,193,318,319,405,429–439] Findings have been ubiquitous as each of the individual indices has been found to be significantly associated with both cognitive function and the structural MRI measure of WMH (Significant effects bolded in above table). Cardiac output (CO) related strongly to attention performance (CPT, Go-No-Go) and also other executive functions.[440] Carotid IMT related to attention/executive measures (particularly processing speed) and WMH.[441] Systolic variability proved to be a positive indicator with greater variability associated with stronger cognitive performance,[442] an effect that we believe reflects healthy endothelial function and vasoreactivity in people with greater variability. IMT emerged as the strongest correlates of cognitive performance. Vascular function indices also were associated with WMH volume when examined simultaneously in hierarchical regression analysis. These two factors were retained in regression analyses suggesting that both systemic vascular function

(Factor 2) and cardiac function (Factor 1) are associated with cognitive performance. Patients with both factors elevated had the most baseline cognitive impairments and WMH.

We also examined the relationship of baseline vascular function to change in cognitive function for patients with IMT and cardiac output data who completed the 36-month assessment ($n = 125$). An executive function index (Composite Z-score) was created, and change scores were generated by subtracting the index at baseline from the index at 36-months. We found a striking relationship between baseline vascular function and executive performance change over 36-months ($R = 0.63$, $p < 0.001$).

Cytokines and Inflammatory Processes[431,435,436,443]

The relationship between cognitive function and specific inflammatory and neuronal markers were studied in our CVD cohort from R01-AG179751. Both C-reactive protein (CRP) and homocysteine were significantly correlated with cognitive performance across multiple measures ($r > 0.40$). CRP was consistently retained as the stronger predictor of the attention-executive-psychomotor ($R^2 = 0.56$, $p < 0.001$), visual-spatial ($R^2 = 0.62$, $p < 0.001$), and memory ($R^2 = 0.42$, $p < 0.01$) performance (composite indices). Patients in the highest and lowest 25th percentile of CRP levels (Low, 0.4 ± 0.1; High, 4.6 ± 1.2) were compared, and elevated CRP was associated with weaker cognitive performance. We next examined the relationship between CRP, WMH and DTI-FA in 12 participants who completed a pilot DTI study. Higher levels of CRP were strongly associated with WMH volume ($r = 0.45$) and reduced FA ($r = 0.52$). We found that brain natriuretic peptide (BNP), brain-derived neurotopic factor (BDNF), and SELP are also associated with cognitive status as well. To obtain preliminary data for the proposed study, we examined whether plasma levels of the three cytokines differed among people with CVD+ MCI. Though not powered to detect small effects, the study suggested that people with CVD+ MCI had elevated mean levels of CRP ($p = 0.09$), BDNF ($p = 0.10$), and TNF-α ($p = 0.11$), with all of these differences in the expected direction and approaching significance. Notably, both CRP ($r = 0.65$) and BDNF ($r = 0.58$) were significantly associated with DLPFC signal intensity ($p < 0.05$), indicating a robust effect in this small sample, providing strong for support for the proposed study hypotheses. Such findings motivate further prospective studies of the role of proinflammatory processes in vascular pathophysiology and brain dysfunction.

Summary and Conceptual Model

Several possible mechanisms may account for the CVD effects on abnormal brain aging that we and other researchers have previously observed.[192,193,225,226,405,406,431,4 37,442-458] Given that these Changes in cerebral hemodynamic homeostasis can occur secondary to perturbations in cardiac function,[459-461] despite autoregulatory mechanisms which normally preserve CBF during systemic hypoperfusion.[462,463] As depicted in the adjacent flow chart, we hypothesize that systemic vascular factors, including reduced cardiac output, increased atherosclerotic burden and endothelial dysfunction interact to alter hemodynamic of the brain, creating a direct pathway of injury between CVD and maladaptive brain aging. These cerebral hemodynamic effects are exacerbated by several complex systemic metabolic mechanisms associated with both CVD and abnormal brain aging, including inflammation,[464-467] and abnormal insulin and glucose metabolism,[468] with these factors impacting brain function in its own right, by causing neurotoxicity and neuronal damage, in addition to affecting cerebral hemodynamic function.[469-473] These systemic factors probably mediate associations between CVD, maladaptive, brain aging, and cognitive decline. Furthermore, these risk factors are strongly associated with systemic vascular dysfunction. In the aging brain, metabolic and vascular disease may interact to affect BBB function[474] and other associated neuropathological processes that contribute to the development of VCI. The neuroimaging approaches discussed in the remainder of this chapter are methods for dissociating the neuropathological processes contributing to CVD-associated brain dysfunction that may provide biomarkers of neurodegenerative brain disease (Fig. 15.5).

Neuroimaging CVD-Associated Brain Dysfunction

A number of neuroimaging methods now exist that can be used for the study and assessment of CVD-associated brain dysfunction. Current neuroimaging approaches are largely based on radiological, magnetic resonance (MR), ultrasound, and electrophysiological techniques. Our focus in this chapter is largely on MR-based techniques, though there is some discussion of radiological methods for assessing CBF and also ultrasound methods for measuring emboli in the context of coronary surgery. Radiological techniques, include CT, single photon emission computed tomography

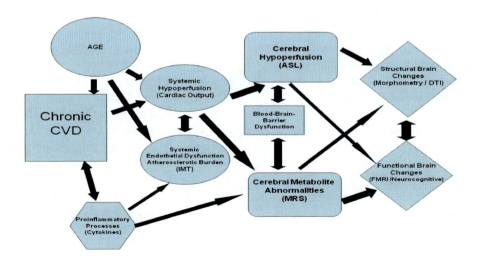

Fig. 15.5 Mechanisms of CVD-associated brain dysfunction. The pathophysiological mechanisms by which chronic CVD affects the brain and neurocognitive functioning are depicted. The resulting cerebral metabolic and hemodynamic disturbances are measurable by neuroimaging methods such as magnetic resonance spectroscopy and arterial spin labeling, while the effects of CVD on brain function and structure can also be assessed by FMRI and morphometric-lesion analysis methods

(SPECT), and positron emission tomography (PET). MR methods include: noninvasive structural imaging methods (e.g., T1, T2, FLAIR), diffusion-weighted imaging (DWI), perfusion-weighted imaging (PWI), functional imaging (FMRI), and magnetic resonance spectroscopy (MRS). Most of these methods are discussed in Part 1 of the book.

Each of these neuroimaging approaches has value and certain advantages over others. For example, EEG and related electrophysiological methods provide measures of the brain's electrical activity and has excellent temporal resolution, while ultrasound methods are useful because they are relatively easy to perform and non-invasive. However, each of these methods tends to yield only a single type of information and some limitations with respect to what can be learned from them. Radiological measures are very useful and powerful in a number in a number of respects. For example, PET provides a gold-standard for measuring cerebral perfusion. However, the use of these methods are somewhat constrained by cost, feasibility, other logistical, as well as the fact that radiation can be harmful with repeated exposure. Our research has largely employed MRI methods for the studies of VCI, CVD, and AD. The rationale for the use of MRI is that most techniques are noninvasive and very feasible to obtain, and extremely powerful in terms of the information that is yielded. MRI lends itself well to multimodal imaging, such that in a single scanning session it is possible to obtain structural anatomic data, information about cerebral perfusion and tissue diffusion, metabolic indices, and functional measures. The ability to obtain both functional and structural data that has high spatial and temporal resolution makes these approaches very compelling. The fact that coregistration of functional and other physiological measures with structural anatomic atlases also facilitates interpretation of MR-based results. Some of our findings from investigations employing MRI methods, as well as radiological and ultrasound, provide examples of methodological approaches to neuroimaging in CVD in the discussion that follows.

Current Routine Clinical Neuroimaging in CVD

In acute care settings, the imaging approaches that are routinely employed for assessing possible CVD-associated brain dysfunction tend to be driven by current stroke center protocols.[475,476] When a cardioembolic stroke is suspected, cranial CT is usually obtained to determine the need for intervention, such as anti-thrombolytic therapy. This typically occurs in the emergency room or in the context of cardiothoracic surgery if there is some sign of an embolic event. The most routine procedure involves non-invasive CT for purposes of detecting evidence of infarction, though increasingly diffusion CT is also performed. These CT methods are discussed in Chap. 18 in greater detail and will not be reviewed here. However, it is important to note that most of the CT based methods used in the first line of acute stroke evaluation can be performed using MRI also, typically with greater spatial resolution and sensitivity. The primary reason that MRI is not used as the initial imaging method for detecting acute stroke in stroke center protocols is that it is not universally available and cannot be used for patients with metal implants. Nonetheless, for research purposes, MRI is generally more powerful.

Structural Brain Abnormalities in CVD

The most basic clinical question for outpatients with CVD is whether there is evidence of infarction indicative of embolic stroke or other cerebrovascular event. If there is no evidence of an acute stroke or in people where a stroke is known to have occurred at some time in the past (greater than 2 weeks ago), evidence of cerebral infarction can generally be obtained through analysis of standard T1, T2 and FLAIR images. During the subacute period (2 days to 2 weeks), low signal on T1 (hypointensity) and high signal on T2-weighted and FLAIR images (hyperintensity) is evident, indicating infarction, that follows the vascular distribution. Revascularization and blood–brain barrier breakdown may cause parenchymal enhancement with contrast agents. After several weeks, the infarction is still evident on T1, T2, and FLAIR, but there is also tissue loss with large infarctions. However, mass effects disappear and enhancement of the parenchyma fades.

In addition to the infarction in cortical areas supplied by the vascular distribution, white matter damage is also typically evident. This presents on MRI as hyperintensities along white matter tracks. There may evidence of loss of white matter, observed as reduced white matter volume. In cases, where a large vessel stroke has occurred secondary to CVD (e.g., middle cerebral artery), functional impairments are often dramatic and the cerebral infarction is the dominant finding. However, many CVD patients do not experience large vessel infarction yet show evidence of cerebrovascular disturbance and brain dysfunction. The basis of this disturbance is not well understood, and is in fact the focus of much of our research, as well as this chapter. However, two general mechanisms are likely to play a role: (1) chronic cerebral hypoperfusion and (2) microvascular infarctions. The second of these mechanisms has received the most research attention, as described below.

White Matter Damage Secondary to Microvascular Disease

Among people with chronic CVD, cerebral microvascular disease is often present even there is no other evidence of prior stroke or clinical evident cerebrovascular disease.[406,477] In fact, WMH on MRI have been associated with hypertension and other vascular risk factors.[478–482] WMH volume tends to increase with age, though this may in part reflect greater vascular disease in the elderly.[430]

Our initial work focused on white matter abnormalities in VaD, using T1 and FLAIR imaging to measure WMH volume. The rationale for these studies was that VaD is thought in occur as a function of microvascular disease among people without large vessel infarction.[483,484] Strong associations were found between WMH volume and cognitive functioning, specifically with psychomotor and information processing speed, executive functioning and learning efficiency.[32,53,406,485] Similar findings were observed among patients with milder VCI, with WMH associated with impairments on symbol digit coding, Stroop, Grooved Pegboard, and CVLT learning performance. However, among patients with VaD, cortical volume was actually much more strongly associated with memory, overall cognitive impairment, and dementia severity (DRS) than was white matter volume, raising the possibility that white matter damage is not the only factor driving cognitive impairments. Given these findings, we shifted focus to on earlier stages of vascular disease, to better understand the basis for cognitive decline and these brain abnormalities (Fig. 15.6).

Our findings in the CVD cohort paralleled those from VCI. WMH volume was associated with psychomotor and information processing speed, executive functioning, and learning efficiency.[192,456] The figure (left) shows the method of quantification of WMH from three regions (periventricular, subcortical, and deep white matter (i.e., corona radiata/cortical white matter). All three regions were associated with performance on attention and psychomotor measures, but not on other cognitive domains. This finding suggests that WMH may not be the only neuroimaging indicator of the CVD-associated cognitive disturbance.

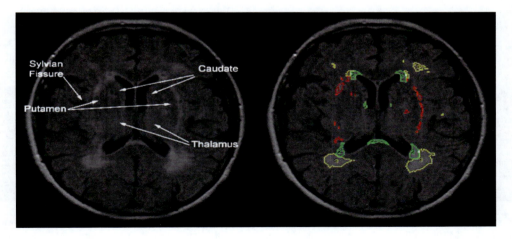

Fig. 15.6 White matter hyperintensities (WMH) as often observed on MRI using a FLAIR protocol. Areas of significant periventricular and deep subcortical WMH have been manually traced

Vascular Function and WMH

In studies that parallel those described earlier on the relationship between systemic vascular function and cognitive impairment in CVD, we also examined whether vascular function to WMH volume. Regression analyses have revealed highly significant associations between the four systemic vascular indices and WMH. Carotid IMT was most strongly associated with WMH ($p<0.01$), suggesting the influence of atherosclerotic burden and reduced vascular distensibility (i.e., inelasticity of vessels) on the development microvascular-associated brain changes.

Altered Functional Brain Response in CVD (FMRI)

A major focus of our current research is change in functional brain response among people with CVD and other neurological disorders. We have over 15 FMRI publications stemming from these efforts to date. We plan to use mean signal intensity data from two FMRI tasks as primary dependent measures of function change: 2-back and continuous visual memory test (CVMT). The 2-back is a widely used FMRI working memory paradigm. The CVMT is an excellent paradigm for examining memory encoding and recognition. Findings of relevance to the current proposal are outlined below (Fig. 15.7).

Identification of 2-Back-Related Networks and ROIs

We have conducted several FMRI studies of attentional/executive networks that demonstrate our capability to examine the BOLD response to the cognitive challenges that we have proposed.[162,163,177–187] These have enabled us to identify relevant brain ROIs for this study. In a series of experiments using the *n*-Back paradigm we have identified an attentional/executive network, including bilateral dorsolateral prefrontal cortex (DLPFC), posterior parietal cortices (PPC), and supplementary motor area (SMA), that is reliably associated with the task across a wide variety of samples, including older adults,[162,163,180,181] cigarette smokers,[187] and Multiple Sclerosis (MS),[177,178] Alzheimer's Disease (AD), and CVD[180–182] (Groups ordered this way in figure). These results demonstrate our ability to obtain consistent, reliable, and valid data from different clinical populations. Among healthy adults and CVD patients, altered response of frontal and parietal regions, and the SMA are associated with successful performance of other tasks requiring high attentional demands and cognitive processing speed.

Aging, CVD, and BOLD

We have examined age effects on the BOLD response to cognitive challenges.[162,163,180] Adults (age >55) had greater activity (signal intensity) in expected regions during the least difficult *n*-Back level (i.e., 1-Back) compared to younger adults (mean age 28). Brain recruitment (volume) in these ROIs was inversely related to age, with increased activation on the least difficult 1-Back condition, and an inverse relationship between BOLD signal intensity and age. These results indicated that age × brain activation effects were more complex than simply underactivation or compensatory overactivation.

We next examined age effects among 15 CVD patients with MCI patients (based on clinical history) The patterns of activation observed on the 2-back were similar to that observed in healthy controls, though

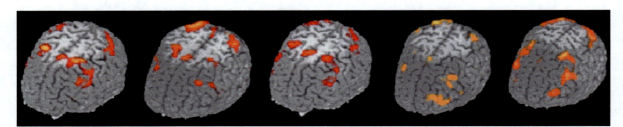

Fig. 15.7 Cortical activation to a 2-back FMRI task of the type used to show abnormalities in functional brain response during verbal working memory among patients CVD, and its relationship to systemic vascular disturbances. Activation is evident across brain ROIs typically involved in working memory including the inferior parietal cortex, dorsolateral prefrontal cortex, and supplementary motor area

people with CVD and MCI exhibited reduced task-associated activity in expected ROIs (DLPFC and PPC) and lower test scores.[31] This preliminary study suggested that less brain activity was associated with worse performance among older people with severe CVD who were experiencing MCI. No compensatory activity was observed.

BOLD Response Alterations in CVD

In order to examine potential impact of vascular health upon brain function during the 2-Back task, we compared CVD patients in good vascular health ($n=10$) to those in poor vascular health ($n=9$) defined by $CO > 0.495$.[181] Those with mild cardiac disease exhibited greater activity in previously observed task-related ROIs (DLPFC, SMA, and PPC bilaterally) and significantly better task performance. A smaller subsample ($n=8$) also performed the SS task. Moderate to severe CVD patients exhibited less DLPFC and PPC activation than healthy control participants ($p<0.05$). CVD patients also had significant activity in unexpected areas (medial and inferior frontal cortices). These results support our hypotheses that vascular health will be positively related to BOLD signal (in expected ROIs) and cognitive performance, and that severe CVD patients will exhibit large alterations in BOLD FMRI signal. These initial findings are promising, but more studies are needed to examine these and links between systemic perfusion, cerebral hypoperfusion, and impaired functional brain response (Figs. 15.8).

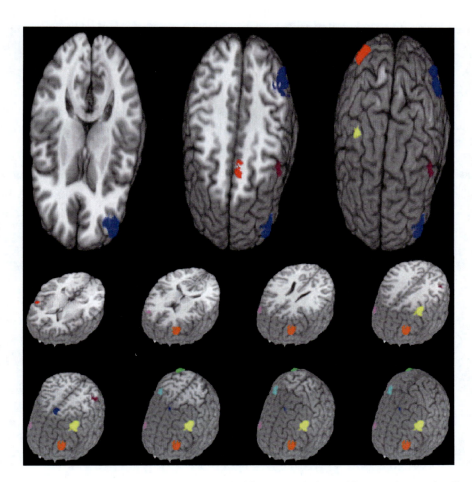

Fig. 15.8 Cortical regions (middle frontal gyrus) showing significant associations with systemic vascular disturbance (IMT) among patients with CVD

Functional Brain Response is Influenced by Systemic Vascular Factors

In a recent series of studies conducted with participants from our two CVD cohorts (RO1-AG179751; HL084178), we examined the relationship of specific systemic vascular indices to functional response on the 2-back. The results were quite striking. Both cardiac output and IMT (a measure of atherosclerotic burden and vascular thickening) were found to be associated with the intensity of activation within the working memory network. IMT was most strongly associated with the intensity of activation in the middle frontal gyrus ($r = -0.71$, $p < 0.05$), with greater vessel thickening (i.e., greater atherosclerotic burden) tied to reduced response on the 2-back compared to the 0-back task.[449] Cardiac output was found to be associated with activation in three brain regions (Insula, SMA, DLPFC; $p < 0.01$). As hypothesized, reduced cardiac output was associated with reduced BOLD response (Fig. 15.9).[404]

Functional imaging of Risk for Vascular Disease

In search of an early marker that may identify individuals predisposed to developing cognitive difficulties, we employed FMRI to test for differences in hemodynamic response to a working memory challenge based on family history of hypertension (HTN).[486] Healthy adults (ages 18–40 years) were assessed on the 2-back paradigm, with half having a positive family HTN, but without HTN themselves. People with HTN family history had reduced 2-Back-related activation in the right inferior parietal lobule and temporal gyrus, and more posterior cingulate deactivation. The results indicate that family history of HTN is associated with subtle changes in brain response to working memory in otherwise healthy adults, suggesting a possible phenotypic effect.

We subsequently piloted FMRI response on the 2-back with several other "at-risk" cohorts, obese, metabolic syndrome, and diabetic adults. Eight adults with metabolic syndrome (ATP-III criteria), and risk factors including insulin resistance, hyperlipidemia, obesity, and HTN were compared to eight age-matched healthy controls on the systemic vascular, ASL, FMRI, cytokine, and cognitive measures proposed for the current project. The metabolic syndrome group exhibited increased mean signal intensity and volume of activation cortex in the DLPFC and SMA, suggesting inefficiencies in their brain response.

Temporal Dynamics of Cortical Recruitment During Working Memory

Our 2-back studies have increasingly focused on differences in the volume of brain activation over time. Young healthy adults show increases in activation

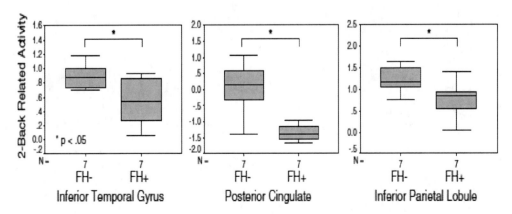

Fig. 15.9 Graphs showing differences in BOLD response on the 2-back task between people with a family history of hypertension (FH+) and people without such history (FS-). Significant differences in mean signal intensity were evident in the inferior temporal, inferior parietal and posterior cingulate regions. People in the FH+ group did not yet have problems with hypertension, so these differences in brain response presumably reflect genetic predisposition

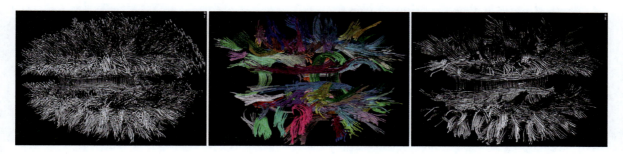

Fig. 15.10 White matter tractography derived from diffusion tensor imaging (DTI) analyses. The three images depict different stages in the derivation of the white matter tracts. The colors show the directionality of specific fiber tracts

over 30 s of working memory performance, most notably in the frontal cortex.[487] Increases in activated cortex over time suggested that recruitment was occurring, and was associated with sustained working memory demands. This conclusion was supported by the fact that 2-back performance declined over the 30 s periods. We are exploring similar analytic methods to examine cortical recruitment over time among people with CVD, with initial results suggesting dramatic increases in activation over time on the 2-back task, suggesting that recruitment on the 2-back task may be an useful measure of working memory inefficiency.

Diffusion Imaging in CVD

Standard structural MRI methods involving T1, T2, and FLAIR scanning are useful for detecting fully developed infarctions and other morphometric abnormalities, including atrophy. They less useful for characterizing the degree of physiological disturbance and tissue damage in brain regions that are not fully infracted. Furthermore, while FLAIR is useful for measuring WMH volume, it is not highly sensitive to microstructural abnormalities in white matter. Diffusion-weighted methods including DWI and DTI provide metrics of tissue experiencing ischemia (DWI and white matter integrity and injury DTI,[488] augmenting the information obtained from FLAIR.[489–491] As discussed in Chap. 18, DWI is now widely used in the assessment of acute stroke.[492–495] Furthermore, diffusion imaging and information obtained by comparing the diffusion and perfusion imaging mismatch have also shown areas of abnormality among patients with white matter disturbance secondary to microvascular disease[496–499] and also lacunar infarctions.[499] DWI abnormalities have been found among people with chronic hypertension.[497,500–510] Delayed diffusion abnormalities have also been shown in the hippocampus and white matter secondary to anoxia,[511] suggesting that this method can be used for detecting physiological changes in neuronal function caused by other factors in addition to infarction. In the context of CVD, DWI has been shown to be sensitive to abnormal brain development in newborns with congenital heart disease.[512] Most studies of DWI in patients with CVD have focused on detecting cerebral ischemic events during cardiothoracic surgery.[513–519] At this point in time, DWI tends not to be a routine used for assessing chronic cerebrovascular effects of CVD in an outpatient context (Fig. 15.10).

Diffusion Tensor Imaging

This imaging method derived from DWI in which diffusivity is measured in a large number of different spatial directions, providing unique data regarding alterations in white matter integrity. For the most part, at this point in time DTI is primarily used clinically by some neurosurgeons for visualizing white matter tracts when performing cranial surgery. However, methods have been developed and are being validated for quantifying the information on white matter tracts that DTI provides.[520–527] The figures below depict DTI methods that provide visualization of DTI from a single study patient showing The processing steps involved in producing fiber bundles based on DTI acquisition are shown. A dense initial pathset representing all regions of linear anisotropy is presented in the first image.

The center image shows paths after culling ambiguous path and noise. The final image shows paths from center after clustering. Through inverse modeling of the underlying DWI data, we will identify individual fiber bundles. These bundles enable determination of metrics (e.g., cross-sectional area, average FA, Trace, Stream Tube number and length) for particular white matter ROIs (e.g. corpus callosum and frontal gray matter (yellow) as shown in the image to the left. These metrics derived from DTI analyses provide evidence of altered white matter in these ROIs. Small white matter lesions can also be detected through visual analysis of DTI tractography. See Chap. 4 for detailed discussion on DTI (Fig. 15.11).

Currently DTI is largely a research tool. It has been used for characterizing abnormalities of the structural integrity of white matter pathways in various neurological brain conditions, including AD, MCI, HIV, and normal aging.[528-531] In the context of cerebrovascular disease, alterations in white matter pathways have been demonstrated.[531-538] To date, there are few DTI studies of CVD.

We piloted DTI for use in CVD, studying 16 CVD patients from the R01-AG17975 cohort (HF=8; no-HF=8). DTI scalar parameters including fractional anisotropy (FA) and apparent diffusivity coefficient (ADC) were measured from the corpus callosum and anterior limb of the internal capsule. . People with severe CVD and HF patients had reduced white matter coherence (FA) in the internal capsule compared to those with mild CVD at the 36-month assessment, associated with attention-executive performance, validating our earlier WMH findings, and supporting a link between white matter damage in CVD and cognitive dysfunction. However, when we examined both WMH and the DTI metric together, WMH volume was retained as the best predictor of cognitive performance ($R^2=0.62$, $p<0.05$). Based on this finding, the overlap between WMH on FLAIR and DTI, and the greater ease of WMH analysis, we decided to collect only FLAIR for WMH in the current study.

Cerebral Perfusion

There are a number of ways that CBF and cerebral hypoperfusion can be assessed. For example, we previously used SPECT to study cerebral perfusion abnormalities in dementia.[58,539] In the first, Ott et al.[437] dissociated WMH from SPECT perfusion in AD. Patients were excluded based on clinical history of

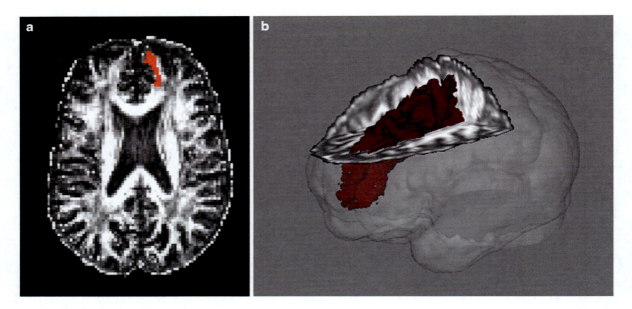

Fig. 15.11 DTI image of the type used to characterize white matter disturbance in our studies of HIV, CVD, and other brain disorders. A left superior frontal white matter ROI for purposes of deriving FA, MD and other scalar metrics that reflect degree of white matter integrity and coherence, or conversely the extent of damages is shown: A) Axial image showing FA in this ROI; B) 3-dimensional rendering of the same ROI

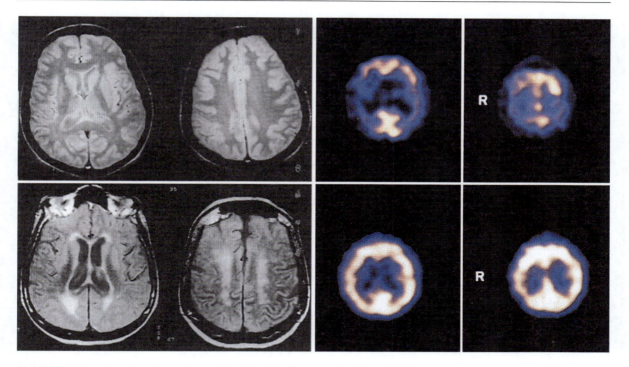

Fig. 15.12 Neuroimaging of a patient with AD. (A) The structural MRI images obtained with FLAIR sequences shows moderate periventricular WMH volume. (B) SPECT obtained from this same person shows global perfusion abnormalities, particularly notable in temporal and parietal regions. The intensity of SPECT activation across cortical ROIs does not correlate with the extent of WMH that is evident. This type of dissociation is characteristic of patients with AD

stroke (see adjacent figure). While both indices related to different aspect of cognitive function, SPECT CBF levels were not correlated with WMH (Fig. 15.12).

In a second study, Cohen et al. quantified SPECT and WMH from FLAIR in 26 VaD patients (NINDS criteria).[58,539] In contrast with our findings from AD patients, WMH significantly correlated with frontal perfusion on SPECT. Interestingly, frontal lobe perfusion did not correlate with performance on measures of executive function, even though global and frontal perfusion, were both associated with other cognitive functions. These results suggested that a functional "disconnection" between the frontal lobes and subcortical structures does not fully account for the global cognitive impairment in VaD, and that a complex relationship seems to exist between cerebral perfusion and cognitive dysfunction, apart from the effects of WMH damage. This was quite remarkable given that enormous effort was made to rule out AD. These results pointed to the possibility that VaD and AD were highly interrelated, and that studies of the vascular contributions to AD development are needed.

A number of studies have employed PET or SPECT imaging to examine cerebral perfusion abnormalities associated with factors related to CVD.[112,353,509,540–547] In one recent study, longitudinal change in rCBF was compared between people with chronic hypertension and healthy controls using PET.[548] The hypertension group had greater rCBF decreases in prefrontal, anterior cingulate, and occipital areas over time, suggesting the susceptibility of these brain areas to hypertension-related dysfunction as they aged. The HTN group also showed worsening of brain response in motor areas, the temporal cortex and hippocampus compared to controls. Pulse pressure, mean arterial pressure, and systolic and diastolic pressure were all associated with longitudinal rCBF changes, while increased duration of hypertension was associated with decreased rCBF in prefrontal and anterior cingulate areas. These results illustrate the effects of hypertension on cerebral perfusion and resting brain function in the elderly over time.

PET and SPECT imaging have also been used to demonstrate diminished rCBF in patients with heart failure.[357,549] Review of the limited number of studies that have been conducted suggests that patients with chronic heart failure exhibit cerebral hypoperfusion that is similar to that observed in AD.[357] However, prospective longitudinal study of changes in perfusion over time using these methods has not been conducted. Several studies have used these methods in conjunction with cardiac surgery.[355,544,550–556] These studies have generally shown some reduction in cerebral perfusion post-cardiac surgery, though that extent of hypoperfusion is modifiable by various neuroprotective interventions during surgery. For example, one study used SPECT to show that neurocognitive impairments among some patients were associated with rCBF reductions post-surgically.[552] Both short-term (68%) and long-term (55%) decreases in rCBF were evident. However, cerebral perfusion and adverse functional outcome could be improved by preventive coronary revascularization of beating heart.

Transcranial Doppler Imaging

CBF abnormalities can also be detected by Transcranial Doppler imaging with ultrasound.[513,557,558] Given the ease of conducting ultrasound measurement, this method is often used to monitor cerebral hemodynamic function during cardiac surgery.[355,559–564] In addition to showing blood flow variations, fusion, Transcranial Doppler imaging can also be used to identify emboli passing through the carotid or other arteries during surgery that have potential to cause cerebral infarction.[565–567] Two microemboli detected on imaging during CABG appear on ultrasound as shown by the arrows in the adjacent figure. However, neurocognitive outcome following cardiac surgery is not necessarily related to the quantity of emboli observed. We previously found that while mild reductions in neurocognitive function occurred in the period following both CABG and valve replacement surgery, these deficits were not strongly associated with intraoperative microemboli count,[181] suggesting that deficits were linked to hypoxia or other factors during surgery, a finding consistent with previous PET results.[550]

The most common methods for assessing regional cerebral perfusion abnormalities in clinical settings, particularly when stroke is suspected involve PWI with either CT or MRI. PWI is typically conducted along with angiography to provide visualization of cerebral vessels that may be dissected or occluded. The perfu-

sion-weighted image is obtained by injecting a contrast agent that enables measurement of blood flow. In the context of stroke, a focal region of diminished CBF can be visualized and its area quantified, providing information on the extent of altered perfusion secondary to the ischemic event. Furthermore, contrasting the mismatch between the perfusion- and diffusion-weighted images provide information on how much of the ischemic region can be salvageable.[568–570] These methods are discussed in detail in Chap. 18.

While a relatively large literature on the use MR-based cerebral perfusion methods for stroke exist, relatively few studies have used these methods to study CVD, or associated risk factors, though a few have focused on the effects of chronic hypertension, carotid atherosclerosis, and cardiac surgery.[568,571–575] For example, one study found that hypertension during 24-h ambulatory blood pressure readings among 80 older adults was associated with slower gait speed, poorer functional outcome, and also reduced cerebral perfusion. A few studies have investigated the use of PWI in the context of cardiac surgery[519,576] or in experimental surgical animal models.[571] Several recent studies have employed a similar strategy to evaluate perfusion and functional brain abnormalities in normal aging, AD, and MCI.[577,578] In one study of normal aging, risk factors for stroke were shown to relate to both BOLD and rCBF differences relative to young controls.[579]

There are relatively few PWI studies of cerebral perfusion among patients with CVD. As part of an ongoing National Institutes of Health sponsored heart failure project, we (Sweet and Cohen) are currently examining cerebral perfusion abnormalities associated with severe CVD and impaired cardiac output in heart failure. This study also aims to bridge the analysis of CBF and functional brain response. This is important given the fact that it is difficult to disentangle the effects of changes in regional blood flow from impaired neuronal response tied to blood oxygen metabolism. This is particularly true when there is a chronic global hypoperfusion, as is the case in heart failure. Noninvasive methods of PWI have been developed in recent years that do not require the administration of a contrast agent. The most widely studied method involves ASL and requires that only particular MR sequences be employed during scanning. While still in its early phases, we are currently simultaneously measuring rCBF using ASL and FMRI during working memory tasks. We also collect systemic vascular measures, as well as FLAIR to measure WMH.

The goal is to determine whether systemic vascular disease effects functional brain response as measured by BOLD beyond its general effect on cerebral perfusion, and to determine whether these effects exist beyond the influence of structural brain changes as reflected by white matter damage on MRI. The rationale for using ASL was fourfold: (1) It could be obtained at the same time as the other MR data; (2) Neuroanatomic coregistration would be relatively easy; (3) ASL could be most readily analyzed relative to the FMRI data from the study; and (4) ASL would provide metrics that could be easily analyzed for specific brain ROIs. This project is an illustration of how two imaging modalities can be simultaneously measured to provide unique information about underlying brain disturbances.

Hemodynamic Influences on the BOLD Response

Given that functional imaging methods such FMRI depend on CBF changes, an important issue is how to disentangle hemodynamic from neuronal contributions to the BOLD response. Hoge and his colleagues have developed methods to examine the relationship of ASL and BOLD during the same scanning session to characterize their relationships over time,[580–584] including in the context of a simple motor paradigm. ASL was carried out using PICORE labeling geometry with Q2TIPS saturation. The correlation between BOLD and HbR was much stronger than the correlations between BOLD and oxyhemoglobin (HbO) or total hemoglobin (HbT). In contrast, the ASL measurement was more strongly correlated with the NIRS HbO and HbT responses than the HbR response. The ASL measured perfusion clearly peaks around 2 s earlier than the BOLD response. While ASL closely follows NIRS measured HbT and HbO, BOLD closely follows HbR. The figures above show the temporal lag between the BOLD and ASL response. The difference between the baseline (magenta arrow) and activated (green arrow) signal levels enabled estimation of rCBF change. Hypercapnia challenge has been used to improve the accuracy and image quality of pulsed ASL, by producing a maximal response with CO_2. The results show that ASL is significantly related to BOLD FMRI signal, with coupling between BOLD FMRI signal and blood perfusion in healthy people and CVD, and that hypercapnia applied with our ASL methods increases the accuracy of rCBF change measures during global periods of global flow increases. Contrasting these imaging measures provides valuable information that enables separation of hemodynamic from BOLD abnormalities related to impaired neuronal response.

Magnetic Resonance Spectroscopy

This MR-based method is potentially valuable for assessing cerebral metabolic abnormalities associated with vascular disease, though to date there is a very limited research literature in CVD. There are a number of methods available for MRS (see Chap. 6), though none are commonly used in routine clinical care at this point in time. The simplest and most studied approach is the single voxel proton MRS method, in which individual ROIs are prescribed in different brain regions (e.g., Frontal gray matter, Frontal white matter, hippocampus), and metabolite concentrations are determined based on the spectrographic MR waveform. As shown in the figure above, several metabolites are typically measured including n-acetyl aspartate (NAA), choline (Cho), creatine (Cr), myoinositol, and glutamine-glutamate (Glx) levels. Ratios are often created, using Cr as a reference metabolite. NAA/Cr is thought to reflect neuronal damage. Cho and MI are markers of cerebral inflammation, while Glx may reflect excitoxicity and other processes associated with GABA metabolism.

MRS has been most widely studied for neurodegenerative brain diseases, including AD/MCI,[585–587] HIV[588–590] and multiple sclerosis.[591–594] The most common finding is decreased NAA levels associated with severity of brain disease, presumably related to neuronal loss. However, increased levels of inflammatory markers (MI, Cho) and other metabolic disturbances have also been found. For example, among patients with HIV-associated cognitive impairments, we have found that Cho and MI ratios were increased in frontal gray matter and the basal ganglia, while NAA was also reduced in frontal gray and white matter compared to controls, and cortical Glx elevations were also evident.

Metabolite abnormalities have also been shown in both experimental and clinical stroke,[595–597] though is generally not performed in routine clinical management of patients. In one of the earliest studies, reduced NAA in the infarct within the first 4 days was related to the clinical stroke syndrome, more extensive infarction, more severely reduced blood supply to the infarct, and the presence of lactate. Lactate was related to large infarcts and reduced NAA. Swelling in the infarct was not associated with reduced NAA, suggesting dissociation between the evolving infarction (reduced NAA levels) and pathophysiological responses to the stroke (e.g., inflammation).[595] In a more recent study, decreased GABA was observed in the brain areas following stroke. In another recent study, NAA levels measured by MRS corresponded with diffusion abnormalities on DWI during the period following acute stroke.[597] There is also evidence of altered cerebral MRS metabolites associated with chronic global ischemia and anoxia in experimental rats,[598] suggesting that effects are not solely attributable to acute infarction. Interestingly, associations have also been shown between MRS abnormalities and migraine aura.[599]

An intriguing application of MRS is for the study of the effects of diabetes, metabolic syndrome, and related risk factors to CVD-associated brain dysfunction. Several studies have employed MRS to study how insulin and glucose metabolic disturbances affect cerebral metabolites.[600–604] In a recent study, Type 2 diabetics showed an increased level of Cho/Cr in the frontal white matter, associated with altered membrane phospholipid metabolism.[600] Increased levels of increase in Glx levels on MRS in the hippocampus of rodents bred to have diabetes, a finding consistent with brain tissue content in human diabetics.[602] In another recent study, a number of MRS abnormalities were observed among people with glucose intolerance and diabetes relative to controls.[603] Frontal cortical Cho/Cr ratios were increased in patients with impaired glucose tolerance compare to controls. Parietal white matter Cho/Cr ratios were also significantly higher in patients with impaired glucose tolerance compared to patients with diabetes, while frontal cortical MI/Cr ratios were increased, and parietal white matter Cho/Cr ratios were decreased when compared to controls. Frontal cortical NAA/Cr and Cho/Cr ratios and parietal white matter Cho/Cr ratio decreases were greatest in diabetic patients with poor glycemic control. One very recent study examined brain metabolism and CBF in young patients with hyperlipidemia. Cho/Cr and NAA/Cr in the occipital region of the brain correlated with excess percentage of body fat and low levels of high density lipoprotein cholesterol. Serum triglyceride levels were also positively correlated with the NAA/Cr and Cho/Cr ratios in the parietal and temporal area.[605] These types of findings have considerable relevance to CVD,

as diabetes and hyperlipidemia often comorbid, and reflect metabolic disturbances that may exacerbate the neuronal impact of hypoperfusion.

MRS has been used to study cerebral metabolite disturbances associated with heart failure.[606] Proton MRS was obtained from localized regions of the occipital gray matter and parietal white matter. Absolute levels of the metabolites NAA, Cr, Cho, and MI were measured. All metabolites were abnormal in the cortical gray matter, but only CR was elevated in the white matter ROI. Interestingly, after heart transplantation, levels of these metabolites normalized to some extent. These findings suggest that cerebral metabolite disturbances occur in associated with chronic heart failure and presumably cerebral hypoperfusion, and raises the possibility that this may contribute to associated brain dysfunction. Another study examined the effects of the drug, MDNA (ecstasy) on cardiac metabolic disturbance, but did not specifically focus on cerebral metabolite effects.[607] A few studies have examined MRS metabolites abnormalities following cardiac surgery.[169,608–613] MRS has also been used to study the effects of apnea and its treatment effects on the brain.[614] These types of studies point to its value as an indicator of impaired cerebral metabolic function in patients with chronic system vascular disease, even in the absence of infarction.

We are beginning to employ MRS in our experimental studies of CVD and heart failure. The measurement of cerebral metabolite abnormalities would be potentially valuable in conjunction with data from other neuroimaging modalities, such as FMRI, structural imaging, and diffusion-perfusion imaging. Together, these approaches may enable determination of: (1) The relative contributions of metabolic disturbance, hemodynamic abnormalities, and structural brain damage to CVD-associated cognitive impairments and brain dysfunction associated with CVD; (2) Worsening over time; (3) Relationships between indices of systemic vascular function and cognitive impairment and brain abnormalities; and (4) Functional brain abnormalities (FMRI) associated with systemic vascular disturbance. We have also shown that: (1) Systemic vascular problems may be tied to cerebrovascular and neuronal disturbances; (2) Regional CBF (ASL) and cerebral metabolite disturbances are likely linked to these brain disturbances; (3) May represent the link between systemic vascular disease and vascular-associated brain dysfunction in the elderly; and (4) These hemodynamic and metabolic factors are also associated with functional brain abnormalities on FMRI. With respect to feasibility, we have shown the ability to successfully conduct large studies of CVD and MCI and to reliably collect and analyze all measure, including the neuroimaging indices ASL, FMRI, systemic vascular function and the cognitive functions of interest in a manner that is very feasible in the context of the current study. We have conducted preliminary studies comparing people with and without CVD and MCI on the planned neuroimaging and vascular measures, with preliminary results that provide compelling support for our the specific aims and hypotheses.

Conclusions

Neuroimaging provides powerful methods for studying CVD-associated cognitive disturbance and brain dysfunction. Some of these methods have future potential to serve as biomarkers of risk for brain dysfunction in people with CVD who are cognitively asymptomatic, but showing early evidence of brain effects. These methods range from approaches that primarily inform about structural brain damage to other like FMRI that provide information on the functional responsiveness of particular regions of the brain suspected of being vulnerable. There are specific methods for measuring brain tissue that is ischemic yet not fully infracted (DWI), as well as areas with decreased perfusion. Furthermore, using MRS it may be possible to identify physiologically vulnerable brain areas among people who are otherwise asymptomatic with respect to cognitive function. In the future some of these methods may prove useful as biomarkers that in the future may provide biomarkers for detecting people with CVD who are at risk for future brain injury and functional decline.

References

1. American Heart Association. Cardiovascular disease statistics: American Heart Association. http://www.americanheart.org: American Heart Association; 2004.
2. Bild DE, Fitzpatrick A, Fried LP, et al. Age-related trends in cardiovascular morbidity and physical functioning in the elderly: the Cardiovascular Health Study. *J Am Geriatr Soc.* 1993;41(10):1047–1056.
3. Smith SM, Mensah GA. Population aging and implications for epidemic cardiovascular disease in Sub-Saharan Africa. *Ethn Dis (Summer).* 2003;13(2 Suppl 2):S77–80.
4. Miller LW, Missov ED. Epidemiology of heart failure. *Cardiol Clin.* 2001;19(4):547–555.
5. Rich MW. Epidemiology, pathophysiology, and etiology of congestive heart failure in older adults. *J Am Geriatr Soc.* 1997;45(8):968–974.
6. Haan MN, Selby JV, Quesenberry CP Jr, Schmittdiel JA, Fireman BH, Rice DP. The impact of aging and chronic disease on use of hospital and outpatient services in a large HMO: 1971–1991. *J Am Geriatr Soc.* 1997;45(6): 667–674.
7. Mangano DT. Cardiovascular morbidity and CABG surgery – a perspective: epidemiology, costs, and potential therapeutic solutions. *J Card Surg.* 1995;10(4 Suppl):366–368.
8. Manton KG. The global impact of noncommunicable diseases: estimates and projections. *World Health Stat Q.* 1988;41(3–4):255–266.
9. Ayanian JZ, Guadagnoli E, Cleary PD. Physical and psychosocial functioning of women and men after coronary artery bypass surgery. *JAMA.* 1995;274(22):1767–1770.
10. Bastone E, Kerns R. Effects of self-efficacy and perceived social support on recovery-related behaviors after coronary artery bypass surgery. *Ann Behav Med.* 1995;17(4):324–330.
11. Jones GE, Jones KR, Cunningham RA, Caldwell JA. Cardiac awareness in infarct patients and normals. *Psychophysiology.* 1985;22(4):480–487.
12. Ruberman W, Weinblatt E, Goldberg JD, Chaudhary BS. Psychosocial influences on mortality after myocardial infarction. *N Engl J Med.* 1984;311(9):552–559.
13. Engebretson T, Clark M, Niaura R, Phillips T, Albrecht A, Tilkemeier P. Quality of life and anxiety in a phase II cardiac rehabilitation program. *Med Sci Sports Exerc.* 1998;31(Suppl 2):216–223.
14. Drexler H, Hayoz D, Munzel T, Just H, Zelis R, Brunner HR. Endothelial function in congestive heart failure. *Am Heart J.* 1993;126(3 Pt 2):761–764.
15. Polidori MC, Marvardi M, Cherubini A, Senin U, Mecocci P. Heart disease and vascular risk factors in the cognitively impaired elderly: implications for Alzheimer's dementia. *Aging (Milano).* 2001;13(3):231–239.
16. Guo Z, Viitanen M, Winblad B. Clinical correlates of low blood pressure in very old people: the importance of cognitive impairment. *J Am Geriatr Soc.* 1997;45(6):701–705.
17. Butler RN, Ahronheim J, Fillit H, Rapoport SI, Tatemichi JK. Vascular dementia: stroke prevention takes on new urgency. *Geriatrics.* 1993;48(11):32–34, 40–32.
18. Caplan L. *Stroke: A Clinical Approach, edn 2.* 2nd ed. Boston: Butterworths; 1993.
19. De Reuck JL. Evidence for chronic ischaemia in the pathogenesis of vascular dementia: from neuroPATH to neuroPET. *Acta Neurol Belg.* 1996;96(3):228–231.
20. Tatemichi TK, Desmond DW, Stern Y, Paik M, Sano M, Bagiella E. Cognitive impairment after stroke: frequency, patterns, and relationship to functional abilities. *J Neurol Neurosurg Psychiatry.* 1994;57(2):202–207.
21. Shuaib A, Boyle C. Stroke in the elderly. *Curr Opin Neurol.* 1994;7(1):41–47.
22. Petty LA, Parker JR, Parker JC Jr. Hypertension and vascular dementia. *Ann Clin Lab Sci.* 1992;22(1):34–39.

23. Phillips SJ, Whisnant JP. Hypertension and the brain. The National High Blood Pressure Education Program. *Arch Intern Med.* 1992;152(5):938–945.

24. Lindsay J, Hebert R, Rockwood K. The Canadian Study of Health and Aging: risk factors for vascular dementia. *Stroke.* 1997;28(3):526–530.

25. Ahto M, Isoaho R, Puolijoki H, Laippala P, Sulkava R, Kivela SL. Cognitive impairment among elderly coronary heart disease patients. *Gerontology.* 1999;45(2):87–95.

26. Aberg T. Effect of open heart surgery on intellectual function. *Scand J Thorac Cardiovasc Surg Suppl.* 1974;15:1–63.

27. Barclay LL, Weiss EM, Mattis S, Bond O, Blass JP. Unrecognized cognitive impairment in cardiac rehabilitation patients. *J Am Geriatr Soc.* 1988;36(1):22–28.

28. Cohen RA, Moser DJ, Clark MM, et al. Neurocognitive functioning and improvement in quality of life following participation in cardiac rehabilitation. *Am J Cardiol.* 1999;83(9):1374–1378.

29. Engebretson Clark MM, Niaura RS, Phillips T, Albrecht A, Tilkemeier P. Quality of life and anxiety in a phase II cardiac rehabilitation program. *Med Sci Sports Exerc.* Feb 1999;31(2):216–223.

30. Ades PA, Huang D, Weaver SO. Cardiac rehabilitation participation predicts lower rehospitalization costs. *Am Heart J.* 1992;123(4 Pt 1):916–921.

31. Cohen RA, Kaplan RF. Neuropsychological aspects of cerebrovascular disease. In: Bogoslovski J, Fisher M, eds. *Current Review of Cerebrovascular Disease.* Philadelphia: Current Medicine; 1995.

32. Cohen RA, Paul RH, Ott BR, et al. The relationship of subcortical MRI hyperintensities and brain volume to cognitive function in vascular dementia. *J Int Neuropsychol Soc.* 2002;8(6):743–752.

33. Cook IL A, Morgan M, et al. Cognitive and physiologic correlates of subclinical structural brain disease in elderly healthy control subjects. *Arch Neurol.* 2002;59: 1612–1620.

34. Tatemichi TK, Desmond DW, Mayeux R, et al. Dementia after stroke: baseline frequency, risks, and clinical features in a hospitalized cohort. *Neurology.* 1992;42(6):1185–1193.

35. Tatemichi T, Desmond D, Paik M. Clinical determinants of dementia related to stroke. *Ann Neurol.* 1994;33: 568–575.

36. Ammash N, Warnes CA. Cerebrovascular events in adult patients with cyanotic congenital heart disease. *J Am Coll Cardiol.* 1996;28(3):768–772.

37. Anderson TJ, Uehata A, Gerhard MD, et al. Close relation of endothelial function in the human coronary and peripheral circulations. *J Am Coll Cardiol.* 1995;26(5):1235–1241.

38. Bracco L, Campani D, Baratti E, et al. Relation between MRI features and dementia in cerebrovascular disease patients with leukoaraiosis: a longitudinal study. *J Neurol Sci.* 1993;120(2):131–136.

39. Brun A. Pathology and pathophysiology of cerebrovascular dementia: pure subgroups of obstructive and hypoperfusive etiology. *Dementia.* 1994;5(3–4):145–147.

40. Jennings JR, Muldoon MF, Ryan CM, et al. Cerebral blood flow in hypertensive patients: an initial report of reduced and compensatory blood flow responses during performance of two cognitive tasks. *Hypertension.* 1998; 31(6):1216–1222.

41. Inzitari D, Diaz F, Fox A, et al. Vascular risk factors and leuko-araiosis. *Arch Neurol.* 1987;44(1):42–47.

42. Haskell WL, Alderman EL, Fair JM, et al. Effects of intensive multiple risk factor reduction on coronary atherosclerosis and clinical cardiac events in men and women with coronary artery disease. The Stanford Coronary Risk Intervention Project (SCRIP). *Circulation.* 1994;89(3):975–990.

43. DeCarli C, Miller B, Swan GE, Reed T, Wolf PA. Cerebrovascular and brain morphometry brain correlates of mild cognitive impairment in the National Heart, Lung, and Blood Twin Study. *Arch Neurol.* 2001;58(4):643–647.

44. Hallevi H, Albright KC, Martin-Schild S, Barreto AD, Grotta JC, Savitz SI. The complications of cardioembolic stroke: lessons from the VISTA database. *Cerebrovasc Dis.* 2008;26(1):38–40.

45. Markus HS, Khan U, Birns J, et al. Differences in stroke subtypes between black and white patients with stroke: the South London Ethnicity and Stroke Study. *Circulation.* 2007;116(19):2157–2164.

46. Lavados PM, Sacks C, Prina L, et al. Incidence, case-fatality rate, and prognosis of ischaemic stroke subtypes in a predominantly Hispanic-Mestizo population in Iquique, Chile (PISCIS project): a community-based incidence study. *Lancet Neurol.* 2007;6(2):140–148.

47. Ohira T, Shahar E, Chambless LE, Rosamond WD, Mosley TH Jr, Folsom AR. Risk factors for ischemic stroke subtypes: the Atherosclerosis Risk in Communities study. *Stroke.* 2006;37(10):2493–2498.

48. Ross MH, Yurgelun-Todd DA, Renshaw PF, et al. Age-related reduction in functional MRI response to photic stimulation. *Neurology.* 1997;48(1):173–176.

49. Schriger DL, Baraff L. Defining normal capillary refill: variation with age, sex, and temperature. *Ann Emerg Med.* 1988;17(9):932–935.

50. Huettel SA, Obembe OO, Song AW, Woldorff MG. The BOLD fMRI refractory effect is specific to stimulus attributes: evidence from a visual motion paradigm. *Neuroimage.* 2004;23(1):402–408.

51. Huettel SA, Singerman JD, McCarthy G. The effects of aging upon the hemodynamic response measured by functional MRI. *Neuroimage.* 2001;13(1):161–175.

52. Taoka T, Iwasaki S, Uchida H, et al. Age correlation of the time lag in signal change on EPI-fMRI. *J Comput Assist Tomogr.* 1998;22(4):514–517.

53. Paul R, Garrett K, Cohen R. Vascular dementia: a diagnostic conundrum for the clinical neuropsychologist. *Appl Neuropsychol.* 2003;10(3):129–136.

54. Paul RH, Cohen RA, Moser D, et al. Performance on the Mattis Dementia Rating Scale in patients with vascular dementia: relationships to neuroimaging findings. *J Geriatr Psychiatry Neurol (Spring).* 2001;14(1):33–36.

55. Paul RH, Cohen RA, Moser DJ, et al. Clinical correlates of cognitive decline in vascular dementia. *Cogn Behav Neurol.* 2003;16(1):40–46.

56. Paul RH, Cohen RA, Moser DJ, et al. The global deterioration scale: relationships to neuropsychological performance and activities of daily living in patients with vascular dementia. *J Geriatr Psychiatry Neurol (Spring).* 2002;15(1):50–54.

57. Paul RH, Cohen RA, Moser DJ, Zawacki TM, Gordon N. The serial position effect in mild and moderately severe vascular dementia. *J Int Neuropsychol Soc.* 2002;8(4):584–587.

58. Cohen RA, Paul RH, Zawacki TM, et al. Single photon emission computed tomography, magnetic resonance imaging hyperintensity, and cognitive impairments in patients with vascular dementia. *J Neuroimaging.* 2001;11(3):253–260.

59. Gunstad J, Brickman AM, Paul RH, et al. Progressive morphometric and cognitive changes in vascular dementia. *Arch Clin Neuropsychol.* 2005;20(2):229–241.

60. Jefferson AL, Cahn-Weiner D, Boyle P, et al. Cognitive predictors of functional decline in vascular dementia. *Int J Geriatr Psychiatry.* 2006;21(8):752–754.

61. Jefferson AL, Paul RH, Ozonoff A, Cohen RA. Evaluating elements of executive functioning as predictors of instrumental activities of daily living (IADLs). *Arch Clin Neuropsychol.* 2006;21(4):311–320.

62. Boyle PA, Cohen RA, Paul R, Moser D, Gordon N. Cognitive and motor impairments predict functional declines in patients with vascular dementia. *Int J Geriatr Psychiatry.* 2002;17(2):164–169.

63. Boyle PA, Paul R, Moser D, Zawacki T, Gordon N, Cohen R. Cognitive and neurologic predictors of functional impairment in vascular dementia. *Am J Geriatr Psychiatry.* 2003;11(1):103–106.

64. Boyle PA, Paul RH, Moser DJ, Cohen RA. Executive impairments predict functional declines in vascular dementia. *Clin Neuropsychol.* 2004;18(1):75–82.

65. Cohen RA, Browndyke JN, Moser DJ, Paul RH, Gordon N, Sweet L. Long-term citicoline (cytidine diphosphate choline) use in patients with vascular dementia: neuroimaging and neuropsychological outcomes. *Cerebrovasc Dis.* 2003;16(3):199–204.

66. Davies CA, Mann DM, Sumpter PQ, Yates PO. A quantitative morphometric analysis of the neuronal and synaptic content of the frontal and temporal cortex in patients with Alzheimer's disease. *J Neurol Sci.* 1987;78(2):151–164.

67. Hamos JE, DeGennaro LJ, Drachman DA. Synaptic loss in Alzheimer's disease and other dementias. *Neurology.* 1989;39(3):355–361.

68. Martin LJ, Pardo CA, Cork LC, Price DL. Synaptic pathology and glial responses to neuronal injury precede the formation of senile plaques and amyloid deposits in the aging cerebral cortex. *Am J Pathol.* 1994;145(6):1358–1381.

69. Glenner GG, Wong CW. Alzheimer's disease: initial report of the purification and characterization of a novel cerebrovascular amyloid protein. *Biochem Biophys Res Commun.* 1984;120(3):885–890.

70. Glenner GG, Wong CW, Quaranta V, Eanes ED. The amyloid deposits in Alzheimer's disease: their nature and pathogenesis. *Appl Pathol.* 1984;2(6):357–369.

71. Masters CL, Multhaup G, Simms G, Pottgiesser J, Martins RN, Beyreuther K. Neuronal origin of a cerebral amyloid: neurofibrillary tangles of Alzheimer's disease contain the same protein as the amyloid of plaque cores and blood vessels. *EMBO J.* 1985;4(11):2757–2763.

72. Masters CL, Simms G, Weinman NA, Multhaup G, McDonald BL, Beyreuther K. Amyloid plaque core protein in Alzheimer disease and Down syndrome. *Proc Natl Acad Sci U S A.* 1985;82(12):4245–4249.

73. Beyreuther K, Masters CL. Amyloid precursor protein (APP) and beta A4 amyloid in the etiology of Alzheimer's disease: precursor-product relationships in the derangement of neuronal function. *Brain Pathol.* 1991;1(4):241–251.

74. Goedert M. Tau protein and the neurofibrillary pathology of Alzheimer's disease. *Ann N Y Acad Sci.* 1996;777:121–131.

75. Hirata-Fukae C, Li HF, Ma L, et al. Levels of soluble and insoluble tau reflect overall status of tau phosphorylation in vivo. *Neurosci Lett.* 2009;450(1):51–55.

76. Sabayan B, Foroughinia F, Mowla A, Borhanihaghighi A. Role of insulin metabolism disturbances in the development of Alzheimer disease: mini review. *Am J Alzheimers Dis Other Demen.* 2008;23(2):192–199.

77. Small SA, Duff K. Linking Abeta and tau in late-onset Alzheimer's disease: a dual pathway hypothesis. *Neuron.* 2008;60(4):534–542.

78. Steinerman JR, Honig LS. Laboratory biomarkers in Alzheimer's disease. *Curr Neurol Neurosci Rep.* 2007;7(5):381–387.

79. Strittmatter WJ, Saunders AM, Goedert M, et al. Isoform-specific interactions of apolipoprotein E with microtubule-associated protein tau: implications for Alzheimer disease. *Proc Natl Acad Sci U S A.* 1994;91(23):11183–11186.

80. Zhou XW, Gustafsson JA, Tanila H, et al. Tau hyperphosphorylation correlates with reduced methylation of protein phosphatase 2A. *Neurobiol Dis.* 2008;31(3):386–394.

81. Roses AD. The Alzheimer diseases. *Curr Opin Neurobiol.* 1996;6(5):644–650.

82. Davies P. The genetics of Alzheimer's disease: a review and a discussion of the implications. *Neurobiol Aging.* 1986;7(6):459–466.

83. Davies P. A very incomplete comprehensive theory of Alzheimer's disease. *Ann N Y Acad Sci.* 2000;924:8–16.

84. Kang J, Lemaire HG, Unterbeck A, et al. The precursor of Alzheimer's disease amyloid A4 protein resembles a cell-surface receptor. *Nature.* 1987;325(6106):733–736.

85. Tanzi RE, McClatchey AI, Lamperti ED, Villa-Komaroff L, Gusella JF, Neve RL. Protease inhibitor domain encoded by an amyloid protein precursor mRNA associated with Alzheimer's disease. *Nature.* 1988;331(6156):528–530.

86. Konig G, Monning U, Czech C, et al. Identification and differential expression of a novel alternative splice isoform of the beta A4 amyloid precursor protein (APP) mRNA in leukocytes and brain microglial cells. *J Biol Chem.* 1992;267(15):10804–10809.

87. Prelli F, Castano E, Glenner GG, Frangione B. Differences between vascular and plaque core amyloid in Alzheimer's disease. *J Neurochem.* 1988;51(2):648–651.

88. Revesz T, Ghiso J, Lashley T, et al. Cerebral amyloid angiopathies: a pathologic, biochemical, and genetic view. *J Neuropathol Exp Neurol.* 2003;62(9):885–898.

89. Attems J, Jellinger KA. Only cerebral capillary amyloid angiopathy correlates with Alzheimer pathology – a pilot study. *Acta Neuropathol (Berl).* 2004;107(2):83–90.

90. Attems J, Lintner F, Jellinger KA. Amyloid beta peptide 1–42 highly correlates with capillary cerebral amyloid angiopathy and Alzheimer disease pathology. *Acta Neuropathol (Berl).* 2004;107(4):283–291.

91. Thal DR, Ghebremedhin E, Rub U, Yamaguchi H, Del Tredici K, Braak H. Two types of sporadic cerebral amyloid angiopathy. *J Neuropathol Exp Neurol.* 2002;61(3):282–293.

92. Borroni B, Akkawi N, Martini G, et al. Microvascular damage and platelet abnormalities in early Alzheimer's disease. *J Neurol Sci.* 2002;203–204:189–193.

93. Buee L, Hof PR, Bouras C, et al. Pathological alterations of the cerebral microvasculature in Alzheimer's disease and related dementing disorders. *Acta Neuropathol.* 1994;87(5): 469–480.

94. Buee L, Hof PR, Delacourte A. Brain microvascular changes in Alzheimer's disease and other dementias. *Ann N Y Acad Sci.* 1997;826:7–24.

95. Perry G, Smith MA, McCann CE, Siedlak SL, Jones PK, Friedland RP. Cerebrovascular muscle atrophy is a feature of Alzheimer's disease. *Brain Res.* 1998;791(1–2):63–66.

96. Mancardi GL, Perdelli F, Rivano C, Leonardi A, Bugiani O. Thickening of the basement membrane of cortical capillaries in Alzheimer's disease. *Acta Neuropathol.* 1980;49(1):79–83.

97. Scheibel AB, Duong TH, Jacobs R. Alzheimer's disease as a capillary dementia. *Ann Med.* 1989;21(2):103–107.

98. Thomas T, Thomas G, McLendon C, Sutton T, Mullan M. beta-Amyloid-mediated vasoactivity and vascular endothelial damage. *Nature.* 1996;380(6570):168–171.

99. Claudio L. Ultrastructural features of the blood–brain barrier in biopsy tissue from Alzheimer's disease patients. *Acta Neuropathol (Berl).* 1996;91(1):6–14.

100. Mancardi GL, Tabaton M, Liwnicz BH. Endothelial mitochondrial content of cerebral cortical capillaries in Alzheimer's disease. An ultrastructural quantitative study. *Eur Neurol.* 1985;24(1):49–52.

101. Perlmutter LS, Myers MA, Barron E. Vascular basement membrane components and the lesions of Alzheimer's disease: light and electron microscopic analyses. *Microsc Res Tech.* 1994;28(3):204–215.

102. Zarow C, Barron E, Chui HC, Perlmutter LS. Vascular basement membrane pathology and Alzheimer's disease. *Ann N Y Acad Sci.* 1997;826:147–160.

103. Kalaria RN. Cerebrovascular degeneration is related to amyloid-beta protein deposition in Alzheimer's disease. *Ann N Y Acad Sci.* 1997;826:263–271.

104. Kalaria RN. Vascular factors in Alzheimer's disease. *Int Psychogeriatr.* 2003;15(Suppl 1):47–52.

105. Perry E, Kay DW. Some developments in brain ageing and dementia. *Br J Biomed Sci.* 1997;54(3):201–215.

106. Snow AD, Mar H, Nochlin D, et al. The presence of heparan sulfate proteoglycans in the neuritic plaques and congophilic angiopathy in Alzheimer's disease. *Am J Pathol.* 1988;133(3):456–463.

107. Snow AD, Sekiguchi R, Nochlin D, et al. An important role of heparan sulfate proteoglycan (Perlecan) in a model system for the deposition and persistence of fibrillar A betaamyloid in rat brain. *Neuron.* 1994;12(1):219–234.

108. Westermark GT, Norling B, Westermark P. Fibronectin and basement membrane components in renal amyloid deposits in patients with primary and secondary amyloidosis. *Clin Exp Immunol.* 1991;86(1):150–156.

109. Roll FJ, Madri JA, Albert J, Furthmayr H. Codistribution of collagen types IV and AB2 in basement membranes and mesangium of the kidney. an immunoferritin study of ultrathin frozen sections. *J Cell Biol.* 1980;85(3):597–616.

110. Liesi P. Laminin-immunoreactive glia distinguish regenerative adult CNS systems from non-regenerative ones. *EMBO J.* 1985;4(10):2505–2511.

111. McGeer PL, Zhu SG, Dedhar S. Immunostaining of human brain capillaries by antibodies to very late antigens. *J Neuroimmunol.* 1990;26(3):213–218.

112. Fujii K, Sadoshima S, Okada Y, et al. Cerebral blood flow and metabolism in normotensive and hypertensive patients with transient neurologic deficits. *Stroke.* 1990;21(2):283–290.

113. Fujii K, Sadoshima S, Yao H, Yoshida F, Iwase M, Fujishima M. Cerebral ischemia in spontaneously hypertensive rats with type 2 (noninsulin-dependent) diabetes mellitus, cerebral blood flow and tissue metabolism. *Gerontology.* 1989;35(2–3):78–87.

114. Shiokawa O, Sadoshima S, Fujii K, Yao H, Fujishima M. Impairment of cerebellar blood flow autoregulation during cerebral ischemia in spontaneously hypertensive rats. *Stroke.* 1988;19(5):615–622.

115. Trollor JN, Sachdev PS, Haindl W, Brodaty H, Wen W, Walker BM. Regional cerebral blood flow deficits in mild Alzheimer's disease using high resolution single photon emission computerized tomography. *Psychiatry Clin Neurosci.* 2005;59(3):280–290.

116. Eberling JL, Reed BR, Baker MG, Jagust WJ. Cognitive correlates of regional cerebral blood flow in Alzheimer's disease. *Arch Neurol.* 1993;50(7):761–766.

117. Eberling JL, Jagust WJ, Reed BR, Baker MG. Reduced temporal lobe blood flow in Alzheimer's disease. *Neurobiol Aging.* 1992;13(4):483–491.

118. Henneman WJ, Sluimer JD, Cordonnier C, et al. MRI biomarkers of vascular damage and atrophy predicting mortality in a memory clinic population. *Stroke.* 2009;40(2): 492–498.

119. Gouw AA, Seewann A, Vrenken H, et al. Heterogeneity of white matter hyperintensities in Alzheimer's disease: postmortem quantitative MRI and neuropathology. *Brain.* 2008;131(Pt 12):3286–3298.

120. van Straaten EC, Harvey D, Scheltens P, et al. Periventricular white matter hyperintensities increase the likelihood of progression from amnestic mild cognitive impairment to dementia. *J Neurol.* 2008;255(9):1302–1308.

121. Frisoni GB, Henneman WJ, Weiner MW, et al. The pilot European Alzheimer's Disease Neuroimaging Initiative of the European Alzheimer's Disease Consortium. *Alzheimers Dement.* 2008;4(4):255–264.

122. Holland CM, Smith EE, Csapo I, et al. Spatial distribution of white-matter hyperintensities in Alzheimer disease, cerebral amyloid angiopathy, and healthy aging. *Stroke.* 2008;39(4):1127–1133.

123. Kang JH, Logroscino G, De Vivo I, Hunter D, Grodstein F. Apolipoprotein E, cardiovascular disease and cognitive function in aging women. *Neurobiol Aging.* 2005;26(4):475–484.

124. Fallon JR, Hall ZW. Building synapses: agrin and dystroglycan stick together. *Trends Neurosci.* 1994;17(11):469–473.

125. Barber AJ, Lieth E. Agrin accumulates in the brain microvascular basal lamina during development of the blood–brain barrier. *Dev Dyn.* 1997;208(1):62–74.

126. Berzin TM, Zipser BD, Rafii MS, et al. Agrin and microvascular damage in Alzheimer's disease. *Neurobiol Aging.* 2000;21(2):349–355.

127. Deyst KA, Bowe MA, Leszyk JD, Fallon JR. The alphadystroglycan-beta-dystroglycan complex. Membrane organization and relationship to an agrin receptor. *J Biol Chem.* 1995;270(43):25956–25959.

128. Deyst KA, Ma J, Fallon JR. Agrin: toward a molecular understanding of synapse regeneration. *Neurosurgery.* 1995;37(1):71–77.

129. Deyst KA, McKechnie BA, Fallon JR. The role of alternative splicing in regulating agrin binding to muscle cells. *Brain Res Dev Brain Res.* 1998;110(2):185–191.

130. Koulen P, Honig LS, Fletcher EL, Kroger S. Expression, distribution and ultrastructural localization of the synapse-organizing molecule agrin in the mature avian retina. *Eur J Neurosci.* 1999;11(12):4188–4196.

131. Kroger S, Schroder JE. Agrin in the developing CNS: new roles for a synapse organizer. *News Physiol Sci.* 2002;17:207–212.

132. Rascher G, Fischmann A, Kroger S, Duffner F, Grote EH, Wolburg H. Extracellular matrix and the blood–brain barrier in glioblastoma multiforme: spatial segregation of tenascin and agrin. *Acta Neuropathol.* 2002;104(1):85–91.

133. Warth A, Kroger S, Wolburg H. Redistribution of aquaporin-4 in human glioblastoma correlates with loss of agrin immunoreactivity from brain capillary basal laminae. *Acta Neuropathol.* 2004;107(4):311–318.

134. Perry G, Siedlak SL, Richey P, et al. Association of heparan sulfate proteoglycan with the neurofibrillary tangles of Alzheimer's disease. *J Neurosci.* 1991;11(11):3679–3683.

135. Small DH, Nurcombe V, Reed G, et al. A heparin-binding domain in the amyloid protein precursor of Alzheimer's disease is involved in the regulation of neurite outgrowth. *J Neurosci.* 1994;14(4):2117–2127.

136. de la Monte SM, Wands JR. Review of insulin and insulin-like growth factor expression, signaling, and malfunction in the central nervous system: relevance to Alzheimer's disease. *J Alzheimers Dis.* 2005;7(1):45–61.

137. de la Monte SM, Wands JR. Alzheimer-associated neuronal thread protein mediated cell death is linked to impaired insulin signaling. *J Alzheimers Dis.* 2004;6(3):231–242.

138. de la Monte SM, Tong M, Lester-Coll N, Plater M Jr, Wands JR. Therapeutic rescue of neurodegeneration in experimental type 3 diabetes: relevance to Alzheimer's disease. *J Alzheimers Dis.* 2006;10(1):89–109.

139. de la Monte SM, Wands JR. Molecular indices of oxidative stress and mitochondrial dysfunction occur early and often progress with severity of Alzheimer's disease. *J Alzheimers Dis.* 2006;9(2):167–181.

140. Steen E, Terry BM, Rivera EJ, et al. Impaired insulin and insulin-like growth factor expression and signaling mechanisms in Alzheimer's disease – is this type 3 diabetes? *J Alzheimers Dis.* 2005;7(1):63–80.

141. Moroz N, Tong M, Longato L, Xu H, de la Monte SM. Limited Alzheimer-type neurodegeneration in experimental obesity and type 2 diabetes mellitus. *J Alzheimers Dis.* 2008;15(1):29–44.

142. Donahue JE, Berzin TM, Rafii MS, et al. Agrin in Alzheimer's disease: altered solubility and abnormal distribution within microvasculature and brain parenchyma. *Proc Natl Acad Sci U S A.* 1999;96(11):6468–6472.

143. Stopa EG, Butala P, Salloway S, et al. Cerebral cortical arteriolar angiopathy, vascular beta-amyloid, smooth muscle actin, Braak stage, and APOE genotype. *Stroke.* 2008;39(3):814–821.

144. Zipser BD, Johanson CE, Gonzalez L, et al. Microvascular injury and blood–brain barrier leakage in Alzheimer's disease. *Neurobiol Aging.* 2007;28(7):977–986.

145. Starr JM, Whalley LJ. Senile hypertension and cognitive impairment: an overview. *J Hypertens Suppl.* 1992;10(2):S31–42.

146. van Swieten JC, Geyskes GG, Derix MM, et al. Hypertension in the elderly is associated with white matter lesions and cognitive decline. *Ann Neurol.* 1991;30(6):825–830.

147. Moser DJ, Cohen RA, Clark MM, et al. Neuropsychological functioning among cardiac rehabilitation patients. *J Cardiopulm Rehabil.* 1999;19(2):91–97.

148. Ferrucci L, Guralnik JM, Salive ME, et al. Cognitive impairment and risk of stroke in the older population. *J Am Geriatr Soc.* 1996;44(3):237–241.

149. Kilander L, Andren B, Nyman H, Lind L, Boberg M, Lithell H. Atrial fibrillation is an independent determinant of low cognitive function: a cross-sectional study in elderly men. *Stroke.* 1998;29(9):1816–1820.

150. DeCarli C, Murphy DG, Tranh M, et al. The effect of white matter hyperintensity volume on brain structure, cognitive performance, and cerebral metabolism of glucose in 51 healthy adults. *Neurology.* 1995;45(11):2077–2084.

151. Lis CG, Gaviria M. Vascular dementia, hypertension, and the brain. *Neurol Res.* 1997;19(5):471–480.

152. Mortel KF, Pavol MA, Wood S, et al. Prospective studies of cerebral perfusion and cognitive testing among elderly normal volunteers and patients with ischemic vascular dementia and Alzheimer's disease. *Angiology.* 1994;45(3):171–180.

153. Fujishima M, Ibayashi S, Fujii K, Mori S. Cerebral blood flow and brain function in hypertension. *Hypertens Res.* 1995;18(2):111–117.

154. Martyn C. Blood pressure and dementia. *Lancet.* 1996;347(9009):1130–1131.

155. Pantoni L, Garcia JH. Cognitive impairment and cellular/vascular changes in the cerebral white matter. *Ann N Y Acad Sci.* 1997;826:92–102.

156. Puddu GM, Zito M, D'Andrea L, Cervone C, Lamanna P, Abate G. Clinical aspects and pathogenetic mechanisms of cognitive impairment in arterial hypertension. *Minerva Cardioangiol.* 1996;44(6):285–297.

157. Elias MF, Wolf PA, D'Agostino RB, Cobb J, White LR. Untreated blood pressure level is inversely related to cognitive functioning: the Framingham Study. *Am J Epidemiol.* 1993;138(6):353–364.

158. Rockwood K, Ebly E, Hachinski V, Hogan D. Presence and treatment of vascular risk factors in patients with vascular cognitive impairment. *Arch Neurol.* 1997;54(1):33–39.

159. Soderlund H, Nyberg L, Adolfsson R, Nilsson LG, Launer LJ. High prevalence of white matter hyperintensities in normal aging: relation to blood pressure and cognition. *Cortex.* 2003;39(4–5):1093–1105.

160. Zuccala G, Onder G, Pedone C, et al. Hypotension and cognitive impairment: selective association in patients with heart failure. *Neurology.* 2001;57(11):1986–1992.

161. Temple RO, Putzke JD, Boll TJ. Neuropsychological performance as a function of cardiac status among heart transplant candidates: a replication. *Percept Mot Skills.* 2000;91(3 Pt 1):821–825.

162. Zuccala G, Onder G, Pedone C, et al. Cognitive dysfunction as a major determinant of disability in patients with heart failure: results from a multicentre survey. On behalf of the GIFA (SIGG-ONLUS) Investigators. *J Neurol Neurosurg Psychiatry.* 2001;70(1):109–112.

163. Putzke JD, Williams MA, Rayburn BK, Kirklin JK, Boll TJ. The relationship between cardiac function and neuropsychological status among heart transplant candidates. *J Card Fail*. 1998;4(4):295–303.
164. Blumenthal JA, Madden DJ, Pierce TW, Siegel WC, Appelbaum M. Hypertension affects neurobehavioral functioning. *Psychosom Med*. 1993;55(1):44–50.
165. de Vos R, de Haes HC, Koster RW, de Haan RJ. Quality of survival after cardiopulmonary resuscitation. *Arch Intern Med*. 1999;159(3):249–254.
166. Emery J. Cognitive functioning among patients in cardiopulmonary rehabilitation patients. *J Cardiopulm Rehabil*. 1997;17:407–410.
167. Guo Z, Viitanen M, Fratiglioni L, Winblad B. Low blood pressure and dementia in elderly people: the Kungsholmen project. *BMJ*. 1996;312(7034):805–808.
168. Guo Z, Viitanen M, Fratiglioni L, Winblad B. Blood pressure and dementia in the elderly: epidemiologic perspectives. *Biomed Pharmacother*. 1997;51(2):68–73.
169. Krep H, Bottiger BW, Bock C, et al. Time course of circulatory and metabolic recovery of cat brain after cardiac arrest assessed by perfusion- and diffusion-weighted imaging and MR-spectroscopy. *Resuscitation*. 2003;58(3): 337–348.
170. Longstreth W. Brain abnormalities in the elderly: frequency and predictors in the United States (the Cardiovascular Health Study). *J Neural Transm Suppl*. 1990;53:9–16.
171. Maeland JG, Havik OE. After the myocardial infarction. A medical and psychological study with special emphasis on perceived illness. *Scand J Rehabil Med Suppl*. 1989;22: 1–87.
172. Roine RO, Kajaste S, Kaste M. Neuropsychological sequelae of cardiac arrest. *JAMA*. 1993;269(2):237–242.
173. Scherr PA, Hebert LE, Smith LA, Evans DA. Relation of blood pressure to cognitive function in the elderly. *Am J Epidemiol*. 1991;134(11):1303–1315.
174. Shaw PJ, Bates D, Cartlidge NE, et al. Early intellectual dysfunction following coronary bypass surgery. *Q J Med*. 1986;58(225):59–68.
175. Skoog I, Lernfelt B, Landahl S, et al. 15-year longitudinal study of blood pressure and dementia. *Lancet*. 1996;347(9009):1141–1145.
176. Tohgi H, Chiba K, Kimura M. Twenty-four-hour variation of blood pressure in vascular dementia of the Binswanger type. *Stroke*. 1991;22(5):603–608.
177. Wilson BA. Cognitive functioning of adult survivors of cerebral hypoxia. *Brain Inj*. 1996;10(12):863–874.
178. Blumenthal JA, Madden DJ, Burker EJ, et al. A preliminary study of the effects of cardiac procedures on cognitive performance. *Int J Psychosom*. 1991;38(1–4):13–16.
179. McKhann GM, Grega MA, Borowicz LM Jr, Selnes OA, Baumgartner WA, Royall RM. Encephalopathy and stroke after coronary artery bypass grafting. *Curr Treat Options Cardiovasc Med*. 2004;6(3):171–178.
180. Newman MF, Kirchner JL, Phillips-Bute B, et al. Longitudinal assessment of neurocognitive function after coronary-artery bypass surgery. *N Engl J Med*. 2001;344(6):395–402.
181. Browndyke JN, Moser DJ, Cohen RA, et al. Acute neuropsychological functioning following cardiosurgical interventions associated with the production of intraoperative cerebral microemboli. *Clin Neuropsychol*. 2002;16(4):463–471.
182. Uekermann J, Suchan B, Daum I, Kseibi S, Perthel M, Laas J. Neuropsychological deficits after mechanical aortic valve replacement. *J Heart Valve Dis*. 2005;14(3):338–343.
183. Zamvar V, Webster S, Falase B. Neurocognitive impairment after minimally invasive aortic valve replacement. *Eur J Cardiothorac Surg*. 2001;20(4):889–890.
184. Herrmann M, Ebert AD, Galazky I, Wunderlich MT, Kunz WS, Huth C. Neurobehavioral outcome prediction after cardiac surgery: role of neurobiochemical markers of damage to neuronal and glial brain tissue. *Stroke*. 2000;31(3):645–650.
185. Massaro AR, Dutra AP, Almeida DR, Diniz RV, Malheiros SM. Transcranial Doppler assessment of cerebral blood flow: effect of cardiac transplantation. *Neurology*. 2006;66(1):124–126.
186. Zuccala G, Cattel C, Manes-Gravina E, Di Niro MG, Cocchi A, Bernabei R. Left ventricular dysfunction: a clue to cognitive impairment in older patients with heart failure. *J Neurol Neurosurg Psychiatry*. 1997;63(4):509–512.
187. Roman GC. Vascular dementia prevention: a risk factor analysis. *Cerebrovasc Dis*. 2005;20(Suppl 2):91–100.
188. Zuccala G, Marzetti E, Cesari M, et al. Correlates of cognitive impairment among patients with heart failure: results of a multicenter survey. *Am J Med*. 2005;118(5):496–502.
189. Clark AP, McDougall G. Cognitive impairment in heart failure. *Dimens Crit Care Nurs*. 2006;25(3):93–100; quiz 101–102.
190. Petrucci RJ, Truesdell KC, Carter A, et al. Cognitive dysfunction in advanced heart failure and prospective cardiac assist device patients. *Ann Thorac Surg*. 2006;81(5):1738–1744.
191. Grubb NR, Fox KA, Smith K, et al. Memory impairment in out-of-hospital cardiac arrest survivors is associated with global reduction in brain volume, not focal hippocampal injury. *Stroke*. 2000;31(7):1509–1514.
192. Paul RH, Gunstad J, Poppas A, et al. Neuroimaging and cardiac correlates of cognitive function among patients with cardiac disease. *Cerebrovasc Dis*. 2005;20(2):129–133.
193. Gunstad J, Macgregor KL, Paul RH, et al. Cardiac rehabilitation improves cognitive performance in older adults with cardiovascular disease. *J Cardiopulm Rehabil*. 2005;25(3): 173–176.
194. Albert MS, Jones K, Savage CR, et al. Predictors of cognitive change in older persons: MacArthur studies of successful aging. *Psychol Aging*. 1995;10(4):578–589.
195. Borozdina LV, Molchanova ON. The quality of self-concept in old age. *Z Gerontol Geriatr*. 1997;30(4):298–305.
196. Corless IB, Bakken S, Nicholas PK, et al. Predictors of perception of cognitive functioning in HIV/AIDS. *J Assoc Nurses AIDS Care*. 2000;11(3):19–26.
197. de Haes JC, de Ruiter JH, Tempelaar R, Pennink BJ. The distinction between affect and cognition in the quality of life of cancer patients–sensitivity and stability. *Qual Life Res*. 1992;1(5):315–322.
198. Diener E, Oishi S, Lucas RE. Personality, culture, and subjective well-being: emotional and cognitive evaluations of life. *Annu Rev Psychol*. 2003;54:403–425.
199. Graves KD. Social cognitive theory and cancer patients quality of life: a meta-analysis of psychosocial intervention components. *Health Psychol*. 2003;22(2):210–219.
200. Jobe JB. Cognitive psychology and self-reports: models and methods. *Qual Life Res*. 2003;12(3):219–227.

201. Joyce CR, Hickey A, McGee HM, O'Boyle CA. A theory-based method for the evaluation of individual quality of life: the SEIQoL. *Qual Life Res.* 2003;12(3):275–280.

202. McAuley E, Elavsky S, Jerome GJ, Konopack JF, Marquez DX. Physical activity-related well-being in older adults: social cognitive influences. *Psychol Aging.* 2005;20(2):295–302.

203. Mitchell AJ, Benito-Leon J, Gonzalez JM, Rivera-Navarro J. Quality of life and its assessment in multiple sclerosis: integrating physical and psychological components of wellbeing. *Lancet Neurol.* 2005;4(9):556–566.

204. Moore SL, Metcalf B, Schow E. The quest for meaning in aging. *Geriatr Nurs.* 2006;27(5):293–299.

205. Pajalic Z, Karlsson S, Westergren A. Functioning and subjective health among stroke survivors after discharge from hospital. *J Adv Nurs.* 2006;54(4):457–466.

206. Pratt SI, Mueser KT, Smith TE, Lu W. Self-efficacy and psychosocial functioning in schizophrenia: a mediational analysis. *Schizophr Res.* 2005;78(2–3):187–197.

207. Prenda KM, Lachman ME. Planning for the future: a life management strategy for increasing control and life satisfaction in adulthood. *Psychol Aging.* 2001;16(2):206–216.

208. Ready RE, Ott BR, Grace J. Insight and cognitive impairment: effects on quality-of-life reports from mild cognitive impairment and Alzheimer's disease patients. *Am J Alzheimers Dis Other Demen.* 2006;21(4):242–248.

209. Sands LP, Ferreira P, Stewart AL, Brod M, Yaffe K. What explains differences between dementia patients' and their caregivers' ratings of patients' quality of life? *Am J Geriatr Psychiatry.* 2004;12(3):272–280.

210. Schimmack U, Radhakrishnan P, Oishi S, Dzokoto V, Ahadi S. Culture, personality, and subjective well-being: integrating process models of life satisfaction. *J Pers Soc Psychol.* 2002;82(4):582–593.

211. Smith SC, Murray J, Banerjee S, et al. What constitutes health-related quality of life in dementia? Development of a conceptual framework for people with dementia and their carers. *Int J Geriatr Psychiatry.* 2005;20(9):889–895.

212. Spector A, Orrell M, Davies S, Woods B. Reality orientation for dementia. *Cochrane Database Syst Rev.* 2000(4):CD001119.

213. Jagger C, Spiers N, Arthur A. The role of sensory and cognitive function in the onset of activity restriction in older people. *Disabil Rehabil.* 2005;27(5):277–283.

214. Njegovan V, Hing MM, Mitchell SL, Molnar FJ. The hierarchy of functional loss associated with cognitive decline in older persons. *J Gerontol A Biol Sci Med Sci.* 2001;56(10):M638–643.

215. Allen SM, Mor V. The prevalence and consequences of unmet need. Contrasts between older and younger adults with disability. *Med Care.* 1997;35(11):1132–1148.

216. Cipher DJ, Clifford PA. Dementia, pain, depression, behavioral disturbances, and ADLs: toward a comprehensive conceptualization of quality of life in long-term care. *Int J Geriatr Psychiatry.* 2004;19(8):741–748.

217. Hellstrom Y, Andersson M, Hallberg IR. Quality of life among older people in Sweden receiving help from informal and/or formal helpers at home or in special accommodation. *Health Soc Care Community.* 2004;12(6):504–516.

218. Hwu YJ. The impact of chronic illness on patients. *Rehabil Nurs.* 1995;20(4):221–225.

219. Newcomer RJ, Clay TH, Yaffe K, Covinsky KE. Mortality risk and prospective medicare expenditures for persons with dementia. *J Am Geriatr Soc.* 2005;53(11):2001–2006.

220. Sloane PD, Zimmerman S, Williams CS, Reed PS, Gill KS, Preisser JS. Evaluating the quality of life of long-term care residents with dementia. *Gerontologist.* 2005;45 Spec No 1(1):37–49.

221. Wu AW, Yasui Y, Alzola C, et al. Predicting functional status outcomes in hospitalized patients aged 80 years and older. *J Am Geriatr Soc.* 2000;48(5 Suppl):S6-S15.

222. Heaton RK, Marcotte TD, Mindt MR, et al. The impact of HIV-associated neuropsychological impairment on everyday functioning. *J Int Neuropsychol Soc.* 2004;10(3):317–331.

223. McCall WV, Dunn AG. Cognitive deficits are associated with functional impairment in severely depressed patients. *Psychiatry Res.* 2003;121(2):179–184.

224. Osowiecki DM, Cohen RA, Morrow KM, et al. Neurocognitive and psychological contributions to quality of life in HIV-1-infected women. *AIDS.* 2000;14(10):1327–1332.

225. Hoth KF, Poppas A, Moser DJ, Paul RH, Cohen RA. Cardiac dysfunction and cognition in older adults with heart failure. *Cogn Behav Neurol.* 2008;21(2):65–72.

226. Hoth KF, Nash J, Poppas A, Ellison KE, Paul RH, Cohen RA. Effects of cardiac resynchronization therapy on health-related quality of life in older adults with heart failure. *Clin Interv Aging.* 2008;3(3):553–560.

227. Okonkwo OC, Cohen RA, Gunstad J, Tremont G, Alosco ML, Poppas A. Longitudinal Trajectories of Cognitive Decline among Older Adults with Cardiovascular Disease. *Cerebrovasc Dis.* 2010;30(4):362–373

228. Bates MC, Campbell JE, Stone PA, Jaff MR, Broce M, Lavigne PS. Factors affecting long-term survival following renal artery stenting. *Catheter Cardiovasc Interv.* 2007;69(7):1037–1043.

229. Chaldakov GN, Fiore M, Tonchev AB, et al. Homo obesus: a metabotrophin-deficient species. Pharmacology and nutrition insight. *Curr Pharm Des.* 2007;13(21):2176–2179.

230. Chow C, Cardona M, Raju PK, et al. Cardiovascular disease and risk factors among 345 adults in rural India – the Andhra Pradesh Rural Health Initiative. *Int J Cardiol.* 2007;116(2):180–185.

231. Cohn JS. Oxidized fat in the diet, postprandial lipaemia and cardiovascular disease. *Curr Opin Lipidol.* 2002;13(1):19–24.

232. Fava F, Lovegrove JA, Gitau R, Jackson KG, Tuohy KM. The gut microbiota and lipid metabolism: implications for human health and coronary heart disease. *Curr Med Chem.* 2006;13(25):3005–3021.

233. Friedlander AH, Weinreb J, Friedlander I, Yagiela JA. Metabolic syndrome: pathogenesis, medical care and dental implications. *J Am Dent Assoc.* 2007;138(2):179–187; quiz 248.

234. Fuller JH, Stevens LK, Wang SL. Risk factors for cardiovascular mortality and morbidity: the WHO Mutinational Study of Vascular Disease in Diabetes. *Diabetologia.* 2001;44(Suppl 2):S54–64.

235. Hlaing WM, Koutoubi S, Huffman FG. Differences in arterial stiffness and its correlates in tri-ethnic young men and women. *Ethn Dis (Autumn).* 2006;16(4):837–843.

236. Karadag O, Calguneri M, Atalar E, et al. Novel cardiovascular risk factors and cardiac event predictors in female

inactive systemic lupus erythematosus patients. *Clin Rheumatol.* 2007;26(5):695–699.

237. Krekoukia M, Nassis GP, Psarra G, Skenderi K, Chrousos GP, Sidossis LS. Elevated total and central adiposity and low physical activity are associated with insulin resistance in children. *Metabolism.* 2007;56(2):206–213.

238. Mozaffarian D. Trans fatty acids – effects on systemic inflammation and endothelial function. *Atheroscler Suppl.* 2006;7(2):29–32.

239. Ruef J, Marz W, Winkelmann BR. Markers for endothelial dysfunction, but not markers for oxidative stress correlate with classical risk factors and the severity of coronary artery disease. (A subgroup analysis from the Ludwigshafen Risk and Cardiovascular Health Study). *Scand Cardiovasc J.* 2006;40(5):274–279.

240. Sitzer M, Markus HS, Mendall MA, Liehr R, Knorr U, Steinmetz H. C-reactive protein and carotid intimal medial thickness in a community population. *J Cardiovasc Risk.* 2002;9(2):97–103.

241. Smith NL, Savage PJ, Heckbert SR, et al. Glucose, blood pressure, and lipid control in older people with and without diabetes mellitus: the Cardiovascular Health Study. *J Am Geriatr Soc.* 2002;50(3):416–423.

242. Tziomalos K, Athyros VG, Karagiannis A, Mikhailidis DP. Endothelial function, arterial stiffness and lipid lowering drugs. *Expert Opin Ther Targets.* 2007;11(9):1143–1160.

243. Wang-Polagruto JF, Villablanca AC, Polagruto JA, et al. Chronic consumption of flavanol-rich cocoa improves endothelial function and decreases vascular cell adhesion molecule in hypercholesterolemic postmenopausal women. *J Cardiovasc Pharmacol.* 2006;47(Suppl 2):S177-S186; discussion S206–S179.

244. Brown DW, Giles WH, Greenlund KJ. Blood pressure parameters and risk of fatal stroke, NHANES II mortality study. *Am J Hypertens.* 2007;20(3):338–341.

245. Conen D, Ridker PM, Buring JE, Glynn RJ. Risk of cardiovascular events among women with high normal blood pressure or blood pressure progression: prospective cohort study. *BMJ.* 2007;335(7617):432.

246. Cordonnier C, van der Flier WM, Sluimer JD, Leys D, Barkhof F, Scheltens P. Prevalence and severity of microbleeds in a memory clinic setting. *Neurology.* 2006;66(9):1356–1360.

247. Franco OH, Peeters A, Bonneux L, de Laet C. Blood pressure in adulthood and life expectancy with cardiovascular disease in men and women: life course analysis. *Hypertension.* 2005;46(2):280–286.

248. Hyman DJ, Pavlik VN. Uncontrolled hypertension as a risk for coronary artery disease: patient characteristics and the role of physician intervention. *Curr Atheroscler Rep.* 2003;5(2):131–138.

249. Kotani K, Osaki Y, Sakane N, Adachi S, Ishimaru Y. Risk factors for silent cerebral infarction in the elderly. *Arch Med Res.* 2004;35(6):522–524.

250. Vermeer SE, Hollander M, van Dijk EJ, Hofman A, Koudstaal PJ, Breteler MM. Silent brain infarcts and white matter lesions increase stroke risk in the general population: the Rotterdam Scan Study. *Stroke.* 2003;34(5):1126–1129.

251. Vermeer SE, Koudstaal PJ, Oudkerk M, Hofman A, Breteler MM. Prevalence and risk factors of silent brain infarcts in

the population-based Rotterdam Scan Study. *Stroke.* 2002;33(1):21–25.

252. Goldstein IB, Bartzokis G, Guthrie D, Shapiro D. Ambulatory blood pressure and brain atrophy in the healthy elderly. *Neurology.* 2002;59(5):713–719.

253. Reitz C, Patel B, Tang MX, Manly J, Mayeux R, Luchsinger JA. Relation between vascular risk factors and neuropsychological test performance among elderly persons with Alzheimer's disease. *J Neurol Sci.* 2007;257(1–2):194–201.

254. Tuomilehto J. Impact of age on cardiovascular risk: implications for cardiovascular disease management. *Atheroscler Suppl.* 2004;5(2):9–17.

255. Tuomilehto J, Piha T, Nissinen A, Geboers J, Puska P. Trends in stroke mortality and in antihypertensive treatment in Finland from 1972 to 1984 with special reference to North Karelia. *J Hum Hypertens.* 1987;1(3):201–208.

256. Yao H, Sadoshima S, Ibayashi S, Kuwabara Y, Ichiya Y, Fujishima M. Leukoaraiosis and dementia in hypertensive patients. *Stroke.* 1992;23(11):1673–1677.

257. Tell GS, Rutan GH, Kronmal RA, et al. Correlates of blood pressure in community-dwelling older adults. The Cardiovascular Health Study. Cardiovascular Health Study (CHS) Collaborative Research Group. *Hypertension.* 1994;23(1):59–67.

258. Kannel WB, Castelli WP, McNamara PM, McKee PA, Feinleib M. Role of blood pressure in the development of congestive heart failure. The Framingham study. *N Engl J Med.* 1972;287(16):781–787.

259. Kannel WB, Wolf PA. Peripheral and cerebral atherothrombosis and cardiovascular events in different vascular territories: insights from the Framingham Study. *Curr Atheroscler Rep.* 2006;8(4):317–323.

260. Tilvis RS, Kahonen-Vare MH, Jolkkonen J, Valvanne J, Pitkala KH, Strandberg TE. Predictors of cognitive decline and mortality of aged people over a 10-year period. *J Gerontol A Biol Sci Med Sci.* 2004;59(3):268–274.

261. Knopman DS, Mosley TH, Catellier DJ, Sharrett AR. Cardiovascular risk factors and cerebral atrophy in a middle-aged cohort. *Neurology.* 2005;65(6):876–881.

262. Pavlik VN, Hyman DJ, Doody R. Cardiovascular risk factors and cognitive function in adults 30–59 years of age (NHANES III). *Neuroepidemiology.* 2005;24(1–2):42–50.

263. Nagata K, Sasaki E, Goda K, et al. Cerebrovascular disease in type 2 diabetic patients without hypertension. *Stroke.* 2003;34(12):e232-e233; author reply e232–e233.

264. Verro P, Levine SR, Tietjen GE. Cerebrovascular ischemic events with high positive anticardiolipin antibodies. *Stroke.* 1998;29(11):2245–2253.

265. Feil D, Marmon T, Unutzer J. Cognitive impairment, chronic medical illness, and risk of mortality in an elderly cohort. *Am J Geriatr Psychiatry.* 2003;11(5):551–560.

266. Kumral E, Ozkaya B, Sagduyu A, Sirin H, Vardarli E, Pehlivan M. The Ege Stroke Registry: a hospital-based study in the Aegean region, Izmir, Turkey. Analysis of 2, 000 stroke patients. *Cerebrovasc Dis.* 1998;8(5):278–288.

267. Klawans HL, Shekelle RB, Ostfeld AM, Tufo HM. Epidemiology of stroke in elderly persons. *Neurology.* 1970;20(4):373–374.

268. Saks K, Kolk H, Allev R, et al. Health status of the older population in Estonia. *Croat Med J.* 2001;42(6):663–668.

269. Verhaegen P, Borchelt M, Smith J. Relation between cardiovascular and metabolic disease and cognition in very old age: cross-sectional and longitudinal findings from the berlin aging study. *Health Psychol.* 2003;22(6):559–569.

270. Posner HB, Tang MX, Luchsinger J, Lantigua R, Stern Y, Mayeux R. The relationship of hypertension in the elderly to AD, vascular dementia, and cognitive function. *Neurology.* 2002;58(8):1175–1181.

271. Landmesser U, Harrison DG, Drexler H. Oxidant stress – a major cause of reduced endothelial nitric oxide availability in cardiovascular disease. *Eur J Clin Pharmacol.* 2006;62(Suppl 13):13–19.

272. Suzuki K, Juo SH, Rundek T, et al. Genetic contribution to brachial artery flow-mediated dilation: The Northern Manhattan Family Study. *Atherosclerosis.* 2008;197(1): 212–216.

273. Constans J, Conri C. Circulating markers of endothelial function in cardiovascular disease. *Clin Chim Acta.* 2006;368(1–2):33–47.

274. Caglayan E, Blaschke F, Takata Y, Hsueh WA. Metabolic syndrome-interdependence of the cardiovascular and metabolic pathways. *Curr Opin Pharmacol.* 2005;5(2):135–142.

275. Kernan WN, Inzucchi SE. Type 2 diabetes mellitus and insulin resistance: stroke prevention and management. *Curr Treat Options Neurol.* 2004;6(6):443–450.

276. Stolar MW, Chilton RJ. Type 2 diabetes, cardiovascular risk, and the link to insulin resistance. *Clin Ther.* 2003;25(Suppl B):B4–B31.

277. Vallbracht KB, Schwimmbeck PL, Seeberg B, Kuhl U, Schultheiss HP. Endothelial dysfunction of peripheral arteries in patients with immunohistologically confirmed myocardial inflammation correlates with endothelial expression of human leukocyte antigens and adhesion molecules in myocardial biopsies. *J Am Coll Cardiol.* 2002;40(3):515–520.

278. Dumont AS, Hyndman ME, Dumont RJ, et al. Improvement of endothelial function in insulin-resistant carotid arteries treated with pravastatin. *J Neurosurg.* 2001;95(3):466–471.

279. Parving HH, Nielsen FS, Bang LE, et al. Macro-microangiopathy and endothelial dysfunction in NIDDM patients with and without diabetic nephropathy. *Diabetologia.* 1996;39(12):1590–1597.

280. Woods SC, Seeley RJ, Baskin DG, Schwartz MW. Insulin and the blood–brain barrier. *Curr Pharm Des.* 2003;9(10):795–800.

281. Watson GS, Craft S. Insulin resistance, inflammation, and cognition in Alzheimer's disease: lessons for multiple sclerosis. *J Neurol Sci.* 2006;245(1–2):21–33.

282. Veneman T, Mitrakou A, Mokan M, Cryer P, Gerich J. Effect of hyperketonemia and hyperlacticacidemia on symptoms, cognitive dysfunction, and counterregulatory hormone responses during hypoglycemia in normal humans. *Diabetes.* 1994;43(11):1311–1317.

283. Vanhanen M, Soininen H. Glucose intolerance, cognitive impairment and Alzheimer's disease. *Curr Opin Neurol.* 1998;11(6):673–677.

284. Vanhanen M, Kuusisto J, Koivisto K, et al. Type-2 diabetes and cognitive function in a non-demented population. *Acta Neurol Scand.* 1999;100(2):97–101.

285. Anthony K, Reed LJ, Dunn JT, et al. Attenuation of insulin-evoked responses in brain networks controlling appetite and reward in insulin resistance: the cerebral basis for impaired control of food intake in metabolic syndrome? *Diabetes.* 2006;55(11):2986–2992.

286. Biessels GJ, Kappelle LJ. Increased risk of Alzheimer's disease in Type II diabetes: insulin resistance of the brain or insulin-induced amyloid pathology? *Biochem Soc Trans.* 2005;33(Pt 5):1041–1044.

287. Enzinger C, Fazekas F, Matthews PM, et al. Risk factors for progression of brain atrophy in aging: six-year follow-up of normal subjects. *Neurology.* 2005;64(10):1704–1711.

288. Park JH, Kwon HM, Roh JK. Metabolic syndrome is more associated with intracranial atherosclerosis than extracranial atherosclerosis. *Eur J Neurol.* 2007;14(4):379–386.

289. Biessels GJ, Gispen WH. The impact of diabetes on cognition: what can be learned from rodent models? *Neurobiol Aging.* 2005;26(Suppl 1):36–41.

290. Burcelin R. The incretins: a link between nutrients and well-being. *Br J Nutr.* 2005;93(Suppl 1):S147–156.

291. Carro E, Spuch C, Trejo JL, Antequera D, Torres-Aleman I. Choroid plexus megalin is involved in neuroprotection by serum insulin-like growth factor I. *J Neurosci.* 2005;25(47):10884–10893.

292. Convit A. Links between cognitive impairment in insulin resistance: an explanatory model. *Neurobiol Aging.* 2005;26(Suppl 1):31–35.

293. Hendrickx H, McEwen BS, Ouderaa F. Metabolism, mood and cognition in aging: the importance of lifestyle and dietary intervention. *Neurobiol Aging.* 2005;26(Suppl 1): 1–5.

294. Messier C, Teutenberg K. The role of insulin, insulin growth factor, and insulin-degrading enzyme in brain aging and Alzheimer's disease. *Neural Plast.* 2005;12(4):311–328.

295. Strachan MW. Insulin and cognitive function in humans: experimental data and therapeutic considerations. *Biochem Soc Trans.* 2005;33(Pt 5):1037–1040.

296. Abbatecola AM, Rizzo MR, Barbieri M, et al. Postprandial plasma glucose excursions and cognitive functioning in aged type 2 diabetics. *Neurology.* 2006;67(2):235–240.

297. McNay EC, Williamson A, McCrimmon RJ, Sherwin RS. Cognitive and neural hippocampal effects of long-term moderate recurrent hypoglycemia. *Diabetes.* 2006;55(4): 1088–1095.

298. Salkovic-Petrisic M, Tribl F, Schmidt M, Hoyer S, Riederer P. Alzheimer-like changes in protein kinase B and glycogen synthase kinase-3 in rat frontal cortex and hippocampus after damage to the insulin signalling pathway. *J Neurochem.* 2006;96(4):1005–1015.

299. Yaffe K, Blackwell T, Whitmer RA, Krueger K, Barrett Connor E. Glycosylated hemoglobin level and development of mild cognitive impairment or dementia in older women. *J Nutr Health Aging.* 2006;10(4):293–295.

300. Craft S. Insulin resistance and Alzheimer's disease pathogenesis: potential mechanisms and implications for treatment. *Curr Alzheimer Res.* 2007;4(2):147–152.

301. Droge W, Schipper HM. Oxidative stress and aberrant signaling in aging and cognitive decline. *Aging Cell.* 2007;6(3):361–370.

302. Fernandez S, Fernandez AM, Lopez-Lopez C, Torres-Aleman I. Emerging roles of insulin-like growth factor-I in the adult brain. *Growth Horm IGF Res.* 2007;17(2):89–95.

303. Gotkine M. Vascular risk factors and cognitive decline among elderly male twins. *Neurology.* 2007;68(21):1871; author reply 1871.

304. Manschot SM, Biessels GJ, de Valk H, et al. Metabolic and vascular determinants of impaired cognitive performance and abnormalities on brain magnetic resonance imaging in patients with type 2 diabetes. *Diabetologia.* 2007;50(11): 2388–2397.

305. Morgan TE, Wong AM, Finch CE. Anti-inflammatory mechanisms of dietary restriction in slowing aging processes. *Interdiscip Top Gerontol.* 2007;35:83–97.

306. Zhao Z, Xiang Z, Haroutunian V, Buxbaum JD, Stetka B, Pasinetti GM. Insulin degrading enzyme activity selectively decreases in the hippocampal formation of cases at high risk to develop Alzheimer's disease. *Neurobiol Aging.* 2007;28(6):824–830.

307. Zhao WQ, Alkon DL. Role of insulin and insulin receptor in learning and memory. *Mol Cell Endocrinol.* 2001;177(1–2):125–134.

308. Dede DS, Yavuz B, Yavuz BB, et al. Assessment of endothelial function in Alzheimer's disease: is Alzheimer's disease a vascular disease? *J Am Geriatr Soc.* 2007;55(10):1613–1617.

309. Simionescu M, Antohe F. Functional ultrastructure of the vascular endothelium: changes in various pathologies. *Handb Exp Pharmacol.* 2006;176(Pt 1):41–69.

310. Hellstrom HR. The altered homeostatic theory: a hypothesis proposed to be useful in understanding and preventing ischemic heart disease, hypertension, and diabetes–including reducing the risk of age and atherosclerosis. *Med Hypotheses.* 2007;68(2):415–433.

311. Takeuchi M, Yamagishi S. Alternative routes for the formation of glyceraldehyde-derived AGEs (TAGE) in vivo. *Med Hypotheses.* 2004;63(3):453–455.

312. Kalaria RN. Small vessel disease and Alzheimer's dementia: pathological considerations. *Cerebrovasc Dis.* 2002;13(Suppl 2):48–52.

313. Kalaria RN. The role of cerebral ischemia in Alzheimer's disease. *Neurobiol Aging.* 2000;21(2):321–330.

314. Perlmutter LS, Chui HC. Microangiopathy, the vascular basement membrane and Alzheimer's disease: a review. *Brain Res Bull.* 1990;24(5):677–686.

315. Kalra PS, Kalra SP. Obesity and metabolic syndrome: long-term benefits of central leptin gene therapy. *Drugs Today (Barc).* 2002;38(11):745–757.

316. Licata G, Scaglione R, Barbagallo M, et al. Effect of obesity on left ventricular function studied by radionuclide angiocardiography. *Int J Obes.* 1991;15(4):295–302.

317. Parrinello G, Scaglione R, Pinto A, et al. Central obesity and hypertension: the role of plasma endothelin. *Am J Hypertens.* 1996;9(12 Pt 1):1186–1191.

318. Gunstad J, Paul RH, Cohen RA, Tate DF, Gordon E. Obesity is associated with memory deficits in young and middle-aged adults. *Eat Weight Disord.* 2006;11(1): e15–19.

319. Gunstad J, Paul RH, Cohen RA, Tate DF, Spitznagel MB, Gordon E. Elevated body mass index is associated with executive dysfunction in otherwise healthy adults. *Compr Psychiatry.* 2007;48(1):57–61.

320. Rodin J, Slochower J, Fleming B. Effects of degree of obesity, age of onset, and weight loss on responsiveness to sensory and external stimuli. *J Comp Physiol Psychol.* 1977;91(3):586–597.

321. Garrow JS, Stalley S. Cognitive thresholds and human body weight. *Proc Nutr Soc.* 1977;36(1):18A.

322. Rodin J, Singer JL. Eye-shift, thought, and obesity. *J Pers.* 1976;44(4):594–610.

323. Wolf PA, Beiser A, Elias MF, Au R, Vasan RS, Seshadri S. Relation of obesity to cognitive function: importance of central obesity and synergistic influence of concomitant hypertension. The Framingham Heart Study. *Curr Alzheimer Res.* 2007;4(2):111–116.

324. Gray J, Yeo GS, Cox JJ, et al. Hyperphagia, severe obesity, impaired cognitive function, and hyperactivity associated with functional loss of one copy of the brain-derived neurotrophic factor (BDNF) gene. *Diabetes.* 2006;55(12): 3366–3371.

325. Pignatti R, Bertella L, Albani G, Mauro A, Molinari E, Semenza C. Decision-making in obesity: a study using the Gambling Task. *Eat Weight Disord.* 2006;11(3):126–132.

326. Kuo HK, Jones RN, Milberg WP, et al. Cognitive function in normal-weight, overweight, and obese older adults: an analysis of the Advanced Cognitive Training for Independent and Vital Elderly cohort. *J Am Geriatr Soc.* 2006;54(1):97–103.

327. Ford ES, Giles WH, Dietz WH. Prevalence of the metabolic syndrome among US adults: findings from the third National Health and Nutrition Examination Survey. *JAMA.* 2002;287(3):356–359.

328. Meigs JB, Wilson PW, Nathan DM, D'Agostino RB Sr, Williams K, Haffner SM. Prevalence and characteristics of the metabolic syndrome in the San Antonio Heart and Framingham Offspring Studies. *Diabetes.* 2003;52(8): 2160–2167.

329. Alexander CM, Landsman PB, Teutsch SM, Haffner SM. NCEP-defined metabolic syndrome, diabetes, and prevalence of coronary heart disease among NHANES III participants age 50 years and older. *Diabetes.* 2003;52(5):1210–1214.

330. Grundy SM. Metabolic syndrome scientific statement by the American Heart Association and the National Heart, Lung, and Blood Institute. *Arterioscler Thromb Vasc Biol.* 2005;25(11):2243–2244.

331. Grundy SM, Brewer HB Jr, Cleeman JI, Smith SC Jr, Lenfant C. Definition of metabolic syndrome: report of the National Heart, Lung, and Blood Institute/American Heart Association conference on scientific issues related to definition. *Arterioscler Thromb Vasc Biol.* 2004;24(2): e13–18.

332. Isomaa B, Almgren P, Tuomi T, et al. Cardiovascular morbidity and mortality associated with the metabolic syndrome. *Diabetes Care.* 2001;24(4):683–689.

333. Lakka HM, Laaksonen DE, Lakka TA, et al. The metabolic syndrome and total and cardiovascular disease mortality in middle-aged men. *JAMA.* 2002;288(21):2709–2716.

334. Bowler JV, Hachinski V. Vascular cognitive impairment: a new approach to vascular dementia. *Baillieres Clin Neurol.* 1995;4(2):357–376.

335. Bowler JV, Steenhuis R, Hachinski V. Conceptual background to vascular cognitive impairment. *Alzheimer Dis Assoc Disord.* 1999;13(Suppl 3):S30–S37.

336. DeCarli C, Miller BL, Swan GE, Reed T, Wolf PA, Carmelli D. Cerebrovascular and brain morphologic correlates of

mild cognitive impairment in the National Heart, Lung, and Blood Institute Twin Study. *Arch Neurol.* 2001;58(4): 643–647.

337. Rockwood K. Vascular cognitive impairment and vascular dementia. *J Neurol Sci.* 2002;203–204:23–27.

338. Choi I, Mikkelsen RB. Plasmodium falciparum: ATP/ADP transport across the parasitophorous vacuolar and plasma membranes. *Exp Parasitol.* 1990;71(4):452–462.

339. Goldberg MP, Choi DW. Intracellular free calcium increases in cultured cortical neurons deprived of oxygen and glucose. *Stroke.* 1990;21(11 Suppl):III75–III77.

340. Simon R, Shiraishi K. *N*-methyl-d-aspartate antagonist reduces stroke size and regional glucose metabolism. *Ann Neurol.* 1990;27(6):606–611.

341. Roman GC. Brain hypoperfusion: a critical factor in vascular dementia. *Neurol Res.* 2004;26(5):454–458.

342. Taylor J, Stott DJ. Chronic heart failure and cognitive impairment: co-existence of conditions or true association? *Eur J Heart Fail.* 2002;4(1):7–9.

343. Lackey J. Cognitive impairment and congestive heart failure. *Nurs Stand.* 2004;18(44):33–36.

344. Rozzini R, Sabatini T, Trabucchi M. Cognitive impairment and mortality in elderly patients with heart failure. *Am J Med.* 2004;116(2):137–138; author reply 138.

345. Stump TE, Callahan CM, Hendrie HC. Cognitive impairment and mortality in older primary care patients. *J Am Geriatr Soc.* 2001;49(7):934–940.

346. Pullicino PM, Hart J. Cognitive impairment in congestive heart failure?: Embolism vs hypoperfusion. *Neurology.* 2001;57(11):1945–1946.

347. Staniforth AD, Kinnear WJ, Cowley AJ. Cognitive impairment in heart failure with Cheyne-Stokes respiration. *Heart.* 2001;85(1):18–22.

348. Riegel B, Bennett JA, Davis A, et al. Cognitive impairment in heart failure: issues of measurement and etiology. *Am J Crit Care.* 2002;11(6):520–528.

349. Di Carlo A, Baldereschi M, Amaducci L, et al. Cognitive impairment without dementia in older people: prevalence, vascular risk factors, impact on disability. The Italian Longitudinal Study on Aging. *J Am Geriatr Soc.* 2000;48(7):775–782.

350. Sabatini T, Barbisoni P, Rozzini R, Trabucchi M. Hypotension and cognitive impairment: selective association in patients with heart failure. *Neurology.* 2002;59(7):1118–1119; author reply 1119.

351. Bornstein RA, Starling RC, Myerowitz PD, Haas GJ. Neuropsychological function in patients with end-stage heart failure before and after cardiac transplantation. *Acta Neurol Scand.* 1995;91(4):260–265.

352. Woo MA, Macey PM, Keens PT, et al. Functional abnormalities in brain areas that mediate autonomic nervous system control in advanced heart failure. *J Card Fail.* 2005;11(6):437–446.

353. Alves TC, Rays J, Fraguas R Jr, et al. Localized cerebral blood flow reductions in patients with heart failure: a study using 99mTc-HMPAO SPECT. *J Neuroimaging.* 2005;15(2):150–156.

354. Cooper ES, West JW, Jaffe ME, Goldberg HI, Kawamura J, McHenry LC Jr. The relation between cardiac function and cerebral blood flow in stroke patients. 1. Effect of CO 2 inhalation. *Stroke.* 1970;1(5):330–347.

355. Gruhn N, Larsen FS, Boesgaard S, et al. Cerebral blood flow in patients with chronic heart failure before and after heart transplantation. *Stroke.* 2001;32(11):2530–2533.

356. Choi BR, Kim JS, Yang YJ, et al. Factors associated with decreased cerebral blood flow in congestive heart failure secondary to idiopathic dilated cardiomyopathy. *Am J Cardiol.* 2006;97(9):1365–1369.

357. Alves TC, Busatto GF. Regional cerebral blood flow reductions, heart failure and Alzheimer's disease. *Neurol Res.* 2006;28(6):579–587.

358. Mathias CJ. Cerebral hypoperfusion and impaired cerebral function in cardiac failure. *Eur Heart J.* 2000;21(5):346.

359. Raiha I, Tarvonen S, Kurki T, Rajala T, Sourander L. Relationship between vascular factors and white matter low attenuation of the brain. *Acta Neurol Scand.* 1993;87(4):286–289.

360. Serrador J, Milberg WP, Lipsitz LA. Cerebral Hemodynamics in the Elderly. In: Paul RC RH, Ott BR, Salloway S, eds. *Vascular Dementia: Cerebrovascular Mechanisms and Clinical Management.* Totowa, NJ: Humana Press Inc.; 2005:75–86.

361. Gokce N. L-arginine and hypertension. *J Nutr.* 2004;134(10 Suppl):2807S-2811S; discussion 2818S–2819S.

362. Tharaux PL. [Effect of sleep apnea syndrome on the vascular endothelium]. *Rev Neurol (Paris).* 2003;159(11 Suppl):6S102–6S106.

363. Nicholls SJ, Tuzcu EM, Crowe T, et al. Relationship between cardiovascular risk factors and atherosclerotic disease burden measured by intravascular ultrasound. *J Am Coll Cardiol.* 2006;47(10):1967–1975.

364. Chien KL, Hsu HC, Sung FC, Su TC, Chen MF, Lee YT. Hyperuricemia as a risk factor on cardiovascular events in Taiwan: the Chin-Shan Community Cardiovascular Cohort Study. *Atherosclerosis.* 2005;183(1):147–155.

365. Chien KL, Hsu HC, Sung FC, Su TC, Chen MF, Lee YT. Metabolic syndrome as a risk factor for coronary heart disease and stroke: an 11-year prospective cohort in Taiwan community. *Atherosclerosis.* 2007;194(1):214–221.

366. Dou XF, Zhang HY, Sun K, et al. [Metabolic syndrome strongly linked to stroke in Chinese]. *Zhonghua Yi Xue Za Zhi.* 2004;84(7):539–542.

367. Friedlander AH, Golub MS. The significance of carotid artery atheromas on panoramic radiographs in the diagnosis of occult metabolic syndrome. *Oral Surg Oral Med Oral Pathol Oral Radiol Endod.* 2006;101(1):95–101.

368. Jeppesen J, Hansen TW, Rasmussen S, Ibsen H, Torp-Pedersen C. Metabolic syndrome, low-density lipoprotein cholesterol, and risk of cardiovascular disease: a population-based study. *Atherosclerosis.* 2006;189(2):369–374.

369. Kawamoto R, Tomita H, Oka Y, Kodama A. Metabolic syndrome as a predictor of ischemic stroke in elderly persons. *Intern Med.* 2005;44(9):922–927.

370. Keller KB, Lemberg L. Obesity and the metabolic syndrome. *Am J Crit Care.* 2003;12(2):167–170.

371. Tamsma JT, Jazet IM, Beishuizen ED, Fogteloo AJ, Meinders AE, Huisman MV. The metabolic syndrome: a vascular perspective. *Eur J Intern Med.* 2005;16(5):314–320.

372. Montalcini T, Gorgone G, Gazzaruso C, Sesti G, Perticone F, Pujia A. Carotid atherosclerosis associated to metabolic syndrome but not BMI in healthy menopausal women. *Diabetes Res Clin Pract.* 2007;76(3):378–382.

373. Zambon A, Pauletto P, Crepaldi G. Review article: the metabolic syndrome – a chronic cardiovascular inflammatory condition. *Aliment Pharmacol Ther.* 2005;22(Suppl 2): 20–23.

374. Singh RB, Pella D, Mechirova V, Otsuka K. Can brain dysfunction be a predisposing factor for metabolic syndrome? *Biomed Pharmacother.* 2004;58(Suppl 1):S56–68.

375. Koren-Morag N, Goldbourt U, Tanne D. Relation between the metabolic syndrome and ischemic stroke or transient ischemic attack: a prospective cohort study in patients with atherosclerotic cardiovascular disease. *Stroke.* 2005;36(7): 1366–1371.

376. Lassen NA. Autoregulation of cerebral blood flow. *Circ Res.* 1964;15(SUPPL):201–204.

377. Lassen NA. Regulation of cerebral circulation. *Acta Anaesthesiol Scand Suppl.* 1971;45:78–80.

378. Lassen NA, Agnoli A. The upper limit of autoregulation of cerebral blood flow – on the pathogenesis of hypertensive encepholopathy. *Scand J Clin Lab Invest.* 1972;30(2):113–116.

379. Celermajer DS, Sorensen KE, Spiegelhalter DJ, Georgakopoulos D, Robinson J, Deanfield JE. Aging is associated with endothelial dysfunction in healthy men years before the age-related decline in women. *J Am Coll Cardiol.* 1994;24(2):471–476.

380. Celermajer DS, Sorensen KE, Bull C, Robinson J, Deanfield JE. Endothelium-dependent dilation in the systemic arteries of asymptomatic subjects relates to coronary risk factors and their interaction. *J Am Coll Cardiol.* 1994;24(6):1468–1474.

381. Clarkson P, Celermajer DS, Donald AE, et al. Impaired vascular reactivity in insulin-dependent diabetes mellitus is related to disease duration and low density lipoprotein cholesterol levels. *J Am Coll Cardiol.* 1996;28(3):573–579.

382. Clarkson P, Celermajer DS, Powe AJ, Donald AE, Henry RM, Deanfield JE. Endothelium-dependent dilatation is impaired in young healthy subjects with a family history of premature coronary disease. *Circulation.* 1997;96(10): 3378–3383.

383. Hassan A, Hunt BJ, O'Sullivan M, et al. Markers of endothelial dysfunction in lacunar infarction and ischaemic leukoaraiosis. *Brain.* 2003;126(Pt 2):424–432.

384. Yataco AR, Corretti MC, Gardner AW, Womack CJ, Katzel LI. Endothelial reactivity and cardiac risk factors in older patients with peripheral arterial disease. *Am J Cardiol.* 1999;83(5):754–758.

385. Dimitrow PP, Krzanowski M, Surdacki A, Nizankowski R, Szczeklik A, Dubiel JS. Impaired response of the forearm resistance but not conductance vessels to reactive hyperemia in hypertrophic cardiomyopathy. *Angiology.* 1999;50(4): 267–272.

386. Corretti MC, Plotnick GD, Vogel RA. Technical aspects of evaluating brachial artery vasodilatation using high-frequency ultrasound. *Am J Physiol.* 1995;268(4 Pt 2): H1397–1404.

387. Uehata A, Lieberman EH, Gerhard MD, et al. Noninvasive assessment of endothelium-dependent flow-mediated dilation of the brachial artery. *Vasc Med.* 1997;2(2):87–92.

388. Leeson P, Thorne S, Donald A, Mullen M, Clarkson P, Deanfield J. Non-invasive measurement of endothelial function: effect on brachial artery dilatation of graded endothelial dependent and independent stimuli. *Heart.* 1997;78(1):22–27.

389. Sinoway LI, Hendrickson C, Davidson WR Jr, Prophet S, Zelis R. Characteristics of flow-mediated brachial artery vasodilation in human subjects. *Circ Res.* 1989;64(1): 32–42.

390. Nakano T, Ohkuma H, Suzuki S. Measurement of ankle brachial index for assessment of atherosclerosis in patients with stroke. *Cerebrovasc Dis.* 2004;17(2–3): 212–217.

391. Nagai K, Akishita M, Machida A, Sonohara K, Ohni M, Toba K. Correlation between pulse wave velocity and cognitive function in nonvascular dementia. *J Am Geriatr Soc.* 2004;52(6):1037–1038.

392. Awad IA, Johnson PC, Spetzler RF, Hodak JA. Incidental subcortical lesions identified on magnetic resonance imaging in the elderly. II. Postmortem pathological correlations. *Stroke.* 1986;17(6):1090–1097.

393. Bonithon-Kopp C, Touboul PJ, Berr C, Magne C, Ducimetiere P. Factors of carotid arterial enlargement in a population aged 59 to 71 years: the EVA study. *Stroke.* 1996;27(4):654–660.

394. Burger PC, Burch JG, Kunze U. Subcortical arteriosclerotic encephalopathy (Binswanger's disease). A vascular etiology of dementia. *Stroke.* 1976;7(6):626–631.

395. Caplan LR, Schoene WC. Clinical features of subcortical arteriosclerotic encephalopathy (Binswanger disease). *Neurology.* 1978;28(12):1206–1215.

396. Chimowitz MI, Estes ML, Furlan AJ, Awad IA. Further observations on the pathology of subcortical lesions identified on magnetic resonance imaging. *Arch Neurol.* 1992;49(7):747–752.

397. Graham DI. Morphologic changes during hypertension. *Am J Cardiol.* 1989;63(6):6C–9C.

398. Ishibashi K, Tanaka K, Nakabayashi T, Nakamura M, Uchiyama M, Okawa M. Latent cerebral artery stenoses on magnetic resonance angiography in a patient diagnosed as probable Alzheimer disease. *Psychiatry Clin Neurosci.* 1998;52(1):93–96.

399. Jogestrand T, Eiken O, Nowak J. Relation between the elastic properties and intima-media thickness of the common carotid artery. *Clin Physiol Funct Imaging.* 2003;23(3): 134–137.

400. Kuwabara Y, Ichiya Y, Sasaki M, et al. Cerebral blood flow and vascular response to hypercapnia in hypertensive patients with leukoaraiosis. *Ann Nucl Med.* 1996;10(3):293–298.

401. Postiglione A, Grossi D, Faccenda F, et al. Non invasive study of carotid arteries by echo-doppler and metabolic abnormalities in patients with dementia. *Angiology.* 1985;36(3):160–164.

402. Parnetti L, Mari D, Mecocci P, Senin U. Pathogenetic mechanisms in vascular dementia. *Int J Clin Lab Res.* 1994;24(1):15–22.

403. Tomonaga M, Yamanouchi H, Tohgi H, Kameyama M. Clinicopathologic study of progressive subcortical vascular encephalopathy (Binswanger type) in the elderly. *J Am Geriatr Soc.* 1982;30(8):524–529.

404. Zeumer H, Hacke W, Hundgen R. Subcortical arteriosclerotic encephalopathy – clinical, CT-morphological and electrophysiological findings (author's transl). *Fortschr Neurol Psychiatr.* 1981;49(6):223–231.

405. Hoth KF, Tate DF, Poppas A, et al. Endothelial function and white matter hyperintensities in older adults with cardiovascular disease. *Stroke*. 2007;38(2):308–312.

406. Cohen RA, Poppas A, Forman DE, et al. Vascular and cognitive functions associated with cardiovascular disease in the elderly. *J Clin Exp Neuropsychol*. 2009;31(1):96–110.

407. Farrar DJ, Bond MG, Riley WA, Sawyer JK. Anatomic correlates of aortic pulse wave velocity and carotid artery elasticity during atherosclerosis progression and regression in monkeys. *Circulation*. 1991;83(5):1754–1763.

408. Gamble G, Zorn J, Sanders G, MacMahon S, Sharpe N. Estimation of arterial stiffness, compliance, and distensibility from M-mode ultrasound measurements of the common carotid artery. *Stroke*. 1994;25(1):11–16.

409. Vietkevicious P, Fleg J, Engel J. Effects of age on aerobic capacity on arterial stiffness in healthy adults. *Circulation*. 1977;56:273–278.

410. Wada T, Kodaira K, Fujishiro K, et al. Correlation of ultrasound-measured common carotid artery stiffness with pathological findings. *Arterioscler Thromb*. 1994;14(3):479–482.

411. Feigenbaum H. Echocardiographic examination of the left ventricle. *Circulation*. 1975;51(1):1–7.

412. Vasan RS, Larson MG, Benjamin EJ, Evans JC, Reiss CK, Levy D. Congestive heart failure in subjects with normal versus reduced left ventricular ejection fraction: prevalence and mortality in a population-based cohort. *J Am Coll Cardiol*. 1999;33(7):1948–1955.

413. Hellermann JP, Jacobsen SJ, Reeder GS, Lopez-Jimenez F, Weston SA, Roger VL. Heart failure after myocardial infarction: prevalence of preserved left ventricular systolic function in the community. *Am Heart J*. 2003;145(4):742–748.

414. Diller PM, Smucker DR, David B, Graham RJ. Congestive heart failure due to diastolic or systolic dysfunction. Frequency and patient characteristics in an ambulatory setting. *Arch Fam Med*. 1999;8(5):414–420.

415. Akosah KO, Moncher K, Schaper A, Havlik P, Devine S. Chronic heart failure in the community: missed diagnosis and missed opportunities. *J Card Fail*. 2001;7(3):232–238.

416. Iwasaka T, Sugiura T, Abe Y, et al. Residual left ventricular pump function following acute myocardial infarction in postmenopausal diabetic women. *Coron Artery Dis*. 1994;5(3):237–242.

417. Kass DA. Age-related changes in venticular-arterial coupling: pathophysiologic implications. *Heart Fail Rev*. 2002;7(1):51–62.

418. Wong M, Bruce S, Joseph D, Lively H. Estimating left ventricular ejection fraction from two-dimensional echocardiograms: visual and computer-processed interpretations. *Echocardiography*. 1991;8(1):1–7.

419. Schiller NB, Shah PM, Crawford M, et al. Recommendations for quantitation of the left ventricle by two-dimensional echocardiography. American Society of Echocardiography Committee on Standards, Subcommittee on Quantitation of Two-Dimensional Echocardiograms. *J Am Soc Echocardiogr*. 1989;2(5):358–367.

420. Herlitz J, Brandrup-Wognsen G, Haglid M, et al. Mortality and morbidity during a period of 2 years after coronary artery bypass surgery in patients with and without a history of hypertension. *J Hypertens*. 1996;14(3):309–314.

421. Aldea GS, Gaudiani JA, Shapira OM, et al. Comparison of risk profile and outcomes in patients undergoing surgical and catheter-based revascularization. *J Card Surg*. 1998;13(2):81–89; discussion 90–92.

422. Boulnois JL, Pechoux T. Non-invasive cardiac output monitoring by aortic blood flow measurement with the Dynemo 3000. *J Clin Monit Comput*. 2000;16(2):127–140.

423. Wang TJ, Evans JC, Benjamin EJ, Levy D, LeRoy EC, Vasan RS. Natural history of asymptomatic left ventricular systolic dysfunction in the community. *Circulation*. 2003;108(8):977–982.

424. Cain AE, Khalil RA. Pathophysiology of essential hypertension: role of the pump, the vessel, and the kidney. *Semin Nephrol*. 2002;22(1):3–16.

425. Okamoto M, Etani H, Yagita Y, Kinoshita N, Nukada T. Diminished reserve for cerebral vasomotor response to L-arginine in the elderly: evaluation by transcranial Doppler sonography. *Gerontology*. 2001;47(3):131–135.

426. Ivanov Iu S, Semin GF. [Cerebrovascular reactivity in the pathogenesis of ischemic brain lesions in patients of different ages]. *Zh Nevropatol Psikhiatr Im S S Korsakova*. 1996;96(5):19–22.

427. Frolkis VV, Bezrukov VV, Shevchuk VG. Hemodynamics and its regulation in old age. *Exp Gerontol*. 1975;10(5):251–271.

428. Higginbotham MB, Morris KG, Williams RS, McHale PA, Coleman RE, Cobb FR. Regulation of stroke volume during submaximal and maximal upright exercise in normal man. *Circ Res*. 1986;58(2):281–291.

429. Brickman AM, Paul RH, Cohen RA, et al. Category and letter verbal fluency across the adult lifespan: relationship to EEG theta power. *Arch Clin Neuropsychol*. 2005;20(5):561–573.

430. Brickman AM, Zimmerman ME, Paul RH, et al. Regional white matter and neuropsychological functioning across the adult lifespan. *Biol Psychiatry*. 2006;60(5):444–453.

431. Gunstad J, Bausserman L, Paul RH, et al. C-reactive protein, but not homocysteine, is related to cognitive dysfunction in older adults with cardiovascular disease. *J Clin Neurosci*. 2006;13(5):540–546.

432. Gunstad J, Cohen RA, Paul RH, Gordon E. Dissociation of the component processes of attention in healthy adults. *Arch Clin Neuropsychol*. 2006;21(7):645–650.

433. Gunstad J, Cohen RA, Paul RH, Luyster FS, Gordon E. Age effects in time estimation: relationship to frontal brain morphometry. *J Integr Neurosci*. 2006;5(1):75–87.

434. Gunstad J, Paul RH, Brickman AM, et al. Patterns of cognitive performance in middle-aged and older adults: a cluster analytic examination. *J Geriatr Psychiatry Neurol*. 2006;19(2):59–64.

435. Gunstad J, Poppas A, Smeal S, et al. Relation of brain natriuretic peptide levels to cognitive dysfunction in adults >55 years of age with cardiovascular disease. *Am J Cardiol*. 2006;98(4):538–540.

436. Gunstad J, Schofield P, Paul RH, et al. BDNF Val66Met polymorphism is associated with body mass index in healthy adults. *Neuropsychobiology*. 2006;53(3):153–156.

437. Jefferson AL, Poppas A, Paul RH, Cohen RA. Systemic hypoperfusion is associated with executive dysfunction in geriatric cardiac patients. *Neurobiol Aging*. 2007;28(3):477–483.

438. Paul RH, Brickman AM, Cohen RA, et al. Cognitive status of young and older cigarette smokers: data from the international brain database. *J Clin Neurosci*. 2006;13(4):457–465.

439. Paul RH, Clark CR, Lawrence J, et al. Age-dependent change in executive function and gamma 40 Hz phase synchrony. *J Integr Neurosci*. 2005;4:63–76.

440. Jefferson AL, Poppas A, Paul RH, Cohen RA. Systemic hypoperfusion is associated with executive dysfunction in geriatric cardiac patients. *Neurobiol Aging*. 2007;28(3): 477–483.

441. Haley AP, Forman DE, Poppas A, et al. Carotid artery intima-media thickness and cognition in cardiovascular disease. *Int J Cardiol*. 2007;121(2):148–154.

442. Gunstad J, Cohen RA, Tate DF, et al. Blood pressure variability and white matter hyperintensities in older adults with cardiovascular disease. *Blood Press*. 2005;14(6):353–358.

443. Hoth KF, Haley AP, Gunstad J, et al. Elevated C-reactive protein is related to cognitive decline in older adults with cardiovascular disease. *J Am Geriatr Soc*. 2008;56(10):1898–1903.

444. Paul RH, Haque O, Gunstad J, et al. Subcortical hyperintensities impact cognitive function among a select subset of healthy elderly. *Arch Clin Neuropsychol*. 2005;20(6): 697–704.

445. Keary TA, Gunstad J, Poppas A, et al. Blood pressure variability and dementia rating scale performance in older adults with cardiovascular disease. *Cogn Behav Neurol*. 2007;20(1):73–77.

446. Jerskey BA, Cohen RA, Jefferson AL, et al. Sustained attention is associated with left ventricular ejection fraction in older adults with heart disease. *J Int Neuropsychol Soc*. 2009;15(1):137–141.

447. Jefferson AL, Tate DF, Poppas A, et al. Lower cardiac output is associated with greater white matter hyperintensities in older adults with cardiovascular disease. *J Am Geriatr Soc*. 2007;55(7):1044–1048.

448. Irani F, Sweet LH, Haley A, et al. An FMRI study of working memory, cardiac output, and ejection fraction in elderly patients with cardiovascular disease. *Brain Imaging Behav*. 2009;3:350–357.

449. Haley AP, Sweet LH, Gunstad J, et al. Verbal working memory and atherosclerosis in patients with cardiovascular disease: an fMRI study. *J Neuroimaging*. 2007;17(3): 227–233.

450. Haley AP, Forman DE, Poppas A, et al. Carotid artery intima-media thickness and cognition in cardiovascular disease. *Int J Cardiol*. 2007;121(2):148–154.

451. Haley A, Gunstad JJ, Cohen RA, Jerskey BA, Mulligan RC, Sweet LH. Neural correlates of visuospatial working memory in healthy young adults at risk for hypertension. *Brain Imaging and Behavior*. 2008;2(3):192–199.

452. Gunstad J, Cohen RA, Paul RH, Tate DF, Hoth KF, Poppas A. Understanding reported cognitive dysfunction in older adults with cardiovascular disease. *Neuropsychiatr Dis Treat*. 2006;2(2):213–218.

453. Gunstad J, Benitez A, Hoth KF, et al. P-selectin 1087G/A polymorphism is associated with neuropsychological test performance in older adults with cardiovascular disease. *Stroke*. 2009;40:2969–2972.

454. Gunstad J, Sweet LH, Paul R, et al. Reduced fMRI activation and task performance in cardiovascular disease. Presentation to the 11th annual meeting of the Organization for Human Brain Mapping, Toronto, Canada, June 2005. *NeuroImage*. 2005;26:S1–S56.

455. Forman DE, Cohen RA, Hoth KF, Poppas A, Moser DJ, Gunstad J, Paul RH, Jefferson AL, Haley AP, Tate DF, Ono M, Wake N, Gerhard-Herman, M. Vascular health and cognitive function in older adults with cardiovascular disease. *Artery Research*. 2008;2(1):35–43.

456. Tate D, Jefferson AL, Brickman AM, et al. Regional white matter signal abnormalities and cognitive correlates among geriatric patients with treated cardiovascular disease. *Brain Imaging Behav*. 2008;2:200–206.

457. Stanek KM, Gunstad J, Paul RH, et al. Longitudinal cognitive performance in older adults with cardiovascular disease: evidence for improvement in heart failure. *J Cardiovasc Nurs*. 2009;24(3):192–197.

458. Jefferson AL, Poppas A, Paul RH, Cohen RA. Systemic hypoperfusion is associated with executive dysfunction in geriatric cardiac patients. *Neurobiol Aging*. Mar 2007;28(3): 477–483.

459. Tranmer B, Keller TS, Kindt GW, Archer D. Loss of cerebral regulation during cardiac output variations in focal cerebral ischemia. *J Neurosurg*. 1992;77:253–259.

460. Gruhn N, Larsen FS, Boesgaard S, et al. Cerebral blood flow in patients with chronic heart failure before and after heart transplantation. *Stroke*. 2001;32:2530–2533.

461. Wanless R, Anand IS, Gurden J, Harris P, Poole-Wilson PA. Regional blood flow and hemodynamics in the rabbit with adriamycin cardiomyopathy: effects of isosorbide dinitrate, dobutamine and captopril. *J Pharmacol Exp Ther*. 1987;243:1101–1106.

462. Saxena P, Schoemaker RG. Organ blood flow protection in hypertension and congestive heart failure. *Am J Med*. 1993;94:4S–12S.

463. Maalikjy-Akkawi N, Borroni B, Agosti C, et al. Volume cerebral blood flow reduction in pre-clinical stage of Alzheimer disease: evidence from an ultrasonographic study. *J Neurol*. 2005;252:559–563.

464. Torre-Amione G, Kapadia S, Benedict C, Oral H, Young JB, Mann DL. Proinflammatory cytokine levels in patients with depressed left ventricular ejection fraction: a report from the Studies of Left Ventricular Dysfunction (SOLVD). *J Am Coll Cardiol*. 1996;27:1201–1206.

465. McGeer P, McGeer EG. Inflammation, autotoxicity and Alzheimer disease. *Neurobiol Aging*. 2001;22: 799–809.

466. Guerreiro R, Santana I, Bras JM, Santiago B, Paiva A, Oliveira C. Peripheral inflammatory cytokines as biomarkers in Alzheimer's disease and mild cognitive impairment. *Neurodegener Dis*. 2007;4:406–412.

467. Alvarez A, Cacabelos R, Sanpedro C, Garcia-Fantini M, Aleixandre M. Serum TNF-alpha levels are increased and correlate negatively with free IGF-I in Alzheimer disease. *Neurobiol Aging*. 2007;28:533–536.

468. Kannel W, Hjortland M, Castelli WP. Role of diabetes in congestive heart failure: the Framingham study. *Am J Cardiol*. 1974;34:29–34.

469. Raher M, Thibault HB, Buys ES, et al. A short duration of high-fat diet induces insulin resistance and predisposes to adverse left ventricular remodeling after pressure overload. *Am J Physiol Heart Circ Physiol*. 2008;295(295): H2495–H2502.

470. Hong E, Jung DY, Ko HJ, et al. Nonobese, insulin-deficient Ins2Akita mice develop type 2 diabetes phenotypes including insulin resistance and cardiac remodeling. *Am J Physiol Endocrinol Metab*. 2007;293:1687–1696.

471. Kim J, Montagnani M, Koh KK, Quon MJ. Reciprocal relationships between insulin resistance and endothelial dysfunction: molecular and pathophysiological mechanisms. *Circulation*. 2006;113(15):1888–1904.

472. Tanne D. Impaired glucose metabolism and cerebrovascular diseases. *Adv Cardiol*. 2008;45:107–113.

473. Watson G, Craft S. The role of insulin resistance in the pathogenesis of Alzheimer's disease: implications for treatment. *CNS Drugs*. 2003;17:27–45.

474. Kim HJ, Pyeun YS, Kim YW, et al. A model for research on the blood–brain barrier disruption induced by unsaturated fatty acid emulsion. *Invest Radiol*. 2005;40(5):270–276.

475. Wintermark M, Albers GW, Alexandrov AV, et al. Acute stroke imaging research roadmap. *AJNR Am J Neuroradiol*. 2008;29(5):e23–30.

476. Wintermark M, Albers GW, Alexandrov AV, et al. Acute stroke imaging research roadmap. *Stroke*. 2008;39(5): 1621–1628.

477. Chalela JA, Wolf RL, Maldjian JA, Kasner SE. MRI identification of early white matter injury in anoxic-ischemic encephalopathy. *Neurology*. 2001;56(4):481–485.

478. Breteler MM, van Swieten JC, Bots ML, et al. Cerebral white matter lesions, vascular risk factors, and cognitive function in a population-based study: the Rotterdam Study. *Neurology*. 1994;44(7):1246–1252.

479. Lazarus R, Prettyman R, Cherryman G. White matter lesions on magnetic resonance imaging and their relationship with vascular risk factors in memory clinic attenders. *Int J Geriatr Psychiatry*. 2005;20(3):274–279.

480. de Leeuw FE, de Groot JC, Oudkerk M, et al. Hypertension and cerebral white matter lesions in a prospective cohort study. *Brain*. 2002;125(Pt 4):765–772.

481. Strassburger TL, Lee HC, Daly EM, et al. Interactive effects of age and hypertension on volumes of brain structures. *Stroke*. 1997;28(7):1410–1417.

482. Swan GE, DeCarli C, Miller BL, et al. Association of midlife blood pressure to late-life cognitive decline and brain morphology. *Neurology*. 1998;51(4):986–993.

483. Roman GC. Vascular dementia. Advances in nosology, diagnosis, treatment and prevention. *Panminerva Med*. 2004;46(4):207–215.

484. Roman GC, Tatemichi TK, Erkinjuntti T, et al. Vascular dementia: diagnostic criteria for research studies. Report of the NINDS-AIREN International Workshop. *Neurology*. 1993;43(2):250–260.

485. Paul R, Cohen R, Navia B, Tashima K. Relationships between cognition and structural neuroimaging findings in adults with human immunodeficiency virus type-1. *Neurosci Biobehav Rev*. 2002;26(3):353–359.

486. Haley A, Gunstad J, Cohen RA, Jerskey B, Mulligan R, Sweet LH. Neural Correlates of Visuospatial Working Memory in Healthy Young Adults at Risk for Hypertension. *Brain Imaging and Behavior*. 2008;2:192–199.

487. Paskavitz J, Sweet LH, Wellen J, Helmer KG, Rao SM, Cohen RA. Recruitment and stabilization of brain activation within a working memory task; an FMRI Study. *Brain Imaging Behav*. 2010;4(1):5–21.

488. Duan JH, Wang HQ, Xu J, et al. White matter damage of patients with Alzheimer's disease correlated with the decreased cognitive function. *Surg Radiol Anat*. 2006;28(2): 150–156.

489. Zhan W, Zhang Y, Mueller SG, et al. Characterization of white matter degeneration in elderly subjects by magnetic resonance diffusion and FLAIR imaging correlation. *Neuroimage*. 2009;47(Suppl 2):T58–T65.

490. Bastin ME. On the use of the FLAIR technique to improve the correction of eddy current induced artefacts in MR diffusion tensor imaging. *Magn Reson Imaging*. 2001;19(7):937–950.

491. Chou MC, Lin YR, Huang TY, et al. FLAIR diffusion-tensor MR tractography: comparison of fiber tracking with conventional imaging. *AJNR Am J Neuroradiol*. 2005;26(3):591–597.

492. Karonen JO, Vanninen RL, Liu Y, et al. Combined diffusion and perfusion MRI with correlation to single-photon emission CT in acute ischemic stroke. Ischemic penumbra predicts infarct growth. *Stroke*. 1999;30(8):1583–1590.

493. Kidwell CS, Saver JL, Mattiello J, et al. Diffusion-perfusion MR evaluation of perihematomal injury in hyperacute intracerebral hemorrhage. *Neurology*. 2001;57(9):1611–1617.

494. Keller E, Flacke S, Urbach H, Schild HH. Diffusion- and perfusion-weighted magnetic resonance imaging in deep cerebral venous thrombosis. *Stroke*. 1999;30(5):1144–1146.

495. Heiss WD, Sobesky J, Hesselmann V. Identifying thresholds for penumbra and irreversible tissue damage. *Stroke*. 2004;35(11 Suppl 1):2671–2674.

496. Chowdhury D, Wardlaw JM, Dennis MS. Are multiple acute small subcortical infarctions caused by embolic mechanisms? *J Neurol Neurosurg Psychiatry*. 2004;75(10): 1416–1420.

497. Nitkunan A, Charlton RA, McIntyre DJ, Barrick TR, Howe FA, Markus HS. Diffusion tensor imaging and MR spectroscopy in hypertension and presumed cerebral small vessel disease. *Magn Reson Med*. 2008;59(3):528–534.

498. Stoeckel MC, Wittsack HJ, Meisel S, Seitz RJ. Pattern of cortex and white matter involvement in severe middle cerebral artery ischemia. *J Neuroimaging*. 2007;17(2):131–140.

499. Wardlaw JM, Doubal F, Armitage P, et al. Lacunar stroke is associated with diffuse blood–brain barrier dysfunction. *Ann Neurol*. 2009;65(2):194–202.

500. Ay H, Buonanno FS, Schaefer PW, et al. Posterior leukoencephalopathy without severe hypertension: utility of diffusion-weighted MRI. *Neurology*. 1998;51(5):1369–1376.

501. Huber R, Aschoff AJ, Ludolph AC, Riepe MW. Transient Global Amnesia. Evidence against vascular ischemic etiology from diffusion weighted imaging. *J Neurol*. 2002;249(11):1520–1524.

502. Seifert T, Enzinger C, Storch MK, Pichler G, Niederkorn K, Fazekas F. Acute small subcortical infarctions on diffusion weighted MRI: clinical presentation and aetiology. *J Neurol Neurosurg Psychiatry*. 2005;76(11):1520–1524.

503. Takahashi M, Fritz-Zieroth B, Chikugo T, Ogawa H. In vivo differentiation of edematous changes after stroke in spontaneously hypertensive rats using diffusion weighted MRI. *Acta Neurochir Suppl (Wien)*. 1994;60:224–227.

504. Raz N, Rodrigue KM. Differential aging of the brain: patterns, cognitive correlates and modifiers. *Neurosci Biobehav Rev*. 2006;30(6):730–748.

505. Huang L, Ling XY, Liu SR. Diffusion tensor imaging on white matter in normal adults and elderly patients with hypertension. *Chin Med J (Engl)*. 2006;119(15): 1304–1307.

506. Owler BK, Higgins JN, Pena A, Carpenter TA, Pickard JD. Diffusion tensor imaging of benign intracranial hypertension: absence of cerebral oedema. *Br J Neurosurg*. 2006;20(2):79–81.

507. Fong CS. Hypertensive encephalopathy involving the brainstem and deep structures: a case report. *Acta Neurol Taiwan*. 2005;14(4):191–194.

508. Alemany M, Stenborg A, Terent A, Sonninen P, Raininko R. Coexistence of microhemorrhages and acute spontaneous brain hemorrhage: correlation with signs of microangiopathy and clinical data. *Radiology*. 2006;238(1): 240–247.

509. Schwartz RB. Hyperperfusion encephalopathies: hypertensive encephalopathy and related conditions. *Neurologist*. 2002;8(1):22–34.

510. Schwartz RB, Mulkern RV, Gudbjartsson H, Jolesz F. Diffusion-weighted MR imaging in hypertensive encephalopathy: clues to pathogenesis. *AJNR Am J Neuroradiol*. 1998;19(5):859–862.

511. Konaka K, Miyashita K, Naritomi H. Changes in diffusion-weighted magnetic resonance imaging findings in the acute and subacute phases of anoxic encephalopathy. *J Stroke Cerebrovasc Dis*. 2007;16(2):82–83.

512. Miller SP, McQuillen PS, Hamrick S, et al. Abnormal brain development in newborns with congenital heart disease. *N Engl J Med*. 2007;357(19):1928–1938.

513. Eifert S, Reichenspurner H, Pfefferkorn T, et al. Neurological and neuropsychological examination and outcome after use of an intra-aortic filter device during cardiac surgery. *Perfusion*. 2003;18(Suppl 1):55–60.

514. Knipp SC, Matatko N, Schlamann M, et al. Small ischemic brain lesions after cardiac valve replacement detected by diffusion-weighted magnetic resonance imaging: relation to neurocognitive function. *Eur J Cardiothorac Surg*. 2005;28(1):88–96.

515. Djaiani G, Fedorko L, Cusimano RJ, et al. Off-pump coronary bypass surgery: risk of ischemic brain lesions in patients with atheromatous thoracic aorta. *Can J Anaesth*. 2006;53(8):795–801.

516. Bendszus M, Stoll G. Silent cerebral ischaemia: hidden fingerprints of invasive medical procedures. *Lancet Neurol*. 2006;5(4):364–372.

517. Pierpaoli C, Alger JR, Righini A, et al. High temporal resolution diffusion MRI of global cerebral ischemia and reperfusion. *J Cereb Blood Flow Metab*. 1996;16(5):892–905.

518. Stolz E, Gerriets T, Kluge A, Klovekorn WP, Kaps M, Bachmann G. Diffusion-weighted magnetic resonance imaging and neurobiochemical markers after aortic valve replacement: implications for future neuroprotective trials? *Stroke*. 2004;35(4):888–892.

519. Wityk RJ, Goldsborough MA, Hillis A, et al. Diffusion- and perfusion-weighted brain magnetic resonance imaging in patients with neurologic complications after cardiac surgery. *Arch Neurol*. 2001;58(4):571–576.

520. Ahrens E, Allman J, Bush E, Laidlaw D, Zhang S. Comparative 3d anatomy of the prosimian brain:DTI and histological studies. In *Proceedings of the Scientific Meeting and Exhibition of the. International Society for Magnetic Resonance in Medicine*; Japan, May 15–21, 2004.

521. Correia S, Zhang S, Laidlaw D, Malloy P, Salloway S. Diffusion-tensor imaging: linear, planar, and spherical diffusion in cadasil. Paper presented In 9th International Conference on Alzheimer's Disease and Related Disorders, 2004; July 17–22, Philadelphia. Abstract P2–232. *Neurobiol Aging*. 2004;25(S2):S298.

522. Laidlaw D, Zhang S, Bastin M, Correia S, Lalloway S, Malloy P. Ramifications of isotropic sampling and acquisition, orientation on DTI analyses. Paper presented at *Scientific Meeting and Exhibition*; Japan, May 15–21, 2004.

523. Zhang S, Bastin ME, Laidlaw DH, Sinha S, Armitage PA, Deisboeck TS. Visualization and analysis of white matter structural asymmetry in diffusion tensor MRI data. *Magn Reson Med*. 2004;51(1):140–147.

524. Zhang S, Demiralp C, Laidlaw D. Visualizing diffusion tensor MR images using streamtubes and streamsurfaces. *IEEE Trans Vis Comput Graph*. 2003;9(4):454–462.

525. Zhang S, Laidlaw, DH. A Model for Some Subcortical DTI Planar and Linear Anisotropy. In: Barillot C, Haynor DR, Hellier P ed. *Medical Image Computing and Computer-Assisted Intervention – MICCAI 2004*. Saint-Malo, France: Springer; 2004:1071–1073.

526. Zhang S, Laidlaw D, Brown M, Miller D. *Visualization of the interaction of multiple sclerosis lesions with adjacent white matter fibers using streamtubes and streamsurfaces*. Washington, DC, USA: IEEE Computer Society; 2004.

527. Zheng J, Ghorpade A, Niemann D, et al. Lymphotropic virions affect chemokine receptor-mediated neural signaling and apoptosis: implications for human immunodeficiency virus type 1-associated dementia. *J Virol*. 1999;73(10):8256–8267.

528. McLaughlin NC, Paul RH, Grieve SM, et al. Diffusion tensor imaging of the corpus callosum: a cross-sectional study across the lifespan. *Int J Dev Neurosci*. 2007;25(4):215–221.

529. Pfefferbaum A, Sullivan EV. Increased brain white matter diffusivity in normal adult aging: relationship to anisotropy and partial voluming. *Magn Reson Med*. 2003;49(5):953–961.

530. Rose SE, Janke AL, Chalk JB. Gray and white matter changes in Alzheimer's disease: a diffusion tensor imaging study. *J Magn Reson Imaging*. 2008;27(1):20–26.

531. Shenkin SD, Bastin ME, Macgillivray TJ, et al. Cognitive correlates of cerebral white matter lesions and water diffusion tensor parameters in community-dwelling older people. *Cerebrovasc Dis*. 2005;20(5):310–318.

532. Fellgiebel A, Wille P, Muller MJ, et al. Ultrastructural hippocampal and white matter alterations in mild cognitive impairment: a diffusion tensor imaging study. *Dement Geriatr Cogn Disord*. 2004;18(1):101–108.

533. Shiraishi A, Hasegawa Y, Okada S, et al. Highly diffusion-sensitized tensor imaging of unilateral cerebral arterial occlusive disease. *AJNR Am J Neuroradiol*. 2005;26(6):1498–1504.

534. Liu Y, D'Arceuil HE, Westmoreland S, et al. Serial diffusion tensor MRI after transient and permanent cerebral ischemia in nonhuman primates. *Stroke*. 2007;38(1):138–145.

535. Guadagno JV, Calautti C, Baron JC. Progress in imaging stroke: emerging clinical applications. *Br Med Bull*. 2003;65:145–157.

536. Jang SH, You SH, Kwon YH, Hallett M, Lee MY, Ahn SH. Cortical reorganization associated lower extremity motor

recovery as evidenced by functional MRI and diffusion tensor tractography in a stroke patient. *Restor Neurol Neurosci.* 2005;23(5–6):325–329.

537. Neumann-Haefelin T, Moseley ME, Albers GW. New magnetic resonance imaging methods for cerebrovascular disease: emerging clinical applications. *Ann Neurol.* 2000;47(5):559–570.

538. Delano-Wood L, Bondi MW, Jak AJ, et al. Stroke risk modifies regional white matter differences in mild cognitive impairment. *Neurobiol Aging.* Oct;31(10):1721–1731.

539. Ott BR, Heindel WC, Whelihan WM, Caron MD, Piatt AL, Noto RB. A single-photon emission computed tomography imaging study of driving impairment in patients with Alzheimer's disease. *Dement Geriatr Cogn Disord.* 2000;11(3):153–160.

540. Schwartz RB, Jones KM, Kalina P, et al. Hypertensive encephalopathy: findings on CT, MR imaging, and SPECT imaging in 14 cases. *AJR Am J Roentgenol.* 1992;159(2): 379–383.

541. Stocchetti N, Chieregato A, De Marchi M, Croci M, Benti R, Grimoldi N. High cerebral perfusion pressure improves low values of local brain tissue O2 tension (PtiO2) in focal lesions. *Acta Neurochir Suppl.* 1998;71:162–165.

542. Semplicini A, Maresca A, Simonella C, et al. Cerebral perfusion in hypertensives with carotid artery stenosis: a comparative study of lacidipine and hydrochlorothiazide. *Blood Press.* 2000;9(1):34–39.

543. Lorberboym M, Lampl Y, Kesler A, Sadeh M, Gadot N. Benign intracranial hypertension: correlation of cerebral blood flow with disease severity. *Clin Neurol Neurosurg.* 2001;103(1):33–36.

544. Hosoda K, Kawaguchi T, Ishii K, et al. Prediction of hyperperfusion after carotid endarterectomy by brain SPECT analysis with semiquantitative statistical mapping method. *Stroke.* 2003;34(5):1187–1193.

545. Moraca R, Lin E, Holmes JH IV, et al. Impaired baseline regional cerebral perfusion in patients referred for coronary artery bypass. *J Thorac Cardiovasc Surg.* 2006;131(3): 540–546.

546. Efimova IY, Efimova NY, Triss SV, Lishmanov YB. Brain perfusion and cognitive function changes in hypertensive patients. *Hypertens Res.* 2008;31(4):673–678.

547. Shin HK, Nishimura M, Jones PB, et al. Mild induced hypertension improves blood flow and oxygen metabolism in transient focal cerebral ischemia. *Stroke.* 2008;39(5): 1548–1555.

548. Beason-Held LL, Moghekar A, Zonderman AB, Kraut MA, Resnick SM. Longitudinal changes in cerebral blood flow in the older hypertensive brain. *Stroke.* 2007;38(6): 1766–1773.

549. Xie A, Skatrud JB, Khayat R, Dempsey JA, Morgan B, Russell D. Cerebrovascular response to carbon dioxide in patients with congestive heart failure. *Am J Respir Crit Care Med.* 2005;172(3):371–378.

550. Jacobs A, Neveling M, Horst M, et al. Alterations of neuropsychological function and cerebral glucose metabolism after cardiac surgery are not related only to intraoperative microembolic events. *Stroke.* 1998;29(3): 660–667.

551. Lee JD, Lee SJ, Tsushima WT, et al. Benefits of off-pump bypass on neurologic and clinical morbidity: a prospective randomized trial. *Ann Thorac Surg.* 2003;76(1):18–25; discussion 25–16.

552. Chernov VI, Efimova NY, Efimova IY, Akhmedov SD, Lishmanov YB. Short-term and long-term cognitive function and cerebral perfusion in off-pump and on-pump coronary artery bypass patients. *Eur J Cardiothorac Surg.* 2006;29(1):74–81.

553. Schaafsma A, de Jong BM, Bams JL, Haaxma-Reiche H, Pruim J, Zijlstra JG. Cerebral perfusion and metabolism in resuscitated patients with severe post-hypoxic encephalopathy. *J Neurol Sci.* 2003;210(1–2):23–30.

554. Hall RA, Fordyce DJ, Lee ME, et al. Brain SPECT imaging and neuropsychological testing in coronary artery bypass patients: single photon emission computed tomography. *Ann Thorac Surg.* 1999;68(6):2082–2088.

555. Degirmenci B, Durak H, Hazan E, et al. The effect of coronary artery bypass surgery on brain perfusion. *J Nucl Med.* 1998;39(4):587–591.

556. Marochnik S, Alexandrov AV, Anthone D, Lewin C, Caldwell CB, Pullicino PM. Feasibility of SPECT for studies of brain perfusion during cardiopulmonary bypass. *J Neuroimaging.* 1996;6(4):243–245.

557. Vogels RL, Oosterman JM, Laman DM, et al. Transcranial Doppler blood flow assessment in patients with mild heart failure: correlates with neuroimaging and cognitive performance. *Congest Heart Fail.* 2008;14(2):61–65.

558. Sugimori H, Ibayashi S, Fujii K, Sadoshima S, Kuwabara Y, Fujishima M. Can transcranial Doppler really detect reduced cerebral perfusion states? *Stroke.* 1995;26(11):2053–2060.

559. Braekken SK, Reinvang I, Russell D, Brucher R, Svennevig JL. Association between intraoperative cerebral microembolic signals and postoperative neuropsychological deficit: comparison between patients with cardiac valve replacement and patients with coronary artery bypass grafting. *J Neurol Neurosurg Psychiatry.* 1998;65(4):573–576.

560. Diegeler A, Hirsch R, Schneider F, et al. Neuromonitoring and neurocognitive outcome in off-pump versus conventional coronary bypass operation. *Ann Thorac Surg.* 2000;69(4):1162–1166.

561. Fearn SJ, Pole R, Wesnes K, Faragher EB, Hooper TL, McCollum CN. Cerebral injury during cardiopulmonary bypass: emboli impair memory. *J Thorac Cardiovasc Surg.* 2001;121(6):1150–1160.

562. Kidwell CS, el-Saden S, Livshits Z, Martin NA, Glenn TC, Saver JL. Transcranial Doppler pulsatility indices as a measure of diffuse small-vessel disease. *J Neuroimaging.* 2001;11(3):229–235.

563. Sloan MA, Alexandrov AV, Tegeler CH, et al. Assessment: transcranial Doppler ultrasonography: report of the Therapeutics and Technology Assessment Subcommittee of the American Academy of Neurology. *Neurology.* 2004;62(9):1468–1481.

564. Razumovsky AY, Gugino LD, Owen JH. Advanced neurologic monitoring for cardiac surgery. *Curr Cardiol Rep.* 2006;8(1):17–22.

565. Fan L, Evans DH, Naylor AR. Automated embolus identification using a rule-based expert system. *Ultrasound Med Biol.* 2001;27(8):1065–1077.

566. Whitaker DC. Apparent reduction of cerebral microemboli during off-pump operations. *Ann Thorac Surg.* 2004;78(4):1513–1514; author reply 1514–1515.

567. Malheiros SM, Massaro AR. Cerebral embolization during coronary artery bypass grafting. *Ann Thorac Surg*. 2005; 79(1):387–388.

568. Neumann-Haefelin T, Wittsack HJ, Fink GR, et al. Diffusion- and perfusion-weighted MRI: influence of severe carotid artery stenosis on the DWI/PWI mismatch in acute stroke. *Stroke*. 2000;31(6):1311–1317.

569. Parsons MW, Barber PA, Chalk J, et al. Diffusion- and perfusion-weighted MRI response to thrombolysis in stroke. *Ann Neurol*. 2002;51(1):28–37.

570. Butcher K, Parsons M, Allport L, et al. Rapid assessment of perfusion-diffusion mismatch. *Stroke*. 2008;39(1):75–81.

571. Szabo K, Gass A, Hennerici MG. Diffusion and perfusion MRI for the assessment of carotid atherosclerosis. *Neuroimaging Clin N Am*. 2002;12(3):381–390.

572. Ducreux D, Meder JF, Fredy D, Bittoun J, Lasjaunias P. MR perfusion imaging in proliferative angiopathy. *Neuroradiology*. 2004;46(2):105–112.

573. Millar SM, Alston RP, Andrews PJ, Souter MJ. Cerebral hypoperfusion in immediate postoperative period following coronary artery bypass grafting, heart valve, and abdominal aortic surgery. *Br J Anaesth*. 2001;87(2):229–236.

574. Murkin JM. Hemodynamic changes during cardiac manipulation in off-CPB surgery: relevance in brain perfusion. *Heart Surg Forum*. 2002;5(3):221–224.

575. Yoda M, Nonoyama M, Shimakura T. Cerebral perfusion during off-pump coronary artery bypass grafting. *Surg Today*. 2004;34(6):501–505.

576. Leary MC, Caplan LR. Technology insight: brain MRI and cardiac surgery – detection of postoperative brain ischemia. *Nat Clin Pract Cardiovasc Med*. 2007;4(7):379–388.

577. Bondi MW, Houston WS, Eyler LT, Brown GG. fMRI evidence of compensatory mechanisms in older adults at genetic risk for Alzheimer disease. *Neurology*. 2005;64(3): 501–508.

578. Restom K, Bangen KJ, Bondi MW, Perthen JE, Liu TT. Cerebral blood flow and BOLD responses to a memory encoding task: a comparison between healthy young and elderly adults. *Neuroimage*. 2007;37(2):430–439.

579. Bangen KJ, Restom K, Liu TT, et al. Differential age effects on cerebral blood flow and BOLD response to encoding: associations with cognition and stroke risk. *Neurobiol Aging*. 2009;30(8):1276–1287.

580. Hoge RD, Atkinson J, Gill B, Crelier GR, Marrett S, Pike GB. Investigation of BOLD signal dependence on cerebral blood flow and oxygen consumption: the deoxyhemoglobin dilution model. *Magn Reson Med*. 1999;42(5): 849–863.

581. Hoge RD, Atkinson J, Gill B, Crelier GR, Marrett S, Pike GB. Linear coupling between cerebral blood flow and oxygen consumption in activated human cortex. *Proc Natl Acad Sci U S A*. 1999;96(16):9403–9408.

582. Hoge RD, Atkinson J, Gill B, Crelier GR, Marrett S, Pike GB. Stimulus-dependent BOLD and perfusion dynamics in human V1. *Neuroimage*. 1999;9(6 Pt 1):573–585.

583. Hoge RD, Franceschini MA, Covolan RJ, Huppert T, Mandeville JB, Boas DA. Simultaneous recording of task-induced changes in blood oxygenation, volume, and flow using diffuse optical imaging and arterial spin-labeling MRI. *Neuroimage*. 2005;25(3):701–707.

584. Hoge RD, Pike GB. Oxidative metabolism and the detection of neuronal activation via imaging. *J Chem Neuroanat*. 2001;22(1–2):43–52.

585. Jessen F, Gur O, Block W, et al. A multicenter (1)H-MRS study of the medial temporal lobe in AD and MCI. *Neurology*. 2009;72(20):1735–1740.

586. Rami L, Gomez-Anson B, Bosch B, et al. Cortical brain metabolism as measured by proton spectroscopy is related to memory performance in patients with amnestic mild cognitive impairment and Alzheimer's disease. *Dement Geriatr Cogn Disord*. 2007;24(4):274–279.

587. Zhang B, Li M, Sun ZZ, et al. Evaluation of functional MRI markers in mild cognitive impairment. *J Clin Neurosci*. 2009;16(5):635–641.

588. Cecil KM, Lenkinski RE. Proton MR spectroscopy in inflammatory and infectious brain disorders. *Neuroimaging Clin N Am*. 1998;8(4):863–880.

589. Ernst T, Chang L, Arnold S. Increased glial metabolites predict increased working memory network activation in HIV brain injury. *Neuroimage*. 2003;19(4):1686–1693.

590. Paul RH, Yiannoutsos CT, Miller EN, et al. Proton MRS and neuropsychological correlates in AIDS dementia complex: evidence of subcortical specificity. *J Neuropsychiatry Clin Neurosci (Summer)*. 2007;19(3):283–292.

591. Bellmann-Strobl J, Stiepani H, Wuerfel J, et al. MR spectroscopy (MRS) and magnetisation transfer imaging (MTI), lesion load and clinical scores in early relapsing remitting multiple sclerosis: a combined cross-sectional and longitudinal study. *Eur Radiol*. 2009;19(8):2066–2074.

592. Caramanos Z, DiMaio S, Narayanan S, Lapierre Y, Arnold DL. (1)H-MRSI evidence for cortical gray matter pathology that is independent of cerebral white matter lesion load in patients with secondary progressive multiple sclerosis. *J Neurol Sci*. 2009;282(1–2):72–79.

593. Bichuetti DB, Rivero RL, de Oliveira EM, et al. White matter spectroscopy in neuromyelitis optica: a case control study. *J Neurol*. 2008;255(12):1895–1899.

594. Cader S, Johansen-Berg H, Wylezinska M, et al. Discordant white matter N-acetylasparate and diffusion MRI measures suggest that chronic metabolic dysfunction contributes to axonal pathology in multiple sclerosis. *Neuroimage*. 2007;36(1):19–27.

595. Wardlaw JM, Marshall I, Wild J, Dennis MS, Cannon J, Lewis SC. Studies of acute ischemic stroke with proton magnetic resonance spectroscopy: relation between time from onset, neurological deficit, metabolite abnormalities in the infarct, blood flow, and clinical outcome. *Stroke*. 1998;29(8):1618–1624.

596. Glodzik-Sobanska L, Slowik A, Kozub J, Sobiecka B, Urbanik A, Szczudlik A. GABA in ischemic stroke. Proton magnetic resonance study. *Med Sci Monit*. 2004;10(Suppl 3):88–93.

597. Walker PM, Ben Salem D, Lalande A, Giroud M, Brunotte F. Time course of NAA T2 and ADC(w) in ischaemic stroke patients: 1H MRS imaging and diffusion-weighted MRI. *J Neurol Sci*. 2004;220(1–2):23–28.

598. Macri MA, D'Alessandro N, Di Giulio C, et al. Regional changes in the metabolite profile after long-term hypoxia-ischemia in brains of young and aged rats: a quantitative proton MRS study. *Neurobiol Aging*. 2006;27(1):98–104.

599. Schulz UG, Blamire AM, Corkill RG, Davies P, Styles P, Rothwell PM. Association between cortical metabolite levels and clinical manifestations of migrainous aura: an MR-spectroscopy study. *Brain*. 2007;130(Pt 12): 3102–3110.

600. Modi S, Bhattacharya M, Sekhri T, Rana P, Tripathi RP, Khushu S. Assessment of the metabolic profile in Type 2 diabetes mellitus and hypothyroidism through proton MR spectroscopy. *Magn Reson Imaging*. 2008;26(3):420–425.

601. Sarac K, Akinci A, Alkan A, Aslan M, Baysal T, Ozcan C. Brain metabolite changes on proton magnetic resonance spectroscopy in children with poorly controlled type 1 diabetes mellitus. *Neuroradiology*. 2005;47(7):562–565.

602. van der Graaf M, Janssen SW, van Asten JJ, et al. Metabolic profile of the hippocampus of Zucker Diabetic Fatty rats assessed by in vivo 1H magnetic resonance spectroscopy. *NMR Biomed*. 2004;17(6):405–410.

603. Sahin I, Alkan A, Keskin L, et al. Evaluation of in vivo cerebral metabolism on proton magnetic resonance spectroscopy in patients with impaired glucose tolerance and type 2 diabetes mellitus. *J Diabetes Complications*. 2008;22(4):254–260.

604. Cameron FJ, Kean MJ, Wellard RM, Werther GA, Neil JJ, Inder TE. Insights into the acute cerebral metabolic changes associated with childhood diabetes. *Diabet Med*. 2005;22(5):648–653.

605. Sinha S, Misra A, Kumar V, et al. Proton magnetic resonance spectroscopy and single photon emission computed tomography study of the brain in asymptomatic young hyperlipidaemic Asian Indians in North India show early abnormalities. *Clin Endocrinol (Oxf)*. 2004;61(2): 182–189.

606. Lee CW, Lee JH, Kim JJ, et al. Cerebral metabolic abnormalities in congestive heart failure detected by proton magnetic resonance spectroscopy. *J Am Coll Cardiol*. 1999; 33(5):1196–1202.

607. Perrine SA, Michaels MS, Ghoddoussi F, Hyde EM, Tancer ME, Galloway MP. Cardiac effects of MDMA on the metabolic profile determined with 1H-magnetic resonance spectroscopy in the rat. *NMR Biomed*. 2009; 22(4):419–425.

608. Bendszus M, Reents W, Franke D, et al. Brain damage after coronary artery bypass grafting. *Arch Neurol*. 2002;59(7): 1090–1095.

609. Harris DN, Wilson JA, Taylor-Robinson SD, Taylor KM. Magnetic resonance spectroscopy of high-energy phosphates and lactate immediately after coronary artery bypass surgery. *Perfusion*. 1998;13(5):328–333.

610. Wilson JA, Taylor-Robinson SD, Bryant DJ, Taylor KM, Harris DN. Localised cerebral phosphorus-31 MR spectroscopy in man before and immediately after coronary bypass surgery with hypothermic cardiopulmonary bypass. *Metab Brain Dis*. 1998;13(3):191–200.

611. Tarasow E, Wiercinska-Drapalo A, Jaroszewicz J, et al. Antiretroviral therapy and its influence on the stage of brain damage in patients with HIV – 1H MRS evaluation. *Med Sci Monit*. 2004;10(Suppl 3):101–106.

612. Bruinsma GJ, Van de Kolk CW, Nederhoff MG, Bredee JJ, Ruigrok TJ, Van Echteld CJ. Brain death-related energetic failure of the donor heart becomes apparent only during storage and reperfusion: an ex vivo phosphorus-31 magnetic resonance spectroscopy study on the feline heart. *J Heart Lung Transplant*. 2001;20(9):996–1004.

613. Nagele T, Seeger U, Pereira P, et al. MR proton spectroscopy to monitor the concentration changes in cerebral metabolites following a TIPS placement. *Rofo*. 1999;170(3): 298–303.

614. Tonon C, Vetrugno R, Lodi R, et al. Proton magnetic resonance spectroscopy study of brain metabolism in obstructive sleep apnoea syndrome before and after continuous positive airway pressure treatment. *Sleep*. 2007;30(3): 305–311.

Chapter 16
Exercise and the Brain

Uraina S. Clark and David Williams

Introduction

It is now widely accepted that regular exercise behavior has numerous health benefits, including enhanced weight control,[217] and reduced risk of cardiovascular disease,[191] type 2 diabetes,[113] and osteoporosis,[205] as well as cancers of the breast[142] and colon.[180] There is also growing evidence that exercise may enhance mood[27,64] and cognitive functioning.[47,75]

There are at least three general types of research questions that require continued pursuit. First, more evidence is needed to illustrate the effects of exercise on various disease states (e.g., cardiovascular disease, diabetes, cancers), including affective (e.g., depression, anxiety) and cognitive (e.g., dementia) disorders. Included in this category are questions regarding the optimal dose (i.e., intensity, frequency, duration) and mode (e.g., aerobic, resistance training, yoga) of exercise. Second, a better understanding of the mechanisms that underlie the effects of exercise on each of these health outcomes is needed. As an example, it will be important not only to know whether exercise can help reduce symptoms of depression or dementia but also how this occurs. Third, it is necessary to increase our understanding of how to best help people adopt and maintain programs of regular exercise that are likely to lead to beneficial health outcomes. This is especially important given that 60% of the US population does not exercise regularly.[197]

The latter two questions are highly relevant to the mission of this book. Thus, with regard to the second type of question, we focus on the mechanisms of the effects of exercise on cognition and affect, since we speculate that these relationships may be more fully mediated by brain processes than the effects of exercise on "physical" disease states, such as heart disease, cancer, and diabetes, which may involve greater and more complex systemic processes. With regard to the third question, we focus on the functional brain response to acute exercise bouts and the implications for successful adoption and adherence to exercise programs. Both of these areas of research are in their infancy, thus much of what we discuss is based on conceptual frameworks and a small, but growing, empirical literature.

Neural Mechanisms of the Effects of Exercise on Cognition

Effects of Exercise on Normal Cognitive Functioning

It has long been posited that exercise may enhance cognitive capabilities. There is growing evidence of improved cognitive functioning in response to exercise among nondepressed adults[47,75] and children.[178] In recent years, increasingly more studies in this area have included randomized controlled examinations of the effects of exercise on cognition, and thus have focused on the effects of specific cardiovascular fitness programs on cognitive function. Notably, there is great variability in the types of physical activity programs examined, and questions remain regarding the level of

---

U.S. Clark (✉)
Department of Neuropsychology,
The Warren Alpert Medical School of Brown University,
The Miriam Hospital, Providence, RI, USA
e-mail: Uraina_Clark@Brown.edu

R.A. Cohen and L.H. Sweet (eds.), *Brain Imaging in Behavioral Medicine and Clinical Neuroscience*,
DOI 10.1007/978-1-4419-6373-4_16, © Springer Science+Business Media, LLC 2011

physical engagement that is most effective. Though the literature contains mixed results, with some studies suggesting that physical fitness may have little to no impact on cognitive function,[93,131] the evidence supporting the benefits of moderate exercise on cognitive function is increasing.

One of the first studies indicating a positive effect of aerobic exercise on cognition in older adults was conducted by Spirduso and Clifford[181] who reported that men who participated regularly in sports activities performed better on cognitive testing compared to a group of sedentary peers. Several cross-sectional studies have replicated these observations and have reported that physically fit older adults demonstrate better performances on tasks of perception, cognition, and motor function (for review, see ref. [75]). In general, results from randomized clinical exercise trials, which some consider the "gold standard" of research designs, also appear to support these initial findings. Such studies are important particularly due to the possibility that participant self-selection effects could bias results from cross-sectional studies. Typically, clinical trials, or intervention studies, involve a group of sedentary adults who are randomized into one of two groups: one that receives the exercise intervention and the other group that either participates in a nonaerobic exercise program (e.g., stretching) or maintains their normal level of activity as part of a waitlist control group. Intervention studies thus allow for a more direct examination of the effects of aerobic fitness training on cognition, without confounding the effects of exercise with participant characteristics (e.g., baseline differences in general health, lifestyle choices, etc.), which may differ between comparison groups in cross-sectional studies. Such studies intervention have borne mixed findings (see ref. [140]); however, interpretation of these differences is complicated by the nuances that differ between studies. For example, there is little consistency between the types of exercise programs employed or cognitive tests assessed. Furthermore, many intervention studies have been based on a small number of participants, which can have a negative impact on the ability to observe group differences. Meta-analyses are helpful in overcoming such shortcomings in the literature, and results from such analyses generally support the idea that aerobic activity in adults is associated with positive effects on cognition.[47,74,75] There is also evidence that executive functions (e.g., task switching, working memory, and response inhibition) may show a greater benefit over other cognitive functions.[47,88,114]

Relatively few studies investigating the relation between physical fitness levels and cognition in children and young adults have been conducted. Still, the evidence to suggest that aerobic fitness levels and exercise behaviors in school-aged children are positively associated with cognitive and academic performance is mounting. A recent meta-analysis showed a positive relation between physical activity and cognitive performance in several domains of functioning, including basic intellectual functioning, verbal abilities, and perceptual skills.[178] In terms of academic performance, physical fitness levels have been shown to correlate positively with scores on standardized measures of academic abilities,[38] general academic performance[41,42,78,109] and on-task behaviors in the classroom.[133]

Like studies in adults, early exercise studies involving children and adolescents were predominated by cross-sectional designs, which are useful in examining correlational relationships; however, such studies do not permit one to evaluate the causal nature of the relation between increases in physical fitness and cognitive function. Fortunately, over the years, more researchers have begun to employ clinical exercise trials to investigate the impact of exercise on cognitive processes in children and younger adults. In such studies, improvements in attention, concentration, and executive functioning skills following acute bouts of exercise[32] as well as prolonged (i.e., multiweek) exercise programs[56] have been observed. Similarly, children and young adults have also been noted to demonstrate improvements in the allocation of attentional resources in studies measuring the P3 component of event-related brain potentials (ERP). In one such study including preadolescent children, larger P3 amplitudes (indicating a facilitation of attentional processes) and better performance on a standardized test of academic achievement was observed following a one-time 20-min exercise session relative to the resting session.[97] These findings parallel those observed in young adults, who also demonstrate larger P3 amplitudes following intense cardiovascular exercise.[98]

Altogether, the literature suggests that moderate levels of physical activity can have positive effects on cognitive functioning in adults. In addition, children also appear to demonstrate benefits from exercise, as improvements in both cognitive and academic functioning are reported. Interestingly, some results indicate that the effects of exercise may be greater in the young. The observed effect size in a meta-analysis of studies investigating the cognitive effects of exercise in children (ages 4–18) was 0.32,[178] whereas the effect size reported in a meta-analysis of the influence of physical activity on cognition across the lifespan was 0.25,[75] suggesting the possibility of a "critical period" or neurodevelopmental window in which exercise may have a greater effect on the brain. Additional research is needed to better examine the possible differential influences of exercise on children and adults. Nevertheless, maintaining an active lifestyle throughout adulthood appears to have long-lasting effects, as studies have shown that regular engagement in moderate exercise during midlife is associated with reduced risk of dementia later in life.[1,169] Such findings highlight the importance of maintaining physical engagement throughout the lifespan, which may benefit cognitive and academic function in the young, and may ultimately prevent or delay the loss of cognitive function associated with aging or neurodegenerative diseases.

Neural Mechanisms and Effects of Exercise on Cognitive Functions

In recent years, much advancement has been made in the study of the neurologic effects of exercise on the central nervous system. As discussed below, the data suggest that the influences that exercise exerts on the brain are remarkable and quite varied. Exercise-related effects are observed on a structural level, a functional level, and a neurochemical level, all of which may impact neurocognitive function. Importantly, one must note that these changes are occurring in a system, and as such they are likely to be highly interrelated. For example, exercise-related neurochemical changes (e.g., increases in neurotrophic factors) likely influence cellular health, which in turn may impact gray matter morphometry and ultimately function.

Some of the effects that exercise has on cognitive function may be mediated by alterations in cerebral vascularization and the development of new neurons, as evidence from animal studies suggests that aerobic exercise increases angiogenesis and neurogenesis.[26,31,112,126,189,202] Although some studies have noted that exercise-induced changes in angiogenesis and neurogenesis occur throughout the brain,[26,112,126,189] greater attention is turning toward the impact of exercise on cells in the hippocampus, and in the dentate gyrus more specifically,[31,116,168,201,202] due in part to the importance of this brain region to learning and memory and the implication of this region in cognitive aging. For example, van Praag et al.[202] reported that exercise resulted in improved vascular architecture in the dentate gyrus of young mice that were housed with a running wheel compared to sedentary mice. These researchers also found that voluntary running in young and older mice resulted in the development of significantly more new cells in the dentate gyrus compared to age-matched control mice. Further, the number of new cells in the dentate gyrus of older mice in the running group did not differ from that of the younger sedentary group, suggesting that exercise might act to reverse age-related reductions in neurogenesis. Notably, the mice in both the younger and older running groups performed better on a task of learning and memory than their age-matched controls. Such results imply a possible link between exercise-induced improvements in hippocampal integrity and increased learning abilities across the lifespan and may help explain the reported effects of exercise on memory function.

Findings from a recent magnetic resonance imaging (MRI) study suggest that a similar process of exercise-induced neurogenesis may occur in human hippocampi and that these changes may be at least partly responsible for memory improvements. In an investigation of middle-aged adults who participated in a 3-week aerobic exercise intervention, Pereira et al.[157] observed an increase in cerebral blood volume in the dentate gyrus, while no other subregion of the hippocampus showed this effect. Dentate gyrus blood volumes were positively correlated with improvements in physical fitness levels as well as with verbal memory abilities at the end of the 3-week program. Based on their finding that exercise-induced cerebral blood volume changes in the dentate gyrus of mice correlated with neurogenesis in this region,[157] the authors suggested that the observed blood volume changes may be a marker of neurogenesis in humans. This is a notion that should be explored further given the evidence for generalized increases in cerebral blood flow in relation to exercise.[166]

MRI has also been utilized to examine the effects of exercise on brain volume and structure. In studies of middle-aged and older adults, aerobic exercise and physical fitness levels have been associated with greater volumes in cortical regions and in white matter tracts. Colcombe et al.[45] reported that higher cardiovascular fitness levels in healthy middle-aged and older adults were related to greater brain volumes in prefrontal, superior parietal, and temporal cortices, as well as increased white matter volumes in tracts communicating between the frontal cortices and posterior parietal lobes. These findings are notable given the relation of the affected cortical regions to tasks of executive functioning (e.g., task switching, working memory, and response inhibition) and higher-order cognitive functions (e.g., visuoperception), which decline with age[36] and also show improvement in response to cardiovascular fitness training.[47,114] Moreover, the volume sparing effects observed by Colcombe et al.[45] occur in those brain regions specifically affected by the aging process,[36,45] suggesting that ongoing aerobic exercise may serve to offset structural declines associated with aging. With only a few exceptions,[159] more recent studies[46,85] have supported these initial findings, and similar exercise-related effects have also been observed in the hippocampi of healthy older adults.[73] Relatively few studies have investigated volume changes in younger adults, with newly emerging findings suggesting a relation between aerobic fitness and right anterior insula volumes.[158]

Although the study of Colcombe et al.[45] reported above was somewhat limited in assessing the casual nature of the relation between exercise and brain structure due to its cross-sectional design, a later study conducted by this group indicated a more direct and acute effect of exercise on brain volumes. In this more recent study, Colcombe et al.[46] found that healthy older adults who participated in a 6-month aerobic training program demonstrated greater volumes in frontal and temporal lobe regions following the exercise intervention, as well as greater white matter volumes in the anterior corpus callosum, compared to age-matched nonaerobic control group.[46] While these findings will need to be replicated by additional research teams, the results are quite striking as they imply that in older adults exercise interventions of relatively short duration may actually increase brain volumes in several neural regions sensitive to age-related decline. More studies are needed to determine the mechanisms that underlie these effects, as well as the stability and functional significance of these effects over time.

Neurophysiological studies have revealed robust exercise-related differences in brain function. The most well investigated phenomenon has been the influence of exercise on the amplitude and latency of the P3 component of the ERP, which has been observed in preadolescent children,[95-97] young adults,[98,162] and older adults.[94,105] Generation of the P3 component is thought to involve a network of structures in the frontal, temporal, and parietal lobes.[160] It has been suggested[94] that physical activity may improve cognitive function by affecting the P3 amplitude, which has been related to improvements in memory and attentional processes, and by decreasing P3 latency, which has been associated with increased speed of cognitive processing.[160] Several researchers have posited that alterations in the P3 component might reflect an effect of exercise on general arousal states.[132,161] One hypothesis, as suggested by Hillman et al.[98] is that the observed changes in P3 amplitude and latency may result from fundamental changes in baseline electrocortical activity [19,65,66,117,118,121] supported by alterations in underlying neurobiology, such as possible increases in cerebral vascularization[26,112,126] and improved neurotransmitter functioning.[39,63]

Surprisingly, very few studies have been conducted that utilize functional MRI (FMRI) methodologies in the assessment of exercise-induced changes in cognitive function. Yet, results from one of the FMRI studies found in the current literature[48] are quite promising. Colcombe et al.[48] reported that, in older adults who completed a 6-month exercise program (i.e., walking), cardiovascular fitness training was associated with increased performance on a task of attention and inhibition, as well as with increased brain activation in a neural network involved in the allocation of spatial attention, including the middle and superior frontal gyri and superior parietal lobe. This was also associated with a decrease in activation of the anterior cingulate,[48] a brain region in which deactivation suggests reduced resources were necessary for conflict resolution.[35] Similar activation patterns were observed in a complementary cross-sectional analysis of older adults of various fitness levels.[48] Because FMRI techniques measure changes in cerebral blood flow, and exercise is known to improve cerebral perfusion in humans,[157,166] one could posit that these findings are simply a marker of improved cerebral vascularization. However, as Colcombe et al. noted,[48] both increases and decreases in cerebral blood flow were observed in relation to improvements in cardiovascular fitness. This would suggest that the reported results do not merely arise due to exercise-induced vascular improvements but instead reflect changes in cortical function. The authors suggested that their FMRI results indicate that aerobic fitness training can lead to improved cognitive and neurologic function in older adults. Moreover, their results indicate that the positive effects of exercise can develop over a relatively short period of time, consistent with previous findings.[46] Follow-up studies will be helpful in further interpretation and elaboration of these findings. In particular, it will be necessary to compare FMRI activation patterns of high-fit and low-fit older adults to those of younger adults, as greater brain activation in older adults can sometimes suggest reduced efficiency (i.e., compensation strategies or dedifferentiation).[155]

Various neurochemical changes are associated with increases in aerobic exercise, including alterations in brain-derived neurotrophic factor (BDNF) and neurotransmitter functions, which may underlie exercise-related functional brain changes and may play a role in improved cognitive function. BDNF is a protein associated with the growth and survival of new neurons, synaptic formation, and synaptic activity.[16,219] It is also critical to hippocampal function, synaptic plasticity, and learning.[119] In animal studies, BDNF levels have been observed to increase with exercise, particularly in the hippocampus.[20,50,149,203] In rats, improvements in memory and learning abilities have been related to increases in hippocampal BDNF levels.[203] In humans, increased serum concentrations of BDNF are noted after acute exercise training, though correlations between BDNF serum concentrations and cognitive function have yet to be observed.[77] In terms of neurotransmitter functions, exercise has been shown to impact monoamine neurotransmitter systems,[39,63,129,130] as well as the cholinergic system,[79,80] which has long been implicated in age-related cognitive decline.[17,18] There is also evidence of an up-regulation of genes related to the excitatory glutamatergic system and a down-regulation of those related to the inhibitory GABAergic system in response to exercise.[145] Interestingly, in rodents, long-term potentiation (LTP), a form of long-lasting synaptic plasticity, in the dentate gyrus has been shown to increase in response to running.[76,200] It has been suggested that increased expression of specific glutamate receptor subtypes (NR2B and Glu5) and BDNF mRNA in new dentate gyrus neurons may underlie the changes in LTP induced by exercise.[76] Improvements in synaptic function may also result from an increase in dendritic spine density in the dentate gyrus[67,165,187] and entorhinal cortex.[187]

The majority of research findings suggest that exercise is accompanied by numerous changes in the brain, including alterations in cytoarchitecture, neuronal proliferation, cerebral vascularization, cerebral blood flow, gray and white matter morphometry, neurophysiology, and neurochemistry. The interplay between each of these effects has yet to be completely understood, and it is likely that several of these events are interconnected. Nevertheless, taken as a whole, the current data suggest that exercise results in a more plastic and effective brain, which may maintain greater functional capability over time.

Effects of Exercise in Treating Cognitive and Neurological Pathology

Recent research indicates that exercise may help prevent the onset of neurodegenerative disease in healthy individuals. In addition, there is evidence to suggest that, in people with dementia, exercise may help slow the progression of the disease and reduce symptom severity. In particular, the question of whether exercise can be used to treat or slow the onset of neurodegenerative diseases, such as Alzheimer's disease, has received increased attention in recent years, based in part on findings that the hippocampus is specifically affected in Alzheimer's disease,[103] combined with reports that exercise promotes neuronal growth in the hippocampus.[201,202] Several studies have demonstrated the beneficial effects of exercise in animal models of neurodegenerative diseases, including a reduction in the neuropathological processes[2] and cognitive impairments[151] associated with Alzheimer's disease, and a delay in symptom onset and memory impairment in a model of Huntington's disease.[154] While there are some inconsistent findings in the literature,[29,216] in humans, several studies show that regular participation in exercise during midlife may reduce the risk of dementia later in life.[1,122,124,169,174] Moreover, individuals with a genotype associated with increased risk for developing Alzheimer's disease (APOE ε4 carriers) may receive greater benefit from regular midlife exercise.[169] A recent meta-analysis has indicated that individuals with Alzheimer's disease and other cognitive impairments receive multiple benefits from exercise training, such as improved cognitive, physical, and behavioral functioning.[92] Similar findings are reported for patients with Parkinson's disease who are noted to demonstrate improvements in movement initiation[21] and daily functioning[52] secondary to aerobic exercise training. There is also evidence indicating that exercise may slow the rate of cognitive decline in individuals with Alzheimer's disease.[185] Consistent with this notion, a recent structural MRI study indicated that higher levels of physical fitness were associated with reduced brain atrophy in patients with early Alzheimer's disease.[33] Findings from a positron emission tomography (PET) study involving patients with mild Alzheimer's dementia indicated that history of exercise, along with other daily leisure activities, was negatively correlated with cerebral blood flow in the temporal lobe and in temporal-parietal-occipital association areas, when controlling for disease severity.[175] That is, greater levels of daily activity were associated with greater cerebral blood flow deficit. The authors suggested that this association reflected a protective effect (i.e., increased cognitive reserve), conferred by exercise and leisure activities, which allowed patients with greater brain pathology to better cope with their neurologic impairments and thus present with less severe clinical symptoms.

Data from both animal models of stroke and studies of stroke patients provide evidence that exercise may have positive effects on poststroke recovery. Findings from an experimental model of focal cerebral ischemia in rats suggest that engagement in voluntary poststroke exercise can lead to improved neuronal survival in the dentate gyrus and recovery of spatial memory function.[128] In addition, engagement in regular exercise prior to an ischemic event appears to impart a protective influence on brain tissue.[57] Similar effects are apparent in humans, as one study reported that history of pre-stroke exercise might help reduce stroke severity and improve poststroke outcomes.[115] Furthermore, studies suggest that for individuals who have suffered a stroke, participation in poststroke aerobic exercise programs may improve functional rehabilitation.[164] It is likely that neural network reorganization may be partially responsible for exercise-related functional recovery in stroke patients. FMRI results indicate that aerobic treadmill training in posthemiparetic stroke patients results in improved ambulation that is associated with activation in both cortical and subcortical structures, reflecting possible neural modifications to exercise training.[127] Notably, the adaptations in neural networks associated with limb movements (i.e., greater cortico-subcortical network activation) were specific to the paretic leg only, and were not present in the control group. These findings,

together with similar reports in the literature[72] indicating possible reorganization in neural networks associated with poststroke exercise training, suggest that exercise may trigger changes in neural systems plasticity following stroke, which may have significant functional implications for patients.

In summary, most findings to date indicate that exercise may be a useful agent that can be employed to help delay the onset of neurodegenerative diseases and to aid in the management of cognitive and behavioral difficulties associated with dementia. Considering the relatively inactive lifestyles of many dementia patients in long-term care,[10] at the very least, increased implementation of exercise programs would likely have a positive impact on patients' quality of life.[11] Yet, research findings suggest a more hopeful picture, in that exercise may even improve cognitive function in dementia patients. In addition, exercise may be useful in helping patients recover from neurological insults such as stroke and possibly traumatic brain injury as well.[86,87] Some of the most appealing aspects of exercise are its accessibility and affordability, which combined with the findings noted above, make exercise a very attractive instrument with which we can improve public health. We are only just beginning to understand the potential of exercise to foster functional reorganization of brain networks. Future research will likely unearth more focused and effective exercise programs for treating cognitive and neurological impairments. As such, the use of neuroimaging techniques in these pursuits will become increasingly important.

Neural Mechanisms of the Effects of Exercise on Affect

Effects of Exercise on Normal Affective Functioning

Exercise has been shown to have positive effects on normal affective function, and has been suggested to be a practical and inexpensive means of defending against the development of some mental health issues.[146] In psychologically healthy individuals, exercise is associated with increases in mood, affect, and self-esteem, as well as a higher reported quality of life.[22,24] These effects are not limited by age, as both young and older individuals appear to benefit from the mood-enhancing effects of exercise. Physical activity levels have been associated with emotional well-being in adolescents[184] as well as adults.[183]

Effects of Exercise in Treating Affective Pathology

Major Depressive Disorder

Most of the research on the effects of exercise in treating affective disorders has focused on major depressive disorder (MDD). MDD is a pervasive, debilitating, and costly disorder.[108,147,186] Recent 12-month prevalence estimates of MDD for US adults are 6.7%,[108] with lifetime prevalence of 16.6%.[107] The effects of depression are severe, with 2–15% of those diagnosed with MDD committing suicide[147] and $44 billion in lost work time alone.[186]

Clinical and experimental data obtained over the past 25 years have provided overwhelming evidence that MDD involves a neurobiological disturbance that affects specific brain systems, including subcortical regions, such as the amygdala, and hippocampus, as well as the ventral striatum (including nucleus accumbens) and cortical regions, such as the ventromedial prefrontal cortex (VMPFC), lateral orbital prefrontal cortex (LOPFC), dorsolateral prefrontal cortex (DLPFC), and anterior cingulate cortex (ACC).[53,134] These regions are consistent with three broad areas of dysfunction, including emotional, cognitive, and sustained effort.

The hallmark symptoms of MDD include increased negative affect and decreased positive affect.[5] The amygdala is known to play a major role in emotional experience.[54,60,90,91,176,221] Other limbic structures such as the hippocampus and nucleus accumbens have been implicated in negative and positive affect, respectively,[90,120,188] and have shown abnormalities in patients with MDD.[49,134,150,173,177,204] Cortical structures, including the DLPFC and ACC, are also related to the manifestation of positive and negative affect[4,34,55,81,125,137,222] and MDD symptomotology.[61,62,135]

In addition to emotional dysfunction, another notable symptom of MDD includes "cognitive slowing" or difficulty with concentration.[5] Cortical structures often associated with cognitive functioning or working memory, such as the DLPFC, inferior parietal cortex, and posterior cingulate have shown abnormalities in patients with MDD.[9,59,70,100] Capacity for sustained effort is often diminished among depressed people who are experiencing negative and vegetative symptoms including reduced motivation and fatigue.[5] Cortical areas, such as the DLPFC,[7,14,106,123] ACC,[4,34,37] and LOPFC,[71,99] have been implicated in motivation and ability to sustain effort and attention.

In sum, there is compelling evidence that MDD involves disruption of multiple brain regions including, limbic, frontal-striatal, and frontal lobe systems.[134] These brain regions are known to have distinct roles in emotional, cognitive, and sustained effort processes,[43] which likely account for the variety of psychological disturbances associated with MDD. While specific brain regions have been implicated in the emotional, cognitive, and sustained effort manifestations of MDD, it is the interaction among these brain regions[135,207] and their behavioral manifestations[44] that may be most critical in understanding the mechanisms of MDD. For example, functional imaging studies have shown poor "communication" between amygdala and ACC in depressed patients, potentially resulting in failure of the ACC to regulate emotion.[6,207] Moreover, neuropsychological studies have shown an interrelated pattern among these three areas of functioning, relating depressed mood to poor concentration and inability to sustain cognitive effort and attention.[44]

Exercise as an Alternative Treatment for MDD

Pharmacological intervention is the standard of care for MDD [153]; however, many patients do not respond or obtain only partial relief of symptoms as a result of pharmacological treatment.[194] Moreover, recent research has shown that over 60% of US adults with diagnosable MDD did not receive treatment in the past 12 months.[206] This may, in part, reflect the fact that existing behavioral and pharmacological treatments are costly, often have numerous negative side effects, and require medical insurance coverage that many do not have.

Exercise is a promising alternative treatment for MDD that is less costly than pharmacological or psychological therapy, available to almost everyone, and has mostly positive rather than negative side effects.[196] Recent reviews note effects for exercise as a treatment for depression similar to that for cognitive therapy and antidepressant medication.[30,179,182] For example, Dunn et al.[64] found that a dose of exercise consistent with public health guidelines[196] resulted in greater reduction of depressive symptoms among mild to moderately depressed adults (aged 20–45 years) than a low dose of exercise or a contact control condition. Additionally, Blumenthal et al.[8,27] found no differences between treatment with exercise and antidepressant medication in clinical outcomes among older adults diagnosed with MDD. Moreover, in a recent study, exercise was rated as the treatment for depression (including cognitive or behavioral therapy and drug treatment) with the highest benefit-to-burden ratio among adults with previous depressive episodes.[156]

Effects of Exercise on Neural Structures Implicated in MDD

Acutely, exercise causes sympathetic nervous system activation and the release of various neurotransmitters into the blood stream, as well as increases in vascular tone, enhanced vascular function, and increased cerebral perfusion.[58,143,210,215] Our understanding of the effects of physical exertion and exercise on specific brain systems is increasing. Most notably, greater activation of the insular cortex and ACC has been shown to occur both immediately following exercise and also as a function of overall level of physical activity.[51,152,193,211-214] Additionally, animal studies have shown responses to exercise in subcortical regions to be similar to responses to antidepressant medication.[25,40,82,83,101,102,157,171,172,223] Thus, many of the brain areas shown to have changes in activation in response to exercise coincide with those that have been implicated in MDD. Although no studies have yet been conducted that directly examine these brain systems as a function of exercise in patients with MDD, the findings among nondepressed humans and animal studies indicate that exercise may result in functional brain response in depressed humans in many of the same brain systems impacted by antidepressant drugs.

While exercise may impact the brain in some ways that are consistent with the effects of antidepressant medication, it may also elicit response in some brain regions that are not as readily influenced by medication. As Mayberg's study[136] shows, alterations in frontal and ACC response occur later in treatment with selective serotonin reuptake inhibitors (SSRIs). This raises the possibility that responses in these areas occur as a secondary response to earlier limbic and striatal changes (i.e., alterations in systems involving emotional experience and reward). In contrast, there are emerging data that exercise may produce direct increases in frontal lobe activation.[51,152,193,211-214] These results indicate that exercise may produce more rapid changes in ACC and prefrontal brain regions, which could improve cognitive function in depressed patients. Thus, such findings in MDD patients suggest a possible mechanism of symptom improvement in which increased activation in prefrontal circuits and associated enhanced attention and executive control could provide an additional route by which depression can be improved. It is clear that more studies are needed to further elucidate the impact of exercise on brain function in MDD patients as well as in individuals with other psychological disorders.

The Role of Neural Processes in the Adoption and Maintenance of Exercise Programs

Exercise, Affect, and Adherence

Understanding of physical activity mechanisms to aid in the design of effective physical activity interventions is a national priority.[196] To date, studies attempting to identify determinants of exercise adherence have focused on cognitive,[138] social,[28] and more recently, environmental factors,[195] consistent with prevailing theoretical models.[3,12,110,163,167] These studies have consistently explained a modest percent of the variance in exercise behavior.[13] As such, further understanding is necessary to produce far-reaching, meaningful, and sustainable physical activity change. In comparison to cognitive, social, and environmental factors, affective processes as determinants of adoption and maintenance of exercise behavior have received considerably less attention (for notable exceptions see, refs. [111,198]). A useful model on which we may develop our understanding of exercise-related affective changes and their relation to exercise adherence is the Hedonic Theory,[220] which posits that behaviors that lead to more positive affective responses are more likely to be repeated and maintained.

A significant body of research has examined changes from preexercise to postexercise in distinct positive affective states, such as positive engagement, tranquility, revitalization, and positive well-being, and in distinct negative affective states, such as tension, depression, anger, fatigue, and psychological distress in response to acute bouts of exercise.[23,84,139] Studies assessing affective responses before and after exercise generally support the conclusion that acute bouts of exercise improve affective states.[218]

The above findings appear to create a paradox, as Learning Theory[192] and Hedonic Theory[220] would predict that behaviors that lead to positive affective states and decrease negative affective states would reinforce the behavior; yet, rates of regular physical activity participation are quite low,[15] especially among overweight and obese adults.[144] Hall et al.[89] have pointed out that this apparent paradox can be explained by the fact that assessments of affect are often administered prior to and following, but not during the exercise task (for a review see, ref. [69]). According to Learning Theory, immediate consequences of behavior are more predictive of future behavior than delayed consequences.[148] The subjective affective response experienced during exercise is more immediate than feelings experienced after the exercise has been completed which may also include the affective response to completing exercise.[89] Indeed, in a review of studies that assessed affective response before, during, and immediately following exercise among previously sedentary adults, Ekkekakis[68] found that affective response to moderate intensity exercise is highly variable (see also, ref. [199]), while affective response is more uniformly positive immediately following exercise. Thus, consistent with Hedonic Theory, the interpersonal variability shown in affective response during exercise may be more important (versus affect experienced after exercise) in understanding whether or not people will continue to exercise.[89]

Indeed, research has shown that those who report greater enjoyment of physical activity are more likely to engage in physical activity[170] and more likely to benefit from physical activity promotion interventions.[209] This suggests that affective response to exercise plays a role in exercise adherence, and is consistent with Hedonic Theory. In support of this idea, data from a recently completed physical activity promotion trial have indicated that affective response to an acute bout of moderate intensity exercise at baseline predicts future physical activity behavior.[208]

Neural Mechanisms of Behavioral Change and Exercise Adherence

The above findings suggest that there may be reward centers in the brain that may respond to exercise differently in individuals, and thus may promote or inhibit exercise differentially. Although such pathways have yet to be studied directly in relation to exercise, this hypothesis mirrors similar research into nicotine reward centers that may lead to greater chances of nicotine addiction and inhibit cessation in some individuals. For example, McClernon et al.[141] reported that genetic variations in the dopamine D4 receptor (DRD4) gene were associated with differences in brain responses to smoking cues in smokers in withdrawal. The authors found that compared to smokers who were homozygous for the short DRD4 allele, smokers who possessed the long DRD4 allele (DRD4 L) demonstrated greater activation in the insula and superior frontal gyrus (BA 10), regions that have been previously related to smoking cue reactivity and craving. One interpretation of these data, discussed by the authors, is that the DRD4 L allele may serve to enhance the signaling of potential reward cues; thus increased activation in the prefrontal cortex (i.e., in BA 10) of DRD4 L carriers might reflect increased attentional and cognitive processing of the smoking cues due to the heightened perception of their reward. Notably, exercise can have a modulating effect on cigarette craving and withdrawal symptoms in smokers[190] consistent with data indicating that exercise may directly influence neural systems involved in motivation and affect (as discussed above). Related to this notion, a recent FMRI study has revealed common circuits that may be implicated in the neural response to acute exercise, as well as smoking maintenance behaviors. Janse Van Rensburg et al.[104] observed that smokers in withdrawal who engaged in an acute bout of exercise reported reduced cigarette cravings and demonstrated modulated brain activation patterns in response to smoking cues. Specifically, smokers displayed reduced activation in regions of the frontal cortex (incorporating BA 10) after exercise, which the authors suggested might be associated with the reported reduction in craving sensations. This finding, together with that of McClernon et al.,[141] suggests that exercise can modulate the brain's response to rewarding stimuli (e.g., activity levels in BA 10) and that the effectiveness of this modulation could vary based on the genotype of the individual. However, this area of research is in its infancy, and substantially, more research is needed to understand the neural underpinnings of the effects of exercise on motivation, reward perception, and behavioral change. Such research will improve our understanding of exercise's utility in promoting healthy behaviors (e.g., smoking cessation), as well as our understanding of individual differences in neurological function that underlie exercise adherence.

Conclusions and Future Directions

There is a growing consensus that regular exercise is critical to healthy living. Moreover, emerging research indicates that exercise may also play a key role in treating brain-related diseases. However, we have only begun to understand why exercise is so critical to cognitive and emotional health and through what neural mechanisms it operates. Better understanding of such mechanisms will allow us to design more effective and broad-based treatments involving exercise therapy. For example, such research will help us identify optimal intensity, duration, frequency, and mode of exercise for treating and preventing neuropsychiatric and neurological disorders. Additionally, research into such mechanisms may uncover additional diseases for which exercise treatment may be beneficial. Finally, it is reasonable to assume that understanding the neurological mechanisms of exercise-related treatments will also aid in the development and refinement of nonexercise-related treatments, as key neural pathways are discovered that can be manipulated through other treatment modalities.

In order for exercise programs – designed for purposes of improving general health, increasing disease prevention, and treating specific disorders – to be of public health significance, we must also better understand the mechanisms that lead to successful adoption and maintenance of regular exercise behavior. To this end, individual variability in the neurological response to acute exercise behavior must be better understood and exploited to help shape sustainable exercise programs for each individual. For example, further research is needed into the interaction of genetic and environmental factors that lead people to experience exercise as either pleasurable or aversive.

In summary, gaining a better understanding of the brain mechanisms that underlie exercise-induced cognitive and emotional change is critical to improving our ability to impact healthy living throughout the lifespan. Clearly, studies involving neuroimaging techniques will play a major role in further elucidating the brain effects of exercise. As such, it will be important to build a greater body of knowledge regarding the acute and long-term effects of exercise through integrating various neuroimaging techniques (e.g., structural, FMRI, PET) with ongoing and developing studies. While much is known about the effects of exercise on the brain, there is still a substantial amount of work to be done. As discussed above, some of the research questions that would benefit from further investigation include the following: Which types of exercise programs benefit individuals the most, and further, what role do individual characteristics (e.g., genetic profiles, disease states, health factors) play in determining the level of benefit observed? What are the specific brain regions that demonstrate enhanced growth and/or spared degeneration in response to exercise across the lifespan, and what are the biological and neurochemical mechanisms that underlie these processes? What are the mechanisms through which cognitive and affective processing are enhanced secondary to exercise in healthy individuals of various ages, and in patients with neurological or neuropsychiatric disorders (e.g., Alzheimer's disease, MDD, stroke, ADHD, schizophrenia, substance abuse)? Are the neural pathways involved in this enhancement the same for neurologically healthy and unhealthy individuals? What are the neural processes associated with increases in exercise maintenance and exercise aversion, and do these processes change over time or with intervention? When possible, an emphasis should be placed on developing studies that utilize randomized clinical trials methodologies to compare these findings to those originating from the body of work that has relied on cross-sectional designs. Overall, such studies will best be completed utilizing a cross-disciplinary approach. Most important, the findings generated from this work will have the potential to impact social policy and produce significant improvements in public health.

References

1. Abbott RD, White LR, Ross GW, Masaki KH, Curb JD, Petrovitch H. Walking and dementia in physically capable elderly men. *JAMA.* 2004;292(12):1447–1453.
2. Adlard PA, Perreau VM, Pop V, Cotman CW. Voluntary exercise decreases amyloid load in a transgenic model of Alzheimer's disease. *J Neurosci.* 2005;25(17):4217–4221.
3. Ajzen I. The theory of planned behavior. *Organ Behav Hum Decis Process.* 1991;50:179–211.
4. Allman JM, Hakeem A, Erwin JM, Nimchinsky E, Hof P. The anterior cingulate cortex. The evolution of an interface between emotion and cognition. *Ann N Y Acad Sci.* 2001;935:107–117.
5. American Psychiatric Association. *Diagnostic and Statistical Manual of Mental Disorders.* 4th ed. Washington, DC: APA; 1994.
6. Anand A, Li Y, Wang Y, et al. Activity and connectivity of brain mood regulating circuit in depression: a functional magnetic resonance study. *Biol Psychiatry.* 2005;57(10): 1079–1088.
7. Asahi S, Okamoto Y, Okada G, Yamawaki S, Yokota N. Negative correlation between right prefrontal activity during response inhibition and impulsiveness: a fMRI study. *Eur Arch Psychiatry Clin Neurosci.* 2004;254(4): 245–251.
8. Babyak M, Blumenthal JA, Herman S, et al. Exercise treatment for major depression: maintenance of therapeutic benefit at 10 months. *Psychosom Med.* 2000;62(5): 633–638.
9. Baker SC, Frith CD, Dolan RJ. The interaction between mood and cognitive function studied with PET. *Psychol Med.* 1997;27(3):565–578.
10. Ballard C, Fossey J, Chithramohan R, et al. Quality of care in private sector and NHS facilities for people with dementia: cross sectional survey. *BMJ.* 2001;323(7310):426–427.
11. Ballard C, O'Brien J, James I, et al. Quality of life for people with dementia living in residential and nursing home care: the impact of performance on activities of daily living, behavioral and psychological symptoms, language skills, and psychotropic drugs. *Int Psychogeriatr.* 2001;13(1):93–106.
12. Bandura A. *Social Foundations of Thought and Action: A Social Cognitive Theory.* Englewood Cliffs, NJ: Prentice-Hall; 1986.
13. Baranowski T, Anderson C, Carmack C. Mediating variable framework in physical activity interventions. How are we doing? How might we do better? *Am J Prev Med.* 1998;15(4):266–297.
14. Barber AD, Carter CS. Cognitive control involved in overcoming prepotent response tendencies and switching between tasks. *Cereb Cortex.* 2005;15(7):899–912.
15. Barnes PM, Schoenborn CA. *Physical Activity Among Adults: United States, 2000.* Hyattsville, MD: U.S. Department of Health and Human Services, Centers for Disease Control and Prevention, National Center for Health Statistics; 2000.
16. Bartrup JT, Moorman JM, Newberry NR. BDNF enhances neuronal growth and synaptic activity in hippocampal cell cultures. *Neuroreport.* 1997;8(17):3791–3794.
17. Bartus RT. On neurodegenerative diseases, models, and treatment strategies: lessons learned and lessons forgotten a generation following the cholinergic hypothesis. *Exp Neurol.* 2000;163(2):495–529.
18. Bartus RT, Dean RL 3rd, Beer B, Lippa AS. The cholinergic hypothesis of geriatric memory dysfunction. *Science.* 1982;217(4558):408–414.
19. Bashore TR. Age, physical fitness, and mental processing speed. *Annu Rev Gerontol Geriatr.* 1989;9:120–144.
20. Berchtold NC, Chinn G, Chou M, Kesslak JP, Cotman CW. Exercise primes a molecular memory for brain-derived neurotrophic factor protein induction in the rat hippocampus. *Neuroscience.* 2005;133(3):853–861.
21. Bergen JL, Toole T, Elliott RG 3rd, Wallace B, Robinson K, Maitland CG. Aerobic exercise intervention improves aerobic capacity and movement initiation in Parkinson's disease patients. *NeuroRehabilitation.* 2002;17(2):161–168.
22. Berger BG. Psychological benefits of an active lifestyle: what we know and what we need to know. *Quest.* 1996;48(3): 330–353.
23. Berger BG, Motl RW. Exercise and mood: a selective review and synthesis of research employing the profile of mood states. *J Appl Sport Psychol.* 2000;12:69–92.
24. Biddle SJH, Fox KR, Boutcher SH. *Physical Activity and Psychological Well-Being.* London: Routledge; 2000.
25. Bjornebekk A, Mathe AA, Brene S. The antidepressant effect of running is associated with increased hippocampal cell proliferation. *Int J Neuropsychopharmacol.* 2005;8(3): 357–368.
26. Black JE, Isaacs KR, Anderson BJ, Alcantara AA, Greenough WT. Learning causes synaptogenesis, whereas motor activity causes angiogenesis, in cerebellar cortex of adult rats. *Proc Natl Acad Sci U S A.* 1990;87(14):5568–5572.
27. Blumenthal JA, Babyak MA, Moore KA, et al. Effects of exercise training on older patients with major depression. *Arch Intern Med.* 1999;159(19):2349–2356.
28. Brassington GS, Atienza AA, Perczek RE, DiLorenzo TM, King AC. Intervention-related cognitive versus social mediators of exercise adherence in the elderly. *Am J Prev Med.* 2002;23(suppl 2):80–86.
29. Broe GA, Creasey H, Jorm AF, et al. Health habits and risk of cognitive impairment and dementia in old age: a prospective study on the effects of exercise, smoking and alcohol consumption. *Aust N Z J Public Health.* 1998;22(5):621–623.
30. Brosse AL, Sheets ES, Lett HS, Blumenthal JA. Exercise and the treatment of clinical depression in adults: recent findings and future directions. *Sports Med.* 2002;32(12):741–760.
31. Brown J, Cooper-Kuhn CM, Kempermann G, et al. Enriched environment and physical activity stimulate hippocampal but not olfactory bulb neurogenesis. *Eur J Neurosci.* 2003;17(10):2042–2046.
32. Budde H, Voelcker-Rehage C, Pietrabyk-Kendziorra S, Ribeiro P, Tidow G. Acute coordinative exercise improves attentional performance in adolescents. *Neurosci Lett.* 2008;441(2): 219–223.
33. Burns JM, Cronk BB, Anderson HS, et al. Cardiorespiratory fitness and brain atrophy in early Alzheimer disease. *Neurology.* 2008;71(3):210–216.
34. Bush G, Luu P, Posner MI. Cognitive and emotional influences in anterior cingulate cortex. *Trends Cogn Sci.* 2000;4(6):215–222.

35. Carter CS, van Veen V. Anterior cingulate cortex and conflict detection: an update of theory and data. *Cogn Affect Behav Neurosci.* 2007;7(4):367–379.
36. Caserta MT, Bannon Y, Fernandez F, Giunta B, Schoenberg MR, Tan J. Normal brain aging clinical, immunological, neuropsychological, and neuroimaging features. *Int Rev Neurobiol.* 2009;84:1–19.
37. Casey BJ, Trainor R, Giedd J, et al. The role of the anterior cingulate in automatic and controlled processes: a developmental neuroanatomical study. *Dev Psychobiol.* 1997;30(1):61–69.
38. Castelli DM, Hillman CH, Buck SM, Erwin HE. Physical fitness and academic achievement in third- and fifth-grade students. *J Sport Exerc Psychol.* 2007;29(2):239–252.
39. Chaouloff F. Physical exercise and brain monoamines: a review. *Acta Physiol Scand.* 1989;137(1):1–13.
40. Chen MJ, Russo-Neustadt AA. Running exercise- and antidepressant-induced increases in growth and survival-associated signaling molecules are IGF-dependent. *Growth Factors.* 2007;25(2):118–131.
41. Chomitz VR, Slining MM, McGowan RJ, Mitchell SE, Dawson GF, Hacker KA. Is there a relationship between physical fitness and academic achievement? Positive results from public school children in the northeastern United States. *J Sch Health.* 2009;79(1):30–37.
42. Coe DP, Pivarnik JM, Womack CJ, Reeves MJ, Malina RM. Effect of physical education and activity levels on academic achievement in children. *Med Sci Sports Exerc.* 2006;38(8):1515–1519.
43. Cohen R. *Neuropsychology of Attention.* New York: Plenum; 1993.
44. Cohen R, Lohr I, Paul R, Boland R. Impairments of attention and effort among patients with major affective disorders. *J Neuropsychiatry Clin Neurosci.* 2001;13(3):385–395.
45. Colcombe SJ, Erickson KI, Raz N, et al. Aerobic fitness reduces brain tissue loss in aging humans. *J Gerontol A Biol Sci Med Sci.* 2003;58(2):176–180.
46. Colcombe SJ, Erickson KI, Scalf PE, et al. Aerobic exercise training increases brain volume in aging humans. *J Gerontol A Biol Sci Med Sci.* 2006;61(11):1166–1170.
47. Colcombe SJ, Kramer AF. Fitness effects on the cognitive function of older adults: a meta-analytic study. *Psychol Sci.* 2003;14(2):125–130.
48. Colcombe SJ, Kramer AF, Erickson KI, et al. Cardiovascular fitness, cortical plasticity, and aging. *Proc Natl Acad Sci U S A.* 2004;101(9):3316–3321.
49. Colla M, Kronenberg G, Deuschle M, et al. Hippocampal volume reduction and HPA-system activity in major depression. *J Psychiatr Res.* 2007;41(7):553–560.
50. Cotman CW, Berchtold NC. Exercise: a behavioral intervention to enhance brain health and plasticity. *Trends Neurosci.* 2002;25(6):295–301.
51. Critchley HD, Corfield DR, Chandler MP, Mathias CJ, Dolan RJ. Cerebral correlates of autonomic cardiovascular arousal: a functional neuroimaging investigation in humans. *J Physiol.* 2000;523(pt 1):259–270.
52. Crizzle AM, Newhouse IJ. Is physical exercise beneficial for persons with Parkinson's disease? *Clin J Sport Med.* 2006;16(5):422–425.
53. Davidson RJ. Affective neuroscience and psychophysiology: toward a synthesis. *Psychophysiology.* 2003;40(5):655–665.
54. Davidson RJ, Irwin W. The functional neuroanatomy of emotion and affective style. *Trends Cogn Sci.* 1999;3(1):11–21.
55. Davidson RJ, Lewis DA, Alloy LB, et al. Neural and behavioral substrates of mood and mood regulation. *Biol Psychiatry.* 2002;52(6):478–502.
56. Davis CL, Tomporowski PD, Boyle CA, et al. Effects of aerobic exercise on overweight children's cognitive functioning: a randomized controlled trial. *Res Q Exerc Sport.* 2007;78(5):510–519.
57. Ding YH, Mrizek M, Lai Q, et al. Exercise preconditioning reduces brain damage and inhibits TNF-alpha receptor expression after hypoxia/reoxygenation: an in vivo and in vitro study. *Curr Neurovasc Res.* 2006;3(4):263–271.
58. Dishman RK, Berthoud HR, Booth FW, et al. Neurobiology of exercise. *Obesity (Silver Spring).* 2006;14(3):345–356.
59. Dolan RJ, Bench CJ, Scott LC, Frackowiak RSJ. Neuropsychological dysfunction in depression: the relationship to regional cerebral blood flow. *Psychol Med.* 1994;24:180–182.
60. Drevets WC. Neuroimaging abnormalities in the amygdala in mood disorders. *Ann N Y Acad Sci.* 2003;985:420–444.
61. Drevets WC, Price JL, Simpson JR, Todd RD, Reich T, Vannier M. Subgenual prefrontal cortex abnormailities in mood disorders. *Nature.* 1997;386:824–827.
62. Drevets WC, Raichle ME. Reciprocal suppression of regional blood flow during emotional versus higher cognitive processes: implications for interactions between emotion and cognition. *Cogn Emot.* 1998;12:353–385.
63. Dunn AL, Reigle TG, Youngstedt SD, Armstrong RB, Dishman RK. Brain norepinephrine and metabolites after treadmill training and wheel running in rats. *Med Sci Sports Exerc.* 1996;28(2):204–209.
64. Dunn AL, Trivedi MH, Kampert JB, Clark CG, Chambliss HO. Exercise treatment for depression: efficacy and dose response. *Am J Prev Med.* 2005;28(1):1–8.
65. Dustman RE, Emmerson RY, Ruhling RO, Shearer DE. Age and fitness effects on EEG, ERPs, visual sensitivity, and cognition. *Neurobiol Aging.* 1990;11(3):193–200.
66. Dustman RE, LaMarche JA, Cohn NB, Shearer DE, Talone JM. Power spectral analysis and cortical coupling of EEG for young and old normal adults. *Neurobiol Aging.* 1985;6(3): 193–198.
67. Eadie BD, Redila VA, Christie BR. Voluntary exercise alters the cytoarchitecture of the adult dentate gyrus by increasing cellular proliferation, dendritic complexity, and spine density. *J Comp Neurol.* 2005;486(1):39–47.
68. Ekkekakis P. Pleasure and displeasure from the body: perspectives from exercise. *Cogn Emot.* 2003;17:213–239.
69. Ekkekakis P, Petruzzello SJ. Acute aerobic exercise and affect: current status, problems and prospects regarding dose-response. *Sports Med.* 1999;28(5):337–374.
70. Elliott R, Baker SC, Rogers RD, et al. Prefrontal dysfunction in depressed patients performing a complex planning task: a study using positron emission tomography. *Psychol Med.* 1997;27(4):931–942.
71. Elliott R, Dolan RJ, Frith CD. Dissociable functions in the medial and lateral orbitofrontal cortex: evidence from human neuroimaging studies. *Cereb Cortex.* 2000;10(3):308–317.
72. Enzinger C, Dawes H, Johansen-Berg H, et al. Brain activity changes associated with treadmill training after stroke. *Stroke.* 2009;40(7):2460–2467.

73. Erickson KI, Prakash RS, Voss MW, et al. Aerobic fitness is associated with hippocampal volume in elderly humans. *Hippocampus*. 2009;19(10):1030–1039.

74. Etnier JL, Nowell PM, Landers DM, Sibley BA. A meta-regression to examine the relationship between aerobic fitness and cognitive performance. *Brain Res Rev*. 2006;52(1):119–130.

75. Etnier JL, Salazar W, Landers DM, Petruzzello SJ, Han M, Nowell PM. The influence of physical fitness and exercise upon cognitive functioning: a meta–analysis. *J Sport Exerc Psychol*. 1997;19:249–277.

76. Farmer J, Zhao X, van Praag H, Wodtke K, Gage FH, Christie BR. Effects of voluntary exercise on synaptic plasticity and gene expression in the dentate gyrus of adult male Sprague–Dawley rats in vivo. *Neuroscience*. 2004;124(1):71–79.

77. Ferris LT, Williams JS, Shen CL. The effect of acute exercise on serum brain-derived neurotrophic factor levels and cognitive function. *Med Sci Sports Exerc*. 2007;39(4):728–734.

78. Field T, Diego M, Sanders CE. Exercise is positively related to adolescents' relationships and academics. *Adolescence*. 2001;36(141):105–110.

79. Fordyce DE, Farrar RP. Enhancement of spatial learning in F344 rats by physical activity and related learning-associated alterations in hippocampal and cortical cholinergic functioning. *Behav Brain Res*. 1991;46(2):123–133.

80. Fordyce DE, Farrar RP. Physical activity effects on hippocampal and parietal cortical cholinergic function and spatial learning in F344 rats. *Behav Brain Res*. 1991;43(2):115–123.

81. Galynker II, Cai J, Ongseng F, Finestone H, Dutta E, Serseni D. Hypofrontality and negative symptoms in major depressive disorder. *J Nucl Med*. 1998;39(4):608–612.

82. Garcia C, Chen MJ, Garza AA, Cotman CW, Russo-Neustadt A. The influence of specific noradrenergic and serotonergic lesions on the expression of hippocampal brain-derived neurotrophic factor transcripts following voluntary physical activity. *Neuroscience*. 2003;119(3):721–732.

83. Garza AA, Ha TG, Garcia C, Chen MJ, Russo-Neustadt AA. Exercise, antidepressant treatment, and BDNF mRNA expression in the aging brain. *Pharmacol Biochem Behav*. 2004;77(2):209–220.

84. Gauvin L, Rejeski W, Reboussin B. Contributions of acute bouts of vigorous physical activity to explaining diurnal variations in feeling states in active, middle-aged women. *Health Psychol*. 2000;19(4):365–375.

85. Gordon BA, Rykhlevskaia EI, Brumback CR, et al. Neuroanatomical correlates of aging, cardiopulmonary fitness level, and education. *Psychophysiology*. 2008;45(5):825–838.

86. Griesbach GS, Hovda DA, Gomez-Pinilla F. Exercise-induced improvement in cognitive performance after traumatic brain injury in rats is dependent on BDNF activation. *Brain Res*. 2009;1288:105–115.

87. Griesbach GS, Hovda DA, Molteni R, Wu A, Gomez-Pinilla F. Voluntary exercise following traumatic brain injury: brain-derived neurotrophic factor upregulation and recovery of function. *Neuroscience*. 2004;125(1):129–139.

88. Hall CD, Smith AL, Keele SW. The impact of aerobic activity on cognitive function in older adults: a new synthesis based on the concept of executive control. *Eur J Cogn Psychol*. 2001;13(1):279–300.

89. Hall EE, Ekkekakis P, Petruzzello SJ. The affective beneficence of vigorous exercise revisited. *Br J Health Psychol*. 2002;7(pt 1):47–66.

90. Hamann S, Mao H. Positive and negative emotional verbal stimuli elicit activity in the left amygdala. *Neuroreport*. 2002;13(1):15–19.

91. Hamann SB, Ely TD, Hoffman JM, Kilts CD. Ecstasy and agony: activation of the human amygdala in positive and negative emotion. *Psychol Sci*. 2002;13(2):135–141.

92. Heyn P, Abreu BC, Ottenbacher KJ. The effects of exercise training on elderly persons with cognitive impairment and dementia: a meta-analysis. *Arch Phys Med Rehabil*. 2004;85(10):1694–1704.

93. Hill RD, Storandt M, Malley M. The impact of long-term exercise training on psychological function in older adults. *J Gerontol*. 1993;48(1):12–17.

94. Hillman CH, Belopolsky AV, Snook EM, Kramer AF, McAuley E. Physical activity and executive control: implications for increased cognitive health during older adulthood. *Res Q Exerc Sport*. 2004;75(2):176–185.

95. Hillman CH, Buck SM, Themanson JR, Pontifex MB, Castelli DM. Aerobic fitness and cognitive development: event-related brain potential and task performance indices of executive control in preadolescent children. *Dev Psychol*. 2009;45(1):114–129.

96. Hillman CH, Castelli DM, Buck SM. Aerobic fitness and neurocognitive function in healthy preadolescent children. *Med Sci Sports Exerc*. 2005;37(11):1967–1974.

97. Hillman CH, Pontifex MB, Raine LB, Castelli DM, Hall EE, Kramer AF. The effect of acute treadmill walking on cognitive control and academic achievement in preadolescent children. *Neuroscience*. 2009;159(3):1044–1054.

98. Hillman CH, Snook EM, Jerome GJ. Acute cardiovascular exercise and executive control function. *Int J Psychophysiol*. 2003;48(3):307–314.

99. Horn NR, Dolan M, Elliott R, Deakin JF, Woodruff PW. Response inhibition and impulsivity: an fMRI study. *Neuropsychologia*. 2003;41(14):1959–1966.

100. Hugdahl K, Rund BR, Lund A, et al. Brain activation measured with fMRI during a mental arithmetic task in schizophrenia and major depression. *Am J Psychiatry*. 2004;161(2):286–293.

101. Hunsberger JG, Newton SS, Bennett AH, et al. Antidepressant actions of the exercise-regulated gene VGF. *Nat Med*. 2007;13(12):1476–1482.

102. Ivy AS, Rodriguez FG, Garcia C, Chen MJ, Russo-Neustadt AA. Noradrenergic and serotonergic blockade inhibits BDNF mRNA activation following exercise and antidepressant. *Pharmacol Biochem Behav*. 2003;75(1):81–88.

103. Jack CR Jr, Petersen RC, Xu Y, et al. Rate of medial temporal lobe atrophy in typical aging and Alzheimer's disease. *Neurology*. 1998;51(4):993–999.

104. Janse Van Rensburg K, Taylor A, Hodgson T, Benattayallah A. Acute exercise modulates cigarette cravings and brain activation in response to smoking-related images: an fMRI study. *Psychopharmacology (Berl)*. 2009;203(3):589–598.

105. Kamijo K, Hayashi Y, Sakai T, Yahiro T, Tanaka K, Nishihira Y. Acute effects of aerobic exercise on cognitive function in older adults. *J Gerontol B Psychol Sci Soc Sci*. 2009;64(3):356–363.

106. Kelly AM, Hester R, Murphy K, Javitt DC, Foxe JJ, Garavan H. Prefrontal-subcortical dissociations underlying inhibitory control revealed by event-related fMRI. *Eur J Neurosci*. 2004;19(11):3105–3112.

107. Kessler RC, Berglund P, Demler O, et al. The epidemiology of major depressive disorder: results from the National Comorbidity Survey Replication (NCS-R). *JAMA*. 2003;289(23):3095–3105.

108. Kessler RC, Berglund P, Demler O, Jin R, Merikangas KR, Walters EE. Lifetime prevalence and age-of-onset distributions of DSM-IV disorders in the National Comorbidity Survey Replication. *Arch Gen Psychiatry*. 2005;62(6):593–602.

109. Kim HY, Frongillo EA, Han SS, et al. Academic performance of Korean children is associated with dietary behaviours and physical status. *Asia Pac J Clin Nutr*. 2003;12(2):186–192.

110. King A, Stokols D, Talen E, Brassington G, Killingsworth R. Theoretical approaches to the promotion of physical activity: forging a transdisciplinary paradigm. *Am J Prev Med*. 2002;23(2):15–25.

111. Kiviniemi MT, Voss-Humke AM, Seifert AL. How do I feel about the behavior? The interplay of affective associations with behaviors and cognitive beliefs as influences on physical activity behavior. *Health Psychol*. 2007;26(2):152–158.

112. Kleim JA, Cooper NR, VandenBerg PM. Exercise induces angiogenesis but does not alter movement representations within rat motor cortex. *Brain Res*. 2002;934(1):1–6.

113. Knowler WC, Barrett-Connor E, Fowler SE, et al. Reduction in the incidence of type 2 diabetes with lifestyle intervention or metformin. *N Engl J Med*. 2002;346(6):393–403.

114. Kramer AF, Hahn S, Cohen NJ, et al. Ageing, fitness and neurocognitive function. *Nature*. 1999;400(6743): 418–419.

115. Krarup LH, Truelsen T, Gluud C, et al. Prestroke physical activity is associated with severity and long-term outcome from first-ever stroke. *Neurology*. 2008;71(17):1313–1318.

116. Kronenberg G, Bick-Sander A, Bunk E, Wolf C, Ehninger D, Kempermann G. Physical exercise prevents age-related decline in precursor cell activity in the mouse dentate gyrus. *Neurobiol Aging*. 2006;27(10):1505–1513.

117. Kubitz KA, Mott AA. EEG power spectral densities during and after cycle ergometer exercise. *Res Q Exerc Sport*. 1996;67(1):91–96.

118. Kubitz KA, Pothakos K. Does aerobic exercise decrease brain activation? *J Sport Exerc Psychol*. 1997;19(3):291–301.

119. Kuipers SD, Bramham CR. Brain-derived neurotrophic factor mechanisms and function in adult synaptic plasticity: new insights and implications for therapy. *Curr Opin Drug Discov Devel*. 2006;9(5):580–586.

120. Lane RD, Reiman EM, Bradley MM, et al. Neuroanatomical correlates of pleasant and unpleasant emotion. *Neuropsychologia*. 1997;35(11):1437–1444.

121. Lardon MT, Polich J. EEG changes from long-term physical exercise. *Biol Psychol*. 1996;44(1):19–30.

122. Larson EB, Wang L, Bowen JD, et al. Exercise is associated with reduced risk for incident dementia among persons 65 years of age and older. *Ann Intern Med*. 2006;144(2): 73–81.

123. Lavric A, Pizzagalli DA, Forstmeier S. When 'go' and 'nogo' are equally frequent: ERP components and cortical tomography. *Eur J Neurosci*. 2004;20(9):2483–2488.

124. Li G, Shen YC, Chen CH, Zhau YW, Li SR, Lu M. A three-year follow-up study of age-related dementia in an urban area of Beijing. *Acta Psychiatr Scand*. 1991;83(2):99–104.

125. Liotti M, Mayberg HS, Brannan SK, McGinnis S, Jerabek P, Fox PT. Differential limbic–cortical correlates of sadness and anxiety in healthy subjects: implications for affective disorders. *Biol Psychiatry*. 2000;48(1):30–42.

126. Lopez-Lopez C, LeRoith D, Torres-Aleman I. Insulin-like growth factor I is required for vessel remodeling in the adult brain. *Proc Natl Acad Sci U S A*. 2004;101(26): 9833–9838.

127. Luft AR, Macko RF, Forrester LW, et al. Treadmill exercise activates subcortical neural networks and improves walking after stroke: a randomized controlled trial. *Stroke*. 2008;39(12):3341–3350.

128. Luo CX, Jiang J, Zhou QG, et al. Voluntary exercise-induced neurogenesis in the postischemic dentate gyrus is associated with spatial memory recovery from stroke. *J Neurosci Res*. 2007;85(8):1637–1646.

129. MacRae PG, Spirduso WW, Cartee GD, Farrar RP, Wilcox RE. Endurance training effects on striatal D2 dopamine receptor binding and striatal dopamine metabolite levels. *Neurosci Lett*. 1987;79(1–2):138–144.

130. MacRae PG, Spirduso WW, Walters TJ, Farrar RP, Wilcox RE. Endurance training effects on striatal D2 dopamine receptor binding and striatal dopamine metabolites in presenescent older rats. *Psychopharmacology (Berl)*. 1987;92(2):236–240.

131. Madden DJ, Blumenthal JA, Allen PA, Emery CF. Improving aerobic capacity in healthy older adults does not necessarily lead to improved cognitive performance. *Psychol Aging*. 1989;4(3):307–320.

132. Magnie MN, Bermon S, Martin F, et al. P300, N400, aerobic fitness, and maximal aerobic exercise. *Psychophysiology*. 2000;37(3):369–377.

133. Mahar MT, Murphy SK, Rowe DA, Golden J, Shields AT, Raedeke TD. Effects of a classroom-based program on physical activity and on-task behavior. *Med Sci Sports Exerc*. 2006;38(12):2086–2094.

134. Maletic V, Robinson M, Oakes T, Iyengar S, Ball SG, Russell J. Neurobiology of depression: an integrated view of key findings. *Int J Clin Pract*. 2007;61(12): 2030–2040.

135. Mayberg HS. Modulating dysfunctional limbic-cortical circuits in depression: towards development of brain-based algorithms for diagnosis and optimised treatment. *Br Med Bull*. 2003;65:193–207.

136. Mayberg HS, Brannan SK, Tekell JL, et al. Regional metabolic effects of fluoxetine in major depression: serial changes and relationship to clinical response. *Biol Psychiatry*. 2000;48(8):830–843.

137. Mayberg HS, Liotti M, Brannan SK, et al. Reciprocal limbic-cortical function and negative mood: converging PET findings in depression and normal sadness. *Am J Psychiatry*. 1999;156(5):675–682.

138. McAuley E, Blissmer B. Self-efficacy determinants and consequences of physical activity. *Exerc Sport Sci Rev*. 2000;28(2):85–88.

139. McAuley E, Courneya KS. The subjective exercise experiences scale (SEES): development and preliminary validation. *J Sport Exerc Psychol*. 1994;16:163–177.

140. McAuley E, Kramer AF, Colcombe SJ. Cardiovascular fitness and neurocognitive function in older adults: a brief review. *Brain Behav Immun*. 2004;18(3):214–220.
141. McClernon FJ, Hutchison KE, Rose JE, Kozink RV. DRD4 VNTR polymorphism is associated with transient fMRI-BOLD responses to smoking cues. *Psychopharmacology (Berl)*. 2007;194(4):433–441.
142. McTiernan A, Kooperberg C, White E, et al. Recreational physical activity and the risk of breast cancer in postmenopausal women: the Women's Health Initiative Cohort Study. *J Am Med Assoc*. 2003;290(10):1331–1336.
143. Meeusen R. Exercise and the brain: insight in new therapeutic modalities. *Ann Transplant*. 2005;10(4):49–51.
144. MMWR. Prevalence of leisure-time physical activity among overweight adults – United States, 1998. *MMWR Morb Mortal Wkly Rep*. 2000;49(15):326–330.
145. Molteni R, Ying Z, Gomez-Pinilla F. Differential effects of acute and chronic exercise on plasticity-related genes in the rat hippocampus revealed by microarray. *Eur J Neurosci*. 2002;16(6):1107–1116.
146. Morgan WP. *Physical Activity and Mental Health*. Philadelphia, PA: Taylor & Francis; 1997.
147. National strategy for suicide prevention: a collaborative effort of SAMSHA, C., NIH, HRSA, &HIS. Available at http://mentalhealth.samsha.gov/suicideprevention/suicide-facts.asp; 2007.
148. Neef NA, Shade D, Miller MS. Assessing influential dimensions of reinforcers on choice in students with serious emotional disturbance. *J Appl Behav Anal*. 1994;27(4):575–583.
149. Neeper SA, Gomez-Pinilla F, Choi J, Cotman C. Exercise and brain neurotrophins. *Nature*. 1995;373(6510):109.
150. Neumeister A, Wood S, Bonne O, et al. Reduced hippocampal volume in unmedicated, remitted patients with major depression versus control subjects. *Biol Psychiatry*. 2005;57(8):935–937.
151. Nichol KE, Parachikova AI, Cotman CW. Three weeks of running wheel exposure improves cognitive performance in the aged Tg2576 mouse. *Behav Brain Res*. 2007;184(2):124–132.
152. Nowak M, Olsen KS, Law I, Holm S, Paulson OB, Secher NH. Command-related distribution of regional cerebral blood flow during attempted handgrip. *J Appl Physiol*. 1999;86(3):819–824.
153. Olfson M, Marcus SC, Druss B, Elinson L, Tanielian T, Pincus HA. National trends in the outpatient treatment of depression. *JAMA*. 2002;287(2):203–209.
154. Pang TY, Stam NC, Nithianantharajah J, Howard ML, Hannan AJ. Differential effects of voluntary physical exercise on behavioral and brain-derived neurotrophic factor expression deficits in Huntington's disease transgenic mice. *Neuroscience*. 2006;141(2):569–584.
155. Park DC, Polk TA, Mikels JA, Taylor SF, Marshuetz C. Cerebral aging: integration of brain and behavioral models of cognitive function. *Dialogues Clin Neurosci*. 2001;3(3):151–165.
156. Parker G, Crawford J. Judged effectiveness of differing antidepressant strategies by those with clinical depression. *Aust N Z J Psychiatry*. 2007;41(1):32–37.
157. Pereira AC, Huddleston DE, Brickman AM, et al. An in vivo correlate of exercise-induced neurogenesis in the adult dentate gyrus. *Proc Natl Acad Sci U S A*. 2007;104(13):5638–5643.

158. Peters J, Dauvermann M, Mette C, et al. Voxel-based morphometry reveals an association between aerobic capacity and grey matter density in the right anterior insula. *Neuroscience*. 2009;163(4):1102–1128.
159. Podewils LJ, Guallar E, Beauchamp N, Lyketsos CG, Kuller LH, Scheltens P. Physical activity and white matter lesion progression: assessment using MRI. *Neurology*. 2007;68(15):1223–1226.
160. Polich J. Updating P300: an integrative theory of P3a and P3b. *Clin Neurophysiol*. 2007;118(10):2128–2148.
161. Polich J, Kok A. Cognitive and biological determinants of P300: an integrative review. *Biol Psychol*. 1995;41(2):103–146.
162. Polich J, Lardon MT. P300 and long-term physical exercise. *Electroencephalogr Clin Neurophysiol*. 1997;103(4):493–498.
163. Prochaska J, DiClemente C. *The Transtheoretical Approach: Crossing the Traditional Boundaries of Therapy*. Homewood, IL: Dow-Jones, Irwin; 1984.
164. Rabadi MH. Randomized clinical stroke rehabilitation trials in 2005. *Neurochem Res*. 2007;32(4–5):807–821.
165. Redila VA, Christie BR. Exercise-induced changes in dendritic structure and complexity in the adult hippocampal dentate gyrus. *Neuroscience*. 2006;137(4):1299–1307.
166. Rogers RL, Meyer JS, Mortel KF. After reaching retirement age physical activity sustains cerebral perfusion and cognition. *J Am Geriatr Soc*. 1990;38(2):123–128.
167. Rogers RW. Cognitive and physiological processes in fear appeals and attitude change: a revised theory of protection motivation. In: Cacioppo JT, Petty RE, eds. *Social Psychophysiology: A Sourcebook*. New York: Guilford; 1983:153–176.
168. Rolls A, Schori H, London A, Schwartz M. Decrease in hippocampal neurogenesis during pregnancy: a link to immunity. *Mol Psychiatry*. 2008;13(5):468–469.
169. Rovio S, Kareholt I, Helkala EL, et al. Leisure-time physical activity at midlife and the risk of dementia and Alzheimer's disease. *Lancet Neurol*. 2005;4(11):705–711.
170. Rovniak LS, Anderson ES, Winett RA, Stephens RS. Social cognitive determinants of physical activity in young adults: a prospective structural equation analysis. *Ann Behav Med*. 2002;24(2):149–156.
171. Russo-Neustadt AA, Alejandre H, Garcia C, Ivy AS, Chen MJ. Hippocampal brain-derived neurotrophic factor expression following treatment with reboxetine, citalopram, and physical exercise. *Neuropsychopharmacology*. 2004;29(12):2189–2199.
172. Russo-Neustadt AA, Beard RC, Huang YM, Cotman CW. Physical activity and antidepressant treatment potentiate the expression of specific brain-derived neurotrophic factor transcripts in the rat hippocampus. *Neuroscience*. 2000;101(2):305–312.
173. Saxena S, Brody AL, Ho ML, et al. Cerebral metabolism in major depression and obsessive-compulsive disorder occurring separately and concurrently. *Biol Psychiatry*. 2001;50(3):159–170.
174. Scarmeas N, Levy G, Tang MX, Manly J, Stern Y. Influence of leisure activity on the incidence of Alzheimer's disease. *Neurology*. 2001;57(12):2236–2242.
175. Scarmeas N, Zarahn E, Anderson KE, et al. Association of life activities with cerebral blood flow in Alzheimer disease: implications for the cognitive reserve hypothesis. *Arch Neurol*. 2003;60(3):359–365.

176. Schaefer SM, Jackson DC, Davidson RJ, Aguirre GK, Kimberg DY, Thompson-Schill SL. Modulation of amygdalar activity by the conscious regulation of negative emotion. *J Cogn Neurosci.* 2002;14(6):913–921.

177. Sheline YI, Gado MH, Kraemer HC. Untreated depression and hippocampal volume loss. *Am J Psychiatry.* 2003;160(8):1516–1518.

178. Sibley BA, Etnier JL. The relationship between physical activity and cognition in children: a meta-analysis. *Pediatr Exerc Sci.* 2003;15(3):243–256.

179. Sjosten N, Kivela SL. The effects of physical exercise on depressive symptoms among the aged: a systematic review. *Int J Geriatr Psychiatry.* 2006;21(5):410–418.

180. Slattery ML. Physical activity and colorectal cancer. *Sports Med.* 2004;34(4):239–252.

181. Spirduso WW, Clifford P. Replication of age and physical activity effects on reaction and movement time. *J Gerontol.* 1978;33(1):26–30.

182. Stathopoulou G, Powers MB. Exercise interventions for mental health: a quantitative and qualitative review. *Clin Psychol Sci Pract.* 2006;13:179–193.

183. Stephens T. Physical activity and mental health in the United States and Canada: evidence from four population surveys. *Prev Med.* 1988;17(1):35–47.

184. Steptoe A, Butler N. Sports participation and emotional well-being in adolescents. *Lancet.* 1996;347(9018):1789–1792.

185. Stevens J, Killeen M. A randomised controlled trial testing the impact of exercise on cognitive symptoms and disability of residents with dementia. *Contemp Nurse.* 2006;21(1):32–40.

186. Stewart WF, Ricci JA, Chee E, Hahn SR, Morganstein D. Cost of lost productive work time among US workers with depression. *JAMA.* 2003;289(23):3135–3144.

187. Stranahan AM, Khalil D, Gould E. Running induces widespread structural alterations in the hippocampus and entorhinal cortex. *Hippocampus.* 2007;17(11):1017–1022.

188. Sutton SK. Asymmetry in prefrontal glucose metabolism during appetitive and aversive emotional states: an FDG-PET study. *Psychophysiology.* 1997;34:S89.

189. Swain RA, Harris AB, Wiener EC, et al. Prolonged exercise induces angiogenesis and increases cerebral blood volume in primary motor cortex of the rat. *Neuroscience.* 2003;117(4):1037–1046.

190. Taylor AH, Ussher MH, Faulkner G. The acute effects of exercise on cigarette cravings, withdrawal symptoms, affect and smoking behaviour: a systematic review. *Addiction.* 2007;102(4):534–543.

191. Thompson PD, Buchner D, Pina IL, et al. Exercise and physical activity in the prevention and treatment of atherosclerotic cardiovascular disease: a statement from the Council on Clinical Cardiology (Subcommittee on Exercise, Rehabilitation, and Prevention) and the Council on Nutrition, Physical Activity, and Metabolism (Subcommittee on Physical Activity). *Circulation.* 2003;107(24):3109–3116.

192. Thorndike EL. The law of effect. *Am J Psychol.* 1927;39:212–222.

193. Thornton JM, Guz A, Murphy K, et al. Identification of higher brain centres that may encode the cardiorespiratory response to exercise in humans. *J Physiol.* 2001;533(Pt 3):823–836.

194. Trivedi MH, Rush AJ, Wisniewski SR, et al. Evaluation of outcomes with citalopram for depression using measurement-based care in STAR*D: implications for clinical practice. *Am J Psychiatry.* 2006;163(1):28–40.

195. Trost SG, Owen N, Bauman AE, Sallis JF, Brown W. Correlates of adults' participation in physical activity: review and update. *Med Sci Sports Exerc.* 2002;34(12):1996–2001.

196. U.S. Department of Health and Human Services. *Physical Activity and Health: A Report of the Surgeon General.* Atlanta, GA: Centers for Disease Control and Prevention, National Center for Chronic Disease Prevention and Health Promotion; 1996.

197. U.S. Department of Health and Human Services. *Healthy People 2010: Understanding and Improving Health.* 2nd ed. Washington, DC, USA: U.S. Government Printing Office; 2000.

198. van der Pligt J, De Vries NK. Expectancy-value models of health behavior: the role of salience and anticipated affect. *Psychol Health.* 1998;13:289–305.

199. Van Landuyt LM, Ekkekakis P, Hall EE, Petruzzello SJ. Throwing the mountains into the lakes: on the perils of nomothetic conceptions of the exercise-affect relationship. *J Sport Exerc Psychol.* 2000;22:208–234.

200. van Praag H, Christie BR, Sejnowski TJ, Gage FH. Running enhances neurogenesis, learning, and long-term potentiation in mice. *Proc Natl Acad Sci U S A.* 1999;96(23):13427–13431.

201. van Praag H, Kempermann G, Gage FH. Running increases cell proliferation and neurogenesis in the adult mouse dentate gyrus. *Nat Neurosci.* 1999;2(3):266–270.

202. van Praag H, Shubert T, Zhao C, Gage FH. Exercise enhances learning and hippocampal neurogenesis in aged mice. *J Neurosci.* 2005;25(38):8680–8685.

203. Vaynman S, Ying Z, Gomez-Pinilla F. Hippocampal BDNF mediates the efficacy of exercise on synaptic plasticity and cognition. *Eur J Neurosci.* 2004;20(10):2580–2590.

204. Videbech P, Ravnkilde B. Hippocampal volume and depression: a meta-analysis of MRI studies. *Am J Psychiatry.* 2004;161(11):1957–1966.

205. Vuori IM. Health benefits of physical activity with special reference to interaction with diet. *Public Health Nutr.* 2001;4((2B)):517–528.

206. Wang PS, Berglund P, Olfson M, Pincus HA, Wells KB, Kessler RC. Failure and delay in initial treatment contact after first onset of mental disorders in the National Comorbidity Survey Replication. *Arch Gen Psychiatry.* 2005;62(6):603–613.

207. Whittle S, Allen NB, Lubman DI, Yucel M. The neurobiological basis of temperament: towards a better understanding of psychopathology. *Neurosci Biobehav Rev.* 2006;30(4):511–525.

208. Williams DM, Dunsiger S, Ciccolo JT, Lewis BA, Albrecht AE, Marcus BH. Acute affective response to a moderate-intensity exercise stimulus predicts physical activity participation 6 and 12 months later. *Psychol Sport Exerc.* 2008;9(3):231–245.

209. Williams DM, Papandonatos GD, Napolitano MA, Lewis BA, Whiteley JA, Marcus BH. Perceived enjoyment moderates the efficacy of an individually tailored physical activity intervention. *J Sport Exerc Psychol.* 2006;28:300–309.

210. Williamson JW, Fadel PJ, Mitchell JH. New insights into central cardiovascular control during exercise in humans: a central command update. *Exp Physiol.* 2006;91(1):51–58.

211. Williamson JW, McColl R, Mathews D. Evidence for central command activation of the human insular cortex during exercise. *J Appl Physiol.* 2003;94(5):1726–1734.

212. Williamson JW, McColl R, Mathews D, Ginsburg M, Mitchell JH. Activation of the insular cortex is affected by the intensity of exercise. *J Appl Physiol.* 1999;87(3):1213–1219.

213. Williamson JW, McColl R, Mathews D, Mitchell JH, Raven PB, Morgan WP. Hypnotic manipulation of effort sense during dynamic exercise: cardiovascular responses and brain activation. *J Appl Physiol.* 2001;90(4):1392–1399.

214. Williamson JW, McColl R, Mathews D, Mitchell JH, Raven PB, Morgan WP. Brain activation by central command during actual and imagined handgrip under hypnosis. *J Appl Physiol.* 2002;92(3):1317–1324.

215. Williamson JW, Morgan WP. Cardiovascular regulation: SPECT neuroimaging. *Int J Sport Exerc Psychol.* 2005;3:352–362.

216. Wilson RS, Mendes De Leon CF, Barnes LL, et al. Participation in cognitively stimulating activities and risk of incident Alzheimer disease. *JAMA.* 2002;287(6):742–748.

217. Wing RR, Hill JO. Successful weight loss maintenance. *Annu Rev Nutr.* 2001;21:323–341.

218. Yeung RR. The acute effects of exercise on mood state. *J Psychosom Res.* 1996;40(2):123–141.

219. Ying SW, Futter M, Rosenblum K, et al. Brain-derived neurotrophic factor induces long-term potentiation in intact adult hippocampus: requirement for ERK activation coupled to CREB and upregulation of Arc synthesis. *J Neurosci.* 2002;22(5):1532–1540.

220. Young PT. The role of hedonic processes in the organization of behavior. *Psychol Rev.* 1952;59(4):249–262.

221. Zald DH. The human amygdala and the emotional evaluation of sensory stimuli. *Brain Res Brain Res Rev.* 2003;41(1): 88–123.

222. Zald DH, Mattson DL, Pardo JV. Brain activity in ventromedial prefrontal cortex correlates with individual differences in negative affect. *Proc Natl Acad Sci U S A.* 2002;99(4):2450–2454.

223. Zheng H, Liu Y, Li W, et al. Beneficial effects of exercise and its molecular mechanisms on depression in rats. *Behav Brain Res.* 2006;168(1):47–55.

Chapter 17
Neuroimaging of Pain: A Psychosocial Perspective

Tamara J. Somers, G. Lorimer Moseley, Francis J. Keefe, and Sejal M. Kothadia

The past 60 years has witnessed major changes in the way that pain is conceptualized and treated. In the 1950s, pain was generally conceptualized using a sensory model that maintained that pain is a simple sensory event that warned of tissue damage. Treatments for pain were biomedical and consisted mainly of attempts to identify underlying tissue damage and treat it medically or surgically. In the 1960s, clinicians and researchers expressed growing dissatisfaction with the sensory model of pain. In particular, it became increasingly clear that the sensory model failed to explain phenomena often seen in patients experiencing chronic pain: pain persisting despite multiple medical and surgical treatments aimed at correcting underlying tissue damage, reports of pain showing poor correlation with underlying evidence of tissue damage, and pain being modified by psychosocial factors such as anxiety, social support, or expectations. Melzack and Wall's gate control theory was one of the first to maintain that pain was complex in that it not only had a sensory component, but also affective, cognitive, and behavioral components.[1] A key tenet of the gate control theory was that the brain could play a major role in modulating nociceptive signals at the spinal cord, through descending pathways from brain areas thought to be involved in affect, cognition, and behavior. The gate control theory also led to renewed interest in expanding pain treatments beyond traditional medical and surgical approaches to a wide array of interventions that could alter pain by modifying sensation (e.g., transcutaneous nerve stimulation, massage), or affective (e.g., anti- anxiety and antidepressant medications), cognitive (e.g., cognitive therapy, distraction techniques), and behavioral processes (e.g., exercise, graded activation).

The advent and progress of brain imaging have provided important corroboration of the complexity of pain. Early imaging studies, for example, demonstrated that delivery of a noxious stimulus to the skin of the body activated not only sensory areas of the brain but also a wide variety of other brain regions. Findings of these imaging studies fit well with the neuromatrix theory of pain developed by Melzack.[2,3] This theory maintains that the experience of pain reflects the coordinated interaction of neurons that are widely distributed in the brain (e.g., in the thalamus, cortex, and limbic systems, which he collectively called the "pain neuromatrix"). It posited that in each individual there is a specific neural "pain neurosignature" that reflects the repetitive cycling and processing of neural inputs (i.e., those responsible for sensory, cognitive-evaluative, and motivational-affect inputs) and neural outputs (i.e., those brain programs responsible for perception, action, and stress regulation). According to the theory, it is this repetitive cycling and processing that is responsible for the experience of pain.

The impact of the neuromatrix theory on the field of pain research has been substantial. This theory generated increased interest in the role that brain imaging can play in understanding the pain experience. It also introduced the terms "pain neuromatrix" and "pain neurosignature," each of which has been adopted by a number of brain imaging researchers. The neuromatrix theory has also provided a conceptual basis for understanding the effects of psychosocial factors and psychosocial interventions on pain.

F.J. Keefe (✉)
Duke University Medical Center, Durham, NC, USA
e-mail: keefe003@mc.duke.edu

Over the past 2 decades, the field of brain imaging of pain has grown enormously. Exciting, new findings are emerging at a rapid pace and these findings are impacting not only pain theory but also research and clinical practice. The purpose of this chapter is to provide a brief review of psychosocial research in this field. The chapter is divided into four sections. The first section highlights research on the neural correlates of pain. The second section provides a summary of studies that have examined the effects of psychological factors on pain using brain imaging. The third section describes psychosocial interventions for pain, on which imaging studies have been undertaken. In the final section, we consider important future directions for research on this topic.

The Neural Correlates of Pain

Exactly how pain emerges from the brain is not clear, but much can be gained by better understanding the structural and functional anatomy of the specific parts of the nervous system that are involved in pain. Broadly speaking, there are two approaches to elucidate pain's neural substrate: (1) To identify the neurons in the tissues of the body that are selectively activated in response to a (normally) painful stimulus and to follow these neurons and their synaptic connections, in vitro, all the way to the brain; (2) to measure changes in activity of neural structures in vivo, for example, through localized fluctuations in blood flow or electric activity – these fluctuations are taken as reflections of fluctuating activity of brain cells.

Conceptualizing a Structural Anatomy of Nociception and Pain

There are several classes of neurons that have their peripheral terminals in the tissues of the body. Many neurons are specifically suited to respond to particular modes of stimulation, for example, light touch or changes in temperature. The class of neurons most obviously, although by no means exclusively, pertinent to the pain system are called nociceptors – "danger receptors." It is critical at the outset to make very clear that these neurons are in no way "pain receptors" or "pain fibers." As pointed out earlier, pain is a conscious experience that is dependent on the brain, not an external stimulus that can be detected, transformed, or transmitted by the body. Unfortunately, the dominant paradigm of pain fails to make this distinction between pain and nociception which leaves our clinical reasoning fundamentally flawed, a situation lamented over more than 20 years ago: "The labeling of nociceptors as pain fibers was not an admirable simplification but an unfortunate trivialization" (p. 255).[4] The nociceptive system, then, is responsible for alerting one's brain to a dangerous stimulus or situation that is threatening the tissues of the body. The first line of defense in this protective alerting system is the peripheral nociceptor.

Peripheral nociceptors have their distal ends in the tissues of the body. Almost all the tissues of our body are innervated by peripheral nociceptors, a notable exception being the brain itself, which is why brain surgery can be performed on a conscious and unanesthetised patient. C fibers, the unmyelinated and thinnest peripheral sensory fibers, and A-δ fibers, which are the thinnest of the myelinated sensory neurons, have conventionally become known as nociceptors. These neurons run from the tissues to the spinal cord, terminating in synaptic connections in laminae I and V of the dorsal horn.[5] From there, second order or "spinal" nociceptive neurons project to the thalamus via the spinothalamic tract. A functional distinction emerges at this level, with spinal nociceptive neurons from lamina I, being biased in their projections toward one part of the thalamus (the ventromedial thalamic nucleus), and those from lamina V being biased toward another part of the thalamus (the ventrolateral thalamic nucleus). This functional distinction is important because the medial and lateral thalamus then project to what have come to be known as distinct nociceptive processing systems within the brain. One system, which projects from the medial thalamus, is termed the sensory-discriminative system because it incorporates parts of the brain known to be involved in representation of the sensory characteristics of a stimulus, for example, its size, location, and duration. The other system, which projects from the lateral thalamus, is termed the affective-emotional system because it incorporates parts of the brain known to be involved in the representation of how one feels about a stimulus, for example its unpleasantness or horribleness.[6] Conceptually, this neuroanatomical distinction between systems is appealing because it makes a clear delineation between the supposedly factual aspect of pain on the one hand and the supposedly personal aspect on the other. The appeal is enhanced by functional imaging studies in awake humans that suggest activity in the sensory-discriminative system more closely relates to pain intensity ratings and activity in the affective-emotional system more closely relates to pain unpleasantness ratings. However, the majority of studies are not able to tease apart pain's intensity and unpleasantness, and the complex arborizations within the human brain suggest that the notion of separate systems is almost certainly simplistic.

The prevailing view then is to conceptualize the neural substrate of pain as encompassing brain areas from both of these "systems." However, the most invariable finding from pain imaging studies is, in fact, the variability in brain activity, between individuals, between studies, and even between identical stimuli within subjects and within studies. This is not altogether surprising because variability is fundamental to biological systems, and the ability to produce the same output in different ways is integral to adaptation and learning.[7]

Consequent to the inherent variability in the cortical neural substrate of pain, current notions of what brain areas subserve pain are really notions of what brain areas are most often activated when an individual is in pain. Certainly, some brain areas are active far more often than others – the primary and secondary sensory, insular, anterior cingulate and prefrontal cortices (see below).[8] Together with the thalamus, these areas have been called the "pain matrix," but not without criticism. For example, it has been argued that activation of these areas may reflect, in part, a "salience network" rather than a pain matrix because novel nonnoxious input from across modalities results in similar activation.[9] Further, much of the pain matrix can be activated, in the absence of noxious input, via hypnosis,[10,11] or while watching your loved one in pain (i.e., an empathetic response).[12]

In order to marry the neuroanatomical and theoretical perspectives on how pain emerges from the human brain, it is helpful to gain a basic understanding the concept of representation in the human brain. Consider a "cortical representation," with three characteristics – (1) it is a physical network of neurons distributed across different brain areas, (2) its activation evokes a response in one or more bodily systems, or into consciousness, or both, (3) it *represents* something else – for example, a movement, a patch of skin, a belief, an immune response, a memory. According to this line of

thinking, everything within one's world is in some way represented in the human brain, and these representations are analogous to "neurosignatures"[13] or "neurotags."[14] Because the brain is so terrifically complex, many neurotags can modulate many others. This modulatory capacity provides a mechanism by which anything relevant to the evaluation of threat to body tissue can modulate activity of the pain neurotag which will modulate the output of that neurotag, namely, pain. For example, the belief that one's back is inherently vulnerable to injury, which is immediately pertinent to the apparent safety of one's back, should upregulate the back pain neurotag. Functional imaging can elucidate the neuroanatomy of some of these modulations in two ways: (1) by experimentally manipulating cognitive factors relevant to the evaluation of threat to body tissues and determining the effect that has on brain activity in response to a noxious stimulus (although, notably, a noxious stimulus is not critical to evoke pain), and (2) by comparing brain activity in response to a noxious stimulus across participants between whom the cognitive variable of interest is variable. The former approach has the advantage of implying a causative relationship between the manipulation of variable one (cognitive factor, for example, anxiety; see Anxiety and Depression section below) and the change in another [functional magnetic resonance imaging (fMRI) signal]. The latter approach has the advantage of investigating implicit cognitive states rather than transient cognitive manipulations that may be less relevant to "the real world." The disadvantage, however, is that one cannot conclude a causative relationship between the two variables.

Identifying the Functional Anatomy of Nociception and Pain

Although there are many methods used to investigate brain activity (see ref. [15] for one review focused on pain), the bulk of functional imaging studies into pain have used electroencephalography (EEG), magnetoencephalography (MEG), fMRI, or positron emission tomography (PET). EEG and MEG investigate electrical or magnetic field changes on the surface of the skull, which limits their spatial acuity, but they have very high temporal acuity (that is, one can interpret when the event occurred but may not be sure exactly where it occurred). PET and fMRI have excellent spatial resolution but the delay between the shift in activity and the resulting change in blood flow or oxygenation is between 6 and 9 s (that is, one can interpret where the event occurred but not be sure exactly when it occurred, which makes statements about relative order of activations very problematic).

PET involves injection of radioactive material (or "tracer") into the blood stream and detection of gamma rays emitted by the tracer. The underlying assumption is that by imaging the location of the tracer, one gains an indirect measure of blood flow. On the principle that neural activity requires changes in blood flow, the resultant image is thought to reflect activity of brain cells.

fMRI involves using a magnetic field to align the cells of the body and then another magnetic field to flip a proportion of cells. Each type of molecule has a certain speed at which it inverts back to its original orientation, or "relaxes," after it has been flipped. By "tuning in" a radiofrequency coil to the relaxation speed of the target molecule, it is possible to identify fluctuations in the location of the target molecule. By tuning the radiofrequency coil to oxygenated hemoglobin, fMRI can provide an indication of where in the brain there is an increase in oxygenated hemoglobin. On the basis of synaptic activity being associated with an overshoot in oxygenated hemoglobin, the resultant image is assumed to reflect synaptic activity. Statistical tests are run on each voxel (a volume of known dimensions, for example 3 mm × 3 mm × 3 mm), and the statistical strength of the comparison is color-coded to yield statistical maps, or "blobs." A limitation of both approaches is that it is not possible to determine from the images that are obtained whether the supposed changes in blood flow or oxygenation reflect excitatory or inhibitory activation – an unknown that is of obvious functional relevance.

Using Experimentally Induced Pain to Image the Pain Matrix

Acute experimentally induced pain is most commonly associated with activation of the primary and secondary somatosensory cortices, the insular cortex, the anterior cingulate cortex, the prefrontal cortex, and the thalamus.[8,15,16] We iterate that this does not imply that they hold the representation of pain, nor that their

removal would eliminate pain (of course, their removal would be associated with severe functional and cognitive impairment!), but most studies of pharmacologically induced analgesia demonstrate reduced activation of these areas, which imply a central role in pain processing – perhaps a kind of "core network."[17–20]

Another key area that is often activated during experimentally induced pain is the brainstem – most often the periaqueductal gray (PAG) and the nucleus cuneiformis.[16] These areas, along with the rostroventral medulla, have long been regarded as important in descending inhibitory mechanisms[21] but recently have also been implicated in descending facilitation too,[22] which makes interpretation of imaging results difficult particularly if they are not considered in light of psychophysical, behavioral, and clinical data. Notably, several other regions are often activated during experimentally induced pain. Cerebellum, basal ganglia, hippocampus, amygdala, posterior parietal areas are cited in some reviews,[15] and primary motor cortex, premotor cortex, insular, operculum, orbitofrontal cortex have also been reported.[23–25]

It is perhaps a little daunting to see the variability in results of studies that induce pain in healthy volunteers because such studies intentionally eliminate contextual factors that are important modulators of pain in the real world but are considered confounders in experiments. Contextual factors can be powerful yet subtle – for example, placing a very cold rod on the back of one hand is substantially more painful if one is simultaneously shown a red light than if one is simultaneously shown a blue light.[26] More pertinent perhaps are the differences in meaning between pain experienced by patients and for which they seek treatment and pain transiently induced as part of an experiment. For example, in experimentally induced pain, one has been informed by scientists who at least seem as though they know what they are doing, about the nature of the stimulus, and the intensity and quality of the pain it is likely to evoke, that there will be no associated tissue damage, no lasting effects, and that they are free to withdraw from the experiment at any time.

The vast distinction between experimental and clinical pain has led to attempts to image patients with persistent pain while their pain is modulated, via provocation or analgesia. Although the core network of primary and secondary somatosensory, insular, anterior cingulate, prefrontal cortex, and thalamus is still commonly involved, differences have emerged. There are subtle shifts in the common distribution of brain areas involved when pain persists. The most consistent shifts concern the insula cortex and the prefrontal cortex. For example, in a meta-analysis including studies of neuropathic pain, angina pectoris, cluster headache and complex regional pain syndrome, insular activation during provocation of clinical pain occurs rostral to that during experimentally induced pain in healthy volunteers.[27] Those authors proposed that this shift might reflect altered emotional processing or heightened vigilance to somatic input in people with chronic painful disorders. A separate meta-analysis reported that prefrontal cortex is more often activated in clinical pain studies than in experimental pain studies.[8] Many studies that modulate cognitive factors demonstrate related activation in prefrontal cortices (see Section III) which suggests that the increased activation in clinical states might relate to a greater import of cognitive and higher order processes in such patients.

Less subtle and arguably more important differences relate to the upregulation of the nociceptive and pain neurotags and downregulation of antinociceptive mechanisms. This means that pain is provoked with less threatening inputs – for example, imagined movements alone can evoke pain [28] and visual input that implies that a painful limb is being touched can evoke pain even though the limb has not in fact been touched, a phenomenon known as dysynchiria.[29] Nuclei in the brainstem have been implicated in this process,[30] but Hebb's learning rule[31] – neurons that fire together, wire together – would predict that persistent activation of nociception and pain neurotags in the brain will result in them becoming sensitized. Dysfunction of antinociceptive mechanisms also contributes to enhanced sensitivity of pain neurotags as pain persists. For example, dysfunction of opioid[32–35] and dopaminergic[35–38] antinociceptive pathways have been reported.

A metaphorical illustration of what occurs in the brain as pain persists is that of the brain as an orchestra. Under normal circumstances, the orchestra plays the pain tune appropriately, when tissues of the body are, in fact, in danger and need to be protected by a concerted behavioral response. However, the more the orchestra plays the pain tune, the better it gets at doing so, such that the pain tune becomes more and more easily activated (see refs. [39] and [14] for further exploration of this idea within a clinical context).

When the pain neurotag is sensitized, so too are the modulatory effects of inputs that relate to the apparent danger faced by the tissues of the painful body part – cognitive, behavioral, and sensory cues become more important and their impact on pain increases.

Psychological Factors and Brain Imaging of Pain

One of the challenges of documenting the neuronal activity of pain is that pain is always impacted by psychological factors.[40] For example, a patient with advanced cancer is likely to respond to disease-related pain with sadness or depression about pain's persistence and/or anxiety about the meaning of the pain (e.g., does it mean my disease is getting worse?). This section examines recent work in this area with a particular focus on the psychological factors of pain catastrophizing, anxiety and depression, anticipation of pain, attention and distraction, and empathy.

Pain Catastrophizing

Pain catastrophizing has been defined as the tendency to magnify the threat value of a painful stimulus and negatively evaluate one's own ability to deal with pain.[41] Over the past 25 years, studies of patients experiencing persistent pain have shown that pain catastrophizing is one of most robust predictors of pain, psychological distress, and physical disability.[42,43] In studies of pain-free volunteers, pain catastrophizing has also been found to relate to higher pain report in response to experimental noxious stimuli.[44]

To date, there have been two studies that have examined the neural correlates of pain catastrophizing. The first study examined brain activation in patients with fibromyalgia, in response to a standardized and noxious blunt pressure stimulus, which evokes pain that is similar to that reported by patients with fibromyalgia.[45] Patients were grouped according to their scores on a pain catastrophizing measure. Brain activation was compared between groups, and results controlled for depression. A number of interesting findings emerged. First, while all patients showed activation of the ipsalateral secondary somatosensory cortex (S2) in response the pressure stimuli, the high pain catastrophizers showed nearly twice as much activation in S2 as low catastrophizers. Second, the level of pain catastrophizing was associated with activation of the cerebellum and the medial frontal gyrus, areas reportedly involved in the anticipation of pain.[46] Third, pain catastrophizing was correlated with activation of the premotor cortex and lentiform nuclei, areas reported to be involved in behavioral and emotional expression of pain. Finally, high pain catastrophizers showed significant increases in activation of the contralateral anterior portion of the anterior cingulated cortex, an area important in the attention and emotional processing of pain. Gracely et al concluded that catastrophizing is significantly associated with increased activity in brain regions related to anticipation of pain, attention to pain, emotional aspects of pain, and motor control.[45]

Seminowicz[47] investigated the relationship between pain catastrophizing and brain activation in 22 healthy volunteers who received two levels of noxious median nerve stimulation.[47] During mild pain, higher pain catastrophizing was related to greater activity in brain areas related to attention, affective, and motor aspects of pain (i.e., increased activity in the dorsolateral prefrontal, insula, rostral anterior cingulate, premotor, and parietal cortices). During intense pain, higher pain catastrophizing related to less activity in the dorsolateral prefrontal cortex and medial frontal cortex, areas believed to be related to descending control of pain. The authors interpret their findings to suggest that during mild pain, catastrophizers are more likely to engage cortical processes related to vigilance and attention to pain, and that during intense pain, these individuals may less able than low catastrophizers to recruit inhibitory or antinociceptive mechanisms.

Anxiety and Depression

Patients who experience persistent pain often report more depressive and anxiety symptoms than patients who do not experience persistent pain. Anxiety, or distress, is potentially very problematic because pain can lead to distress and distress can lead to pain, which sets up a vicious circle of increasing pain and distress.[48–51] Several brain regions have been implicated in anxiety, depression and pain.

The neural substrate of the effect of anxiety on pain was elegantly investigated by Ploghaus et al, who modified cues of impending pain to manipulate pain-related anxiety in their participants.[52] To do this, they first presented a visual signal that was always followed by a mild thermal nociceptive stimulus, thus making that particular cue induce low anxiety. A separate visual signal was followed by a mild nociceptive stimulus on most trials, but occasionally it was followed by a very intense thermal noxious stimulus, thus making that visual cue induce high anxiety. That study showed (1) a clear affect of cue (and thus anxiety) on pain induced by the mild noxious stimulus, (2) that this effect was associated with activation of the entorhinal cortex, and (3) that entorhinal cortex activity correlated closely to activity in perigenual cingulated and midinsular cortices. Interpretation of such studies is not without problems, but it seems reasonable to suggest that entorhinal cortex activity may prime protective neurotags (in this case the neurotag for pain) to facilitate their recruitment if the provocative stimulus occurs.

The neural correlate of the relationship between anxiety and pain has also been investigated by inducing pain in subjects who report different levels of pain-related anxiety and fear of pain,[53] and the results are slightly different. In response to a noxious thermal stimulus, higher anxiety sensitivity was related to higher pain and also to greater activation of medial prefrontal cortex, which is considered important in self-focused attention and self-monitoring.[53–55] One cannot draw a causative link between anxiety sensitivity and pain on the basis of this study, but that attention to pain increases levels of physical and psychological disability has been suggested,[56] and seems intuitively sensible on the basis of the paradigm of pain advocated here – that pain depends on the brain's evaluation of danger and the need for action. Brain activation after a noxious stimulus was also related to fear of pain. Participants completed a questionnaire in which they rated how fearful they were of the pain associated with reasonably common injuries (e.g., breaking a leg, the pulling of a tooth). Data analyses revealed that fear of pain (as assessed by questionnaire scores) was related to activation in the anterior and posterior cingulate cortices and the ventral lateral frontal cortex. Cingulate regions have elsewhere been related to monitoring and affective response evaluation,[53,57] and ventral lateral frontal cortex has been related to the ability to use distraction techniques (e.g., relaxation) and to cope with pain.[58,59] Again, one cannot make causative links with these data, but they raise the possibility that a causative link does exist between fear of pain and pain and that the link involves specific brain areas.

Posttraumatic stress disorder (PTSD) is an anxiety disorder that may occur in individuals who are exposed to traumatic events. Often, the traumatic event (e.g., assault, combat, motor-vehicle accidents) also causes musculoskeletal injury, and there is some correlational evidence to suggest that PTSD and chronic pain may exacerbate one another, for example, persistent and intense pain is more common in people with PTSD than in the general population.[60–64] The relationship between experimentally induced pain and PTSD was investigated by Geuze et al: brain activity in response to standardized and participant-determined painful thermal stimuli was evaluated in participants with PTSD and in healthy controls, with intriguing results: (1) there were clear differences in brain activation between the groups – the PTSD group had greater activation of the left hippocampus, right putamen, and bilateral insula, less activation of the bilateral ventrolateral prefrontal cortex, right precentral gyrus, and the right amygdala; (2) the PTSD group reported less pain than the control group.[65] These results seem surprising because epidemiological data would predict increased sensitivity to noxious stimuli in the PTSD group, whereas these results clearly show the opposite, as well as less activation of classic threat-related areas (e.g., the amygdala). Perhaps the protective role of PTSD intrusions competes with the protective role for pain, although the opposite effect has been demonstrated for thirst – increased pain in response to noxious stimulation (Farrell 2006)[134].

Depression and pain also commonly occur together. Giesecke et al examined the relationship between depressive symptoms and experimentally induced pressure pain patients with fibromyalgia.[66] Depressive symptoms were positively related with tissue pressure-evoked activation of affective brain areas. Specifically, higher levels of depressive symptoms were associated with activation of the amygdala and contralateral anterior insula. Furthermore, patients' ratings of their usual pain due to fibromyalgia correlated with activation of the contralateral anterior insula, anterior cingulate cortex, and prefrontal cortex. Schweinhardt et al examined the relationship between depressive symptoms and provoked joint pain in patients with rheumatoid arthritis (RA).[67] They showed activation that correlated with depressive symptoms and pain in medial prefron-

tal cortex activity and that medial prefrontal cortex mediated an effect of pain evoked by joint squeezing. Others have shown strong projections from the medial prefrontal cortex to nociceptive modulating nuclei in the brain stem (e.g., the PAG),[68] which raises the possibility that depression imparts an effect on pain via pronociceptive modulation at the spinal cord. This is still somewhat speculative, but there seems to be a strong case to suggest that depression upregulates pain via a frontal cortex activation. Regardless, the importance that has been placed on assessing and managing depressive symptoms in people with pain seems vindicated by these imaging data.

Anticipation of Pain

While anticipating pain can certainly serve a purpose – to remove oneself from harm's way – it may also lead to increased fear and anxiety, which are themselves distressing and increase pain.[69] This is particularly important when the anticipation of pain is not accurate (i.e., one's anticipation of pain is poorly related to the likelihood of pain occurring) or the pain and nociceptive systems are sensitized, in which case the facilitatory effect on pain of anticipating pain has a large impact. Empirical work has indicated that an individual's past experience with pain, the memory of that pain, and recurrent episodes of pain can heighten anticipation of pain.[70] Clinically, a very high level of anticipation of pain is also problematic because it promotes fear of pain and behavioral avoidance– both of which contribute to increased levels of pain, physical disability, and psychological disability.[71]

In an innovative study, Ploghaus et al conditioned 12 healthy volunteers to expect either a painfully hot stimulus or a nonpainful warm stimulus on the basis of which of two different colored lights preceded the stimulus.[46] fMRI does not have the temporal resolution to differentiate between brain blood flow changes associated with a stimulus or the cue, but the investigators included catch trials in which the cue was not followed with the stimulus. This allowed them to compare brain activation between the anticipation of pain and the anticipation of warm. They reported that the anticipation of pain was associated with activation of the anterior medial frontal cortex, insular cortex, and cerebellum, all areas associated with affective pain processes. As would be expected, several brain areas were activated during both pain and its anticipation, including the thalamus, premotor cortex, right anterior cingulate cortex, and PAG.

Wise et al[72] used a methodological paradigm similar to that used by Ploghaus and colleagues[46] to examine the selective modulation by midzolam (i.e., a short acting anxiety medication) on brain activity associated with anticipation of pain and pain. They hypothesized that brain activity associated with anticipation of pain would be reduced when participants were administered midazolam (compared to administration of saline) but that the brain activity associated with pain stimulus would not change. They found that midazolam administration did modulate the brain activity associated with anticipation of pain. The three brain regions (i.e., contralateral anterior insula, anterior cingulate, and ipsilateral S2) associated with pain anticipation showed decreases in activity when anticipating pain under midazolam application, but not under saline application. While some trends toward decreased pain-related brain activity were observed with midazolam application, it did not produce a consistent or significant effect on pain-related brain activity. Interestingly, stimulus intensity ratings for the painful stimulus were significantly lower when participants received midazolam versus saline administration. This suggests that while midazolam produced some analgesic effect evidenced by pain report, it did not significantly alter brain activity related to pain. This study is important because it demonstrates that pharmacological agents can have a differential neural effect on the anticipation of pain and pain. Further, it demonstrates that it is possible to further examine brain activity in regards to anticipation of pain and actual pain using pharmacological agents. Alternatively, these findings may suggest that anxiety increases pain report via its effect on anticipation of pain.

In another study, Fairhurst et al examined the functional significance of anticipation of pain and the involvement of brainstem structures in its underlying neurobiological mechanisms.[73] Specifically, they studied responses to pain signaling cues (anticipation induced by visual signaling) and the application of noxious stimuli in healthy subjects. First, as would be expected, these investigators found that pain anticipation scores were associated with pain ratings, suggesting that anticipating more intense pain leads to more intense pain. They reported that the ventral tegmental

area and the enthorhinal cortex were important in imparting this effect. Activity in these areas also related positively to insular cortex activation during pain.

Attention and Distraction

Experimental studies have shown that participants who are directed to pay close attention to pain stimuli report more intense and unpleasant pain than participants who are instructed to direct their attention away from the pain.[74] It is thought that the brain region that modulates attention to pain is the anterior cingulate cortex. Some work has suggested that there are distinct regions in the anterior cingulate cortex that are active during attention to pain and pain.[75,76] Bantick et al used fMRI to examine attention-induced changes in pain.[58] In this study, participants were first asked to identify the temperature at which thermal noxious stimuli applied to their hand became "strong pain." Then, participants were given a challenging cognitive task that involved motor movement of the hand (a modified Stroop task)[77] or a neutral, nonchallenging task. During the cognitive tasks, participants were asked to pay attention to the task but remain aware that painful thermal stimuli were going to be applied and that they would need to rate them. Participants in this study rated the same degree of thermal stimuli as less painful while being occupied with a challenging cognitive task than when engaging in a neutral task. While participants were distracted during painful stimuli, they reported lower pain and demonstrated increased activation in brain regions associated with affective parts of the perigenual cingulate and orbitofrontal regions. Interestingly, during distraction, decreases in brain activity were seen in other areas of the pain matrix including the thalamus, insula, hippocampus, and the midcingulate cortex. This study provides insight into the neural bases of intervention techniques such as pain coping skills training that use distraction as a primary strategy to decrease patients' pain. This study was completed in healthy volunteers – it remains unknown whether the same results would occur in those suffering from clinical pain.

Seminowicz et al[78] used a counting Stroop task[79] that was either neutral or demanding, while pain was induced via stimulation of the median nerve. Some participants performed better on the cognitive task when subjected to painful stimuli, and other participants performed worse when subjected to painful stimuli. Interestingly, participants who performed better on the cognitive task when they were subjected to painful stimuli demonstrated decreased pain-related activity in the primary and secondary somatosensory cortices and anterior insula cortex. Participants who performed more poorly on the cognitive task when subjected to pain did not demonstrate this pain-related neuronal activity. The results of this study indicate that cognitive engagement modulates pain and suggest that the effect probably involves the sensory-discrimination component of pain. Further, while some individuals may be able to distract themselves from pain by increasing their attention to other activities, other individuals may not able to distract themselves from pain and they perform their activities worse. Of interest, these results may be important in understanding individual differences in response to distraction. While distraction techniques are a key coping strategy, for some patients, it may be necessary to focus more on other techniques such as altering thoughts about pain and its implications.

Empathy

Empathy can be defined as the reactions of one individual to the observed experiences of another.[80] Several fields of research, including neuroscience, posit that empathy is necessary for survival.[81–83] Empathy is a central component in moral reasoning, prosocial behaviors, inhibiting aggression toward others, and it is a crucial social tie.[84] Empathy for others' pain may enable us to understand what it feels like when someone else experiences pain and to respond effectively. Recent research in brain imaging has begun to elucidate the neural substrates for empathy for pain. Some studies suggest that empathy for pain triggers affective components of the pain matrix, but not sensory components.[12,85,86] Singer et al assessed brain activity while participants experienced painful stimuli and compared it to brain activity when they observed a signal indicating that their loved one was receiving similar painful stimuli.[12] Investigators found that both affective components and sensory components of the pain matrix were activated in response to pain stimuli delivered to self, while only affective components of the pain matrix (anterior insula, anterior cingulate cortex) were activated in response a loved one receiving a painful

stimuli. That work was corroborated by Morrison et al who compared brain activation during a pinprick to that during video observation of another individual (someone the participant did not know) receiving a pinprick.[86] This study also found that the affective components of the pain matrix (anterior cingulate cortex) were activated even when an individual viewed painful stimulation in an unknown model. These findings suggest that empathy for pain may be a general response to human pain and not limited to loved ones.

These findings have been extended using transcranial magnetic stimulation (TMS) to evaluate the effect of observing someone getting a needle stick injury on motor cortex excitability.[87] Corticospinal excitability was reduced but only for the muscle directly implicated in the observed scenario (that is, the effect is anatomically specific).[87,88] Interestingly, observers who estimated that the pain experienced by the model was more intense showed greater stimulus-induced modulation of motor cortex excitability.[87]

While empathy appears to be an important human attribute, it would be interesting to more fully understand the similarities and differences in brain activation for (1) seeing pain in others and (2) anticipating pain in oneself. It is possible that similar brain activation patterns seen between one's own pain and others' pain is actually a reaction to anticipation of pain in oneself or serves as a warning to avoid stimulus that evoked others' pain.[85] This would suggest that similar neuronal activity in response to one's own and another's pain is not empathy, but a self-protective response.

Effects of Psychological Interventions

Over the past 30 years, numerous research and clinical studies have examined the effects of psychological interventions on pain. In this section, we review several commonly used psychological interventions that have been investigated using functional imaging.

Placebo

Placebo analgesia has long intrigued pain clinicians and researchers. In particular, there has been keen interest in the mechanisms that underpin placebo analgesia.

Over the past 15 years, imaging studies have sought to identify the neural correlates and mechanisms of placebo analgesia. Petrovic et al were among the first to use PET to pinpoint areas of the brain related to placebo analgesia.[89] In their study, they collected self-report ratings of pain and data on regional cerebral blood flow from nine healthy volunteers during painful heat stimuli and mild warm stimuli while participants were receiving either a placebo or fast-acting opioid. When receiving placebo, participants evidenced increased activation in the right anterior cingulated cortex, the orbitofrontal cortex, and the anterior insula. During both opioid analgesia and placebo analgesia, there was a significant correlation between increased activity in the rostral ACC (rACC) and activity in areas close to the PAG and in the pons. Taken together, these findings suggest that placebo effects may involve activation of an endogenous opioid pain modulation pathway that involve connections between the rACC (a region having numerous opioid receptors) and key brainstem areas related to opioid analgesia (i.e., the PAG and pons). The authors argued that the increased activation in the orbitofrontal cortex may indicate that cognitive cues (e.g., a warning that a pain stimulus is about to occur) play a role in activating this pathway.

In an early report using fMRI methodology, Wager et al examined the effects of expectations on placebo analgesia.[90] During noxious stimulation, they found that placebo reduced activation in pain matrix areas (the rACC, contralateral insula, and contralateral thalamus). There was a significant correlation between the amount of pain relief reported and the reductions in activation in these brain areas. These findings underscore the notion that placebo effects have a neural basis and are not simply a manifestation of altered reporting on behalf of the patient. During anticipation of pain, these investigators found that placebo was associated with increased activity in the prefrontal cortex. Based on these findings, they suggested that the anticipation of pain relief from a placebo might trigger neural mechanisms (e.g., release of endogenous opioids in the midbrain) that, in turn, inhibit activity in pain-processing regions.

Zubieta et al used molecular imaging techniques (PET and a mμ-opioid tracer) to further test the notion that placebo effects might be related to endogenous opioid activity.[91] In this study, 14 right-handed pain-free volunteers were studied under two conditions: sustained pain versus sustained pain plus placebo.

The placebo condition produced significant activation of the mμ-opioid system in the left prefrontal cortex, dorsolateral prefrontal cortex, rostral right anterior cingulated cortex, right anterior insular cortex, and left nucleus accumbens. Correlational analyses showed that the magnitude of pain relief reported with placebo was correlated with lower ratings of pain. These findings lend support to the notion that activation of the endogenous opioid system may be one key mechanism responsible for placebo effects.

In an fMRI study using connectivity analysis, Bingel et al examined the hypothesis that, during placebo, the rACC interacts with other brain areas to produce endogenous opioid-dependent analgesia.[92] Prior to noxious stimulation, each participant had one hand treated with a placebo cream that was described as an analgesic, while the other hand was left untreated. During the imaging session, participants first were given a warning stimulus and then received controlled noxious stimulus (laser heat) to the back of both hands. Two key findings emerged. First, as in prior studies, the investigators found that the placebo manipulation produced increases in activation in the rACC confirming the importance of this area in placebo effects. Second, the investigators found that, during placebo, there was a significant correlation between activation in the rACC and activity in the bilateral amygdala and PAG. The authors argued that their findings are consistent with the notion that the rACC activates subcortical areas that produce endogenous pain relief.

Price et al criticized prior imaging studies on the grounds that the placebo effects reported are relatively small and that the reductions in activation levels reported were found after stimulus offset, a period during which participants are rating their pain.[93] To address these limitations, they conducted an fMRI study that examined patterns of placebo-related neural activation that occurred during rectal stimulation (bowel distention), in patients suffering from irritable bowel syndrome (IBS). To enhance placebo effects, the saline jelly applied to the rectal balloon used for bowel distention was described as an agent that powerfully reduced pain. Results indicated that, in contrast to prior imaging studies, the placebo manipulation used by Price et al produced large reductions in pain report.[93] This underscores the clinical significance of the placebo manipulation they used. This manipulation also decreased activation in areas of the pain matrix – anterior cingulate cortex, insula, somatosensory cortices, and thalamus. Regional connectivity analysis, whereby the pattern of brain activation over time is correlated to that in a particular area (or "seed"), was undertaken on brain regions conventionally associated with the cognitive-affective component of pain, and thus most likely to be involved in placebo analgesia.[94] That analysis suggested that, when people had received the placebo cream, activity in the anterior insula cortex was negatively correlated with that in the dorsal anterior cingulate cortex and supplementary motor area. These data suggest that placebo analgesia, when evoked by a preemptive intervention (rather than an intervention applied in response to pain, which is obviously a more common situation clinically), decreases the intensity of expected pain, which "preemptively" downregulates the pain matrix via a specific interaction between the insula, anterior cingulated, and supplementary motor areas.

Similar to the pain literature, a consistent aspect of the placebo literature is, in fact, the inconsistency of response. Scott et al proposed the variability between individuals in their tendency to respond to reward might relate to the analgesia they experience in response to a placebo.[95] They targeted an area of the brain previously implicated in reward, the nucleus accumbens, and found it to be activated in response to a placebo. They, then, demonstrated that the anticipation of a monetary reward activated the nucleus accumbens. Finally, they correlated nucleus accumbens activity associated with monetary reward to analgesia after placebo and demonstrated the former to explain 28% of the variance in the latter. These data might seem consistent with the hypothesis that placebo analgesia is related to reward-based systems in the human brain, but it is notable that 72% of the variance in placebo analgesia was not explained by reward-based brain processing, which indicates that other factors certainly contribute.

It is relevant, when trying to disentangle the contributions to placebo analgesia and its neural substrate, to revisit the conceptualization of pain suggested by the neuromatrix theory, which we introduced at the start of this chapter. If one accepts that pain emerges from the human brain when the "pain neurosignature" is activated and that *any* neural representation relevant to the evaluation of threat to body tissue can modulate activity of the pain neurosignature, then placebo analgesia can be conceptualized as corroborating evidence of this theory. As has been noted elsewhere, the fact that

placebos can invoke analgesia is not mysterious and clinically unhelpful. Rather, it demonstrates that there are other aspects of a therapeutic intervention that downregulate the brain's evaluation of danger to body tissues and that, obviously, this downregulation must have a neural substrate somewhere in the human brain.[96]

Cognitive Behavioral Therapy

Cognitive behavioral therapy (CBT) utilizes both cognitive and behavioral techniques to address psychosocial issues that are interfering with an individual's functioning. One major goal of CBT is to identify irrational and problematic thinking styles (i.e., cognitions) that maintain distress or discomfort. The other major goal of CBT is to identify maladaptive behaviors that maintain distress or discomfort and replace them with new behaviors that lead to better functioning.[97] CBT has been applied to a wide range of psychological disorders, including anxiety disorders (e.g., panic disorder, generalized anxiety disorder, specific phobias) and depressive disorders (e.g., major depressive disorder, dysthymia).[98–102] Several meta-analyses have provided support for the efficacy of CBT with large effect sizes seen for depression, generalized anxiety disorder, panic disorder, social phobia, and post traumatic stress disorder.[103] Investigation into brain activity changes following CBT has largely focused on its application to anxiety disorders and depression.[104–106] Though different regions of the brain are implicated in several disorders (e.g., depression, obsessive compulsive disorder, panic disorder) activity in the anterior cingulate cortex is a common point of interest. CBT has been associated with changes in activity in the anterior cingulate cortex, and these changes may be a result of adaptive changes in cognitions and behaviors that result from CBT.[105]

Pain coping skills training is an intervention based on CBT principles that systematically teaches patients with persistent pain to more effectively cope with pain and pain-related psychological and physical disability. Keefe et al outline three basic components of pain coping skills training: (1) patients are provided with an educational rationale using the gate control theory to better understand how their thoughts and behaviors influence pain and how they can learn to alter their thoughts and behaviors to manage pain; (2) a therapist guides patients in learning cognitive and behavioral strategies for pain management such as progressive muscle relaxation, brief relaxation methods, goal setting, activity pacing, imagery, and strategies for changing overly negative thoughts related to pain; and (3) patients are encouraged to engage in home practice of these skills and to learn how to apply these skills in pain-related situations.[107] Pain coping skills training is efficacious for several painful conditions including osteoarthritis, rheumatoid arthritis, cancer pain, and chronic low back pain.[108–111]

Investigation of the neural substrate for the effect of CBT or coping skills training on pain is in its infancy. Lackner et al compared brain activation before and after CBT, in patients with severe IBS.[112] CBT consisted of ten weekly sessions that focused on teaching patients to identify and correct maladaptive beliefs and information processing errors. CBT was associated with reduced pain, anxiety, and gastrointestinal symptoms. Improvements in these symptoms were related to reduced activation of the amygdala and the subgenual part of the perigenual anterior cingulate cortex, in response to inflation of a rectal balloon during imaging. These findings support the notion that CBT is associated with changes in brain processesing of noxious input and corroborate the significant body of work that shows CBT and coping skills training to be effective in the management of chronic pain disorders.[108]

Reconceptualizing Pain

A fundamental tenet of CBT for chronic pain is that a patient's pain is not an accurate indication of the true threat to the tissues of the body. That hurt does not equal harm and that it is OK to move despite pain are key messages. The efficacy of an approach based on such messages depends, in part, on whether or not the patient believes those messages. If the underlying schema by which patients makes sense of their pain adheres to a structural-pathology model of pain, then those messages are counterintuitive. Reconceptualization of pain, then, becomes a potentially important aspect of pain rehabilitation. One approach to reconceptualization of pain is to explain the biological processes that underpin pain to patients. Intriguingly, most clinicians tend to think that patients are not able to understand modern pain biology. Notably, they are wrong – patients demonstrate marked increases in knowledge of modern pain biology from as little as a single seminar.[113] In fact, randomized controlled trials demonstrate that teaching patients about pain biology ("explaining pain" – see ref. [14]) results in immediate increases in pain threshold during functionally relevant tasks,[114] decreased catastrophizing, decreased conviction that hurt equals harm, and increased pain-related self-efficacy[115] – the very conceptual shifts that are targeted in CBT for pain. Furthermore, integrating explaining pain within a multimodal CBT-based approach to rehabilitation reduces pain and disability in people with chronic pain in as little as 4 weeks, resulting in gains that are maintained for at least a year.[116,117]

Psychophysical and self-report data suggest that explaining pain reduces pain and disability by reconceptualizing for a patient, the cause and meaning of their pain. The neural substrate of such high-order cognitive shifts are difficult to determine, but initial single-case data suggest explaining pain reduces threat-related activation in the human brain, most notably in the amygdala and anterior-cingulate cortex.[118] Other preliminary work suggests that the analgesic effect of explaining pain on pain threshold may be mediated by increased activation of the medial prefrontal cortex and its antinociceptive projection to midbrain nociception modulatory nuclei.[119] Such studies lay the ground work for further work which should elucidate the neuranatomical context of explaining pain. That work should suggest better approaches and optimal integration with other psychological and possibly pharmacological approaches. Of course, the key findings of such studies really relate to their positive effect on pain and function, and those outcomes should remain primary consideration.

Hypnosis

Hypnosis for the management of pain often includes an induction phase and a suggestion phase. During the induction phase, patients are led through a sequence of calming images or statements (e.g., a peaceful lake, "everything is just right"). Then, they are given suggestions of experiencing less pain, less stress, more energy, and/or more control.[120] Hypnosis has been utilized in both acute and chronic pain settings to produce an analgesic effect.[121,122] Evidence from controlled trials suggests that hypnosis can be helpful for managing pain-related conditions in patients with sickle-cell disease, advanced stage cancer pain, osteoarthritis pain, and disability-related pain.[123–126]

Rainville et al examined how hypnosis impacts brain activity in response to a noxious stimulus in healthy volunteers, using PET.[127] They showed that hypnotic suggestion could specifically modulate pain unpleasantness and that this was associated with correlated modulation of anterior cingulate activity. There was no effect of hypnotic suggestion on activity of the primary or secondary somatosensory cortices. A limbic-specific effect corroborates the notion of distinct neural substrates for the affective and sensory components of pain. Derbyshire et al took a different approach by comparing brain response to a noxious stimulus, brain activation during a suggested painful state in the absence of noxious input, and imagined pain.[11] Brain activity during pain in response to a noxious stimulus and pain via hypnotic suggestion were similar – the thalamus, anterior cingulate cortex, midanterior insula, and parietal and prefrontal cortices showed similar activity in the two conditions. Imagined pain did not involve the same degree or pattern of activation. The former result is important because it both highlights that noxious stimulation is not necessary for pain and corroborates patient report findings by using physiological data not dependent on participant report.

An analgesic effect of hypnosis has also been reported in people with clinical pain. For example, Wik et al examined differences in cerebral blood flow during states of hypnosis and resting wakefulness patients with fibromyalgia.[128] Patients reported less pain during hypnosis than at rest. The effect was associated with increased activity of orbitofrontal cortex, the right thalamus, and the left inferior parietal cortex and decreased activity in the cingulate cortex. Derbyshire et al also investigated brain activity in patients with fibromyalgia, but they modulated pain by suggestion with and without hypnotic induction.[129] Both conditions were associated with changes in reported pain, but the hypnosis group reported bigger changes, as well as a stronger conviction that they could control their pain. Regardless of condition, changes in pain correlated with activation in the midbrain, cerebellum, thalamus, midcingulate, primary and secondary sensory, inferior parietal, insula, and prefrontal cortices – the bulk of which reflect the conventional "pain matrix," providing a strong corroboration of patient report, but not offering the system-specific findings reported in experimental studies. It is difficult at this stage to reconcile the variability in the neural effects of hypnosis across paradigms and studies. Suffice at this stage to highlight that hypnosis, and suggestion not under hypnosis, modulate pain in an intuitive manner and that this modulation is associated with changes in brain areas commonly conceptualized as belonging to the pain matrix.

Meditation

Meditation has also been shown to reduce both acute pain and persistent pain,[130,131] although the mechanism(s) by which analgesia occurs is not well understood. Possible explanations include distraction, reduced noxious input because of a tissue-based effect, or reduction of anxiety. Each of these potential mechanisms would suggest discrete neuronanatomy, but imaging studies of meditation for pain relief are in their infancy. One study hypothesized that participation in a meditation program would reduce activation of the affective components of the pain matrix.[132] Healthy, pain-free participants who had either been practicing meditation for several years or who had not undergone experimentally induced pain. The participants who had been practicing meditation demonstrated 40–50% less activity in the thalamus, prefrontal cortex, and anterior cingulate cortex than the other group. When the other group was subsequently taught meditation techniques and practiced for 5 months, they reduced activation of the very same areas.

Issues and Future Research Direction

Brain imaging has clearly made important contributions to our understanding of pain. It is now apparent that pain activates a neural network that typically includes the primary and secondary somatosensory, insular, anterior cingulate, prefrontal cortex, and thalamus. Furthermore, the importance of brainstem nuclei, most notably the PAG, has been iterated by brain imaging studies. A growing literature of brain imaging studies suggests that the neural substrates of psychological factors known to affect experimental and clinical pain (e.g., pain catastrophizing, depression and anxiety, anticipation of pain, attention and distraction, and empathy) can be identified. Not surprisingly, there is already some imaging data that support clinical assessment data in suggesting that psychosocial treatment interventions such as placebo, cognitive-behavioral treatment, reconceptualizing pain, hypnosis, and meditation can alter pain and therefore activation of pain-related neural representations or neurotags in the human brain.

It is notable that most pain-related imaging studies are robust and well reported. Experimental pain studies minimize variability by using within-subject designs. Both experimental and clinical pain studies use the best self-report measures, and by utilizing both designs, researchers can identify relationships and then interrogate their causal nature. However, imaging studies also have the limitations we have highlighted throughout, for example, spatial or temporal resolution limitations, inability for current approaches to differential facilitation of inhibition of the spinal cord, limited generalizability, artificially homogeneous samples due to screening out of potential confounders that are in fact common clinical factors (e.g., depression, anxiety).

Brain imaging studies of pain-related processes almost always feature an analysis of neural activations achieved during exposure to a pain stimulus versus a nonpainful stimulus. The pain stimuli used are carefully controlled, typically brief, and can be terminated at the participant's request. Investigators need to be careful about drawing clinical implications in this situation. These stimuli differ markedly from clinical situation where pain can last for hours, days, or months, may not be well controlled, may not be avoidable, and/or the noxious stimulus is seldom precisely known. Encouraging trends are the use of more clinically relevant stimuli (e.g., delivering pressure to an arthritic joint) in brain imaging studies and the use of clinical samples. An important future direction is developing better ways to capture the neural processes related to how individuals deal with complex, and often persistent, clinical pain phenomena.

One of the most interesting and important uses of brain imaging in the pain area is to study the effects of psychosocial pain treatments. However, with few notable exceptions[112] the psychological interventions studied are atypical of what is provided in clinical settings. These interventions are delivered by an experimenter, often quite brief (e.g., limited to a single session), and place few demands on the participant (e.g., a hypnosis manipulation). The fact that these brief interventions have been shown to have effects on brain activity is encouraging because in a clinical situation, psychosocial treatments for pain (e.g., CBT) are typically delivered by a highly trained psychologist, over a series of sessions, and involve extensive in-session and home practice, and tailored to the exact requirements of the patient. It is possible that these more intensive treatments will have larger effect sizes than those observed in prior, more experimental studies of psychological interventions. It is also possible that clinically based psychological treatments produce a somewhat different pattern of pain-related brain activation. Along these lines, an interesting direction for future treatment research would be to conduct brain imaging studies to directly compare the effects of different psychological treatments (e.g., hypnosis versus CBT) for a common persistent pain condition (e.g., osteoarthritis). Finally, although persistent pain is often treated with a combination of a psychosocial intervention and medication (e.g., a combined behavioral and abortive pharmacological treatment for vascular headache[133]) studies have yet to examine cortical mechanisms related to the effects of such treatment combinations.

Acknowledgment Preparation of this chapter was supported by grants from the National Institutes of Health (P01 AR50245, R01 AR049059, T32 MH019109, R01 AR054626, R01 NR010777, R01CA131148, R34AR056727, R01 NS053759, R01 CA107477, R01 CA 122704), the Department of Defense (W81XWH-07-1-0091), and the American College of Rheumatology (*Within Our Reach,* Rheumatoid Arthritis Research Grant).

References

1. Melzack R, Wall PD. Pain mechanisms: a new theory. *Science.* 1965;150(699):971–979.
2. Melzack R. Pain: past, present and future. *Can J Exp Psychol.* 1993;47(4):615–629.
3. Melzack R. Pain and the neuromatrix in the brain. *J Dent Educ.* 2001;65(12):1378–1382.
4. Wall P, McMahon S. The relationship of perceived pain to afferent nerve impulses. *Trends Neurosci.* 1986;9(6):254–255.
5. Doubell TP, Mannion RJ, Woolf CJ. The dorsal horn: state-dependent sensory processing, placticity and the

generation of pain. In: Wall P, Melzack R, eds. *The Textbook of Pain*. 4th ed. Edinburgh: Churchill Livingstone; 1999: 165–181.

6. Price DD. *Psychological Mechanisms of Pain and Analgesia*, vol. 15. Seattle: IASP Press; 2000.

7. Moseley GL, Hodges PW. Reduced variability of postural strategy prevents normalization of motor changes induced by back pain: a risk factor for chronic trouble? *Behav Neurosci*. 2006;120(2):474–476.

8. Apkarian AV, Bushnell MC, Treede RD, Zubieta JK. Human brain mechanisms of pain perception and regulation in health and disease. *Eur J Pain*. 2005;9(4):463–484.

9. Iannetti GD, Hughes NP, Lee MC, Mouraux A. Determinants of laser-evoked EEG responses: pain perception or stimulus saliency? *J Neurophysiol*. 2008;100(2):815–828.

10. Rainville P, Carrier B, Hofbauer RK, Bushnell MC, Duncan GH. Dissociation of sensory and affective dimensions of pain using hypnotic modulation. *Pain*. 1999;82(2):159–171.

11. Derbyshire SWG, Whalley MG, Stenger VA, Oakley DA. Cerebral activation during hypnotically induced and imagined pain. *Neuroimage*. 2004;23(1):392–401.

12. Singer T, Seymour B, O'Doherty J, Kaube H, Dolan RJ, Frith CD. Empathy for pain involves the affective but not sensory components of pain. *Science*. 2004;303(5661): 1157–1162.

13. Melzack R. Phantom limbs and the concept of a neuromatrix. *Trends Neurosci*. 1990;13:88–92.

14. Butler D, Moseley GL. *Explain Pain*. Adelaide: NOI Group Publishing; 2003.

15. Tracey I. Imaging pain. *Br J Anaesth*. 2008;101(1):32–39.

16. Brooks J, Tracey I. From nociception to pain perception: imaging the spinal and supraspinal pathways. *J Anat*. 2005;207(1):19–33.

17. Casey KL, Svensson P, Morrow TJ, Raz J, Jone C, Minoshima S. Selective opiate modulation of nociceptive processing in the human brain. *J Neurophysiol*. 2000;84(1): 525–533.

18. Rushworth MFS, Kennerley SW, Walton ME. Cognitive neuroscience: resolving conflict in and over the medial frontal cortex. *Curr Biol*. 2005;15(2):R54–R56.

19. Wagner KJ, Sprenger T, Kochs EF, Tolle TR, Valet M, Willoch F. Imaging human cerebral pain modulation by dose-dependent opioid analgesia – a positron emission tomography activation study using remifentanil. *Anesthesiology*. 2007;106(3):548–556.

20. Witting N, Kupers RC, Svensson P, Jensen TS. A PET activation study of brush-evoked allodynia in patients with nerve injury pain. *Pain*. 2006;120(1–2):145–154.

21. Reynolds DV. Surgery in the rat during electrical analgesia induced by focal brain stimulation. *Science*. 1969; 164(3878):444–445.

22. Vanegas H, Schaible HG. Descending control of persistent pain: inhibitory or facilitatory? *Brain Res Rev*. 2004;46(3): 295–309.

23. Hsieh JC, Hannerz J, Ingvar M. Right-lateralised central processing for pain of nitroglycerin-induced cluster headache. *Pain*. 1996;67(1):59–68.

24. Macefield VG, Gandevia SC, Henderson LA. Discrete changes in cortical activation during experimentally induced referred muscle pain: a single-trial fMRI study. *Cereb Cortex*. 2007;17(9):2050–2059.

25. Lorenz J, Casey KL. Imaging of acute versus pathological pain in humans. *Eur J Pain*. 2005;9(2):163–165.

26. Moseley GL, Arntz A. The context of a noxious stimulus affects the pain it evokes. *Pain*. 2007;133:64–71.

27. Schweinhardt P, Glynn C, Brooks J, et al. An fMRI study of cerebral processing of brush-evoked allodynia in neuropathic pain patients. *NeuroImage*. 2006;32(1):256–265.

28. Moseley GL, Zalucki N, Birklein F, Marinus J, van Hilten JJ, Luomajoki H. Thinking about movement hurts: the effect of motor imagery on pain and swelling in people with chronic arm pain. *Arthritis Care Res*. 2008;59(5): 623–631.

29. Acerra NE, Moseley GL. Dysynchiria: watching the mirror image of the unaffected limb elicits pain on the affected side. *Neurology*. 2005;65(5):751–753.

30. Zambreanu L, Wise RG, Brooks JCW, Iannetti GD, Tracey I. A role for the brainstem in central sensitisation in humans. Evidence from functional magnetic resonance imaging. *Pain*. 2005;114(3):397–407.

31. Hebb D. *The Organization of Behavior*. New York: Wiley; 1949.

32. Jones AKP, Kitchen ND, Watabe H, et al. Measurement of changes in opioid receptor binding in vivo during trigeminal neuralgic pain using [C-11] diprenorphine and positron emission tomography. *J Cereb Blood Flow Metab*. 1999;19(7):803–808.

33. Jones AKP, Watabe H, Cunningham VJ, Jones T. Cerebral decreases in opioid receptor binding in patients with central neuropathic pain measured by [C-11] diprenorphine binding and PET. *Eur J Pain*. 2004;8(5):479–485.

34. Willoch F, Schindler F, Wester HE, et al. Central poststroke pain and reduced opioid receptor binding within pain processing circuitries: a [C-11] diprenorphine PET study. *Pain*. 2004;108(3):213–220.

35. Altier N, Stewart J. The role of dopamine in the nucleus accumbens in analgesia. *Life Sci*. 1999;65(22):2269–2287.

36. Hagelberg N, Jaaskelainen SK, Martikainen IK, et al. Striatal dopamine D2 receptors in modulation of pain in humans: a review. *Eur J Pharmacol*. 2004;500(1–3): 187–192.

37. Scott DJ, Heitzeg MM, Koeppe RA, Stohler CS, Zubieta JK. Variations in the human pain stress experience mediated by ventral and dorsal basal ganglia dopamine activity. *J Neurosci*. 2006;26(42):10789–10795.

38. Wood PB, Patterson JC, Sunderland JJ, Tainter KH, Glabus MF, Lilien DL. Reduced pre-synaptic dopamine activity in fibromyalgia syndrome demonstrated with positron emission tomography: a pilot study. *J Pain*. 2007;8(1):51–58.

39. Moseley GL. *Painful Yarns. Metaphors and Stories to Help Understand the Biology of Pain*. Canberra: Dancing Giraffe Press; 2007.

40. Eccleston C, Crombez G. Pain demands attention: a cognitive affective model of the interruptive function of pain. *Psychol Bull*. 1999;125(3):356–366.

41. Rosenstiel AK, Keefe FJ. The use of coping strategies in chronic low back pain patients: relationship to patient characteristics and current adjustment. *Pain*. 1983;17(1): 33–44.

42. Sullivan MJ, Thorn B, Haythornthwaite JA, et al. Theoretical perspectives on the relation between catastrophizing and pain. *Clin J Pain*. 2001;17(1):52–64.

43. Quartana PJ, Campbell CM, Edwards RR. Pain catastrophizing: a critical review. *Expert Rev Neurother*. 2009;9(5): 745–758.

44. Rhudy JL, Maynard LJ, Russell JL. Does in vivo catastrophizing engage descending modulation of spinal nociception? *J Pain*. 2007;8(4):325–333.

45. Gracely RH, Geisser ME, Giesecke T, et al. Pain catastrophizing and neural responses to pain among persons with fibromyalgia. *Brain.* 2004;127(Pt 4):835–843.

46. Ploghaus A, Tracey I, Gati JS, et al. Dissociating pain from its anticipation in the human brain. *Science.* 1999; 284(5422):1979–1981.

47. Seminowicz DA, Davis KD. Cortical responses to pain in healthy individuals depends on pain catastrophizing. *Pain.* 2006;120(3):297–306.

48. Fishbain DA, Cutler R, Rosomoff HL, Rosomoff RS. Chronic pain-associated depression: antecedent or consequence of chronic pain? A review. *Clin J Pain.* 1997;13(2): 116–137.

49. Fishbain DA. The pain-depression relationship. *Psychosomatics.* 2002;43(4):341, author re- ply 341–342.

50. Mee S, Bunney BG, Reist C, Potkin SG, Bunney WE. Psychological pain: a review of evidence. *J Psychiatr Res.* 2006;40(8):680–690.

51. Williams LS, Jones WJ, Shen J, Robinson RL, Weinberger M, Kroenke K. Prevalence and impact of depression and pain in neurology outpatients. *J Neurol Neurosurg Psychiatry.* 2003;74(11):1587–1589.

52. Ploghaus A, Narain C, Beckmann CF, et al. Exacerbation of pain by anxiety is associated with activity in a hippocampal network. *J Neurosci.* 2001;21(24):9896–9903.

53. Ochsner KN, Ludlow DH, Knierim K, et al. Neural correlates of individual differences in pain-related fear and anxiety. *Pain.* 2006;120(1–2):69–77.

54. Gusnard DA, Raichle ME. Searching for a baseline: functional imaging and the resting human brain. *Nat Rev Neurosci.* 2001;2(10):685–694.

55. Kelley WM, Macrae CN, Wyland CL, Caglar S, Inati S, Heatherton TF. Finding the self? An event-related fMRI study. *J Cogn Neurosci.* 2002;14(5):785–794.

56. McCracken LM. "Attention" to pain in persons with chronic pain: a behavioral approach. *Behav Ther.* 1997;28(2):271–284.

57. Coghill RC, Sang CN, Maisog JM, Iadarola MJ. Pain intensity processing within the human brain: a bilateral, distributed mechanism. *J Neurophysiol.* 1999;82(4):1934–1943.

58. Bantick SJ, Wise RG, Ploghaus A, Clare S, Smith SM, Tracey I. Imaging how attention modulates pain in humans using functional MRI. *Brain.* 2002;125(Pt 2):310–319.

59. Petrovic P, Petersson KM, Ghatan PH, Stone-Elander S, Ingvar M. Pain-related cerebral activation is altered by a distracting cognitive task. *Pain.* 2000;85(1–2):19–30.

60. Smith MY, Egert J, Winkel G, Jacobson J. The impact of PTSD on pain experience in persons with HIV/AIDS. *Pain.* 2002;98(12):9–17.

61. Asmundson GJ, Coons MJ, Taylor S, Katz J. PTSD and the experience of pain: research and clinical implications of shared vulnerability and mutual maintenance models. *Can J Psychiatry.* 2002;47(10):930–937.

62. Beckham JC, Crawford AL, Feldman ME, et al. Chronic post-traumatic stress disorder and chronic pain in Vietnam combat veterans. *J Psychosom Res.* 1997;43(4):379–389.

63. McWilliams LA, Goodwin RD, Cox BJ. Depression and anxiety associated with three pain conditions: results from a nationally representative sample. *Pain.* 2004;111(1–2): 77–83.

64. Jenewein J, Moergeli H, Wittmann L, Buchi S, Kraemer B, Schnyder U. Development of chronic pain following severe accidental injury. Results of a 3-year follow-up study. *J Psychosom Res.* 2009;66(2):119–126.

65. Geuze E, Westenberg HG, Jochims A, et al. Altered pain processing in veterans with post traumatic stress disorder. *Arch Gen Psychiatry.* 2007;64(1):76–85.

66. Giesecke T, Gracely RH, Williams DA, Geisser ME, Petzke FW, Clauw DJ. The relationship between depression, clinical pain, and experimental pain in a chronic pain cohort. *Arthritis Rheum.* 2005;52(5):1577–1584.

67. Schweinhardt P, Kalk N, Wartolowska K, Chessell I, Wordsworth P, Tracey I. Investigation into the neural correlates of emotional augmentation of clinical pain. *Neuroimage.* 2008;40(2):759–766.

68. Hadjipavlou G, Dunckley P, Behrens TE, Tracey I. Determining anatomical connectivities between cortical and brainstem pain processing regions in humans: a diffusion tensor imaging study in healthy controls. *Pain.* 2006;123(1–2):169–178.

69. Crombez G, Vlaeyen JW, Heuts PH, Lysens R. Pain-related fear is more disabling than pain itself: evidence on the role of pain-related fear in chronic back pain disability. *Pain.* 1999;80(1–2):329–339.

70. Al-Obaidi SM, Nelson RM, Al-Awadhi S, Al-Shuwaie N. The role of anticipation and fear of pain in the persistence of avoidance behavior in patients with chronic low back pain. *Spine.* 2000;25(9):1126–1131.

71. Vlaeyen JW, Kole-Snijders AM, Boeren RG, van Eek H. Fear of movement/(re)injury in chronic low back pain and its relation to behavioral performance. *Pain.* 1995;62(3): 363–372.

72. Wise RG, Lujan BJ, Schweinhardt P, Peskett GD, Rogers R, Tracey I. The anxiolytic effects of midazolam during anticipation to pain revealed using fMRI. *Magn Reson Imaging.* 2007;25(6):801–810.

73. Fairhurst M, Wiech K, Dunckley P, Tracey I. Anticipatory brainstem activity predicts neural processing of pain in humans. *Pain.* 2007;128(1–2):101–110.

74. Miron D, Duncan GH, Bushnell MC. Effects of attention on the intensity and unpleasantness of thermal pain. *Pain.* 1989;39(3):345–352.

75. Davis KD, Taylor SJ, Crawley AP, Wood ML, Mikulis DJ. Functional MRI of pain- and attention-related activations in the human cingulate cortex. *J Neurophysiol.* 1997;77(6): 3370–3380.

76. Hsieh JC, Belfrage M, Stone-Elander S, Hansson P, Ingvar M. Central representation of chronic ongoing neuropathic pain studied by positron emission tomography. *Pain.* 1995;63(2):225–236.

77. Bush G, Whalen PJ, Rosen BR, Jenike MA, McInerney SC, Rauch SL. The counting Stroop: an interference task specialized for functional neuroimaging – validation study with functional MRI. *Hum Brain Mapp.* 1998;6(4):270–282.

78. Seminowicz DA, Mikulis DJ, Davis KD. Cognitive modulation of pain-related brain responses depends on behavioral strategy. *Pain.* 2004;112(1–2):48–58.

79. Reisberg D, Baron J, Kemler DG. Overcoming Stroop interference: the effects of practice on distractor potency. *J Exp Psychol Hum Percept Perform.* 1980;6(1):140–150.

80. Decety J, Jackson PL. The functional architecture of human empathy. *Behav Cogn Neurosci Rev.* 2004;3(2):71–100.

81. Batson CD, Polycarpou MP, Harmon-Jones E, et al. Empathy and attitudes: can feeling for a member of a stigmatized

group improve feelings toward the group? *J Pers Soc Psychol*. 1997;72(1):105–118.

82. Meltzoff A. Imitation as a mechanism of social cognition: origins of empathy, theory of mind, and the representation of action. In: Goswami U, ed. *Blackwell Handbook of Childhood Cognitive Development*. Oxford: Blackwell Publishers; 2002:6–25.

83. Preston SD, de Waal FB. Empathy: its ultimate and proximate bases. *Behav Brain Sci*. 2002;25(1):1–20; discussion 20–71.

84. Williams AC de C. Facial expression of pain: an evolutionary account. *Behav Brain Sci*. 2002;25:439–488.

85. Jackson PL, Meltzoff AN, Decety J. How do we perceive the pain of others? A window into the neural processes involved in empathy. *Neuroimage*. 2005;24(3):771–779.

86. Morrison I, Lloyd D, di Pellegrino G, Roberts N. Vicarious responses to pain in anterior cingulate cortex: is empathy a multisensory issue? *Cogn Affect Behav Neurosci*. 2004;4(2):270–278.

87. Avenanti A, Bueti D, Galati G, Aglioti SM. Transcranial magnetic stimulation highlights the sensorimotor side of empathy for pain. *Nat Neurosci*. 2005;8(7):955–960.

88. Fecteau S, Pascual-Leone A, Theoret H. Psychopathy and the mirror neuron system: preliminary findings from a non-psychiatric sample. *Psychiatry Res*. 2008;160(2):137–144.

89. Petrovic P, Kalso E, Petersson KM, Ingvar M. Placebo and opioid analgesia – imaging a shared neuronal network. *Science*. 2002;295(5560):1737–1740.

90. Wager TD, Rilling JK, Smith EE, et al. Placebo-induced changes in FMRI in the anticipation and experience of pain. *Science*. 2004;303(5661):1162–1167.

91. Zubieta JK, Bueller JA, Jackson LR, et al. Placebo effects mediated by endogenous opioid activity on mu-opioid receptors. *J Neurosci*. 2005;25(34):7754–7762.

92. Bingel U, Lorenz J, Schoell E, Weiller C, Buchel C. Mechanisms of placebo analgesia: rACC recruitment of a subcortical antinociceptive network. *Pain*. 2006;120(1–2):8–15.

93. Price DD, Craggs J, Verne GN, Perlstein WM, Robinson ME. Placebo analgesia is accompanied by large reductions in pain-related brain activity in irritable bowel syndrome patients. *Pain*. 2007;127(1–2):63–72.

94. Craggs JG, Price DD, Verne GN, Perlstein WM, Robinson MM. Functional brain interactions that serve cognitive-affective processing during pain and placebo analgesia. *Neuroimage*. 2007;38(4):720–729.

95. Scott DJ, Stohler CS, Egnatuk CM, Wang H, Koeppe RA, Zubieta JK. Individual differences in reward responding explain placebo-induced expectations and effects. *Neuron*. 2007;55(2):325–336.

96. Moseley GL. Reconceptualising placebo. *BMJ*. 2008; 336(7653):1086.

97. Gatchel RJ, Rollings KH. Evidence-informed management of chronic low back pain with cognitive behavioral therapy. *Spine J*. 2008;8(1):40–44.

98. Durham R, Fisher P, Dow M, et al. Cognitive behaviour therapy for good and poor prognosis generalized anxiety disorder: a clinical effectiveness study. *Clin Psychol Psychother*. 2004;11:145–157.

99. Barlow DH. *Clinical Handbook of Psychological Disorders*. New York, NY: Guilford Press; 2001.

100. Reynolds WM, Coats KI. A comparison of cognitive-behavioral therapy and relaxation training for the treatment of depression in adolescents. *J Consult Clin Psychol*. 1986; 54(5):653–660.

101. Lynch D, Laws KR, McKenna PJ. Cognitive behavioural therapy for major psychiatric disorder: does it really work? A meta-analytical review of well-controlled trials. *Psychol Med*. 2010;40(1):9–24.

102. Kiropoulos L, Klein B, Austin D, et al. Is internet-based CBT for panic disorder and agoraphobia as effective as face-to-face CBT? *J Anxiety Disord*. 2008;22:1273–1284.

103. Butler AC, Chapman JE, Forman EM, Beck AT. The empirical status of cognitive-behavioral therapy: a review of meta-analyses. *Clin Psychol Rev*. 2006;26(1):17–31.

104. Fu CH, Williams SC, Cleare AJ, et al. Neural responses to sad facial expressions in major depression following cognitive behavioral therapy. *Biol Psychiatry*. 2008;64(6):505–512.

105. Sakai Y, Kumano H, Nishikawa M, et al. Changes in cerebral glucose utilization in patients with panic disorder treated with cognitive-behavioral therapy. *Neuroimage*. 2006;33(1):218–226.

106. Saxena S, Gorbis E, O'Neill J, et al. Rapid effects of brief intensive cognitive-behavioral therapy on brain glucose metabolism in obsessive-compulsive disorder. *Mol Psychiatry*. 2009;14(2):197–205.

107. Keefe FJ, Somers TJ, Martire LM. Psychologic interventions and lifestyle modifications for arthritis pain management. *Rheum Dis Clin North Am*. 2008;34(2): 351–368.

108. Abernethy AP, Keefe FJ, McCrory DC, Scipio CD, Matchar DB. Behavioral therapies for the management of cancer pain: a systematic review. In: Flor H, Kalso E, Dostrovsky JO, eds. *Proceedings of the 11th World Congress on Pain*. Seattle: IASP Press; 2006.

109. Emery CF, Keefe FJ, France CR, et al. Effects of a brief coping skills training intervention on nociceptive flexion reflex threshold in patients having osteoarthritic knee pain: a preliminary laboratory study of sex differences. *J Pain Symptom Manage*. 2006;31(3):262–269.

110. Carson JW, Keefe FJ, Affleck G, et al. A comparison of conventional pain coping skills training and pain coping skills training with a maintenance training component: a daily diary analysis of short- and long-term treatment effects. *J Pain*. 2006;7(9):615–625.

111. van Tulder MW, Ostelo R, Vlaeyen JW, Linton SJ, Morley SJ, Assendelft WJ. Behavioral treatment for chronic low back pain: a systematic review within the framework of the Cochrane Back Review Group. *Spine*. 2000;25(20):2688–2699.

112. Lackner JM, Lou Coad M, Mertz HR, et al. Cognitive therapy for irritable bowel syndrome is associated with reduced limbic activity, GI symptoms, and anxiety. *Behav Res Ther*. 2006;44(5):621–638.

113. Moseley GL. Unravelling the barriers to reconceptualisation of the problem in chronic pain: the actual and perceived ability of patients and health professionals to understand the neurophysiology. *J Pain*. 2003;4(4):184–189.

114. Moseley GL. Evidence for a direct relationship between cognitive and physical change during an education intervention in people with chronic low back pain. *Eur J Pain*. 2004;8(1):39–45.

115. Moseley GL, Nicholas MK, Hodges PW. A randomized controlled trial of intensive neurophysiology education in chronic low back pain. *Clin J Pain*. 2004;20(5):324–330.

116. Moseley GL. Combined physiotherapy and education is effective for chronic low back pain. A randomised controlled trial. *Aust J Physioth.* 2002;48:297–302.

117. Moseley GL. Joining forces – combining cognition-targeted motor control training with group or individual pain physiology education: a successful treatment for chronic low back pain. *J Man Manip Ther.* 2003;11:88–94.

118. Moseley GL. Widespread brain activity during an abdominal task markedly reduced after pain physiology education – fMRI evaluation of a single patient with chronic low back pain. *Aust J Physioth.* 2005;51:49–52.

119. Moseley GL. Cortical issues with rehabilitation and learning. *Paper Presented at: 8th International Congress of the Australian Physiotherapy Association.* Adelaide, Australia; 2004.

120. Keefe FJ, Abernethy AP, Wheeler JL, Somers TJ. Psychological approaches to managing cancer pain. In: Bruera E, Portenoy R, eds. *Cancer Pain: Assessment and Management.* New York: Cambridge University Press; in press.

121. Barber J, ed. *Hypnosis and Suggestion in the Treatment of Pain: A Clinical Guide.* New York: Norton; 1996.

122. Crawford HJ, Gur RC, Skolnick B, Gur RE, Benson DM. Effects of hypnosis on regional cerebral blood flow during ischemic pain with and without suggested hypnotic analgesia. *Int J Psychophysiol.* 1993;15(3):181–195.

123. Dinges DF, Whitehouse WG, Orne EC, et al. Self-hypnosis training as an adjunctive treatment in the management of pain associated with sickle cell disease. *Int J Clin Exp Hypn.* 1997;45(4):417–432.

124. Elkins G, Marcus J, Palamara L, Stearns V. Can hypnosis reduce hot flashes in breast cancer survivors? A literature review. *Am J Clin Hypn.* 2004;47(1):29–42.

125. Gay MC, Philippot P, Luminet O. Differential effectiveness of psychological interventions for reducing osteoarthritis pain: a comparison of Erikson [correction of Erickson]

hypnosis and Jacobson relaxation. *Eur J Pain.* 2002;6(1): 1–16.

126. Jensen MP, Hanley MA, Engel JM, et al. Hypnotic analgesia for chronic pain in persons with disabilities: a case series. *Int J Clin Exp Hypn.* 2005;53(2):198–228.

127. Rainville P, Duncan GH, Price DD, Carrier B, Bushnell MC. Pain affect encoded in human anterior cingulate but not somatosensory cortex. *Science.* 1997;277(5328): 968–971.

128. Wik G, Fischer H, Bragee B, Finer B, Fredrikson M. Functional anatomy of hypnotic analgesia: a PET study of patients with fibromyalgia. *Eur J Pain.* 1999;3(1):7–12.

129. Derbyshire SW, Whalley MG, Oakley DA. Fibromyalgia pain and its modulation by hypnotic and non-hypnotic suggestion: an fMRI analysis. *Eur J Pain.* 2009;13(5): 542–550.

130. Carson JW, Carson KM, Porter LS, Keefe FJ, Shaw H, Miller JM. Yoga for women with metastatic breast cancer: results from a pilot study. *J Pain Symptom Manage.* 2007; 33(3):331–341.

131. Kabat-Zinn J. An outpatient program in behavioral medicine for chronic pain patients based on the practice of mindfulness meditation: theoretical considerations and preliminary results. *Gen Hosp Psychiatry.* 1982;4(1): 33–47.

132. Orme-Johnson DW, Schneider RH, Son YD, Nidich S, Cho ZH. Neuroimaging of meditation's effect on brain reactivity to pain. *Neuroreport.* 2006;17(12):1359–1363.

133. Holroyd KA, Holm JE, Hursey KG, et al. Recurrent vascular headache: home-based behavioral treatment versus abortive pharmacological treatment. *J Consult Clin Psychol.* 1988;56(2):218–223.

134. Farrell MJ, Egan Zamarripa F, Shade R, Blair-West J, Fox P, Denton DA. Unique, common, and interacting cortical of thirst and pain. *Proc Nalt Acad Sci.* 2006;103:2416–2421.

Chapter 18
Neuroimaging in Acute Ischemic Stroke

Shashidhara Nanjundaswamy, Ronald A. Cohen, and Marc Fisher

Stroke, the third leading cause of death is a medical emergency.[1] The phrase "Time is Brain" has been coined to emphasize the urgency of rapid intervention for stroke.[2] For each minute, the stroke is untreated, more than two million neurons, 14 billion synapses, and 12 km (7.5 miles) of myelinated fibers may be lost.[3] Intravenous tissue plasminogen activator (tPA) is the only FDA approved treatment for a nonhemorrhagic stroke. Currently, it must be administered within 3–4.5 h of stroke onset for it to be effective in reducing infarction volume and its functional impact.[4] Other non-FDA treatment approaches have been developed, including intraarterial tPA, mechanical removal of the embolus, penumbra endovascular system devices that suction the embolus through a catheter, anti-platelet and anticoagulant medications, and neuroprotective agents.[5] All of these approaches are time sensitive and depend on the initiation of intervention soon after ischemic onset. Accordingly, there is an obvious need for a reliable and rapid means of detecting and diagnosing acute ischemic stroke to offer timely and appropriate treatment.

Neuroimaging provides a powerful method for both detecting and diagnosing stroke, and measuring and monitoring the evolution of the penumbra and infarction. In the field of clinical neurology, neuroimaging is now well established as part of the standard of care for patients suspected of having a stroke. In fact, cerebral infarction and neoplasm are among the primary conditions that are tested for when routine neuroimaging is conducted. When considering brain approaches that may have value in the future in clinical neuroscience and behavioral medicine, it is useful to consider how neuroimaging is currently being employed in the assessment of stroke, and also current experimental methods that are being explored. When combined, these methods provide for a sequential approach for dissociating various pathophysiological processes associated with stroke and the evolution of infarction.

Current neuroimaging methods generally involve two primary approaches: computed tomography (CT) and magnetic resonance imaging (MRI). For purposes of identification of infarctions resulting from stroke occurring in the more distant past, CT and MRI can typically be conducted in a noninvasive manner to obtain structural neuroanatomic data on the size and location of lesions. When assessing acute stroke, these noninvasive methods are often combined with perfusion imaging methods that in some cases involve the administration of contrast agents, such as gadolinium for magnetic resonance angiography (MRA), especially for the neck, and iodinated contrast agents for computerized tomography angiogram (CTA). While invasive, the intravenous delivery of these agents is relatively safe for most patients. Other neuroimaging methods are derived using specialized CT or MRI scanning sequences that provide for analysis of diffusion and perfusion of fluid in the area of cerebral ischemia, including perfusion weighted (PWI) and diffusion weighted (DWI) imaging. The multimodal neuroimaging approach currently being employed for stroke provides a model for what may occur in the future for other brain and behavioral disorders.

M. Fisher (✉)
UMASS-Memorial Medical Center, Belmont St.,
Worcester, MA 01506, USA
e-mail: fisherm@ummhc.org

R.A. Cohen and L.H. Sweet (eds.), *Brain Imaging in Behavioral Medicine and Clinical Neuroscience*,
DOI 10.1007/978-1-4419-6373-4_18, © Springer Science+Business Media, LLC 2011

Rationale for Stroke Neuroimaging

The standard imaging protocol for Stroke performed at most centers includes performing an urgent noncontrast (NCCT) head CT, and if negative for a bleed, to continue with CT angiography (CTA) of the brain and neck to look for a large artery occlusion. CT perfusion scans (CTP) are performed for stroke onset beyond 3 h to look for a salvageable ischemic penumbra, which requires intravenous tPA with or without additional thrombectomy. The CT protocol is standard because not all hospitals have access to MRI, though increasingly this technology is now available at most stroke centers. When MRI is available, perfusion and diffusion weighted MRI is also performed, as these methods provide increased sensitivity to early effects of cerebral ischemia. The general rationale for imaging is to obtain evidence of: (1) localized cerebral hypoperfusion (PWI), (2) occlusion and/or dissection of specific cerebral vessels (MRA); (3) altered fluid diffusion in brain tissue in the affected vascular territory (DWI), and (4) permanent infarction (T1, T2, FLAIR, etc.).

The fact that some brain some brain tissue may be recoverable if reperfusion occurs rapidly via one of the treatment approaches mentioned earlier makes it important to distinguish between the areas of the brain that experience physiological alterations (i.e., the penumbra), from the areas that have become infracted, and are likely to have permanent functional impairments.[6,7] A penumbra is defined as a shadowy, indefinite, or marginal area, such as the partial or imperfect shadow outside the complete shadow of an opaque body, where the light from the source of illumination is only partly cut off. The fact that this definition has been applied to the evolution of ischemic brain tissue reflects the importance of information obtained from neuroimaging in characterizing the processes occurring during stroke. In the context of stroke, the shadow refers to differences in the characteristics of the abnormal cerebral areas as seen on the brain perfusion scans.

Stroke stage	Time course
Hyperacute	<6 h
Acute	6–48 h
Subacute	2 days to 2 weeks
Chronic	>2 weeks

Evolution of Cerebral Infarction (Fig. 18.9)

When considering the temporal dynamics of the evolution of cerebral infarction, clinicians in the stroke field have found that it is important to distinguish between four stages. The first "hyperacute" stage refers to a period of generally less than 6 h during which there is localized hypoperfusion indicative of cerebral ischemia, and physiological disturbance in affected brain tissue, but in many cases only limited infarction. This is the ideal period for intervention. The next subacute period extends from about 6 h to 2 days and is a period during which the effects of cerebral ischemia and its secondary physiological effects are resulting in infarction that is more permanent in nature. During the acute period that follows, the infarction is for the most part fully developed, but some degree of recovery of brain tissue may be possible. After 2 weeks, chronic injury is usually evident and minimal recovery of infracted tissue is likely.

Normal Oxygen and glucose delivery to brain is dependent upon a normal cerebral blood flow (CBF), which is maintained by a normal cerebral autoregulation. Cerebral ischemia results when brain perfusion falls below critical levels causing loss of neuronal function electrically and lead to neurological deficits that are seen clinically. When the perfusion deficit is prolonged, it leads to neuronal and glial death with ensuing irreversible cerebral infarction. Normal CBF is 50–55 mL/100 g brain tissue/min. Severe perfusion defect with a CBF <10 mL/100 g/min leads to infarction within minutes. Moderate levels of perfusion deficit, CBF 10–20 mL/100 g /min causes neuronal electrical failure with loss of function.

These effects may be reversible for a period of hours from the onset of the ischemic insult. However, a severe perfusion defect causes additional hypoxic/anoxic cellular injury. The sodium-potassium ATPase pump fails, cell membrane gets depolarized, and glutamate is released into the extracellular space. This activates the NMDA, AMPA, and kainite receptors leading to influx of sodium and calcium into the cells. Water follows passively with resultant cytotoxic edema. Intracellular calcium accumulation activates proteolytic mechanisms with oxygen free radicals causing further cell damage. This anoxic depolarization occurs with severe perfusion deficits only. Thus, there could be two thresholds, initially a moderate perfusion deficit with CBF less than 10–20 mL/100 g/min causing electrical failure as seen in the ischemic penumbra that could be potentially salvageable.[8-10] Second, a severe perfusion deficit with CBF <10 mL/100 g/min that causes anoxic membrane depolarization, activating the inevitable cascade resulting in lipolysis, cell necrosis, inflammation, and eventual apoptosis, cell death.

Pathologically, within the first 6 h, in the hyperacute stage, the brain appears normal on gross examination, despite irreversible cellular damage at the microscopic level. Soon after, within 8–48 h, of the acute stage, there is indistinct differentiation between the gray and the white matter. In the subacute stage, 2 days to 2 weeks after the infarction there is swelling and softening of the brain tissue with evidence of mass effect and the boundaries of the infracted territory is more prominent. The chronic period is marked by liquefaction of the infarct and development of a CSF-filled cystic area or an encephalomalacia. Histologically, after 6–12 h the infarcted cell cytoplasm becomes eosinophilic, nucleus shrinks and the nucleolus disappears.[11] Endothelial swelling of the capillaries along with vasogenic and cytotoxic edema with some extravasation of RBCs is seen. Glia along with the neurons shows ischemic damage. There is emigration of neutrophils between 24 and 48 h, after which macrophages replace them. Liquefaction begins after 10 days, and from third week onward, cavitation becomes evident.[11]

Neuroimaging of Stroke

In sections that follow, the use of specific imaging methods in the assessment of evolving cerebral infarction and the type of clinical information that is obtained from each method are reviewed. We begin with assessment conducted during the hyperacute stage and proceed to the assessment of stroke during later stages of its evolution.

Noncontrast CT

Currently, Noncontrast CT (NCCT) scan of the head is widely available for neuroimaging in acute stroke.

Hemorrhage can be reliably ruled out and IV tPA could be administered if there are no other contraindications. In stroke centers, CTA and CTP are routinely performed, which helps in deciding neuro interventional procedures including IA tPA with or without thrombectomy. MRI diffusion and perfusion imaging is not widely available even in designated stroke centers.

In order to quickly rule out an acute hemorrhagic event, cranial NCCT is done. Acute hemorrhage is a contraindication for tPA, so determining whether this is a hemorrhagic stroke is essential. If hemorrhage is ruled, then other earlier indicators of cerebral ischemia are explored. (Figs. 18.1 and 18.2) Either early signs of infarction or a hyperdense MCA or a Basilar artery can also be demonstrated. Signs of cerebral infarction, hypodensity more than 1/3 of an arterial territory indicate the possibility of a stroke onset >3 h and predict increased bleeding risk with thrombolysis and hence preclude thrombolytics. A hyperdense MCA sign may suggest that the recanalization success with IV tPA is low and may push toward treating with IA tPA much earlier, even within the 3 h window. The hypodensity on a NCCT head indicates an irreversible process of cytotoxic edema with failure of the Na+K+ATPase pumps, thereby allowing accumulation of Na+ and water inside the neurons causing cell death.

Early signs of infarction on a NCCT
Loss of gray-white matter differentiation
Fullness of the sulci
Obliteration of the basal ganglia density
Loss of insular ribbon sign

CT Perfusion Imaging (Figs. 18.3–18.5)

The commonly employed dynamic perfusion CT employs an iodinated contrast, which is injected at a certain rate.[12-15] Two regions of interest (ROIs), one involving the unaffected artery – Anterior cerebral artery and the other involving the Superior Sagittal Sinus for a venous outflow is used to study arterial and venous outflow functions. The cerebral parenchymal density increases over time with contrast infusion, plateaus and then rises slightly higher than the baseline due to recirculation of the contrast. The time density curve is used to calculate the cerebral blood flow parameters. Peak arterial enhancement CT perfusion is

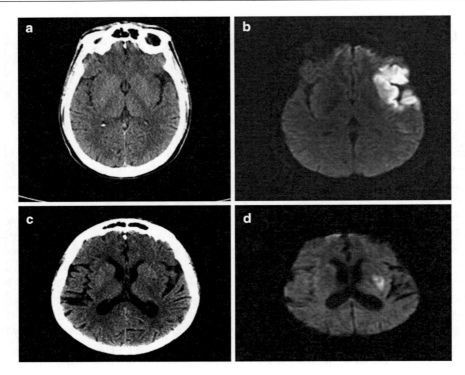

Fig. 18.1 Stroke in the anterior division of the left middle cerebral artery (MCA) as evident on Computed Tomography (CT) and diffusion-weighted (DWI) Magnetic Resonance Imaging (MRI) which is seen much better on diffusion MRI (**b**, **d**) versus CT (**a**, **c**). One of the early signs of developing infarction is the loss of definition of the gray–white interface in the lateral margins of the insula, referred to as an insular ribbon sign. This is apparent on CT, but to an even greater extent on the MRI images. There is also obliteration of the lenticular density

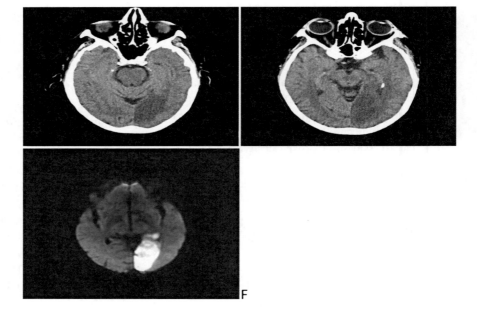

Fig. 18.2 Left Posterior Cerebral Artery (PCA) infarction on MRI. The image on *bottom* shows the full extent of the infarction, better visualized than on noncontrast CT

18 Neuroimaging in Acute Ischemic Stroke

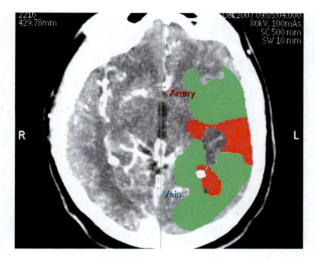

Fig. 18.3 Summary maps perfusion based on CT perfusion imaging. The summary maps are color-coded. *Green* and *Red* – total area of reduced blood flow; *Green* – reduced blood flow with relatively preserved blood volume (Penumbra); *Red* – reduced blood flow with severely reduced volume (likely infarction). This type of contrast enables delineation of infracted area from penumbra that may be recoverable

analyzed pixel by pixel with respect to the inflow and outflow characteristics as there is a linear relationship between the dye concentration and the signal intensity.[16] CBF=CBV/MTT. (CBF – cerebral blood flow; CBV – cerebral blood volume; MTT – mean transit time). MTT is the time elapsed between the arterial inflow and the venous outflow. TTP is the time taken by the contrast to achieve maximum enhancement in the ROI. CBV is the volume of blood per unit of brain tissue.

$$CBF = \frac{\text{Maximal slope of tissue time density cur}}{\text{Peak arterial enhancement}}$$

Severe perfusion deficits with a CBF below 10 mL/100 g/min may lead to infarction within minutes. Moderate levels of ischemia (10–20 mL/100 g/min) may be reversible for a period of hours. CT perfusion imaging is helpful especially when the exact time of stroke onset is unknown,[17] as in wake up strokes and also dominant MCA territory stroke when the patient

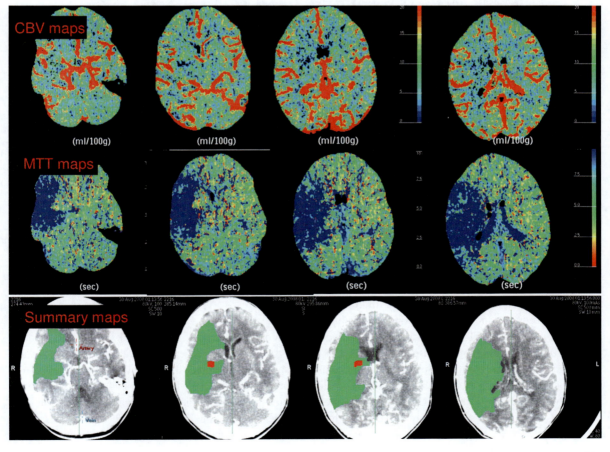

Fig. 18.4 CT perfusion imaging, including cerebral blood volume (CBV), Cerebral Blood Flow (CBF), mean transit time (MTT), and Summary (TTP) maps. CBF=CBV/MTT

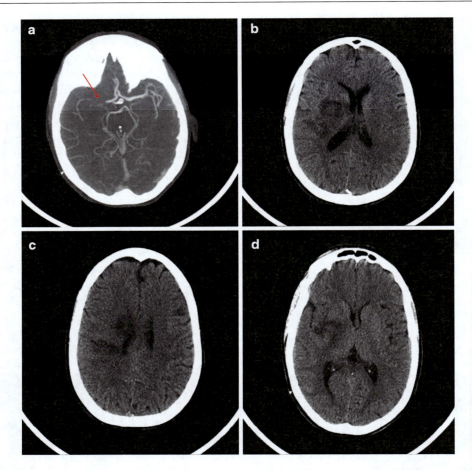

Fig. 18.5 CT imaging showing recovery of brain tissue following neurointervention (clot retrieval). CT angiography shows left MCA stroke. (*Arrow* points to vessel that is occluded.) There is a local intraarterial thrombolysis in M2 divisions. Subsequent scans show follow-up CT results with significant sparing of brain tissue, with final infarction size shown in figure on the *bottom right*

cannot give the exact time of onset because of aphasia. CTP helps in decision making for consideration of thrombolytics. Previously, tPA could not be offered without knowing the exact time of onset.

CT perfusion demonstrates the central infarct core, which is irreversible and is surrounded by a penumbra, which is salvageable tissue with reperfusion. Without timely reperfusion this zone becomes an infarct. CBV is severely reduced in the infarct core. Penumbra is depicted by increased MTT with moderately reduced CBF (>60%) and normal or increased CBV (80–100%) secondary to cerebral auto regulatory mechanisms. Penumbra is also depicted by increased MTT and markedly decreased CBF (>30%) and moderately reduced CBV (>60%). The following criteria have been suggested for defining the infarct core and penumbra on perfusion CT: cerebral blood volume should be less than 2.0 mL/100 g for the infarct core but more than 2.0 mL/100 g for the penumbra, and the mean transit time should be more than 145% of that of the contra lateral side for the penumbra.

CT Angiography (Fig. 18.6)

CTA of the circle of Willis and Neck is performed to demonstrate a large vessel occlusion, within the 3-h window and also up to 8 h. After the 3-h window, if the occlusion can be demonstrated and a CT Perfusion study shows a large mismatch indicating a large potentially salvageable penumbra, further interventional procedures are contemplated. CTA also identifies intracranial aneurysms of >3 mm size. They

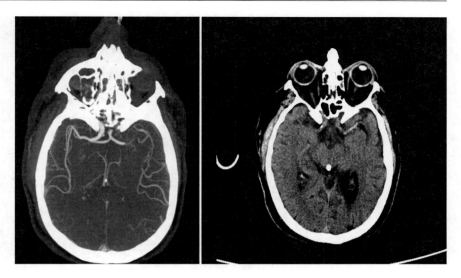

Fig. 18.6 Occlusion of MCA shown on angiography (*left*). Dense infarction left hemisphere MCA territory infarction is evident

can show the stenosis, as well as the adequacy or lack of the intracranial collateral circulation. MCA/Basilar artery stenosis or occlusions can be easily diagnosed. In the neck, extracranially, it reliably demonstrates the carotid stenosis, carotid dissections, vertebral artery stenosis and dissections. CTA requires administration of an iodinated contrast and hence significant renal dysfunction precludes CTA.

MR-Based Methods (Figs. 18.2, 18.7–18.14)

The stroke imaging protocol for MRI brain consists of obtaining Diffusion weighted images (DWI), Apparent diffusion coefficient (ADC) images in addition to the routine T1, T2, Gradient refocused echo (GRE) and fluid attenuated inversion recovery (FLAIR) images with or without proton density (PD) images.

Diffusion Weighted Imaging

The most sensitive method for acute stroke is Diffusion Weighted Imaging (DWI). It typically shows a positive response as early as a few minutes of an ischemic stroke and tends to remain positive for 10–14 days and shows up as bright lesion(s) in an acute ischemic stroke.

ADC sequences in the corresponding areas to the DWI lesion are dark in an acute stroke and remain dark up to 10–14 days. FLAIR shows early stroke changes but is negative for at least a few hours of stroke onset. T2 images can be negative up to 8 h after a stroke. DWI positivity, the light bulb sign, usually indicates an irreversible cerebral injury, that is, the core of the infarct. GRE or the MultiPlanar Gradient sequence (MPGR) shows blood products and is as sensitive as a NCCT for acute blood, and more sensitive than a CT for old blood products. Multiple bleeds of various ages seen in the GRE may indicate amyloid angiopathy, where thrombolytics can increase the risk of intra cerebral bleeds. MRI shows the vascular distribution more clearly and is more sensitive for posterior circulation strokes, unlike CT where streak artifacts due to the dense bones mask the posterior circulation stroke changes. Gyral swelling and sulcal obliteration along with gyral pattern enhancement as well as intravascular contrast enhancement can be seen. Arterial flow voids can be absent. A diagnosis of Large Artery atherosclerosis, Small vessel disease –lacunar stroke, and Border zone or watershed infarctions can be more easily made out with MRI. Subacute cortical infarcts can look isointense to the surrounding brain tissue, from the second to the sixth week of cerebral infarction, a phenomenon of MRI fogging, which is also observed with noncontrast head CT. The previously hyperintense/hyperdense

Fig. 18.7 Acute L. PCA infarct seen only on diffusion weighted images

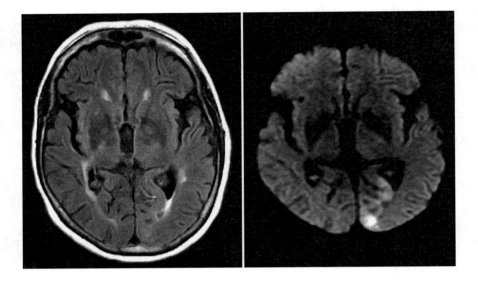

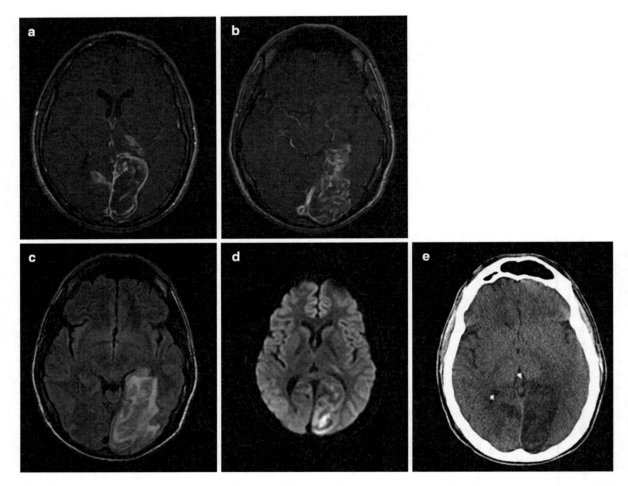

Fig. 18.8 Subacute infarction from stroke several days ago. CT images (**a**, **b**) show characteristics of the infarction soon after its onset. MRI images (*below*) conducted several days show subacute infarction on MRI and impaired diffusion characteristics on MRI based DWI

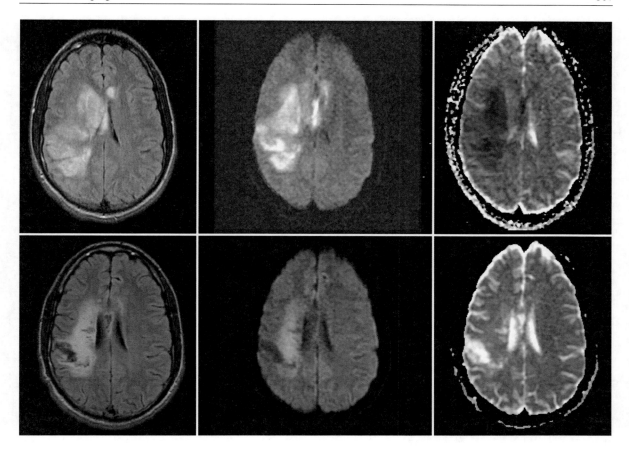

Fig. 18.9 Evolution of infarction over several days as seen across MRI images

lesion will look isointense/isodense. This area enhances after intravenous administration of a contrast agent. The corresponding ADC lesion also normalizes (pseudo-normalization) during the subacute stage. Chronic infarcts show up as dark on DWI and bright on ADC and are associated with volume loss, sulcal widening and ipsilateral ventricle horn dilatation.[4]

MR imaging abnormalities depend upon abnormal accumulation of water after the onset of brain injury.[4] Water accumulates intracellularly within minutes of stroke onset once there is membrane depolarization, water entering passively with influx of sodium ions. Additionally, there is alteration of the morphology and function of the cerebral vasculature. The integrity of the blood brain barrier (BBB) is lost beginning 4–6 h after the insult and lasts 4–5 days after the start of the infarction. This results in vasogenic edema and mass effect with much higher brain tissue water retention and brain swelling. This is more intense in areas with some residual cerebral blood flow. Gradual resolution of the edema and mass effect occurs with resorption of water and proteins. With liquefactive necrosis, there is further water accumulation in the chronic stage resulting in an encephalomalacia.

Small vessel diseases (lacunar strokes) are 2–20 mm in size, seen mainly in the basal ganglia, internal capsule, brain stem, and deep white matter of the cerebral hemispheres. The pathology is lipohyalinosis most often secondary to hypertension, diabetes, and dyslipidemia resulting in obliteration of the deep penetrating or perforator arteries.

Advantages of MRI are that it can detect a stroke much earlier than a CT scan, multiplanar imaging is possible, edema is easily imaged and the posterior fossa beam hardening artifacts seen on the CT scan is not a concern. The disadvantage of MRI is that it is time consuming and difficult to perform in very sick, agitated, and ventilated patients. MRI is contraindicated in patients with pacemakers, aneurysm clips, and other nonremovable ferromagnetic metallic objects in their bodies.

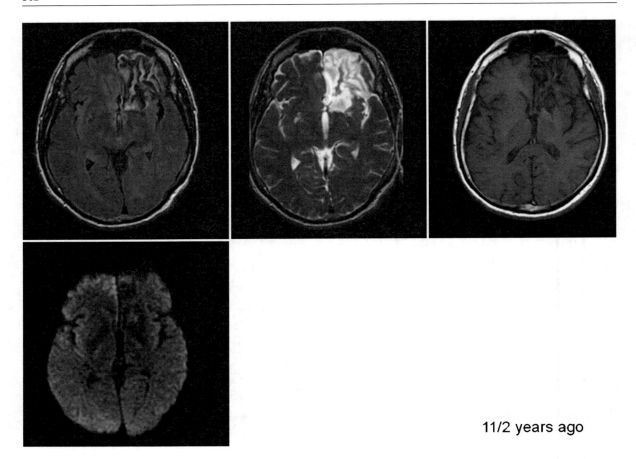

Fig. 18.10 Chronic infarct in anterior cerebral artery (ACA) territory from stroke that occurred approximately 1.5 years ago. Standard MRI (T1, T2, FLAIR, etc.) now show large infarction, where diffusion abnormality has largely cleared, and DWI is relatively normal

Magnetic Resonance Angiography (Figs. 18.12 and 18.13)

MRA of the brain does not require a contrast agent. However, MRA of the neck yields better information with administration of a contrast agent such as gadolinium and the sensitivity reaches that of CTA. Gadolinium cannot be administered in the presence of significant renal dysfunction for fear of nephrogenic systemic fibrosis. In those instances, a noncontrast MRA can be obtained which depends on flow signal characteristics. T1 weighted axial images with fat suppression demonstrates the false lumen with the clot in dissections. The degree of stenosis can also be reliably measured.

MR Perfusion-Weighted Imaging (Fig. 18.15)

Perfusion Weighted Imaging (PWI) is similar to dynamic CT perfusion imaging and needs intravenous injection of a bolus of gadolinium (Gd). Dynamic Susceptibility MRI images provide quantitative relative and absolute measures of perfusion and are used to calculate CBV, CBF, and MTT maps. There is increase in the MTT, and reduction in CBF and CBV. Delayed MTT means delay in cerebral perfusion. A color-coded map is constructed as in CT perfusion imaging depicting the area of irreversible infarct, core; and the DWI/PWI mismatch, which depicts the ischemic penumbra, a potentially salvageable area with reperfusion procedures. Time to Peak (TTP) can be quantified and a delayed TTP ≥6 s has been shown more often to progress into an infarct.

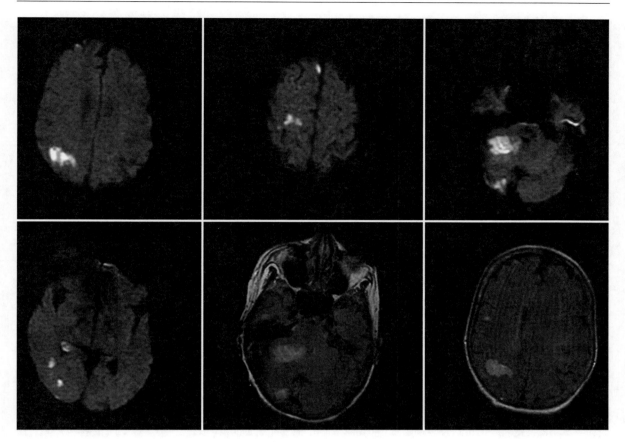

Fig. 18.11 MRI imaging showing multiple embolic infarctions

Continuous Arterial Spin Labelling Perfusion MRI

This noninvasive technique obviates the need for a contrast agent, as the arterial water is electromagnetically labeled proximal to the cerebral flow as a diffuse tracer. Images with and without arterial spin labeling are compared. Quantitative perfusion maps can be calculated. However, this technique is not widely available for clinical use.[18]

Stable Xenon CT

Xe-CT allows measurement of CBF using inhaled radioiodine Xenon. It quantifies CBF well, but does not depict cytotoxic injury in the posterior fossa unlike MRI-DWI images. Good cooperation from the patient is necessary. Moreover, some patients are sensitive to the anesthetic properties of xenon and experience transient paresthesias and altered sensorium. Headaches, nausea, vomiting, and even seizures have been reported.[19]

Positron Emission Tomography

Though PET is the gold standard for CBF measurements, the lack of universal availability, its expense, and other logistical considerations makes it unlikely to be used in clinical practice in the near future.[20]

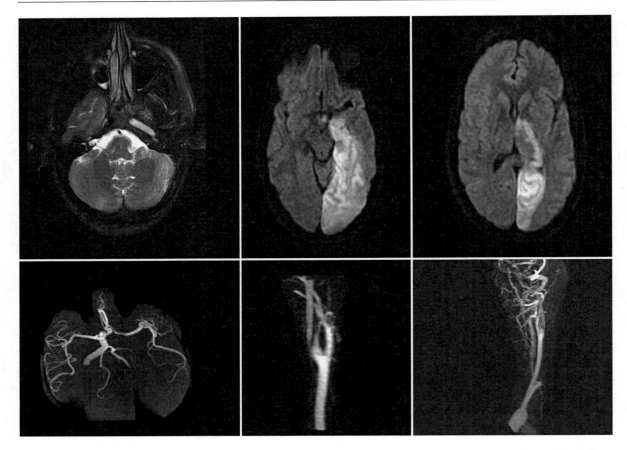

Fig. 18.12 Dissection of ICA and PCA infarct due to disrupted fetal supply. This could be caused by a tear in the intima media of a carotid artery, resulting blood collapsing the cerebral vessel. The *top images* show resulting infarctions on MRI, the *bottom images* show vessel causing the stroke

Brain Spect W/ Diamox

Demonstration of cerebrovascular reserve is necessary before contemplating surgical revascularization procedures in patients with chronic cerebrovascular ischemia. Brain SPECT scan is obtained using HMPAO labeled with Technetium m 99. Brain SPECT scans pre- and postadministration of Acetazolamide (Diamox) a weak carbonic anhydrase inhibitor helps in demonstration of the same. The resultant accumulation of CO_2, which is a cerebral arterial vasodilator, should increase CBF up to 30% over the baseline. However, if the stenotic lesion is severe and progressive, the brain cannot compensate any further, and there is limited or no increase in CBF, thereby indicating need for such procedures.[21]

Future Directions

Advances in neuroimaging have clearly helped the clinician in diagnosing the various types of stroke reliably, which is essential for timely and appropriate management. The ability to demonstrate a salvageable ischemic penumbra when the time of stroke onset is unknown, as in wake up stroke and in aphasic patients who are unable to tell the time of onset has been of great help in deciding to offer thrombolytics. The future of neuroimaging in acute stroke will depend on much quicker and reliable imaging demonstrating the early signs of infarction, the intracranial and extracranial vasculature, rule-out of hemorrhage, and quickly determining salvageable ischemic penumbra without the need to administer IV contrast or MR imaging.

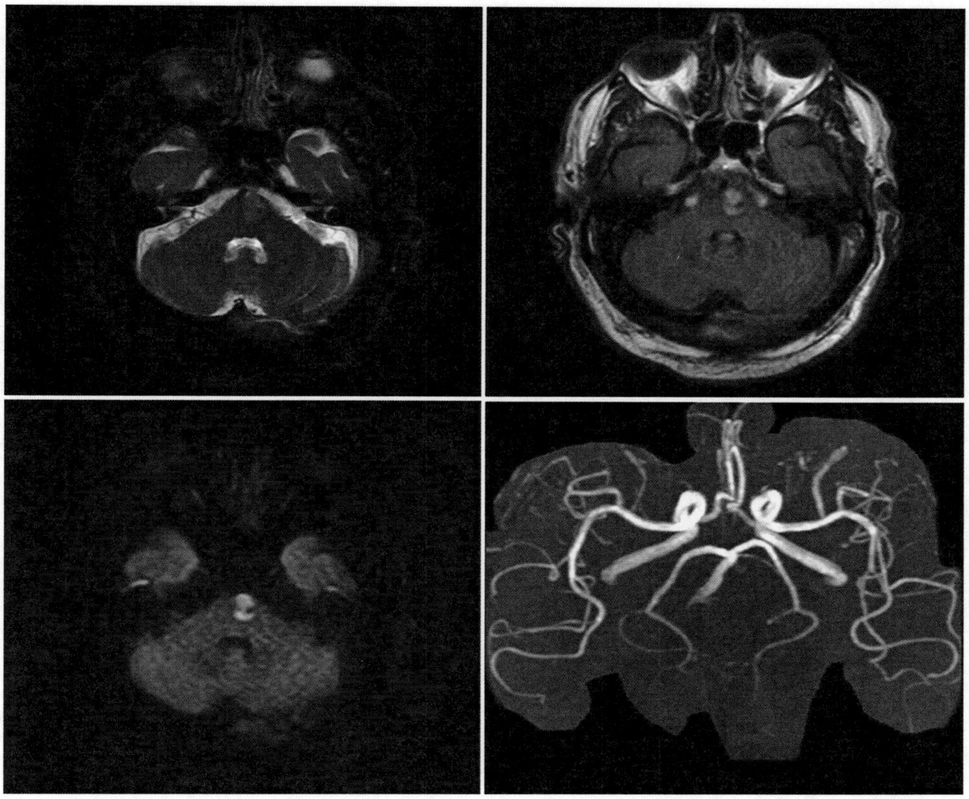

Fig. 18.13 Pontine infarction seen through different types of MR imaging. T2 and FLAIR structural images are shown on the *top*. The DWI image is shown on *bottom left*, with angiography to the *right*. The comparison of these different types of images enables a more complete understanding of the vascular abnormality and its brain effects

The quicker the imaging is performed, the sooner the treatment can be instituted. Time is brain and every minute counts.

Acute stroke imaging is increasingly important for evaluating such patients and for making treatment decisions. Documentation of an arterial occlusion by CTA or MRA provides direction as to whether a patient may be a candidate for intraarterial therapy with tPA or a mechanical clot removal device. Imaging of the ischemic penumbra with either diffusion/perfusion MRI or CT perfusion will identify patients who are more likely to respond to such therapies. Preliminary case series and a few small clinical trials support the concept that penumbral identification with diffusion/perfusion MRI can reliably identify ischemic stroke patients more likely to respond to therapy and provide a mechanism to extend the benefits of IV. tPA and I A. therapies beyond the currently proven 4.5 h for i.v. therapy.[22-24] However, definitive proof that penumbral identification

can identify treatment responders remains elusive and a large, successful, phase III clinical trial with enrollment criteria based upon the presence of an extensive penumbra on diffusion/perfusion MRI is clearly needed.

Many issues concerning the use of diffusion/perfusion MRI for the identification of the ischemic penumbra remain unresolved. The principal unresolved issue is how best to identify the perfusion region of reduced cerebral blood flow highly predictive of ischemic tissue likely to evolve into infarction without timely reperfusion therapy.[25] Currently, using a T_{max} threshold of 5–6 s compared to the normal hemisphere is used to identify such a perfusion lesion.

CT perfusion is widely used in clinical practice for the identification of an approximation of the ischemic penumbra.[6,7,15] The ischemic region is identified on mean transit time and/or time to peak maps, while the ischemic core is approximated by that region with low

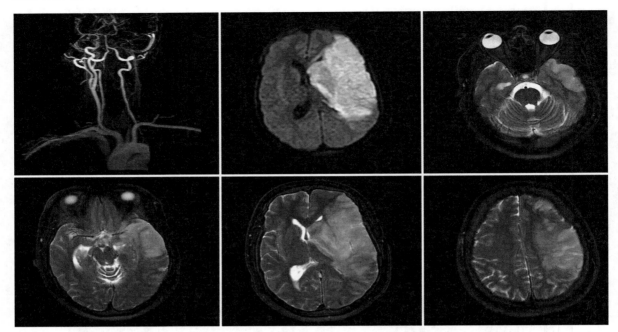

Fig. 18.14 MCA territory infarct resulting from common carotid artery occlusion, probably dissection. Again the nature of the infarction and its diffusion characteristics can be determined by analysis of data from multiple MRI methods

cerebral blood volume values. Unfortunately, the thresholds used on these maps are not well validated, and concerns exist regarding their accuracy and predictability. In clinical trials, diffusion/perfusion MRI will likely be used for the foreseeable future, not CT perfusion. However, efforts are underway to enhance the accuracy of CT perfusion thresholds and to provide comparability to diffusion/perfusion MRI identification of the ischemic penumbra. If current and future trials confirm the utility of MRI penumbral identification as a predictor of response to therapy, especially over a longer therapeutic time window, then it is likely that CT perfusion which is more widely available will also be useful for future patient selection. In the future, acute stroke imaging with both diffusion/perfusion MRI and perfusion CT will be of increasing importance for identifying patients who are potential candidates for a variety of acute therapies over and expanding therapeutic time window.

Acknowledgments The authors wish to thank Dr. Satish Dundamadappa, MD Asst. Prof of Radiology, UMASS Medical School, for providing the images.

Appendix

Neuroimaging Protocols for Acute Stroke: University of Massachusetts Medical Center

Hyperacute Period

Plain CT head and CTA brain and neck (unless known renal insufficiency)

- IV rtPA if there are no contraindications.

Large Artery occlusion on CTA (ICA, Main stem BA, MCA)

- Direct IA tPA if Angiogram can be done within 1 h
- If angiogram is delayed for >1 h – IV tPA+IA rescue

MRI (DWI) and MRA if unable to do a CTA in the following situations

- Suspected ischemic stroke with seizures at the onset

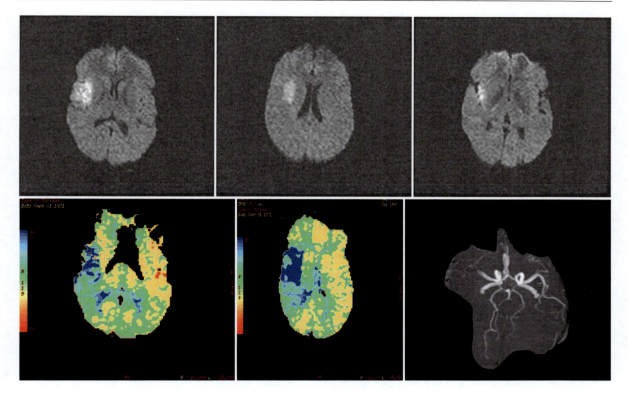

Fig. 18.15 Diffusion–perfusion mismatch. This method has become an important aspect of the assessment of acute stroke. By comparing the volume of abnormal diffusion on DWI (*top*) to the volume of abnormal perfusion on PWI (*bottom*), determination of the discrepancy between the larger volume of ischemia (PWI) and the smaller brain region showing physiological damage (DWI) is possible. This information helps in determining the extent of tissue that may be permanently damaged and the area that is likely recoverable with reperfusion

- Suspected dissection of the carotid or vertebral system
- Large vessel stroke syndrome clinically, demonstrating some improvement
- Uncertainty in clinical diagnosis of a lacunar stroke

Perfusion CT is more widely available and may be substituted for MRI and MRA protocols if the MRI is not immediately or when MRI is contraindicated.

Acute Stage (3–12 h Postsymptom Onset)

MRI with DWI-PWI and MRA (using short prespecified 20 min protocol).

Intraarterial thrombolysis for Large vessel occlusion and DWI-PWI mismatch

- Anterior circulation stroke presenting within 6 h.
- Posterior circulation stroke presenting within 12 h.

Suspected Dissection. MRI, MRA and MRI C-Spine with T1 fat suppressed images performed.

References

1. Lloyd-Jones D, Adams R, Carnethon M, et al. Heart disease and stroke statistics – 2009 update: a report from the American Heart Association Statistics Committee and Stroke Statistics Subcommittee. *Circulation*. 2009;119(3):480–486.
2. Gomez C. Time is brain. *J Stroke Cerebrovasc Dis*. 1993; 3:12.
3. Saver JL. Time is brain – quantified. *Stroke*. 2006;37(1): 263–266.
4. Bluhmki E, Chamorro A, Davalos A, et al. Stroke treatment with alteplase given 3.0–4.5 h after onset of acute ischaemic stroke (ECASS III): additional outcomes and subgroup analysis of a randomised controlled trial. *Lancet Neurol*. 2009;8(12):1095–1102.
5. Fisher M, Feuerstein G, Howells DW, et al. Update of the stroke therapy academic industry roundtable preclinical recommendations. *Stroke*. 2009;40(6):2244–2250.

6. Paciaroni M, Caso V, Agnelli G. The concept of ischemic penumbra in acute stroke and therapeutic opportunities. *Eur Neurol*. 2009;61(6):321–330.
7. Procter AW. Can we reverse ischemic penumbra? Some mechanisms in the pathophysiology of energy-compromised brain tissue. *Clin Neuropharmacol*. 1990;13(Suppl 3): S34–S39.
8. Astrup J, Siesjo BK, Symon L. Thresholds in cerebral ischemia – the ischemic penumbra. *Stroke*. 1981;12(6):723–725.
9. Astrup J, Sorensen PM, Sorensen HR. Oxygen and glucose consumption related to Na+-K+ transport in canine brain. *Stroke*. 1981;12(6):726–730.
10. Atlas SW, ed. *MRI Imaging of the Brain and Spine*, vol. 1. 3rd ed. Philadelphia: Lippincott Williams & Wilkins; 2008.
11. Gray F et al. *Escourolle and Poirier's Manual of Basic Neuropathology*. 4th ed. Philadelphia: Butterworth Heinemann; 2004.
12. Metting Z, Rodiger LA, De Keyser J, van der Naalt J. Structural and functional neuroimaging in mild-to-moderate head injury. *Lancet Neurol*. 2007;6(8):699–710.
13. Lopes L, Sousa R, Ruivo J, Reimao S, Sequeira P, Campos J. The contribution of perfusion CT in stroke. *Acta Med Port*. 2006;19(6):484–488.
14. Murphy BD, Chen X, Lee TY. Serial changes in CT cerebral blood volume and flow after 4 hours of middle cerebral occlusion in an animal model of embolic cerebral ischemia. *AJNR Am J Neuroradiol*. 2007;28(4):743–749.
15. Pepper EM, Parsons MW, Bateman GA, Levi CR. CT perfusion source images improve identification of early ischaemic change in hyperacute stroke. *J Clin Neurosci*. 2006;13(2): 199–205.
16. Meuli RA. Imaging viable brain tissue with CT scan during acute stroke. *Cerebrovasc Dis*. 2004;17(Suppl 3):28–34.
17. Hellier KD, Hampton JL, Guadagno JV, et al. Perfusion CT helps decision making for thrombolysis when there is no clear time of onset. *J Neurol Neurosurg Psychiatry*. 2006;77(3):417–419.
18. Detre JA, Alsop DC, Vives LR, Maccotta L, Teener JW, Raps EC. Noninvasive MRI evaluation of cerebral blood flow in cerebrovascular disease. *Neurology*. 1998;50(3):633–641.
19. Latchaw RE, Yonas H, Pentheny SL, Gur D. Adverse reactions to xenon-enhanced CT cerebral blood flow determination. *Radiology*. 1987;163(1):251–254.
20. Powers WJ, Zazulia AR. The use of positron emission tomography in cerebrovascular disease. *Neuroimaging Clin N Am*. 2003;13(4):741–758.
21. Yamauchi H, Okazawa H, Kishibe Y, Sugimoto K, Takahashi M. Oxygen extraction fraction and acetazolamide reactivity in symptomatic carotid artery disease. *J Neurol Neurosurg Psychiatry*. 2004;75(1):33–37.
22. Albers GW, Thijs VN, Wechsler L, et al. Magnetic resonance imaging profiles predict clinical response to early reperfusion: the diffusion and perfusion imaging evaluation for understanding stroke evolution (DEFUSE) study. *Ann Neurol*. 2006;60(5):508–517.
23. Davis SM, Donnan GA, Parsons MW, et al. Effects of alteplase beyond 3 h after stroke in the Echoplanar Imaging Thrombolytic Evaluation Trial (EPITHET): a placebo-controlled randomised trial. *Lancet Neurol*. 2008;7(4): 299–309.
24. Schellinger PD, Thomalla G, Fiehler J, et al. MRI-based and CT-based thrombolytic therapy in acute stroke within and beyond established time windows: an analysis of 1210 patients. *Stroke*. 2007;38(10):2640–2645.
25. Kane I, Carpenter T, Chappell F, et al. Comparison of 10 different magnetic resonance perfusion imaging processing methods in acute ischemic stroke: effect on lesion size, proportion of patients with diffusion/perfusion mismatch, clinical scores, and radiologic outcomes. *Stroke*. 2007;38(12): 3158–3164.

Chapter 19
Neuroimaging of Alzheimer's Disease, Mild Cognitive Impairment, and Other Dementias

Shannon L. Risacher and Andrew J. Saykin

Introduction

The goal of the present chapter is to provide an overview of the major findings from studies of neuroimaging in dementia, particularly from patients with Alzheimer's disease (AD). The major emphasis is on findings from a variety of imaging modalities and the use of these measures for early diagnosis and as biomarkers of disease progression. In this chapter, we first describe the basic neurobiological changes and clinical symptoms associated with AD and related cognitive decline. Next, we discuss results from studies in AD utilizing structural neuroimaging techniques, including computerized tomography (CT), traditional structural magnetic resonance imaging (MRI), and other MRI techniques [diffusion tensor imaging (DTI), perfusion MRI, magnetic resonance spectroscopy (MRS)]. We also explore findings from functional MRI studies, including task-related activation studies and resting and functional connectivity research. Then, we discuss results from the use of nuclear medicine techniques in AD, including single-photon emission computerized tomography (SPECT) and positron emission tomography

A.J. Saykin (✉)
IU Center for Neuroimaging, Department of Radiology and Imaging Sciences, Indiana University School of Medicine, 950 West Walnut Street, R2, E124, Indianapolis, IN 46202, USA
and
Indiana Alzheimer Disease Center, Indiana University School of Medicine, 950 West Walnut Street, R2, E124, Indianapolis, IN, USA
and
Medical Neuroscience Program, Stark Neurosciences Research Institute, Indiana University School of Medicine, 950 West Walnut Street, R2, E124, Indianapolis, IN, USA
e-mail: asaykin@iupui.edu

(PET) studies. Neuroimaging in other dementias is also briefly discussed, with particular emphasis on differential diagnosis of dementia type. Finally, we explore future directions for neuroimaging of early AD and dementia.

Background

AD is the most common form of age-related dementia. As of 2000, nearly 25 million individuals worldwide aged 60 or older suffered from AD and that number is expected to more than double by 2030.[1] The annual cost for AD-related treatment and care in the United States is over $100 billion.[2] In addition to the social and economic implications of AD, this devastating disorder robs millions of elderly individuals of their memories, ability to function independently, and ultimately their lives. Early detection of AD is an important goal because the efficacy of future treatments is likely to be maximal in the prodromal stages of the disease. Neuroimaging is a unique set of tools that have shown promise in early detection of AD-related brain changes, predicting the course and speed of disease progression, and monitoring effects of treatment.

The most common form of AD is sporadic or late-onset AD (LOAD), which primarily affects people over the age 65. Less than 5% of AD cases are caused by dominantly inherited mutations in three genes including the amyloid precursor protein (APP) gene, and presenilin 1 and 2 (PS1, PS2) genes.[3] Genetic factors are also likely to be important in LOAD. Apolipoprotein E (APOE) is the most commonly reported genetic variation associated with AD. Patients with an APOE epsilon 4 (ε4) allele are predisposed to developing AD, with a fivefold increased risk for patients with one ε4

R.A. Cohen and L.H. Sweet (eds.), *Brain Imaging in Behavioral Medicine and Clinical Neuroscience*,
DOI 10.1007/978-1-4419-6373-4_19, © Springer Science+Business Media, LLC 2011

allele and an even higher risk in patients with two ε4 alleles.[3-5] On the other hand, the APOE epsilon 2 (ε2) allele is potentially protective against the development of AD.[6] Numerous other candidate genes have also been identified for AD (see www.alzgene.org for an updated list of candidate genes). Future developments in the genetic basis of LOAD are likely to play an important role in early diagnosis. Studies in AD that combine neuroimaging and genomics are briefly explored at the end of this chapter.

Neurobiology & Neuropathology of AD

Both the inherited and sporadic forms of AD feature two neuropathological hallmarks: amyloid plaques and neurofibrillary tangles. Amyloid plaques are extracellular aggregations of the Aβ peptide and are found throughout the AD brain. Aβ is formed from dysfunctional processing of the APP, featuring cleavage by β-secretase and γ-secretase to form a neurotoxic peptide ranging from 36 to 42 amino acids in length. The most common forms of Aβ are composed of 40 and 42 amino acids (Aβ40 and Aβ42), with the Aβ42 form most likely to show formation of the amyloid plaques found in AD.[7-9] Neurofibrillary tangles result from the hyperphosphorylation of a microtubule-associated protein known as "tau". The underlying cause of this abnormal phosphorylation is unknown but is likely due to alterations in the balance between the kinases and phosphatases regulating tau. The formation of neurofibrillary tangles of hyperphosphorylated tau is strongly associated with the neurodegeneration and neuronal death in AD. The link between amyloid plaques and neurofibrillary tangles is complex and not completely understood, but many researchers believe that oxidative stress, inflammatory responses, altered ionic homeostasis following Aβ accumulation, and other changes, upset the balance of tau phosphorylation.[10,11] Ultimately, the accumulation of amyloid and the formation of neurofibrillary tangles results in neuronal loss throughout the brain.

The stages of neurodegeneration in AD are described in detail by Braak & Braak.[12] The first regions of the brain to show neuronal loss associated with AD are in the medial temporal lobe (MTL), including the entorhinal cortex (EC), hippocampus, amygdala, and parahippocampal cortex. Additionally, extensive degeneration of the cholinergic innervations to the neocortex from the basal nucleus of Mynert and the medial septal nucleus occurs early in the disease process.[13] By the time a patient has reached a diagnosis of full-blown AD, neurodegeneration is usually found throughout the neocortex and in subcortical regions, with significant atrophy of the temporal, parietal, and frontal cortices with relative sparing of the occipital cortex and primary sensory-motor regions.[12,14]

Clinical Symptoms of AD

The earliest clinical symptoms associated with AD are a direct result of the brain regions to first degenerate, namely, the MTL. Memory impairments, particularly in the episodic and semantic domains, as well as deficits in language and executive functioning are common symptoms early in the disease course.[15] Attempts at early diagnosis of AD have led to the development of a clinical syndrome termed "mild cognitive impairment" (MCI).[16-19] MCI is characterized by impairments in one or more cognitive domains (memory, executive, semantic, and/or visuospatial) beyond that which is expected as a part of normal aging, but with no dementia or significant disruption in daily functioning. MCI featuring memory impairments is termed "amnestic MCI" and is widely considered to be a prodromal form of AD. In fact, nearly 10–15% of amnestic MCI patients convert to AD each year, relative to only 1–2% of the general elderly population.[19] On the other hand, nonamnestic MCI patients may be more likely to progress to other forms of dementia. Recently, researchers and clinicians have been attempting to detect AD related changes even earlier than MCI (i.e., "pre-MCI") using subjective reports of cognitive complaints, APOE status, and family history of dementia to predict the development of AD.[20-24] This research is discussed in further detail at the end of this chapter.

Imaging and AD

Currently, few treatments are available for patients with early AD which have been found to slow the progression of disease and improve cognitive function in some individuals. However, efficacy of these treatments is limited. A number of new treatments are currently in the process of development for MCI and AD. Future treatments are likely to have optimal efficacy early in the disease course when cognitive function is only minimally impaired. Biological markers of disease severity are desperately needed to detect early AD and effectively monitor the outcome of new treatments. Neuroimaging is an exceptional tool for measuring *in vivo* brain atrophy associated with MCI and AD, as well as for predicting disease progression, even in patients with relatively minor cognitive impairments (i.e., pre-MCI patients).

An exciting opportunity to evaluate the utility of neuroimaging biomarkers in AD is a consortium study that is currently underway known as the Alzheimer's Disease Neuroimaging Initiative (ADNI, www.adni-info.org). As part of this study, 800 patients, including 200 patients with early AD, 400 patients with MCI, and 200 healthy elderly controls (HC) are being followed longitudinally for 2–3 years with repeat structural MRI scans and extensive clinical evaluations on a 6–12 month basis. Additionally, subsets of ADNI patients also receive longitudinal PET imaging and cerebral spinal fluid (CSF) biomarker collection (Aβ and tau levels). All data is made publically available to the research community, allowing for extensive and widespread investigation of the largest imaging dataset of AD, MCI, and HC to date. Numerous studies have already been published regarding the ADNI purpose and protocols,[25-27] analyses of the baseline[28-44] and longitudinal[39,40,45-47] MRI scans, and investigations of the PET[48-52] and CSF[29,43,47,53-55] biomarkers. Additionally, two journals have recently published special issues containing additional information about ADNI, as well as a number of research reports using the ADNI data (Alzheimer's & Dementia, Vol. 6, Issue 3, May 2010 and Neurobiology of Aging, Volume 31, Issue 8, August 2010).

Structural Imaging in AD and MCI

Computed Tomography

Because of limited resolution, CT is not widely used in the diagnosis of AD except to rule out alternative causes for dementia. A few studies have examined brain changes using CT in patients with AD by scanning thin slices covering the MTL, including the hippocampus. CT scans of patients with AD show enlarged ventricles,[56] particularly of the temporal horn of the lateral ventricle, and general cortical atrophy.[57-59]

Other studies with CT have shown significantly greater rate of whole-brain atrophy[60] and wider hippocampal fissure[61-63] in patients with AD relative to HCs.

Structural Magnetic Resonance Imaging

The most widely used neuroimaging technique to investigate structural changes and neurodegeneration in MCI and AD patients is MRI. Numerous studies have investigated differences between AD patients, MCI patients and HCs on measures of global and local brain volume, tissue morphology, and rate of atrophy using a variety of manually applied and automated techniques. The most widely used techniques are manually applied methods such as manual tracing of regions of interest (ROIs), in which an anatomically trained scientist traces a border around a specific brain structure on sequential MRI slices to extract a three-dimensional representation that can be used to extract volumetric and morphometric characteristics,[64,65] and medial temporal atrophy (MTA) scores, in which a trained neuroradiologist scores the amount of MTL atrophy.[66,67] More recently, automated techniques to extract volumes of interest (VOIs) and cortical thickness values for numerous neocortical regions,[68-70] as well as semiautomated whole-brain morphometry techniques, including voxel-based morphometry (VBM[71,72]) and other techniques,[32,36] which determine the density of grey matter (GM), white matter (WM), and CSF on a voxel-by-voxel basis, have been developed and utilized in studies of brain aging and AD.

MRI estimates of regional volumes, extracted using either manual or automated techniques, show significant brain atrophy in AD and MCI patients, following an anatomical distribution similar to the pattern reported in Braak and Braak[12] according to disease severity.[73] The most commonly reported and most significant differences between AD and MCI patients and HCs are in the MTL (Fig. 19.1). Numerous studies have reported that AD patients have significantly smaller whole brain,[74] hippocampal,[64,65,75-77] EC,[65,78-81] and amygdalar volumes,[82-84] and significantly enlarged ventricles,[85,86] particularly in the temporal horn of the lateral ventricle,[87] relative to HCs. MCI patients tend to have intermediate volumetric estimates between AD patients and HCs, supporting this as an intermediate stage between healthy aging

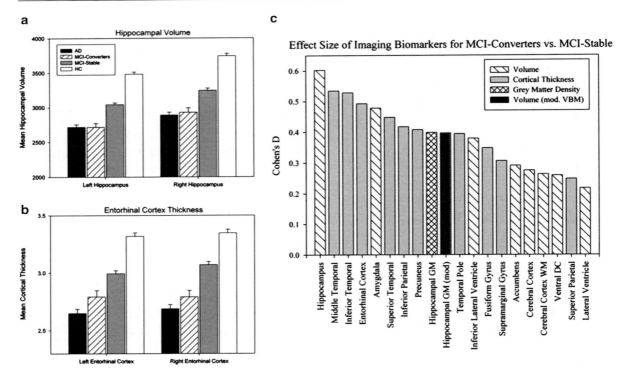

Fig. 19.1 Structural MRI – hippocampal volume and EC thickness differences between AD, MCI-converters, MCI-stable, HCs from the ADNI cohort. *Figure adapted with permission from ref.* [42]. Patients with AD and those who converted from MCI to probable AD within 12 months [MCI-Converters (MCI-C)] have significantly reduced baseline hippocampal volume (**a**) and EC thickness (**b**) relative to both HCs and patients who have a stable MCI diagnosis [MCI-Stables (MCI-S)]. Patients with MCI-S also show significant hippocampal and EC atrophy relative to HCs. All values are extracted using an automated parcellation technique[69,70] of scans from the ADNI database (www.loni.ucla.edu/ADNI). (**c**) A comparison of the effect sizes of selected structural MRI biomarkers demonstrates significantly greater utility of MTL and lateral temporal lobe measures in distinguishing between MCI-C and MCI-S patients at baseline.

and AD.[88-94] AD patients have also been shown to have extensive cortical atrophy throughout the brain, particularly in later stages of the disease. The frontal, parietal, and temporal lobes of AD patients show significantly reduced volume and thickness relative to HCs,[82,95-99] while MCI patients have intermediate atrophy in these regions. The occipital lobe and primary sensory-motor regions show minimal atrophy until late in the disease. A number of studies have also shown that measures of hippocampal and EC volume can correctly classify AD patients and HCs with an overall accuracy of between 85 and 95%[65,81,82,94,100-103] and MCI patients and HC with an overall accuracy of between 75 and 85%.[81,89,90,94,104-106]

Similar differences between AD, MCI, and HCs are also seen in studies evaluating global and regional tissue morphometry. AD patients show reduced GM density and volume in the MTL and throughout the frontal, parietal, and temporal neocortex.[107-115] MCI patients tend to have a more focal GM density reduction in the MTL, particularly in the EC and hippocampus, supporting the early degeneration of these regions in the disease process (Fig. 19.2).[108,110,116-118] This technique has also been shown to effectively monitor progression over the course of 3 years, showing the expected expansion of atrophy as the disease progresses from MCI to probable AD.[119] Changes in global and local tissue morphometry have also been shown to correctly classify AD patients and HC with an overall accuracy of approximately 85–90%[112,117] and MCI patients and HCs with an overall accuracy of 87%.[117]

Longitudinal structural MRI with multiple scanning sessions has also been collected to evaluate the rate of whole brain and regional atrophy in AD and MCI patients and healthy elderly. Numerous studies have

19 Neuroimaging of Alzheimer's Disease, Mild Cognitive Impairment, and Other Dementias

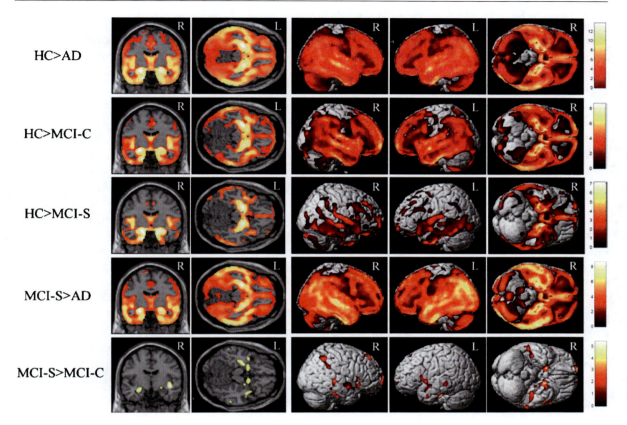

Fig. 19.2 Structural MRI – Global GM density differences between AD, MCI-converters, MCI-stable, HCs from the ADNI cohort. *Figure adapted with permission from ref.* [42]. AD and MCI-C patients show significant GM atrophy relative to MCI-S and HC. Relative to HC and MCI-S, AD patients show global reductions GM density throughout the neocortex with maximal differences in the MTL. MCI-C show significant atrophy throughout the cortex relative to HCs, but focal GM atrophy in the MTL relative to MCI-S. MCI-S patients also show significant GM atrophy relative to HCs, although the pattern is more focal than for either ADs or MCI-Cs. No significant differences were observed between AD and MCI-C participants. These comparisons were done using standard VBM methods[42,71,72,480] and all statistical maps are displayed at a threshold of $p<0.005$ [false discovery rate (FDR) correction for multiple comparisons] and a minimal cluster size of 27 voxels

shown accelerated rates in AD and MCI patients of whole-brain atrophy,[120-122] as well as regional atrophy in the MTL.[100,120,122-125] Patients with AD show an approximate annual hippocampal decline of −4.5%, while MCI patients and HCs show annual hippocampal declines of approximately −3 and −1%, respectively (for meta-analysis, see ref.[126]). The annual rates of ventricular enlargement and cortical atrophy in multiple regions have also been shown to be significantly greater in patients with AD and MCI relative to healthy elderly.[120,122,127-131]

MRI measures of volume, morphometry, and rates of brain atrophy have also shown promise in predicting the course of AD progression. In fact, numerous studies have demonstrated significantly reduced hippocampal and EC volume in patients destined to convert from MCI to probable AD ("MCI-Converters"), up to 2 years prior to clinical conversion, relative to MCI patients that remain at a stable MCI diagnosis ("MCI-Stable", Fig. 19.1).[79,91,93,127,132-136] Additionally, MCI-Converters show significantly reduced cortical thickness in regions of the MTL, lateral temporal cortex, and parietal cortex relative to MCI-Stables.[42,137-139] Techniques assessing global and local tissue morphometry have also shown significantly reduced GM density and volume in MCI-Converters relative to MCI-Stables (Fig. 19.2).[108,116,118,140,141] In a recent study by our group using data from ADNI, we have found a significantly reduced hippocampal and amygdalar volume, EC thickness, reduced lateral temporal and parietal lobe cortical thicknesses in patients who converted from MCI to AD within 12 months relative to those who remained stable using the largest sample to date of patients with imaging data (62 MCI-Converters, 277 MCI-Stables). Interestingly, the MCI-Converters showed equivalent brain atrophy (hippocampal volume, EC thickness, etc.) as seen in the AD patients, suggesting that neuroimaging markers of neurodegeneration could detect AD up to 12 months prior to clinical conversion (Figs. 19.1 and 19.2).[42] Rates of brain atrophy, including annualized whole brain, hippocampal, and EC volume decline, as well as rates of ventricular enlargement, are also accelerated in patients who are rapidly converting from MCI to AD.[122,125,142-145] In addition to detecting differences in MCI-Converters, baseline and rate of hippocampal atrophy have been used to predict MCI to probable AD conversion. Using Cox proportional hazard models, reduced baseline hippocampal volume and increased annual hippocampal atrophy rates accurately predicted MCI to probable AD conversion.[91,133,134,146,147] Baseline hippocampal volume also correctly classified MCI-Converters and MCI-Stables with an overall accuracy of between 75 and 90%.[80,81,92,132,137,138]

Other Structural MRI Techniques

Diffusion Weighted and Diffusion Tensor Imaging

Diffusion weighted and diffusion tensor imaging (DWI/DTI) techniques measure the integrity of WM tracts using two types of measures: (1) fractional anisotropy (FA), which reflects the diffusion direction of water in the fiber tracts and is thought to be a general measure of axonal integrity; (2) mean diffusivity (MD) or apparent diffusion coefficient (ADC), which measures the overall diffusivity. Reduced FA and increased MD/ADC are considered to be markers of neuronal fiber loss and WM atrophy. Numerous studies have employed DWI and DTI techniques to evaluate WM degeneration associated with AD and MCI. Patients with AD show reduced FA relative to HCs in many WM structures throughout the brain, including in the corpus callosum (CC), temporal, parietal, and frontal WM, cingulum bundles, posterior cingulate, internal capsule, thalamus, superior longitudinal fasiculus, uncinate fasiculus, hippocampal

WM, and parahippocampal subgyral WM.[148-162] MCI patients also show intermediate reductions in FA relative to ADs and HCs, with significantly smaller FA values than HCs in the CC, temporal WM, hippocampus, cingulum bundles, superior longitudinal fasiculus, thalamus, parahippocampal subgyral WM, posterior uncinate fasiculus, and posterior cingulate.[152,153,155,158,162-165] Increased ADC and MD values are also seen in patients with AD and MCI relative to HCs, with higher MD/ADC values in the CC, hippocampus, EC, centrum semiovale, parietal and temporal WM, and uncinate fasiculus in both AD and MCI patients,[149-152,154,156,158,164-170] and in the frontal WM and posterior cingulate in AD patients only.[156] FA and MD have also been shown to correctly distinguish AD patients and HCs with 80–90% accuracy,[162,164,166,170] as well as to predict future conversion from MCI to probable AD.[171] Overall, DWI/DTI studies of AD and MCI patients have confirmed widespread changes in WM microarchitecture in both cortical and subcortical regions, particularly as the disease progresses. Thus, diffusion may prove to be a useful biomarker to detect and predict progression of AD.

Magnetic Resonance Spectroscopy

Magnetic resonance spectroscopy (MRS) is a noninvasive technique allowing the measurement of biological metabolites in target tissue and has been used in studies of brain aging and AD. Two major metabolites that consistently show alterations in patients with AD and MCI include: (1) N-acetylaspartate (NAA), which is found primarily in neurons and considered to be a measure of neuronal health[172,173] and (2) myoinositol (mIns), which is considered to be a marker of glial cells and gliosis.[174,175] These levels are often reported as ratios relative to the level of creatine (Cr; i.e., NAA/Cr, mIns/Cr) because the level of Cr is typically constant in tissue.[176] AD patients show decreased NAA levels (or decreased NAA/Cr) relative to HCs throughout the brain, with the most significant changes in the temporal lobe and hippocampus (~15% reduction),[177-182] and relatively uniform reductions in the rest of the brain (~10% reductions).[180,183-187] MCI patients also show reductions in NAA, with relatively intermediate levels reported relative to AD and HCs.[179,184,185,187] The reductions in NAA are thought to reflect ongoing atrophy, decreased metabolism, and neuronal loss.

mIns levels are also found to be altered in AD and MCI patients, with AD and MCI patients showing significantly greater mIns (mIns/Cr) throughout the brain relative to HCs.[179-181,183-190] Increased mIns levels are thought to represent increased gliosis in the brains of AD and MCI patients. MRS measures of NAA and mIns levels may also be useful biomarkers in AD and MCI patients, showing AD vs. HC classification of 80–90%.[182,188,191,192] Additionally, NAA/Cr has been shown to correlate with cognitive performance[177,189,193,194] and to predict future MCI to AD conversion.[195,196]

Perfusion MRI

Changes in cerebral blood flow (CBF) and regional cerebral blood volume (rCBV) have also been reported in patients with MCI and AD relative to HCs. Two MRI methods have been employed to measure cerebral perfusion, including dynamic susceptibility contrast enhanced MRI (DSC-MRI), which involves the injection of contrast agents to measure CBF and rCBV, and a relatively new technique called arterial spin labeling (ASL), which measures CBF without any external contrast agents by using magnetic pulses to "label" blood entering the brain. Nuclear medicine techniques are also commonly used to measure brain perfusion and are discussed in a later section. Studies of brain perfusion with MRI have consistently demonstrated decreased perfusion or "hypoperfusion" in patients with AD and MCI. DSC-MRI studies show significant hypoperfusion in AD and MCI patients relative to HCs in temporoparietal regions,[197-202] as well as frontal, parietal, and temporal cortices.[202] ASL studies have reported similar temporoparietal hypoperfusion in patients with AD relative to HCs,[203] as well as reduced CBF in the parietal lobe, frontal lobe, temporal lobe, posterior cingulate, MTL, and precuneus.[203-207] MCI patients also show decreased perfusion in the parietal lobe using ASL techniques.[205] Hypoperfusion in the temporoparietal cortex, parietooccipital cortex, and posterior cingulate has also been shown to correlate to cognitive performance and dementia severity.[203,204]

Functional MRI

Although structural MRI measures have proven extremely useful in studies of brain aging and AD,

these tools do not provide any direct measure of brain function, beside the assumption that brain atrophy will lead to decreased function. Additional techniques have been developed for use in MRI which can measure brain function during activated and resting states, specifically functional MRI (fMRI) and functional and resting connectivity techniques. The primary outcome measured in fMRI studies is a blood-oxygenation level-dependent (BOLD) signal in which regional brain activity is measured via changes in local blood flow and oxygenation.[208,209] Given that activity-related brain metabolism is tightly coupled to regional blood oxygenation and flow (i.e., blood flow increases to keep the regional blood oxygen level high during brain activation and associated increases metabolic demand), the BOLD signal is a useful measure for brain activation.[210-212] However, changes in the regional coupling of neuronal metabolism and blood flow due to brain atrophy, as well as the reported hypoperfusion in patients with AD and MCI (see previous section), may cause alterations in the BOLD signal. In fact, recent studies have demonstrated a delayed BOLD response in AD and MCI patients,[213] as well as decreased BOLD amplitude associated with normal aging.[214-216] Therefore, studies in older patient populations with brain atrophy (i.e., MCI and AD) should be evaluated and interpreted with these considerations in mind.

Task-Related fMRI

The first and most significant cognitive domain disrupted in AD is episodic memory. Therefore, the majority of task-related fMRI studies of brain aging and AD have investigated brain activity during episodic memory and learning tasks. Memory function can broadly be divided into two domains, encoding, in which new information is converted for short or long-term storage, and retrieval, in which stored memories are accessed.[217] Both processes can be evaluated with fMRI using functional tasks designed to probe each of these domains.

Results from fMRI studies in AD and MCI patients have shown conflicting results. Most studies with AD patients have shown decreased or even absent activation relative to HCs in the hippocampus, MTL, posterior cingulate, parietal lobe, and frontal lobe during episodic memory encoding (Fig. 19.3a)[218-230] and recall tasks.[218-222,231,232] However, other studies have suggested increased activation during episodic memory encoding and recall in the posterior cingulate, precuneus, parietal lobe, and frontal lobe.[219,222,226,230,231] Similar conflicting results have been shown in patients with MCI. Some studies have shown decreased activation during episodic memory encoding[218,227,233-236] and recall tasks,[218,232,234,236,237] while others show increased activation relative to HCs,[218,223,225,236,238,239] in the hippocampus (Fig. 19.3a), parahippocampal gyrus, other MTL regions, posterior cingulate, precuneus, parietal lobe, and frontal lobe. Authors of these studies suggest that these conflicting results may be due to differences in patient populations, including differences in the

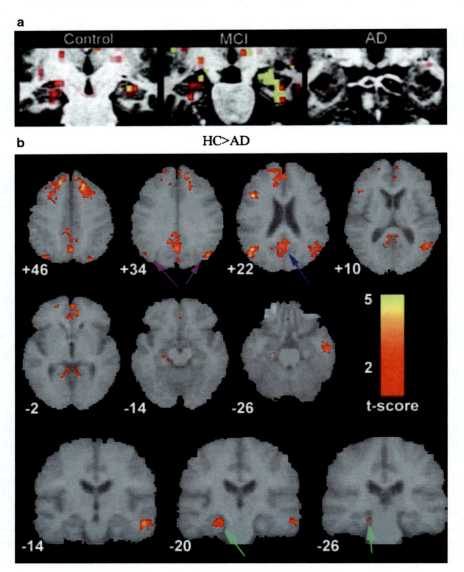

Fig. 19.3 Functional MRI – differences in hippocampal activation during episodic memory tasks in AD, MCI, and HC; DMN connectivity alterations in AD relative to HCs. (**a**) *Adapted with permission from ref.*[223]. Differences in hippocampal activation during a memory encoding task were observed between representative AD, MCI, and HC participants. The AD patient shows significantly decreased hippocampal activation, while the MCI patient shows significantly increased activation in the hippocampus. These differences may be related to compensatory changes associated with MCI. Results are a contrast of new vs. repeated responses and significantly activated voxels (*yellow & red*) within the hippocampus and EC (ROI mask) are overlaid on each participant's T1-weighted structural MRI scan. (**b**) *Adapted with permission from ref.*[289]. Resting-state connectivity in the DMN is significantly reduced in AD patients relative to HCs in the inferior parietal lobe (*magenta arrows*), the posterior cingulate (*blue arrow*), and left hippocampus (*green arrow*)

severity of symptoms. Patients who are minimally impaired tend to show increased activation, which is believed to be a compensatory mechanism to assist with successful completion of the task. However, more impaired MCI and AD patients likely have advanced atrophy that can no longer support increased or compensatory neuronal activity and thus these patients may show decreased activation during tasks. A recent study provides evidence supporting this theory, demonstrating that more impaired MCI and AD patients showed decreased hippocampal activation, while less impaired MCI patients showed increased hippocampal activation during an episodic memory encoding task.[218] Other types of cognitive tasks, including semantic, working memory, and phonological tasks, also show significantly different patterns of activation in MCI and AD patients relative to HCs.[222,240-242]

Functional activation patterns may have potential as biomarkers for the early detection of cognitive changes associated with AD, as well as for the prediction of disease course, yet this research is still at an early stage. Some encouraging resulting suggest that in addition to detecting differences between patients and HCs in brain activation, fMRI responses during memory tasks may distinguish patients who convert from MCI to AD from those who have a stable MCI diagnosis. In fact, increased activation in the hippocampus during encoding memory task has been correlated with a greater degree of decline and a faster rate of progression in MCI patients in two reports.[238,243]

Altered hippocampal activation during encoding and recall tasks has also been observed in young, middle-aged, and elderly cognitively normal controls with increased risk for the development of AD because of genetic status (i.e., APOE ε4 positive) and/or a positive family history for dementia.[244-254] Performance on visuospatial, working memory, fluency, and naming tasks were also shown to be significantly altered in APOE ε4 positive and family history positive HCs.[255-260] Increased hippocampal activation during memory tasks has also been shown to predict the extent and rate of future cognitive decline in HC patients with a predisposition to develop AD (APOE ε4 or family history positive), with increased activation associated with more significant and rapid declines.[246,250,258] Therefore, task-related fMRI activations may be useful in detecting AD related changes in memory and other cognitive functions prior to clinical impairments.

Functional and Resting-State Connectivity

Traditional fMRI studies have focused on the independent activation relative to baseline in one or more ROIs or in a whole-brain approach. However, these estimates do not assess the relationship between multiple brain regions that are activated (or deactivated) during a task. Given that most cognitive tasks are likely processed in functionally connected brain networks, quantification of these networks can provide a unique measure of brain activity. Techniques for quantifying brain connectivity from fMRI data have recently been developed and applied in studies of brain aging during functional activation (i.e., during performance of tasks), as well as during "resting" state.[261-266] Briefly, these techniques select a particular ROI based either on a priori assumptions of importance in the cognitive process under study or based on experimentally determined regional activation patterns and correlate the temporal pattern of activation in this region with others throughout the brain. This process results in the extraction of networks of functionally connected regions showing positively or negatively associated activation patterns, suggesting synchronized and/or connected activation during tasks or at rest.

Functional connectivity studies evaluating brain regions showing correlated responses during task-induced brain activation have shown decreased connectivity in patients with AD and MCI. Specifically, studies evaluating episodic encoding and recall tasks have found decreased whole brain connectivity, as well as decreased connectivity of the hippocampus, in patients with MCI and AD.[218,267-274] Additionally, a number of functional connectivity studies in patients and HCs have shown significant functional connectivity during memory tasks between activation in the hippocampus and MTL, activation in the prefrontal cortex and superior parietal lobe, and deactivation in the posterior cingulate and precuneus. These results suggest the presence of two functional networks, the memory network activated during tasks (MTL-frontal-parietal) and a resting-state network (default mode network, see next section) deactivated during tasks (precuneus, cingulate, other regions).[275] Similar to the activation fMRI studies, MCI patients with minimal impairment show increased connectivity between the memory network and the resting-state network, suggesting compensatory changes.[218,268-272,276] However, more severely impaired AD and MCI patients show decreased or absent connectivity between these regions.[218] This decreased functional connectivity is consistent with DTI studies showing decreased structural connectivity (i.e., impaired integrity of WM tracts) within and between the memory and resting-state networks.[274] These observed changes in functional connectivity in AD and MCI patients have also been shown to be significantly correlated with disease severity and impaired cognition.[268,272]

In addition to studies of functional connectivity, connectivity has also been evaluated during baseline brain activity (i.e., nontask related activity). The connectivity of brain regions activated during rest is referred to as "resting-state connectivity".[265,277-282] Studies of resting state connectivity have identified multiple distinct networks including a motor network, visual processing network, auditory processing network, executive functional network, memory network, an attentional/readiness network, and the previously discussed resting-state network or "default mode network" (DMN), which is active when the brain is at rest and deactivated during task related activities.[263,265,278,281,283-286] The DMN is of particular interest in studies of brain aging because the connected regions, including the MTL, posterior cingulate, precuneus, retrosplenial gyrus, and medial frontal lobe, have been shown to have significant amyloid deposits in MCI and AD patients, as well as significant hypometabolism (see PET sections). Studies have shown significant alterations in DMN function and decreased DMN connectivity in patients with AD and MCI (Fig. 19.3b). Specifically, AD and MCI patients have shown decreased activity in the posterior cingulate and hippocampus at rest, as well as impaired deactivation of the DMN (anterior and medial frontal, posterior cingulate, precuneus) during tasks.[218,270,272,273,276,285,287] Additionally, AD and MCI patients show altered connectivity of the DMN to other regions, including impaired connectivity between the hippocampus (episodic memory network) and DMN, at rest.[273,278,288-294] The resting-state connectivity or "coherence" of the DMN regions has been shown to directly correlate with cognitive performance.[290] The activity of the DMN and the extent of DMN deactivation upon task initiation have also been shown to distinguish AD and MCI patients from HCs, as well as to distinguish between AD and MCI patients.[273,275,289,291]

Nuclear Medicine Techniques

Positron emission tomography (PET) and single-photon emission computerized tomography (SPECT) allow for measurement of physiological and/or neurochemical processes in the brain by injecting a tracer molecule labeled with a radioactive isotope and monitoring global and regional uptake, distribution, and retention. SPECT is primarily used to monitor CBF and perfusion. PET has the advantage of higher resolution and is used to measure a variety of targets, including cerebral metabolism, neurotransmission, and the presence, distribution, and quantity of target proteins for which an effective and safe PET tracer can be created. Both techniques have been widely employed in studies of brain aging and AD.

SPECT

SPECT studies of brain aging and AD have shown similar results as those using MRI-based perfusion techniques (ASL, DSC-MRI), which have been discussed in a previous section. Specifically, AD and MCI patients show significant hypoperfusion in temporoparietal regions, the lateral and medial temporal lobes, hippocampus, posterior cingulate, and frontal and parietal lobes.[202,295-301] Temporoparietal hypoperfusion has also been shown to correlate with disease severity and cognitive performance.[295,296] Additionally, SPECT measures of MTL and temporoparietal hypoperfusion have some predictive value for MCI to probable AD conversion.[297,302]

Positron Emission Tomography

PET studies of AD and MCI have primarily focused on four target measures: (1) cerebral metabolism at rest and during functional tasks, (2) amyloid pathology, (3) neurotransmission and (4) neuroinflammation and activated microglia. Cerebral metabolism is primarily assessed using an altered form of glucose tagged with a fluorine-18 isotope [^{18}F-deoxyglucose (FDG),[303,304]]. Amyloid pathology, specifically the presence of insoluble amyloid plaques, is most commonly measured using a thioflavin based compound called "Pittsburg

Compound B" or PiB, which is labeled with a carbon-11 isotope (^{11}C-PiB).[305] Additional tracers that have been utilized to measure *in vivo* brain amyloid include ^{18}F-FDDNP, ^{11}C-BL-227, ^{18}F-AV45, and others.[306-309] PET studies of neurotransmitters affect by AD and MCI have focused primarily on acetylcholine (ACh), GABA, dopamine (DA), and serotonin (5-HT), by measuring enzymatic markers [i.e., acetylcholinesterase (AChE)] and neurotransmitter receptors.[310] Finally, studies have also examined the presence and extent of neuroinflammation in AD and MCI patients with tracers that bind to the peripheral benzodiazepine receptor (PBR) or translocator protein (TSPO) (18 kD), a protein expressed on the mitochondria of activated microglia. The main tracers used to assess neuroinflammation in AD and MCI to date are ^{11}C-PK11195 and ^{11}C-DAA1106.[311,312]

Metabolic Measures (FDG-PET)

FDG-PET studies of patients with AD and MCI have shown significant differences in resting cerebral metabolism (CMRglu) between patients and healthy elderly. Specifically, patients with AD and MCI show significantly reduced resting CMRglu relative to HCs in the temporoparietal cortex, posterior cingulate, parietal lobe, temporal lobe, and in the MTL, including the hippocampus (Fig. 19.4).[51,105,278,313-330] In addition, more impaired AD patients also show hypometabolism in the frontal lobe and prefrontal cortex relative to less impaired patients and HCs.[313,314,318,323,325,331] Temporoparietal, posterior cingulate, temporal lobe, parietal lobe, prefrontal cortex, and MTL hypometabolism are associated with disease severity,[319] cognitive performance,[51,314,332,333] and other CSF and MRI biomarkers.[334,335] Hypometabolism in the temporoparietal and parietal cortices has also been shown to distinguish between AD and HCs with 80–90% overall accuracy.[105,326,331,336-341] Although changes in cerebral metabolism could represent a variety of neurochemical alterations, the reductions in CMRglu in AD and MCI patients are thought to be the result of impaired synaptic activity and reduced synaptic density, particularly of glutamatergic synapses.[323,342-344] Longitudinal studies of CMRglu in AD and MCI patients also show a significant rate of annual decline in metabolism in the temporal, parietal, and frontal lobes, as well as the posterior cingulate and precuneus.[345-349]

Alterations in resting CMRglu in an "AD-like" pattern have also been shown in people with an increased risk for developing dementia due to genetic factors (i.e., APOE ε4 positive) and/or a family history of dementia.[348,350-357] Furthermore, temporoparietal and posterior cingulate hypometabolism has been shown to predict cognitive decline, both progression from MCI to probable AD and from healthy cognition to MCI or AD. Cross-sectional measures of reduced CMRglu in the temporoparietal cortex, temporal lobe, parietal lobe, frontal lobe, posterior cingulate, and MTL have shown predictive accuracy for future conversion of HCs to MCI and/or AD of between 75 and 95%, particularly when combined with APOE ε4 genetic status.[324,331,332,350,358-367] Therefore, numerous studies have shown that FDG-PET is a useful biomarker in studies of MCI and AD. Clinical trials of potential treatments, as well as other investigations of drug effects, have used FDG-PET as a secondary measure in studies of AD and MCI.[368-373]

In addition to resting state CMRglu changes, patients with AD and MCI have shown alterations in glucose metabolism during functional tasks. AD and MCI patients show significantly reduced glucose metabolism during memory and other cognitive tasks relative to HCs, particularly in the temporoparietal cortex and MTL.[374-377] In additions to general reductions in functional glucose metabolism, specific differences in regional metabolic patterns have been reported in AD and MCI. For example, one study suggested that AD patients may recruit alternative brain regions as a compensatory change to successfully complete cognitive tasks.[378] Similar to the results from the fMRI studies,[242] these differences are likely related to disease severity.

Amyloid Imaging

One of the most exciting developments in the field of neuroimaging of dementia was the development of specific tracers which bind to amyloid, allowing for *in vivo* assessment of plaque burden and potentially identification of patients at risk for the development of AD before cognitive changes occur. Although multiple tracers have been developed which image amyloid,[306-309] the most widely used and studied is ^{11}C-PiB.[305] First reported in 2004, there are currently hundreds of PiB studies in patients with AD and MCI, familial dementias, other types of dementias, and in animal models of dementia. PiB has been shown to bind to both neuritic and diffuse plaques,[379,380] as well as to cerebral amyloid[381] within the vasculature. The primary signal measured in patient studies with PiB is due to specific binding to amyloid plaques, with a high correlation between the anatomical distribution of PiB binding and postmortem amyloid deposits.[382-384]

In general, PiB studies in patients with MCI and AD have shown significantly higher uptake and binding of PiB than seen in healthy elderly in brain regions known to be affected by amyloid deposition, including the frontal, temporal, and parietal lobes, posterior cingulate, and precuneus, as well as the MTL, including the hippocampus (Fig. 19.4).[52,113,305,385-395] Global measures of "PiB positivity" are often reported as a ratio of global neocortical binding of PiB relative to binding in the cerebellum (assumed to be nonspecific binding due to minimal amyloid plaque presence in the cerebellum). AD and MCI patients have a higher prevalence of PiB positivity than HCs. Some, but not all, studies have demonstrated a significant correlation between PiB binding and dementia severity, as well as cognitive performance.[52,113,391,396-400] Additionally, PiB binding in AD and MCI patients is correlated with other neuroimaging markers, including FDG-PET measures of cerebral metabolism and structural MRI measures of atrophy (i.e., hippocampal volume).[52,113,387,397,401,402] There is also a high correlation ($r > 0.9$) between PiB binding and Aβ levels measured from the CSF, suggesting these markers are near equivalent measures of brain amyloid levels.[403-405] A few longitudinal assessments of PiB in AD and MCI patients have been conducted and have typically shown minimal increases in PiB over 1–2 years in PiB positive patients.[37,397,406] Thus, researchers have tentatively concluded that amyloid deposition occurs earlier in the disease and by the time significant cognitive impairment occurs and a diagnosis of AD or MCI has

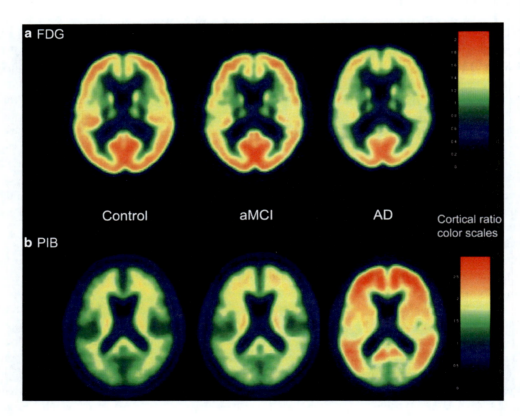

Fig. 19.4 Representative FDG-PET and PIB-PET scans from AD, MCI, and HC participants. (**a**) *Adapted with permission from ref.* [388]. AD participants show significant hypometabolism in the temporal, parietal, and frontal lobe with relative sparing of the occipital lobe, relative to amnestic MCI (aMCI) patients and HCs. aMCI patients also have intermediate metabolism showing hypometabolism in the temporal and parietal lobe relative to HCs. (**b**) AD patients show widespread PiB retention, suggesting significantly greater global amyloid burden than either aMCI patients or HCs. aMCI show intermediate PiB levels, with significantly greater PiB retention in the frontal and parietal lobes than HCs

been made, brain amyloid burden is relatively stable and further deposition is minimal.

Despite the generally intermediate levels of PiB binding in MCI relative to AD and HCs, the presence of significant PiB binding in patients with MCI is variable, with some participants showing an "AD-like" quantity and distribution of PiB and others showing minimal PiB binding.[113,391,393,394,398,405,407,408] Studies have shown that MCI patients who are PiB positive have a higher likelihood of progressing to dementia than PiB negative MCI patients, reflecting PiB's prognostic sensitivity.[398,405,408,409] Interestingly, approximately 25–30% of elderly individuals with normal cognition are also PiB positive.[389,391,393,400,410,411] Although comprehensive longitudinal follow-up studies of HCs with significant PiB binding have not been completed, initial studies suggest that HCs with significant amyloid deposition are more likely to convert to MCI or AD.[389,400] This is currently an active and important area of investigation, and future studies will likely further elucidate these issues.

Neurotransmitter PET

In addition to evaluating cerebral metabolism and the presence of amyloid, researchers have investigated specific alterations in neurotransmitter systems using PET. A number of studies have found significant reductions in ACh neurotransmission.[13,412] Using PET techniques with tracers specific for AChE as a surrogate measure for ACh synaptic density, significant reductions in binding were found in AD patients in the MTL, including the hippocampus and amygdala, as well as in the frontal, parietal, and temporal lobes and cingulate cortex.[413-421] Similar but less extensive changes were also shown in MCI patients.[420,422] These changes in ACh synaptic density correlate with changes in cognitive performance and may predict conversion from MCI to probable AD.[421-423] These techniques have also shown promise in monitoring treatment response to AChE inhibitors, which is a common pharmacological treatment for patients with AD.[423,424] Decreased ACh synaptic density was also shown in the hippocampus and temporal cortex using SPECT and PET tracers specific for nicotinic ACh receptors.[419,425,426]

Neuroimaging of neurotransmitter systems other than ACh has been relatively limited. However, a few studies in AD patients have shown decreases in GABA, serotonin (5-HT), and dopamine (DA) synaptic densities. Specifically, SPECT studies of GABA receptor tracers in moderate to severe AD patients has shown decreased binding in the temporal, parietal, and frontal cortex, with minimal changes in mild AD or MCI patients.[310,427,428] SPECT and PET studies using tracers specific for 5-HT_1 and 5-HT_2 receptors have shown significant decreases in receptor density in the hippocampus and throughout the neocortex, respectively, in patients with AD and MCI.[429-433] Finally, dopamine D_1 and D_2 receptors were shown to be significantly decreased in patients with AD in the caudate and putamen, as well as in the hippocampus.[434-437] In fact, one study demonstrated a significant correlation between reductions in D_2 receptor density and impaired memory performance.[434] Overall, PET techniques measuring changes in neurotransmitter systems have shown significant reductions, particularly in more advanced stages, which are likely due to widespread neuronal atrophy and synaptic loss.

Neuroinflammation PET

In addition to the accumulation of amyloid and hyperphosphorylated tau, AD patients show a large amount of activated microglia, particularly surrounding amyloid plaques.[438] This neuroinflammatory response associated with AD and MCI may be a key factor in disease progression. Recently developed tracers, including $^{11}\text{C-PK11195}$ and $^{11}\text{C-DAA1106}$, show specific binding to activated microglia in vitro, as well as in the living brain.[311,312,439] Studies have shown significantly elevated global and regional binding of both tracers in patients with AD relative to HCs, particularly in the MTL, including the amygdala and EC, as well as in the frontal lobe, parietal lobe, lateral temporal lobe, occipital lobe, anterior cingulate, and cerebellum.[440-445] MCI patients also show elevated binding in the frontal lobe and cingulate.[442] However, a few studies have not shown increased binding of these tracers in AD and MCI patients relative to HCs.[394,446] These differences likely reflect conflicting quantification methodologies, and future studies will likely elucidate the role of neuroinflammation in AD and MCI, as well as utility of this technique as a biomarker.

Imaging of Non-AD Dementias

Although almost 60% of dementias are AD related, other dementias are clinically and biologically important disorders. Neuroimaging is a useful tool in non-AD dementias, both for early diagnosis and for differential diagnosis of dementia type *in vivo*. The most common non-AD dementias include Vascular Dementia (VaD), Dementia with Lewy Bodies (DLB), and Frontotemporal Dementia (FTD). Including AD, these four disorders account for nearly 90% of age-related, sporadic dementias.[447]

Vascular dementia is characterized by significant cerebrovascular pathology that leads to dementia.[448] The definition of vascular dementia is confounded by the high prevalence of vascular pathology in AD, leading to the clinical definition of "mixed dementia." In fact, up to 70% of AD cases are thought to include significant vascular pathology.[449,450] Neuroimaging studies of VaD have primarily investigated WM lesions (WML) by characterizing and quantifying the extent of vascular pathology using T2-weighted MRI scans. Two major forms of WMLs are typically observed on T2-weighted structural MRI scans in patients with VaD including "deep white matter lesions" (DWML), which are often observed as bright spots in the corona radiata and centrum semiovale, and paraventricular hyperintensity (PVH), which are bright spots around the edges of ventricles.[451] Studies of VaD have shown that the presence of DWML on MRI is highly correlated cognitive performance and future cognitive decline.[452,453] Both DWML and PVH are commonly seen in AD patients also, but are significantly more extensive in patients with VaD.

DLB is characterized by cognitive impairment, visual hallucinations, and spontaneous Parkinsonism.[454] Although both DLB and AD show significant brain atrophy on structural MRI scans, DLB patients tend to show primarily subcortical atrophy even in later stages, with a relative sparing of the MTL.[455,456] Additionally, unlike the widespread neocortical pattern seen in AD, SPECT perfusion imaging and FDG-PET imaging of DLB patients show hypoperfusion and hypometabolism in primarily the occipital cortex, primary visual cortices, and posterior parietal lobe.[457,458] Additionally, DLB patients show significant dopaminergic cell loss, so PET imaging with DA specific tracers shows significantly more reduction in DA neurotransmission than is observed in AD.[459-461]

FTD is a collection of disorders, including language related disorders [i.e., semantic dementia (SD), primary progressive aphasia (PPA)], motor disorders [i.e., corticobasal degeneration (CBD), progressive supranuclear palsy (PSP)], and behavioral disorders. These disorders are generally characterized by changes in personality, behavior, and/or difficulties in language or executive function, with relative sparing of memory function.[462] Although there are significant overlaps in neuroimaging findings from AD and FTD patients, some distinguishing features can be seen using both MRI and PET techniques. Motor and behavioral FTDs tend to show atrophy primarily in the frontal lobe. Language related FTD disorders show significant frontal and temporal atrophy with anatomically limited reductions in the anterior temporal lobe relative to AD patients, who typically show widespread temporal atrophy.[101,463-468] In fact, a study of SD and AD patients demonstrated more significant atrophy in the SD patients relative to the AD patients in the lateral temporal lobe and temporal pole.[469] Additionally, SPECT and other perfusion techniques and FDG-PET show significant hypoperfusion and hypometabolism in primarily the frontal lobes in all forms of FTD, relative to the more posterior pattern seen in AD.[206,470] A recent study has demonstrated that frontal hypoperfusion distinguished FTD from AD with about 75% accuracy.[471]

Future Directions

Imaging and Genomics

Genetic factors play a significant role in the development of AD and MCI. Previous studies have suggested a high heritability for AD.[472] Although APOE is currently the major gene associated with late-onset AD,[3-6] future developments in genotyping technology and refinement of disease phenotypes will likely lead to the identification of important loci. The combination of imaging and genetics is a new transdisciplinary field designed to identify new genetic factors in disease by using specific neuroimaging biomarkers as phenotypes. Studies have suggested that using continuous and biologically specific phenotypes may lead to increased power in genetic associations.[473] To date, very few studies have been published in this area, but one study using the ADNI MRI and genetic data showed significant association of a number of candidate genes with hippocampal volume in patients with AD.[474] Future studies in this area will likely help identify important genetic factors underlying MCI and AD, allowing for earlier identification of people at risk for developing AD.

Early Diagnosis and Pre-MCI

A major goal has been to identify patients at high risk for developing AD even earlier than an MCI diagnosis and/or significant cognitive decline. The concept of "pre-MCI" has begun to appear, either defining a group of patients with subjective (i.e., patient given) and/or informant provided cognitive complaints but normal cognitive performance on clinical tests or individuals at high risk for development of AD due to genetic predispositions (APOE ε4 positive) and/or a family history of AD. Studies have shown that pre-MCI patients show measurable changes in neuroimaging biomarker. A study by our group in 2006 demonstrated that patients with subjective cognitive complaints but normal cognitive performance on standard clinical measures had significantly reduced hippocampal GM density relative to HCs with no cognitive complaints (Fig. 19.5).[24]

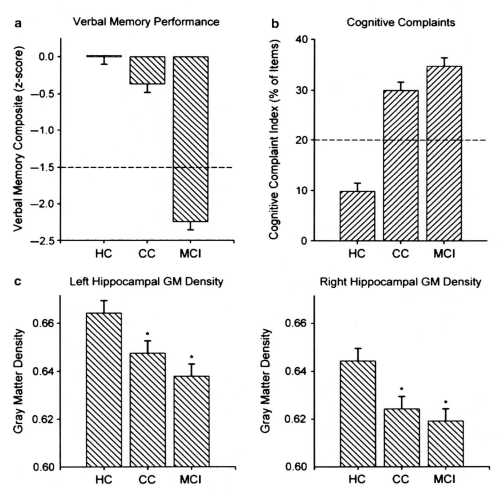

Fig. 19.5 Significant reductions in hippocampal GM in elderly with significant cognitive complaints but normal memory performance. *Adapted with permission from ref.* [24]. Elderly patients showing (**a**) normal memory performance but (**b**) significant cognitive complaints (CC) have significantly reduced (**c**) hippocampal GM density. CC participants show significantly smaller bilateral hippocampal GM density than HC without cognitive complaints, and nearly equivalent atrophy to MCI patients. Thus, elders with normal memory but significant subjective and informant-verified cognitive complaints may represent an earlier stage of AD (*Note: dotted lines represent thresholds for impairment*)

These results have been confirmed by other groups in independent samples.[23] Patients with cognitive complaints but no clinically relevant memory deficits also show significant longitudinal atrophy in the MTL, including significant hippocampal and amygdalar volume loss,[23] as well as an increased decline in global functioning.[475] Similarly, patients with "pre-MCI" defined by the presence of an APOE ε4 allele but normal cognitive testing have accelerated cognitive decline over 2 years,[476] as well as significant hypometabolism in the parietal lobe, posterior cingulate, and prefrontal cortex, as assessed using FDG-PET.[361] As previously discussed, approximately 25–30% of cognitively normal elderly have also been shown to be PiB positive, reflecting significant amyloid burden.[389,391,400] These patients may also constitute a form of "presymptomatic" MCI or AD. Future studies to fully characterize patients at risk for AD before significant cognitive impairments, including longitudinal follow-up of HCs with significant amyloid and patients with cognitive complaints, will be extremely important in early diagnosis of AD related changes.

Clinical Trials Using Imaging

One of the major uses for imaging biomarkers is and will likely continue to be in clinical trials of new therapeutics for the treatment of MCI and AD. MRI and PET measures have already been used in clinical trials of a number of different types of treatments, including AChE inhibitors[369,371-373,477] and Aβ immunization treatments.[478] Due to the biological basis and relatively small measurement error of imaging biomarkers, studies have estimated significantly greater power of these markers relative to only clinical diagnosis and/or psychometric tests.[479] As new disease-modifying treatments are developed, imaging biomarkers will likely play a significant role in sensitive and specific trial outcomes.

Conclusions

In conclusion, neuroimaging studies of AD and MCI have characterized significant alterations in structure and function relative to healthy elderly. AD and MCI patients show pronounced brain atrophy, starting in MTL regions and eventually encompassing the entire brain, which can be accurately and sensitively detected and monitored using structural MRI techniques. Advanced MRI techniques have also shown significant brain alterations in patients with AD and MCI, including significant loss of WM integrity (measured via DTI), hypoperfusion in temporoparietal and other regions (perfusion MRI), alterations in cellular metabolites (MR spectroscopy), changes in brain function (fMRI) during tasks and at rest, and a loss of connectivity between functional networks. Nuclear medicine techniques including SPECT and PET have also shown differences between AD and MCI patients and HCs, including hypoperfusion (SPECT), hypometabolism at rest and during functional tasks (FDG-PET), significant deposition of amyloid (PIB-PET), deficits in neurotransmitter systems (ACh, GABA, 5-HT, DA), and increased neuroinflammation (PK-11195, DAA1106). Neuroimaging tools have also shown clear utility in accurate and early detection and diagnosis, prediction of disease course and rate of decline, and monitoring declines in brain structure and function.

Despite the abundant studies of neuroimaging as a biomarker in AD and MCI, no single technique is considered to be the "gold standard." Future studies, including consortium studies such as ADNI, that have multimodal imaging in the same patients will provide an opportunity to directly compare different types of imaging. By estimating the relative contribution of each imaging technique in early diagnosis and prediction of AD and MCI, the best technique or optimal combination of techniques can be established and implemented in future studies for even earlier detection or in clinical trials. Although AD diagnostic criteria still requires postmortem neuropathology for a conclusive diagnosis, neuroimaging biomarkers are essential tools for the *in vivo* diagnosis of AD and may one day be considered adequate for a conclusive AD diagnosis.

Acknowledgements Preparation of this manuscript was supported in part by grants from the National Institutes of Health (NIA R01 AG19771 to AJS and P30 AG101133-18S1 Core Supplement to Bernardino Ghetti, MD and AJS; CTSI Training Grant, TL1 RR025759 to SLR; and NIBIB R03 EB008674 to Li Shen, PhD), the Indiana Economic Development Corporation (IEDC #87884 to AJS), and by the Alzheimer's Disease Neuroimaging Initiative (PI: Michael Weiner, MD; NIH grant U01 AG024904 and RC2 AG036535-01). ADNI is funded by the National Institute on Aging (NIA), the National Institute of

Biomedical Imaging and Bioengineering (NIBIB), and through generous contribution from the following: Pfizer Inc., Wyeth Research, Bristol-Myers Squibb, Eli Lilly and Company, GlaxoSmithKline, Merck & Co. Inc., AstraZeneca AB, Novartis Pharmaceuticals Corporation, the Alzheimer's Association, Eisai Global Clinical Development, Elan Corporation plc, Forest Laboratories, and the Institute for the Study of Aging, with participation of the U.S. Food and Drug Administration. Industry partnerships are coordinated through the Foundation for the National Institutes of Health. The grantee organization is the Northern California Institute for Research and Education, and the study is coordinated by the Alzheimer's Disease Cooperative Study at the University of California, San Diego. ADNI data are disseminated by the Laboratory of Neuro Imaging at the University of California, Los Angeles.

References

1. Wimo A, Winblad B, Aguero-Torres H, von Strauss E. The magnitude of dementia occurrence in the world. *Alzheimer Dis Assoc Disord.* 2003;17(2):63-67.
2. Newcomer RJ, Fox PJ, Harrington CA. Health and long-term care for people with Alzheimer's disease and related dementias: policy research issues. *Aging Ment Health.* 2001;5(Suppl 1):S124-S137.
3. Bertram L, Tanzi RE. Thirty years of Alzheimer's disease genetics: the implications of systematic meta-analyses. *Nat Rev Neurosci.* 2008;9(10):768-778.
4. Corder EH, Saunders AM, Strittmatter WJ, et al. Gene dose of apolipoprotein E type 4 allele and the risk of Alzheimer's disease in late onset families. *Science.* 1993;261(5123):921-923.
5. Mayeux R, Saunders AM, Shea S, et al. Utility of the apolipoprotein E genotype in the diagnosis of Alzheimer's disease. Alzheimer's Disease Centers Consortium on Apolipoprotein E and Alzheimer's Disease. *N Engl J Med.* 1998;338(8):506-511.
6. Corder EH, Saunders AM, Risch NJ, et al. Protective effect of apolipoprotein E type 2 allele for late onset Alzheimer disease. *Nat Genet.* 1994;7(2):180-184.
7. Masters CL, Cappai R, Barnham KJ, Villemagne VL. Molecular mechanisms for Alzheimer's disease: implications for neuroimaging and therapeutics. *J Neurochem.* 2006;97(6):1700-1725.
8. Minati L, Edginton T, Bruzzone MG, Giaccone G. Current concepts in Alzheimer's disease: a multidisciplinary review. *Am J Alzheimers Dis Other Demen.* 2009;24(2):95-121.
9. Nathalie P, Jean-Noel O. Processing of amyloid precursor protein and amyloid peptide neurotoxicity. *Curr Alzheimer Res.* 2008;5(2):92-99.
10. Brion JP. Neurofibrillary tangles and Alzheimer's disease. *Eur Neurol.* 1998;40(3):130-140.
11. Sorrentino G, Bonavita V. Neurodegeneration and Alzheimer's disease: the lesson from tauopathies. *Neurol Sci.* 2007;28(2):63-71.
12. Braak H, Braak E, Bohl J. Staging of Alzheimer-related cortical destruction. *Eur Neurol.* 1993;33(6):403-408.
13. Whitehouse PJ, Price DL, Clark AW, Coyle JT, DeLong MR. Alzheimer disease: evidence for selective loss of cho-

linergic neurons in the nucleus basalis. *Ann Neurol.* 1981;10(2):122-126.
14. Braak H, Braak E. Evolution of the neuropathology of Alzheimer's disease. *Acta Neurol Scand Suppl.* 1996;165:3-12.
15. Storey E, Kinsella GJ, Slavin MJ. The neuropsychological diagnosis of Alzheimer's disease. *J Alzheimers Dis.* 2001;3(3):261-285.
16. Petersen RC. Mild cognitive impairment as a diagnostic entity. *J Intern Med.* 2004;256(3):183-194.
17. Petersen RC. Mild cognitive impairment: current research and clinical implications. *Semin Neurol.* 2007;27:22-31.
18. Petersen RC, Bennett D. Mild cognitive impairment: is it Alzheimer's disease or not? *J Alzheimers Dis.* 2005;7(3): 241-245. discussion 55-62.
19. Petersen RC, Smith GE, Waring SC, Ivnik RJ, Tangalos EG, Kokmen E. Mild cognitive impairment: clinical characterization and outcome. *Arch Neurol.* 1999;56(3): 303-308.
20. Ahmed S, Mitchell J, Arnold R, Dawson K, Nestor PJ, Hodges JR. Memory complaints in mild cognitive impairment, worried well, and semantic dementia patients. *Alzheimer Dis Assoc Disord.* 2008;22(3):227-235.
21. Dik MG, Jonker C, Comijs HC, et al. Memory complaints and APOE-epsilon4 accelerate cognitive decline in cognitively normal elderly. *Neurology.* 2001;57(12):2217-2222.
22. Kliegel M, Zimprich D, Eschen A. What do subjective cognitive complaints in persons with aging-associated cognitive decline reflect? *Int Psychogeriatr.* 2005;17(3): 499-512.
23. Nunes T, Fragata I, Ribeiro F, et al. The outcome of elderly patients with cognitive complaints but normal neuropsychological tests. *J Alzheimers Dis.* 2009 Sep 11.
24. Saykin AJ, Wishart HA, Rabin LA, et al. Older adults with cognitive complaints show brain atrophy similar to that of amnestic MCI. *Neurology.* 2006;67(5):834-842.
25. Jack CR Jr, Bernstein MA, Fox NC, et al. The Alzheimer's Disease Neuroimaging Initiative (ADNI): MRI methods. *J Magn Reson Imaging.* 2008;27(4):685-691.
26. Mueller SG, Weiner MW, Thal LJ, et al. The Alzheimer's disease neuroimaging initiative. *Neuroimaging Clin N Am.* 2005;15(4):869-877. xi-xii.
27. Mueller SG, Weiner MW, Thal LJ, et al. Ways toward an early diagnosis in Alzheimer's disease: the Alzheimer's Disease Neuroimaging Initiative (ADNI). *Alzheimers Dement.* 2005;1(1):55-66.
28. Chang YL, Jacobson MW, Fennema-Notestine C, et al. Level of executive function influences verbal memory in amnestic mild cognitive impairment and predicts prefrontal and posterior cingulate thickness. *Cereb Cortex.* 2010;20(6):1305-1313.
29. Chou YY, Lepore N, Avedissian C, et al. Mapping correlations between ventricular expansion and CSF amyloid and tau biomarkers in 240 subjects with Alzheimer's disease, mild cognitive impairment and elderly controls. *Neuroimage.* 2009;46(2):394-410.
30. Desikan RS, Cabral HJ, Hess CP, et al. Automated MRI measures identify individuals with mild cognitive impairment and Alzheimer's disease. *Brain.* 2009;132(Pt 8): 2048-2057.
31. Fan Y, Batmanghelich N, Clark CM, Davatzikos C. Spatial patterns of brain atrophy in MCI patients, identified via

high-dimensional pattern classification, predict subsequent cognitive decline. *Neuroimage.* 2008;39(4):1731-1743.

32. Fan Y, Resnick SM, Wu X, Davatzikos C. Structural and functional biomarkers of prodromal Alzheimer's disease: a high-dimensional pattern classification study. *Neuroimage.* 2008;41(2):277-285.

33. Fennema-Notestine C, Hagler DJ Jr, McEvoy LK, et al. Structural MRI biomarkers for preclinical and mild Alzheimer's disease. *Hum Brain Mapp.* 2009;30(10): 3238-3253.

34. Gerardin E, Chetelat G, Chupin M, et al. Multidimensional classification of hippocampal shape features discriminates Alzheimer's disease and mild cognitive impairment from normal aging. *Neuroimage.* 2009;47(4):1476-1486.

35. Hinrichs C, Singh V, Mukherjee L, Xu G, Chung MK, Johnson SC. Spatially augmented LPboosting for AD classification with evaluations on the ADNI dataset. *Neuroimage.* 2009;48(1):138-149.

36. Hua X, Leow AD, Parikshak N, et al. Tensor-based morphometry as a neuroimaging biomarker for Alzheimer's disease: an MRI study of 676 AD, MCI, and normal subjects. *Neuroimage.* 2008;43(3):458-469.

37. Jack CR Jr, Lowe VJ, Weigand SD, et al. Serial PIB and MRI in normal, mild cognitive impairment and Alzheimer's disease: implications for sequence of pathological events in Alzheimer's disease. *Brain.* 2009;132(Pt 5):1355-1365.

38. Kovacevic S, Rafii MS, Brewer JB. High-throughput, fully automated volumetry for prediction of MMSE and CDR decline in mild cognitive impairment. *Alzheimer Dis Assoc Disord.* 2009;23(2):139-145.

39. Leow AD, Yanovsky I, Parikshak N, et al. Alzheimer's Disease Neuroimaging Initiative: A one-year follow up study using Tensor-Based Morphometry correlating degenerative rates, biomarkers and cognition. *Neuroimage.* 2009;45(3):644-655.

40. Misra C, Fan Y, Davatzikos C. Baseline and longitudinal patterns of brain atrophy in MCI patients, and their use in prediction of short-term conversion to AD: results from ADNI. *Neuroimage.* 2009;44(4):1415-1422.

41. Morra JH, Tu Z, Apostolova LG, et al. Validation of a fully automated 3D hippocampal segmentation method using subjects with Alzheimer's disease mild cognitive impairment, and elderly controls. *Neuroimage.* 2008;43(1):59-68.

42. Risacher SL, Saykin AJ, West JD, et al. Baseline MRI predictors of conversion from MCI to probable AD in the ADNI cohort. *Curr Alzheimer Res.* 2009;6:347-361.

43. Vemuri P, Wiste HJ, Weigand SD, et al. MRI and CSF biomarkers in normal, MCI, and AD subjects: diagnostic discrimination and cognitive correlations. *Neurology.* 2009;73(4):287-293.

44. Walhovd KB, Fjell AM, Dale AM, et al. Multi-modal imaging predicts memory performance in normal aging and cognitive decline. *Neurobiol Aging.* 2010;31(7):1107-1121.

45. Risacher SL, Shen L, West JD, et al. Longitudinal MRI atrophy biomarkers: Relationship to conversion in the ADNI cohort. *Neurobiol Aging.* 2010;31(8):1401-1418.

46. Morra JH, Tu Z, Apostolova LG, et al. Automated mapping of hippocampal atrophy in 1-year repeat MRI data from 490 subjects with Alzheimer's disease, mild cognitive impairment, and elderly controls. *Neuroimage.* 2009;45(1 Suppl):S3-S15.

47. Vemuri P, Wiste HJ, Weigand SD, et al. MRI and CSF biomarkers in normal, MCI, and AD subjects: predicting future clinical change. *Neurology.* 2009;73(4):294-301.

48. Haense C, Herholz K, Jagust WJ, Heiss WD. Performance of FDG PET for detection of Alzheimer's disease in two independent multicentre samples (NEST-DD and ADNI). *Dement Geriatr Cogn Disord.* 2009;28(3):259-266.

49. Jagust WJ, Landau SM, Shaw LM, et al. Relationships between biomarkers in aging and dementia. *Neurology.* 2009;73(15):1193-1199.

50. Landau SM, Harvey D, Madison CM, et al. Associations between cognitive, functional, and FDG-PET measures of decline in AD and MCI. *Neurobiol Aging.* 2009 Aug 4.

51. Langbaum JB, Chen K, Lee W, et al. Categorical and correlational analyses of baseline fluorodeoxyglucose positron emission tomography images from the Alzheimer's Disease Neuroimaging Initiative (ADNI). *Neuroimage.* 2009;45(4): 1107-1116.

52. Mormino EC, Kluth JT, Madison CM, et al. Episodic memory loss is related to hippocampal-mediated beta-amyloid deposition in elderly subjects. *Brain.* 2009;132(Pt 5):1310-1323.

53. Leow AD, Yanovsky I, Parikshak N, et al. Alzheimer's disease neuroimaging initiative: a one-year follow up study using tensor-based morphometry correlating degenerative rates, biomarkers and cognition. *Neuroimage.* 2009;45(3): 645-655.

54. Schuff N, Woerner N, Boreta L, et al. MRI of hippocampal volume loss in early Alzheimer's disease in relation to ApoE genotype and biomarkers. *Brain.* 2009;132(Pt 4): 1067-1077.

55. Shaw LM, Vanderstichele H, Knapik-Czajka M, et al. Cerebrospinal fluid biomarker signature in Alzheimer's disease neuroimaging initiative subjects. *Ann Neurol.* 2009;65(4): 403-413.

56. de Leon MJ, George AE, Reisberg B, et al. Alzheimer's disease: longitudinal CT studies of ventricular change. *AJR Am J Roentgenol.* 1989;152(6):1257-1262.

57. Willmer J, Carruthers A, Guzman DA, Collins B, Pogue J, Stuss DT. The usefulness of CT scanning in diagnosing dementia of the Alzheimer type. *Can J Neurol Sci.* 1993;20(3):210-216.

58. LeMay M, Stafford JL, Sandor T, Albert M, Haykal H, Zamani A. Statistical assessment of perceptual CT scan ratings in patients with Alzheimer type dementia. *J Comput Assist Tomogr.* 1986;10(5):802-809.

59. Kido DK, Caine ED, LeMay M, Ekholm S, Booth H, Panzer R. Temporal lobe atrophy in patients with Alzheimer disease: a CT study. *AJNR Am J Neuroradiol.* 1989; 10(3):551-555.

60. DeCarli C, Kaye JA, Horwitz B, Rapoport SI. Critical analysis of the use of computer-assisted transverse axial tomography to study human brain in aging and dementia of the Alzheimer type. *Neurology.* 1990;40(6):872-883.

61. George AE, de Leon MJ, Stylopoulos LA, et al. CT diagnostic features of Alzheimer disease: importance of the choroidal/hippocampal fissure complex. *AJNR Am J Neuroradiol.* 1990;11(1):101-107.

62. de Leon MJ, George AE, Stylopoulos LA, Smith G, Miller DC. Early marker for Alzheimer's disease: the atrophic hippocampus. *Lancet.* 1989;2(8664):672-673.

63. Ambrosetto P, Bacci A. CT diagnostic features of choroidal/hippocampal fissure complex in Alzheimer disease and progressive supranuclear palsy. *AJNR Am J Neuroradiol.* 1991;12(3):583-584.
64. Jack CR Jr, Petersen RC, O'Brien PC, Tangalos EG. MR-based hippocampal volumetry in the diagnosis of Alzheimer's disease. *Neurology.* 1992;42(1):183-188.
65. Jack CR Jr, Petersen RC, Xu YC, et al. Medial temporal atrophy on MRI in normal aging and very mild Alzheimer's disease. *Neurology.* 1997;49(3):786-794.
66. Korf ES, Wahlund LO, Visser PJ, Scheltens P. Medial temporal lobe atrophy on MRI predicts dementia in patients with mild cognitive impairment. *Neurology.* 2004;63(1):94-100.
67. Scheltens P, Pasquier F, Weerts JG, Barkhof F, Leys D. Qualitative assessment of cerebral atrophy on MRI: inter- and intra-observer reproducibility in dementia and normal aging. *Eur Neurol.* 1997;37(2):95-99.
68. Dale A, Fischl B, Sereno M. Cortical surface-based analysis. I. Segmentation and surface reconstruction. *Neuroimage.* 1999;9(2):179-194.
69. Fischl B, Dale AM. Measuring the thickness of the human cerebral cortex from magnetic resonance images. *Proc Natl Acad Sci U S A.* 2000;97(20):11050-11055.
70. Fischl B, Salat D, Busa E, et al. Whole brain segmentation: automated labeling of neuroanatomical structures in the human brain. *Neuron.* 2002;33(3):341-355.
71. Ashburner J, Friston KJ. Voxel-based morphometry – the methods. *Neuroimage.* 2000;11(6 Pt 1):805-821.
72. Good CD, Johnsrude IS, Ashburner J, Henson RN, Friston KJ, Frackowiak RS. A voxel-based morphometric study of ageing in 465 normal adult human brains. *Neuroimage.* 2001;14(1 Pt 1):21-36.
73. Jack CR Jr, Dickson DW, Parisi JE, et al. Antemortem MRI findings correlate with hippocampal neuropathology in typical aging and dementia. *Neurology.* 2002;58(5):750-757.
74. Henneman WJ, Sluimer JD, Barnes J, et al. Hippocampal atrophy rates in Alzheimer disease: added value over whole brain volume measures. *Neurology.* 2009;72(11):999-1007.
75. Convit A, de Leon MJ, Golomb J, et al. Hippocampal atrophy in early Alzheimer's disease: anatomic specificity and validation. *Psychiatr Q.* 1993;64(4):371-387.
76. de Leon MJ, Convit A, DeSanti S, et al. The hippocampus in aging and Alzheimer's disease. *Neuroimaging Clin N Am.* 1995;5(1):1-17.
77. Laakso MP, Lehtovirta M, Partanen K, Riekkinen PJ, Soininen H. Hippocampus in Alzheimer's disease: a 3-year follow-up MRI study. *Biol Psychiatry.* 2000;47(6):557-561.
78. Bobinski M, de Leon MJ, Convit A, et al. MRI of entorhinal cortex in mild Alzheimer's disease. *Lancet.* 1999;353(9146):38-40.
79. De Toledo-Morrell L, Goncharova I, Dickerson B, Wilson RS, Bennett DA. From healthy aging to early Alzheimer's disease: in vivo detection of entorhinal cortex atrophy. *Ann NY Acad Sci.* 2000;911:240-253.
80. Dickerson BC, Goncharova I, Sullivan MP, et al. MRI-derived entorhinal and hippocampal atrophy in incipient and very mild Alzheimer's disease. *Neurobiol Aging.* 2001;22(5):747-754.

81. Killiany RJ, Hyman BT, Gomez-Isla T, et al. MRI measures of entorhinal cortex vs hippocampus in preclinical AD. *Neurology.* 2002;58(8):1188-1196.
82. Laakso MP, Soininen H, Partanen K, et al. Volumes of hippocampus, amygdala and frontal lobes in the MRI-based diagnosis of early Alzheimer's disease: correlation with memory functions. *J Neural Transm Park Dis Dement Sect.* 1995;9(1):73-86.
83. Lehericy S, Baulac M, Chiras J, et al. Amygdalohippocampal MR volume measurements in the early stages of Alzheimer disease. *AJNR Am J Neuroradiol.* 1994;15(5):929-937.
84. Teipel SJ, Pruessner JC, Faltraco F, et al. Comprehensive dissection of the medial temporal lobe in AD: measurement of hippocampus, amygdala, entorhinal, perirhinal and parahippocampal cortices using MRI. *J Neurol.* 2006;253(6):794-800.
85. Carmichael OT, Kuller LH, Lopez OL, et al. Ventricular volume and dementia progression in the Cardiovascular Health Study. *Neurobiol Aging.* 2007;28(3):389-397.
86. Tanna NK, Kohn MI, Horwich DN, et al. Analysis of brain and cerebrospinal fluid volumes with MR imaging: impact on PET data correction for atrophy. Part II. Aging and Alzheimer dementia. *Radiology.* 1991;178(1):123-130.
87. Giesel FL, Hahn HK, Thomann PA, et al. Temporal horn index and volume of medial temporal lobe atrophy using a new semiautomated method for rapid and precise assessment. *AJNR Am J Neuroradiol.* 2006;27(7):1454-1458.
88. Bottino CM, Castro CC, Gomes RL, Buchpiguel CA, Marchetti RL, Neto MR. Volumetric MRI measurements can differentiate Alzheimer's disease, mild cognitive impairment, and normal aging. *Int Psychogeriatr.* 2002;14(1):59-72.
89. Convit A, De Leon MJ, Tarshish C, et al. Specific hippocampal volume reductions in individuals at risk for Alzheimer's disease. *Neurobiol Aging.* 1997;18(2):131-138.
90. Du AT, Schuff N, Amend D, et al. Magnetic resonance imaging of the entorhinal cortex and hippocampus in mild cognitive impairment and Alzheimer's disease. *J Neurol Neurosurg Psychiatry.* 2001;71(4):441-447.
91. Jack CR Jr, Petersen RC, Xu YC, et al. Prediction of AD with MRI-based hippocampal volume in mild cognitive impairment. *Neurology.* 1999;52(7):1397-1403.
92. Killiany RJ, Gomez-Isla T, Moss M, et al. Use of structural magnetic resonance imaging to predict who will get Alzheimer's disease. *Ann Neurol.* 2000;47(4):430-439.
93. Pennanen C, Kivipelto M, Tuomainen S, et al. Hippocampus and entorhinal cortex in mild cognitive impairment and early AD. *Neurobiol Aging.* 2004;25(3):303-310.
94. Xu Y, Jack CR Jr, O'Brien PC, et al. Usefulness of MRI measures of entorhinal cortex versus hippocampus in AD. *Neurology.* 2000;54(9):1760-1767.
95. Apostolova LG, Dinov ID, Dutton RA, et al. 3D comparison of hippocampal atrophy in amnestic mild cognitive impairment and Alzheimer's disease. *Brain.* 2006;129(Pt 11):2867-2873.
96. Ballmaier M, O'Brien JT, Burton EJ, et al. Comparing gray matter loss profiles between dementia with Lewy bodies and Alzheimer's disease using cortical pattern matching: diagnosis and gender effects. *Neuroimage.* 2004;23(1):325-335.

97. Becker JT, Davis SW, Hayashi KM, et al. Three-dimensional patterns of hippocampal atrophy in mild cognitive impairment. *Arch Neurol.* 2006;63(1):97-101.

98. Kaye JA, Swihart T, Howieson D, et al. Volume loss of the hippocampus and temporal lobe in healthy elderly persons destined to develop dementia. *Neurology.* 1997;48(5): 1297-1304.

99. Thompson PM, Hayashi KM, de Zubicaray G, et al. Dynamics of gray matter loss in Alzheimer's disease. *J Neurosci.* 2003;23(3):994-1005.

100. Du AT, Schuff N, Kramer JH, et al. Higher atrophy rate of entorhinal cortex than hippocampus in AD. *Neurology.* 2004;62(3):422-427.

101. Frisoni GB, Laakso MP, Beltramello A, et al. Hippocampal and entorhinal cortex atrophy in frontotemporal dementia and Alzheimer's disease. *Neurology.* 1999;52(1):91-100.

102. Juottonen K, Laakso MP, Insausti R, et al. Volumes of the entorhinal and perirhinal cortices in Alzheimer's disease. *Neurobiol Aging.* 1998;19(1):15-22.

103. Juottonen K, Laakso MP, Partanen K, Soininen H. Comparative MR analysis of the entorhinal cortex and hippocampus in diagnosing Alzheimer disease. *AJNR Am J Neuroradiol.* 1999;20(1):139-144.

104. Convit A, de Leon MJ, Hoptman MJ, Tarshish C, De Santi S, Rusinek H. Age-related changes in brain: I. Magnetic resonance imaging measures of temporal lobe volumes in normal subjects. *Psychiatr Q.* 1995;66(4):343-355.

105. De Santi S, de Leon MJ, Rusinek H, et al. Hippocampal formation glucose metabolism and volume losses in MCI and AD. *Neurobiol Aging.* 2001;22(4):529-539.

106. Wolf H, Grunwald M, Kruggel F, et al. Hippocampal volume discriminates between normal cognition; questionable and mild dementia in the elderly. *Neurobiol Aging.* 2001;22(2):177-186.

107. Baron JC, Chetelat G, Desgranges B, et al. In vivo mapping of gray matter loss with voxel-based morphometry in mild Alzheimer's disease. *Neuroimage.* 2001;14(2):298-309.

108. Bozzali M, Filippi M, Magnani G, et al. The contribution of voxel-based morphometry in staging patients with mild cognitive impairment. *Neurology.* 2006;67(3):453-460.

109. Busatto GF, Garrido GE, Almeida OP, et al. A voxel-based morphometry study of temporal lobe gray matter reductions in Alzheimer's disease. *Neurobiol Aging.* 2003;24(2):221-231.

110. Chetelat G, Desgranges B, De La Sayette V, Viader F, Eustache F, Baron JC. Mapping gray matter loss with voxel-based morphometry in mild cognitive impairment. *Neuroreport.* 2002;13(15):1939-1943.

111. Frisoni GB, Testa C, Zorzan A, et al. Detection of grey matter loss in mild Alzheimer's disease with voxel based morphometry. *J Neurol Neurosurg Psychiatry.* 2002;73(6):657-664.

112. Hirata Y, Matsuda H, Nemoto K, et al. Voxel-based morphometry to discriminate early Alzheimer's disease from controls. *Neurosci Lett.* 2005;382(3):269-274.

113. Jack CR Jr, Lowe VJ, Senjem ML, et al. 11C PiB and structural MRI provide complementary information in imaging of Alzheimer's disease and amnestic mild cognitive impairment. *Brain.* 2008;131(Pt 3):665-680.

114. Karas GB, Burton EJ, Rombouts SA, et al. A comprehensive study of gray matter loss in patients with Alzheimer's disease using optimized voxel-based morphometry. *Neuroimage.* 2003;18(4):895-907.

115. Karas GB, Scheltens P, Rombouts SA, et al. Global and local gray matter loss in mild cognitive impairment and Alzheimer's disease. *Neuroimage.* 2004;23(2):708-716.

116. Hamalainen A, Tervo S, Grau-Olivares M, et al. Voxel-based morphometry to detect brain atrophy in progressive mild cognitive impairment. *Neuroimage.* 2007;37(4): 1122-1131.

117. Trivedi MA, Wichmann AK, Torgerson BM, et al. Structural MRI discriminates individuals with Mild Cognitive Impairment from age-matched controls: a combined neuropsychological and voxel based morphometry study. *Alzheimers Dement.* 2006;2:296-302.

118. Whitwell JL, Shiung MM, Przybelski SA, et al. MRI patterns of atrophy associated with progression to AD in amnestic mild cognitive impairment. *Neurology.* 2008;70(7):512-520.

119. Whitwell JL, Przybelski SA, Weigand SD, et al. 3D maps from multiple MRI illustrate changing atrophy patterns as subjects progress from mild cognitive impairment to Alzheimer's disease. *Brain.* 2007;130(Pt 7):1777-1786.

120. Cardenas VA, Du AT, Hardin D, et al. Comparison of methods for measuring longitudinal brain change in cognitive impairment and dementia. *Neurobiol Aging.* 2003;24(4): 537-544.

121. Fox NC, Freeborough PA. Brain atrophy progression measured from registered serial MRI: validation and application to Alzheimer's disease. *J Magn Reson Imaging.* 1997;7(6):1069-1075.

122. Jack CR Jr, Shiung MM, Gunter JL, et al. Comparison of different MRI brain atrophy rate measures with clinical disease progression in AD. *Neurology.* 2004;62(4):591-600.

123. Barnes J, Lewis EB, Scahill RI, et al. Automated measurement of hippocampal atrophy using fluid-registered serial MRI in AD and controls. *J Comput Assist Tomogr.* 2007;31(4):581-587.

124. Mungas D, Harvey D, Reed BR, et al. Longitudinal volumetric MRI change and rate of cognitive decline. *Neurology.* 2005;65(4):565-571.

125. Stoub TR, Rogalski EJ, Leurgans S, Bennett DA, Detoledo-Morrell L. Rate of entorhinal and hippocampal atrophy in incipient and mild AD: relation to memory function. *Neurobiol Aging.* 2010;31(7):1089-1098.

126. Barnes J, Bartlett JW, van de Pol LA, et al. A meta-analysis of hippocampal atrophy rates in Alzheimer's disease. *Neurobiol Aging.* 2009;30(11):1711-1723.

127. Jack CR Jr, Petersen RC, Xu Y, et al. Rate of medial temporal lobe atrophy in typical aging and Alzheimer's disease. *Neurology.* 1998;51(4):993-999.

128. Scahill RI, Schott JM, Stevens JM, Rossor MN, Fox NC. Mapping the evolution of regional atrophy in Alzheimer's disease: unbiased analysis of fluid-registered serial MRI. *Proc Natl Acad Sci U S A.* 2002;99(7):4703-4707.

129. Thompson PM, Hayashi KM, De Zubicaray GI, et al. Mapping hippocampal and ventricular change in Alzheimer disease. *Neuroimage.* 2004;22(4):1754-1766.

130. Thompson PM, Hayashi KM, Sowell ER, et al. Mapping cortical change in Alzheimer's disease, brain development, and schizophrenia. *Neuroimage.* 2004;23(Suppl 1):S2-S18.

131. Whitwell JL, Jack CR Jr, Pankratz VS, et al. Rates of brain atrophy over time in autopsy-proven frontotemporal dementia and Alzheimer disease. *Neuroimage.* 2008;39(3):1034-1040.

132. deToledo-Morrell L, Stoub TR, Bulgakova M, et al. MRI-derived entorhinal volume is a good predictor of conversion from MCI to AD. *Neurobiol Aging.* 2004;25(9): 1197-1203.

133. Devanand DP, Liu X, Tabert MH, et al. Combining early markers strongly predicts conversion from mild cognitive impairment to Alzheimer's disease. *Biol Psychiatry.* 2008;64(10):871-879.

134. Devanand DP, Pradhaban G, Liu X, et al. Hippocampal and entorhinal atrophy in mild cognitive impairment: prediction of Alzheimer disease. *Neurology.* 2007;68(11):828-836.

135. Eckerstrom C, Olsson E, Borga M, et al. Small baseline volume of left hippocampus is associated with subsequent conversion of MCI into dementia: the Goteborg MCI study. *J Neurol Sci.* 2008;272(1-2):48-59.

136. Visser PJ, Verhey FR, Hofman PA, Scheltens P, Jolles J. Medial temporal lobe atrophy predicts Alzheimer's disease in patients with minor cognitive impairment. *J Neurol Neurosurg Psychiatry.* 2002;72(4):491-497.

137. Convit A, de Asis J, de Leon MJ, Tarshish CY, De Santi S, Rusinek H. Atrophy of the medial occipitotemporal, inferior, and middle temporal gyri in non-demented elderly predict decline to Alzheimer's disease. *Neurobiol Aging.* 2000;21(1):19-26.

138. Teipel SJ, Born C, Ewers M, et al. Multivariate deformation-based analysis of brain atrophy to predict Alzheimer's disease in mild cognitive impairment. *Neuroimage.* 2007;38(1):13-24.

139. Wolf H, Grunwald M, Ecke GM, et al. The prognosis of mild cognitive impairment in the elderly. *J Neural Transm Suppl.* 1998;54:31-50.

140. Chetelat G, Landeau B, Eustache F, et al. Using voxel-based morphometry to map the structural changes associated with rapid conversion in MCI: a longitudinal MRI study. *Neuroimage.* 2005;27(4):934-946.

141. Karas G, Sluimer J, Goekoop R, et al. Amnestic mild cognitive impairment: structural MR imaging findings predictive of conversion to Alzheimer disease. *AJNR Am J Neuroradiol.* 2008;29(5):944-949.

142. Erten-Lyons D, Howieson D, Moore MM, et al. Brain volume loss in MCI predicts dementia. *Neurology.* 2006;66(2):233-235.

143. Jack CR Jr, Petersen RC, Xu Y, et al. Rates of hippocampal atrophy correlate with change in clinical status in aging and AD. *Neurology.* 2000;55(4):484-489.

144. Jack CR Jr, Shiung MM, Weigand SD, et al. Brain atrophy rates predict subsequent clinical conversion in normal elderly and amnestic MCI. *Neurology.* 2005;65(8):1227-1231.

145. Sluimer JD, van der Flier WM, Karas GB, et al. Whole-brain atrophy rate and cognitive decline: longitudinal MR study of memory clinic patients. *Radiology.* 2008;248(2): 590-598.

146. Tapiola T, Pennanen C, Tapiola M, et al. MRI of hippocampus and entorhinal cortex in mild cognitive impairment: a follow-up study. *Neurobiol Aging.* 2008;29(1):31-38.

147. Wang PN, Lirng JF, Lin KN, Chang FC, Liu HC. Prediction of Alzheimer's disease in mild cognitive impairment: a prospective study in Taiwan. *Neurobiol Aging.* 2006;27(12):1797-1806.

148. Bozzali M, Falini A, Franceschi M, et al. White matter damage in Alzheimer's disease assessed in vivo using diffusion tensor magnetic resonance imaging. *J Neurol Neurosurg Psychiatry.* 2002;72(6):742-746.

149. Choi SJ, Lim KO, Monteiro I, Reisberg B. Diffusion tensor imaging of frontal white matter microstructure in early Alzheimer's disease: a preliminary study. *J Geriatr Psychiatry Neurol.* 2005;18(1):12-19.

150. Fellgiebel A, Wille P, Muller MJ, et al. Ultrastructural hippocampal and white matter alterations in mild cognitive impairment: a diffusion tensor imaging study. *Dement Geriatr Cogn Disord.* 2004;18(1):101-108.

151. Ibrahim I, Horacek J, Bartos A, et al. Combination of voxel based morphometry and diffusion tensor imaging in patients with Alzheimer's disease. *Neuro Endocrinol Lett.* 2009;30(1):39-45.

152. Kiuchi K, Morikawa M, Taoka T, et al. Abnormalities of the uncinate fasciculus and posterior cingulate fasciculus in mild cognitive impairment and early Alzheimer's disease: a diffusion tensor tractography study. *Brain Res.* 2009;1287: 184-191.

153. Medina D, DeToledo-Morrell L, Urresta F, et al. White matter changes in mild cognitive impairment and AD: a diffusion tensor imaging study. *Neurobiol Aging.* 2006;27(5):663-672.

154. Naggara O, Oppenheim C, Rieu D, et al. Diffusion tensor imaging in early Alzheimer's disease. *Psychiatry Res.* 2006;146(3):243-249.

155. Parente DB, Gasparetto EL, Da Cruz LC Jr, Domingues RC, Baptista AC, Carvalho AC. Potential role of diffusion tensor MRI in the differential diagnosis of mild cognitive impairment and Alzheimer's disease. *AJR Am J Roentgenol.* 2008;190(5):1369-1374.

156. Rose SE, Janke AL, Chalk JB. Gray and white matter changes in Alzheimer's disease: a diffusion tensor imaging study. *J Magn Reson Imaging.* 2008;27(1):20-26.

157. Stahl R, Dietrich O, Teipel S, Hampel H, Reiser MF, Schoenberg SO. Assessment of axonal degeneration on Alzheimer's disease with diffusion tensor MRI. *Radiologe.* 2003;43(7):566-575.

158. Stahl R, Dietrich O, Teipel SJ, Hampel H, Reiser MF, Schoenberg SO. White matter damage in Alzheimer disease and mild cognitive impairment: assessment with diffusion-tensor MR imaging and parallel imaging techniques. *Radiology.* 2007;243(2):483-492.

159. Sugihara S, Kinoshita T, Matsusue E, Fujii S, Ogawa T. Usefulness of diffusion tensor imaging of white matter in Alzheimer disease and vascular dementia. *Acta Radiol.* 2004;45(6):658-663.

160. Sydykova D, Stahl R, Dietrich O, et al. Fiber connections between the cerebral cortex and the corpus callosum in Alzheimer's disease: a diffusion tensor imaging and voxel-based morphometry study. *Cereb Cortex.* 2007;17(10): 2276-2282.

161. Takahashi S, Yonezawa H, Takahashi J, Kudo M, Inoue T, Tohgi H. Selective reduction of diffusion anisotropy in white matter of Alzheimer disease brains measured by 3.0 Tesla magnetic resonance imaging. *Neurosci Lett.* 2002;332(1):45-48.

162. Zhang Y, Schuff N, Jahng GH, et al. Diffusion tensor imaging of cingulum fibers in mild cognitive impairment and Alzheimer disease. *Neurology.* 2007;68(1):13-19.

163. Fellgiebel A, Muller MJ, Wille P, et al. Color-coded diffusion-tensor-imaging of posterior cingulate fiber tracts in mild cognitive impairment. *Neurobiol Aging.* 2005;26(8):1193-1198.

164. Muller MJ, Greverus D, Weibrich C, et al. Diagnostic utility of hippocampal size and mean diffusivity in amnestic MCI. *Neurobiol Aging.* 2007;28(3):398-403.

165. Rose SE, McMahon KL, Janke AL, et al. Diffusion indices on magnetic resonance imaging and neuropsychological performance in amnestic mild cognitive impairment. *J Neurol Neurosurg Psychiatry.* 2006;77(10):1122-1128.

166. Kantarci K, Jack CR Jr, Xu YC, et al. Mild cognitive impairment and Alzheimer disease: regional diffusivity of water. *Radiology.* 2001;219(1):101-107.

167. Muller MJ, Greverus D, Dellani PR, et al. Functional implications of hippocampal volume and diffusivity in mild cognitive impairment. *Neuroimage.* 2005;28(4):1033-1042.

168. Ray KM, Wang H, Chu Y, et al. Mild cognitive impairment: apparent diffusion coefficient in regional gray matter and white matter structures. *Radiology.* 2006;241(1):197-205.

169. Sandson TA, Felician O, Edelman RR, Warach S. Diffusion-weighted magnetic resonance imaging in Alzheimer's disease. *Dement Geriatr Cogn Disord.* 1999;10(2):166-171.

170. Wang H, Su MY. Regional pattern of increased water diffusivity in hippocampus and corpus callosum in mild cognitive impairment. *Dement Geriatr Cogn Disord.* 2006;22(3):223-229.

171. Kantarci K, Petersen RC, Boeve BF, et al. DWI predicts future progression to Alzheimer disease in amnestic mild cognitive impairment. *Neurology.* 2005;64(5):902-904.

172. D'Adamo AF Jr, Gidez LI, Yatsu FM. Acetyl transport mechanisms. Involvement of N-acetyl aspartic acid in de novo fatty acid biosynthesis in the developing rat brain. *Exp Brain Res.* 1968;5(4):267-273.

173. Simmons ML, Frondoza CG, Coyle JT. Immunocytochemical localization of N-acetyl-aspartate with monoclonal antibodies. *Neuroscience.* 1991;45(1):37-45.

174. Downes CP, Macphee CH. Myo-inositol metabolites as cellular signals. *Eur J Biochem.* 1990;193(1):1-18.

175. Kanfer JN, Sorrentino G, Sitar DS. Phospholipases as mediators of amyloid beta peptide neurotoxicity: an early event contributing to neurodegeneration characteristic of Alzheimer's disease. *Neurosci Lett.* 1998;257(2):93-96.

176. Miller BL, Chang L, Booth R, et al. In vivo 1H MRS choline: correlation with in vitro chemistry/histology. *Life Sci.* 1996;58(22):1929-1935.

177. Bartres-Faz D, Junque C, Clemente IC, et al. Relationship among (1)H-magnetic resonance spectroscopy, brain volumetry and genetic polymorphisms in humans with memory impairment. *Neurosci Lett.* 2002;327(3):177-180.

178. Block W, Traber F, Flacke S, Jessen F, Pohl C, Schild H. In-vivo proton MR-spectroscopy of the human brain: assessment of N-acetylaspartate (NAA) reduction as a marker for neurodegeneration. *Amino Acids.* 2002;23(1-3):317-323.

179. Chantal S, Braun CM, Bouchard RW, Labelle M, Boulanger Y. Similar 1H magnetic resonance spectroscopic metabolic pattern in the medial temporal lobes of patients with mild

cognitive impairment and Alzheimer disease. *Brain Res.* 2004;1003(1-2):26-35.

180. Firbank MJ, Harrison RM, O'Brien JT. A comprehensive review of proton magnetic resonance spectroscopy studies in dementia and Parkinson's disease. *Dement Geriatr Cogn Disord.* 2002;14(2):64-76.

181. Parnetti L, Tarducci R, Presciutti O, et al. Proton magnetic resonance spectroscopy can differentiate Alzheimer's disease from normal aging. *Mech Ageing Dev.* 1997;97(1):9-14.

182. Schuff N, Capizzano AA, Du AT, et al. Selective reduction of N-acetylaspartate in medial temporal and parietal lobes in AD. *Neurology.* 2002;58(6):928-935.

183. Catani M, Cherubini A, Howard R, et al. (1)H-MR spectroscopy differentiates mild cognitive impairment from normal brain aging. *Neuroreport.* 2001;12(11):2315-2317.

184. Kantarci K, Jack CR Jr, Xu YC, et al. Regional metabolic patterns in mild cognitive impairment and Alzheimer's disease: a 1H MRS study. *Neurology.* 2000;55(2):210-217.

185. Kantarci K, Reynolds G, Petersen RC, et al. Proton MR spectroscopy in mild cognitive impairment and Alzheimer disease: comparison of 1.5 and 3 T. *AJNR Am J Neuroradiol.* 2003;24(5):843-849.

186. Moats RA, Ernst T, Shonk TK, Ross BD. Abnormal cerebral metabolite concentrations in patients with probable Alzheimer disease. *Magn Reson Med.* 1994;32(1):110-115.

187. Shonk TK, Moats RA, Gifford P, et al. Probable Alzheimer disease: diagnosis with proton MR spectroscopy. *Radiology.* 1995;195(1):65-72.

188. Antuono PG, Jones JL, Wang Y, Li SJ. Decreased glutamate + glutamine in Alzheimer's disease detected in vivo with (1)H-MRS at 0.5 T. *Neurology.* 2001;56(6):737-742.

189. Chantal S, Labelle M, Bouchard RW, Braun CM, Boulanger Y. Correlation of regional proton magnetic resonance spectroscopic metabolic changes with cognitive deficits in mild Alzheimer disease. *Arch Neurol.* 2002;59(6):955-962.

190. Miller BL, Moats RA, Shonk T, Ernst T, Woolley S, Ross BD. Alzheimer disease: depiction of increased cerebral myo-inositol with proton MR spectroscopy. *Radiology.* 1993;187(2):433-437.

191. Jessen F, Traeber F, Freymann N, et al. A comparative study of the different N-acetylaspartate measures of the medial temporal lobe in Alzheimer's disease. *Dement Geriatr Cogn Disord.* 2005;20(2-3):178-183.

192. Schuff N, Amend D, Ezekiel F, et al. Changes of hippocampal N-acetyl aspartate and volume in Alzheimer's disease. A proton MR spectroscopic imaging and MRI study. *Neurology.* 1997;49(6):1513-1521.

193. Jessen F, Block W, Traber F, et al. Proton MR spectroscopy detects a relative decrease of N-acetylaspartate in the medial temporal lobe of patients with AD. *Neurology.* 2000;55(5):684-688.

194. Pfefferbaum A, Adalsteinsson E, Spielman D, Sullivan EV, Lim KO. In vivo brain concentrations of N-acetyl compounds, creatine, and choline in Alzheimer disease. *Arch Gen Psychiatry.* 1999;56(2):185-192.

195. Metastasio A, Rinaldi P, Tarducci R, et al. Conversion of MCI to dementia: role of proton magnetic resonance spectroscopy. *Neurobiol Aging.* 2006;27(7):926-932.

196. Modrego PJ, Fayed N, Pina MA. Conversion from mild cognitive impairment to probable Alzheimer's disease

predicted by brain magnetic resonance spectroscopy. *Am J Psychiatry.* 2005;162(4):667-675.

197. Bozzao A, Floris R, Baviera ME, Apruzzese A, Simonetti G. Diffusion and perfusion MR imaging in cases of Alzheimer's disease: correlations with cortical atrophy and lesion load. *AJNR Am J Neuroradiol.* 2001;22(6):1030-1036.

198. Harris GJ, Lewis RF, Satlin A, et al. Dynamic susceptibility contrast MRI of regional cerebral blood volume in Alzheimer's disease. *Am J Psychiatry.* 1996;153(5): 721-724.

199. Harris GJ, Lewis RF, Satlin A, et al. Dynamic susceptibility contrast MR imaging of regional cerebral blood volume in Alzheimer disease: a promising alternative to nuclear medicine. *AJNR Am J Neuroradiol.* 1998;19(9):1727-1732.

200. Maas LC, Harris GJ, Satlin A, English CD, Lewis RF, Renshaw PF. Regional cerebral blood volume measured by dynamic susceptibility contrast MR imaging in Alzheimer's disease: a principal components analysis. *J Magn Reson Imaging.* 1997;7(1):215-219.

201. Mattia D, Babiloni F, Romigi A, et al. Quantitative EEG and dynamic susceptibility contrast MRI in Alzheimer's disease: a correlative study. *Clin Neurophysiol.* 2003;114(7):1210-1216.

202. Olazaran J, Alvarez-Linera J, de Santiago R, Escribano J, Benito-Leon J, Morales JM. Regional correlations between MR imaging perfusion and SPECT in Alzheimer's disease. *Neurologia.* 2005;20(5):240-244.

203. Sandson TA, O'Connor M, Sperling RA, Edelman RR, Warach S. Noninvasive perfusion MRI in Alzheimer's disease: a preliminary report. *Neurology.* 1996;47(5):1339-1342.

204. Alsop DC, Detre JA, Grossman M. Assessment of cerebral blood flow in Alzheimer's disease by spin-labeled magnetic resonance imaging. *Ann Neurol.* 2000;47(1):93-100.

205. Johnson NA, Jahng GH, Weiner MW, et al. Pattern of cerebral hypoperfusion in Alzheimer disease and mild cognitive impairment measured with arterial spin-labeling MR imaging: initial experience. *Radiology.* 2005;234(3): 851-859.

206. Du AT, Jahng GH, Hayasaka S, et al. Hypoperfusion in frontotemporal dementia and Alzheimer disease by arterial spin labeling MRI. *Neurology.* 2006;67(7):1215-1220.

207. Hayasaka S, Du AT, Duarte A, et al. A non-parametric approach for co-analysis of multi-modal brain imaging data: application to Alzheimer's disease. *Neuroimage.* 2006;30(3):768-779.

208. Ogawa S, Lee TM, Kay AR, Tank DW. Brain magnetic resonance imaging with contrast dependent on blood oxygenation. *Proc Natl Acad Sci U S A.* 1990;87(24): 9868-9872.

209. Ogawa S, Tank DW, Menon R, et al. Intrinsic signal changes accompanying sensory stimulation: functional brain mapping with magnetic resonance imaging. *Proc Natl Acad Sci U S A.* 1992;89(13):5951-5955.

210. Buxton RB, Uludag K, Dubowitz DJ, Liu TT. Modeling the hemodynamic response to brain activation. *Neuroimage.* 2004;23(Suppl 1):S220-S233.

211. Uludag K, Dubowitz DJ, Yoder EJ, Restom K, Liu TT, Buxton RB. Coupling of cerebral blood flow and oxygen consumption during physiological activation and deactivation measured with fMRI. *Neuroimage.* 2004;23(1):148-155.

212. Logothetis NK, Pauls J, Augath M, Trinath T, Oeltermann A. Neurophysiological investigation of the basis of the fMRI signal. *Nature.* 2001;412(6843):150-157.

213. Rombouts SA, Goekoop R, Stam CJ, Barkhof F, Scheltens P. Delayed rather than decreased BOLD response as a marker for early Alzheimer's disease. *Neuroimage.* 2005;26(4): 1078-1085.

214. Buckner RL, Snyder AZ, Sanders AL, Raichle ME, Morris JC. Functional brain imaging of young, nondemented, and demented older adults. *J Cogn Neurosci.* 2000;12(Suppl 2):24-34.

215. D'Esposito M, Deouell LY, Gazzaley A. Alterations in the BOLD fMRI signal with ageing and disease: a challenge for neuroimaging. *Nat Rev Neurosci.* 2003;4:863-872.

216. Tekes A, Mohamed MA, Browner NM, Calhoun VD, Yousem DM. Effect of age on visuomotor functional MR imaging. *Acad Radiol.* 2005;12(6):739-745.

217. Squire LR, Knowlton B, Musen G. The structure and organization of memory. *Annu Rev Psychol.* 1993;44: 453-495.

218. Celone KA, Calhoun VD, Dickerson BC, et al. Alterations in memory networks in mild cognitive impairment and Alzheimer's disease: an independent component analysis. *J Neurosci.* 2006;26(40):10222-10231.

219. Daselaar SM, Veltman DJ, Rombouts SA, Raaijmakers JG, Jonker C. Neuroanatomical correlates of episodic encoding and retrieval in young and elderly subjects. *Brain.* 2003;126(Pt 1):43-56.

220. Gron G, Bittner D, Schmitz B, Wunderlich AP, Riepe MW. Subjective memory complaints: objective neural markers in patients with Alzheimer's disease and major depressive disorder. *Ann Neurol.* 2002;51(4):491-498.

221. Remy F, Mirrashed F, Campbell B, Richter W. Verbal episodic memory impairment in Alzheimer's disease: a combined structural and functional MRI study. *Neuroimage.* 2005;25(1):253-266.

222. Yetkin FZ, Rosenberg RN, Weiner MF, Purdy PD, Cullum CM. FMRI of working memory in patients with mild cognitive impairment and probable Alzheimer's disease. *Eur Radiol.* 2006;16(1):193-206.

223. Dickerson BC, Salat DH, Greve DN, et al. Increased hippocampal activation in mild cognitive impairment compared to normal aging and AD. *Neurology.* 2005;65(3): 404-411.

224. Golby A, Silverberg G, Race E, et al. Memory encoding in Alzheimer's disease: an fMRI study of explicit and implicit memory. *Brain.* 2005;128(Pt 4):773-787.

225. Hamalainen A, Pihlajamaki M, Tanila H, et al. Increased fMRI responses during encoding in mild cognitive impairment. *Neurobiol Aging.* 2007;28(12):1889-1903.

226. Kato T, Knopman D, Liu H. Dissociation of regional activation in mild AD during visual encoding: a functional MRI study. *Neurology.* 2001;57(5):812-816.

227. Machulda MM, Ward HA, Borowski B, et al. Comparison of memory fMRI response among normal, MCI, and Alzheimer's patients. *Neurology.* 2003;61(4):500-506.

228. Rombouts SA, Barkhof F, Veltman DJ, et al. Functional MR imaging in Alzheimer's disease during memory encoding. *AJNR Am J Neuroradiol.* 2000;21(10):1869-1875.

229. Small SA, Nava AS, Perera GM, Delapaz R, Stern Y. Evaluating the function of hippocampal subregions with

230. high-resolution MRI in Alzheimer's disease and aging. *Microsc Res Tech.* 2000;51(1):101-108.

230. Sperling RA, Bates JF, Chua EF, et al. fMRI studies of associative encoding in young and elderly controls and mild Alzheimer's disease. *J Neurol Neurosurg Psychiatry.* 2003;74(1):44-50.

231. Pariente J, Cole S, Henson R, et al. Alzheimer's patients engage an alternative network during a memory task. *Ann Neurol.* 2005;58(6):870-879.

232. Petrella JR, Prince SE, Wang L, Hellegers C, Doraiswamy PM. Prognostic value of posteromedial cortex deactivation in mild cognitive impairment. *PLoS ONE.* 2007;2(10):e1104.

233. Johnson SC, Baxter LC, Susskind-Wilder L, Connor DJ, Sabbagh MN, Caselli RJ. Hippocampal adaptation to face repetition in healthy elderly and mild cognitive impairment. *Neuropsychologia.* 2004;42(7):980-989.

234. Johnson SC, Schmitz TW, Moritz CH, et al. Activation of brain regions vulnerable to Alzheimer's disease: the effect of mild cognitive impairment. *Neurobiol Aging.* 2006;27(11):1604-1612.

235. Mandzia JL, McAndrews MP, Grady CL, Graham SJ, Black SE. Neural correlates of incidental memory in mild cognitive impairment: an fMRI study. *Neurobiol Aging.* 2009;30(5):717-730.

236. Trivedi MA, Murphy CM, Goetz C, et al. fMRI activation changes during successful episodic memory encoding and recognition in amnestic mild cognitive impairment relative to cognitively healthy older adults. *Dement Geriatr Cogn Disord.* 2008;26(2):123-137.

237. Ries ML, Schmitz TW, Kawahara TN, Torgerson BM, Trivedi MA, Johnson SC. Task-dependent posterior cingulate activation in mild cognitive impairment. *Neuroimage.* 2006;29(2):485-492.

238. O'Brien JL, O'Keefe KM, LaViolette PS, et al. Longitudinal fMRI in elderly reveals loss of hippocampal activation with clinical decline. *Neurology.* 2010;74(24):1969-1976.

239. Kircher TT, Weis S, Freymann K, et al. Hippocampal activation in patients with mild cognitive impairment is necessary for successful memory encoding. *J Neurol Neurosurg Psychiatry.* 2007;78(8):812-818.

240. Grossman M, Koenig P, DeVita C, et al. Neural basis for verb processing in Alzheimer's disease: an fMRI study. *Neuropsychology.* 2003;17(4):658-674.

241. Grossman M, Koenig P, Glosser G, et al. Neural basis for semantic memory difficulty in Alzheimer's disease: an fMRI study. *Brain.* 2003;126(Pt 2):292-311.

242. Saykin AJ, Flashman LA, Frutiger SA, et al. Neuroanatomic substrates of semantic memory impairment in Alzheimer's disease: patterns of functional MRI activation. *J Int Neuropsychol Soc.* 1999;5(5):377-392.

243. Miller SL, Fenstermacher E, Bates J, Blacker D, Sperling RA, Dickerson BC. Hippocampal activation in adults with mild cognitive impairment predicts subsequent cognitive decline. *J Neurol Neurosurg Psychiatry.* 2008;79(6):630-635.

244. Bassett SS, Yousem DM, Cristinzio C, et al. Familial risk for Alzheimer's disease alters fMRI activation patterns. *Brain.* 2006;129(Pt 5):1229-1239.

245. Bondi MW, Houston WS, Eyler LT, Brown GG. fMRI evidence of compensatory mechanisms in older adults at genetic risk for Alzheimer disease. *Neurology.* 2005;64(3):501-508.

246. Bookheimer SY, Strojwas MH, Cohen MS, et al. Patterns of brain activation in people at risk for Alzheimer's disease. *N Engl J Med.* 2000;343(7):450-456.

247. Fleisher AS, Houston WS, Eyler LT, et al. Identification of Alzheimer disease risk by functional magnetic resonance imaging. *Arch Neurol.* 2005;62(12):1881-1888.

248. Han SD, Houston WS, Jak AJ, et al. Verbal paired-associate learning by APOE genotype in non-demented older adults: fMRI evidence of a right hemispheric compensatory response. *Neurobiol Aging.* 2007;28(2):238-247.

249. Johnson SC, Schmitz TW, Trivedi MA, et al. The influence of Alzheimer disease family history and apolipoprotein E epsilon4 on mesial temporal lobe activation. *J Neurosci.* 2006;26:6069-6076.

250. Lind J, Ingvar M, Persson J, et al. Parietal cortex activation predicts memory decline in apolipoprotein E-epsilon4 carriers. *Neuroreport.* 2006;17(16):1683-1686.

251. Lind J, Persson J, Ingvar M, et al. Reduced functional brain activity response in cognitively intact apolipoprotein E epsilon4 carriers. *Brain.* 2006;129(Pt 5):1240-1248.

252. Trivedi MA, Schmitz TW, Ries ML, et al. fMRI activation during episodic encoding and metacognitive appraisal across the lifespan: risk factors for Alzheimer's disease. *Neuropsychologia.* 2008;46(6):1667-1678.

253. Trivedi MA, Schmitz TW, Ries ML, et al. Reduced hippocampal activation during episodic encoding in middle-aged individuals at genetic risk of Alzheimer's disease: a cross-sectional study. *BMC Med.* 2006;4:1.

254. Xu G, McLaren DG, Ries ML, et al. The influence of parental history of Alzheimer's disease and apolipoprotein E epsilon4 on the BOLD signal during recognition memory. *Brain.* 2009;132(Pt 2):383-391.

255. Filbey FM, Slack KJ, Sunderland TP, Cohen RM. Functional magnetic resonance imaging and magnetoencephalography differences associated with APOEepsilon4 in young healthy adults. *Neuroreport.* 2006;17(15):1585-1590.

256. Smith CD, Andersen AH, Kryscio RJ, et al. Altered brain activation in cognitively intact individuals at high risk for Alzheimer's disease. *Neurology.* 1999;53(7):1391-1396.

257. Smith CD, Andersen AH, Kryscio RJ, et al. Women at risk for AD show increased parietal activation during a fluency task. *Neurology.* 2002;58(8):1197-1202.

258. Smith CD, Kryscio RJ, Schmitt FA, et al. Longitudinal functional alterations in asymptomatic women at risk for Alzheimer's disease. *J Neuroimaging.* 2005;15(3):271-277.

259. Wishart HA, Saykin AJ, Rabin LA, et al. Increased brain activation during working memory in cognitively intact adults with the APOE epsilon4 allele. *Am J Psychiatry.* 2006;163(9):1603-1610.

260. Yassa MA, Verduzco G, Cristinzio C, Bassett SS. Altered fMRI activation during mental rotation in those at genetic risk for Alzheimer disease. *Neurology.* 2008;70(20):1898-1904.

261. Biswal B, Yetkin FZ, Haughton VM, Hyde JS. Functional connectivity in the motor cortex of resting human brain using echo-planar MRI. *Magn Reson Med.* 1995;34(4):537-541.

262. Cordes D, Haughton VM, Arfanakis K, et al. Mapping functionally related regions of brain with functional connectivity MR imaging. *AJNR Am J Neuroradiol.* 2000;21(9):1636-1644.

263. Fox MD, Snyder AZ, Vincent JL, Corbetta M, Van Essen DC, Raichle ME. The human brain is intrinsically organized into dynamic, anticorrelated functional networks. *Proc Natl Acad Sci U S A.* 2005;102(27):9673-9678.

264. Friston K. Causal modelling and brain connectivity in functional magnetic resonance imaging. *PLoS Biol.* 2009;7(2):e33.

265. Greicius MD, Krasnow B, Reiss AL, Menon V. Functional connectivity in the resting brain: a network analysis of the default mode hypothesis. *Proc Natl Acad Sci U S A.* 2003;100(1):253-258.

266. Hampson M, Peterson BS, Skudlarski P, Gatenby JC, Gore JC. Detection of functional connectivity using temporal correlations in MR images. *Hum Brain Mapp.* 2002;15(4): 247-262.

267. Allen G, Barnard H, McColl R, et al. Reduced hippocampal functional connectivity in Alzheimer disease. *Arch Neurol.* 2007;64(10):1482-1487.

268. Bai F, Zhang Z, Watson DR, et al. Abnormal functional connectivity of hippocampus during episodic memory retrieval processing network in amnestic mild cognitive impairment. *Biol Psychiatry.* 2009;65(11):951-958.

269. Bokde AL, Lopez-Bayo P, Meindl T, et al. Functional connectivity of the fusiform gyrus during a face-matching task in subjects with mild cognitive impairment. *Brain.* 2006;129(Pt 5):1113-1124.

270. Grady CL, McIntosh AR, Beig S, Keightley ML, Burian H, Black SE. Evidence from functional neuroimaging of a compensatory prefrontal network in Alzheimer's disease. *J Neurosci.* 2003;23(3):986-993.

271. Petrella JR, Krishnan S, Slavin MJ, Tran TT, Murty L, Doraiswamy PM. Mild cognitive impairment: evaluation with 4-T functional MR imaging. *Radiology.* 2006;240(1):177-186.

272. Pihlajamaki M, DePeau KM, Blacker D, Sperling RA. Impaired medial temporal repetition suppression is related to failure of parietal deactivation in Alzheimer disease. *Am J Geriatr Psychiatry.* 2008;16(4):283-292.

273. Rombouts S, Scheltens P. Functional connectivity in elderly controls and AD patients using resting state fMRI: a pilot study. *Curr Alzheimer Res.* 2005;2(2):115-116.

274. Zhou Y, Dougherty JH Jr, Hubner KF, Bai B, Cannon RL, Hutson RK. Abnormal connectivity in the posterior cingulate and hippocampus in early Alzheimer's disease and mild cognitive impairment. *Alzheimers Dement.* 2008;4(4):265-270.

275. Wang K, Jiang T, Liang M, et al. Discriminative analysis of early Alzheimer's disease based on two intrinsically anticorrelated networks with resting-state fMRI. *Med Image Comput Comput Assist Interv.* 2006;9(Pt 2):340-347.

276. Bartres-Faz D, Serra-Grabulosa JM, Sun FT, et al. Functional connectivity of the hippocampus in elderly with mild memory dysfunction carrying the APOE epsilon4 allele. *Neurobiol Aging.* 2008;29(11):1644-1653.

277. Beckmann CF, DeLuca M, Devlin JT, Smith SM. Investigations into resting-state connectivity using independent component analysis. *Philos Trans R Soc Lond B Biol Sci.* 2005;360(1457):1001-1013.

278. Buckner RL, Snyder AZ, Shannon BJ, et al. Molecular, structural, and functional characterization of Alzheimer's disease: evidence for a relationship between default activity, amyloid, and memory. *J Neurosci.* 2005;25(34):7709-7717.

279. Fransson P. Spontaneous low-frequency BOLD signal fluctuations: an fMRI investigation of the resting-state default mode of brain function hypothesis. *Hum Brain Mapp.* 2005;26(1):15-29.

280. Greicius M. Resting-state functional connectivity in neuropsychiatric disorders. *Curr Opin Neurol.* 2008;21(4): 424-430.

281. Gusnard DA, Raichle ME. Searching for a baseline: functional imaging and the resting human brain. *Nat Rev Neurosci.* 2001;2(10):685-694.

282. Guye M, Bartolomei F, Ranjeva JP. Imaging structural and functional connectivity: towards a unified definition of human brain organization? *Curr Opin Neurol.* 2008;21(4): 393-403.

283. Damoiseaux JS, Rombouts SA, Barkhof F, et al. Consistent resting-state networks across healthy subjects. *Proc Natl Acad Sci U S A.* 2006;103(37):13848-13853.

284. Greicius MD, Supekar K, Menon V, Dougherty RF. Resting-state functional connectivity reflects structural connectivity in the default mode network. *Cereb Cortex.* 2009;19(1):72-78.

285. Lustig C, Snyder AZ, Bhakta M, et al. Functional deactivations: change with age and dementia of the Alzheimer type. *Proc Natl Acad Sci U S A.* 2003;100(24):14504-14509.

286. Raichle ME, MacLeod AM, Snyder AZ, Powers WJ, Gusnard DA, Shulman GL. A default mode of brain function. *Proc Natl Acad Sci U S A.* 2001;98(2):676-682.

287. Wagner AD, Shannon BJ, Kahn I, Buckner RL. Parietal lobe contributions to episodic memory retrieval. *Trends Cogn Sci.* 2005;9(9):445-453.

288. Grady CL, Springer MV, Hongwanishkul D, McIntosh AR, Winocur G. Age-related changes in brain activity across the adult lifespan. *J Cogn Neurosci.* 2006;18(2): 227-241.

289. Greicius MD, Srivastava G, Reiss AL, Menon V. Default-mode network activity distinguishes Alzheimer's disease from healthy aging: evidence from functional MRI. *Proc Natl Acad Sci U S A.* 2004;101(13):4637-4642.

290. He Y, Wang L, Zang Y, et al. Regional coherence changes in the early stages of Alzheimer's disease: a combined structural and resting-state functional MRI study. *Neuroimage.* 2007;35(2):488-500.

291. Rombouts SA, Barkhof F, Goekoop R, Stam CJ, Scheltens P. Altered resting state networks in mild cognitive impairment and mild Alzheimer's disease: an fMRI study. *Hum Brain Mapp.* 2005;26(4):231-239.

292. Sorg C, Riedl V, Muhlau M, et al. Selective changes of resting-state networks in individuals at risk for Alzheimer's disease. *Proc Natl Acad Sci U S A.* 2007;104(47): 18760-18765.

293. Wang K, Liang M, Wang L, et al. Altered functional connectivity in early Alzheimer's disease: a resting-state fMRI study. *Hum Brain Mapp.* 2007;28(10):967-978.

294. Wang L, Zang Y, He Y, et al. Changes in hippocampal connectivity in the early stages of Alzheimer's disease: evidence from resting state fMRI. *Neuroimage.* 2006;31(2):496-504.

295. Bartenstein P, Minoshima S, Hirsch C, et al. Quantitative assessment of cerebral blood flow in patients with Alzheimer's disease by SPECT. *J Nucl Med.* 1997;38(7):1095-1101.

296. Bradley KM, O'Sullivan VT, Soper ND, et al. Cerebral perfusion SPET correlated with Braak pathological stage in Alzheimer's disease. *Brain*. 2002;125(Pt 8):1772-1781.

297. Johnson KA, Jones K, Holman BL, et al. Preclinical prediction of Alzheimer's disease using SPECT. *Neurology*. 1998;50:1563-1571.

298. Julin P, Lindqvist J, Svensson L, Slomka P, Wahlund LO. MRI-guided SPECT measurements of medial temporal lobe blood flow in Alzheimer's disease. *J Nucl Med*. 1997;38:914-919.

299. Kogure D, Matsuda H, Ohnishi T, et al. Longitudinal evaluation of early Alzheimer's disease using brain perfusion SPECT. *J Nucl Med*. 2000;41:1155-1162.

300. Scheltens P, Launer LJ, Barkhof F, Weinstein HC, Jonker C. The diagnostic value of magnetic resonance imaging and technetium 99m-HMPAO single-photon-emission computed tomography for the diagnosis of Alzheimer disease in a community-dwelling elderly population. *Alzheimer Dis Assoc Disord*. 1997;11(2):63-70.

301. Silverman DH. Brain 18F-FDG PET in the diagnosis of neurodegenerative dementias: comparison with perfusion SPECT and with clinical evaluations lacking nuclear imaging. *J Nucl Med*. 2004;45(4):594-607.

302. Caroli A, Testa C, Geroldi C, et al. Cerebral perfusion correlates of conversion to Alzheimer's disease in amnestic mild cognitive impairment. *J Neurol*. 2007;254(12): 1698-1707.

303. Phelps ME, Schelbert HR, Mazziotta JC. Positron computed tomography for studies of myocardial and cerebral function. *Ann Intern Med*. 1983;98(3):339-359.

304. Reivich M. Application of the deoxyglucose method to human cerebral dysfunction. The use of [2-18F] fluoro-2-deoxy-D-glucose in man. *Neurosci Res Program Bull*. 1976;14(4):502-504.

305. Klunk WE, Engler H, Nordberg A, et al. Imaging brain amyloid in Alzheimer's disease with Pittsburgh Compound-B. *Ann Neurol*. 2004;55(3):306-319.

306. Kudo Y, Okamura N, Furumoto S, et al. 2-(2-[2-Dimethylaminothiazol-5-yl]ethenyl)-6- (2-[fluoro]ethoxy) benzoxazole: a novel PET agent for in vivo detection of dense amyloid plaques in Alzheimer's disease patients. *J Nucl Med*. 2007;48(4):553-561.

307. Shoghi-Jadid K, Small GW, Agdeppa ED, et al. Localization of neurofibrillary tangles and beta-amyloid plaques in the brains of living patients with Alzheimer disease. *Am J Geriatr Psychiatry*. 2002;10(1):24-35.

308. Small GW, Kepe V, Ercoli LM, et al. PET of brain amyloid and tau in mild cognitive impairment. *N Engl J Med*. 2006;355(25):2652-2663.

309. Verhoeff NP, Wilson AA, Takeshita S, et al. In-vivo imaging of Alzheimer disease beta-amyloid with [11C]SB-13 PET. *Am J Geriatr Psychiatry*. 2004;12(6):584-595.

310. Pappata S, Salvatore E, Postiglione A. In vivo imaging of neurotransmission and brain receptors in dementia. *J Neuroimaging*. 2008;18(2):111-124.

311. Banati RB, Newcombe J, Gunn RN, et al. The peripheral benzodiazepine binding site in the brain in multiple sclerosis: quantitative in vivo imaging of microglia as a measure of disease activity. *Brain*. 2000;123(Pt 11):2321-2337.

312. Chaki S, Funakoshi T, Yoshikawa R, et al. Binding characteristics of [3H]DAA1106, a novel and selective ligand for peripheral benzodiazepine receptors. *Eur J Pharmacol*. 1999;371(2-3):197-204.

313. Choo IH, Lee DY, Youn JC, et al. Topographic patterns of brain functional impairment progression according to clinical severity staging in 116 Alzheimer disease patients: FDG-PET study. *Alzheimer Dis Assoc Disord*. 2007;21(2): 77-84.

314. Desgranges B, Baron JC, de la Sayette V, et al. The neural substrates of memory systems impairment in Alzheimer's disease. A PET study of resting brain glucose utilization. *Brain*. 1998;121(Pt 4):611-631.

315. Drzezga A, Riemenschneider M, Strassner B, et al. Cerebral glucose metabolism in patients with AD and different APOE genotypes. *Neurology*. 2005;64(1):102-107.

316. Foster NL, Chase TN, Mansi L, et al. Cortical abnormalities in Alzheimer's disease. *Ann Neurol*. 1984;16(6): 649-654.

317. Friedland RP, Budinger TF, Ganz E, et al. Regional cerebral metabolic alterations in dementia of the Alzheimer type: positron emission tomography with [18F]fluorodeoxyglucose. *J Comput Assist Tomogr*. 1983;7(4):590-598.

318. Heiss WD, Pawlik G, Holthoff V, Kessler J, Szelies B. PET correlates of normal and impaired memory functions. *Cerebrovasc Brain Metab Rev*. 1992;4(1):1-27.

319. Herholz K. FDG PET and differential diagnosis of dementia. *Alzheimer Dis Assoc Disord*. 1995;9(1):6-16.

320. Hoffman JM, Welsh-Bohmer KA, Hanson M, et al. FDG PET imaging in patients with pathologically verified dementia. *J Nucl Med*. 2000;41(11):1920-1928.

321. Jagust WJ, Eberling JL, Richardson BC, et al. The cortical topography of temporal lobe hypometabolism in early Alzheimer's disease. *Brain Res*. 1993;629(2):189-198.

322. Jelic V, Nordberg A. Early diagnosis of Alzheimer disease with positron emission tomography. *Alzheimer Dis Assoc Disord*. 2000;14(Suppl 1):S109-S113.

323. Mielke R, Heiss WD. Positron emission tomography for diagnosis of Alzheimer's disease and vascular dementia. *J Neural Transm Suppl*. 1998;53:237-250.

324. Minoshima S, Giordani B, Berent S, Frey KA, Foster NL, Kuhl DE. Metabolic reduction in the posterior cingulate cortex in very early Alzheimer's disease. *Ann Neurol*. 1997;42(1):85-94.

325. Mosconi L. Brain glucose metabolism in the early and specific diagnosis of Alzheimer's disease. FDG-PET studies in MCI and AD. *Eur J Nucl Med Mol Imaging*. 2005;32(4): 486-510.

326. Mosconi L, Tsui WH, Herholz K, et al. Multicenter standardized 18F-FDG PET diagnosis of mild cognitive impairment, Alzheimer's disease, and other dementias. *J Nucl Med*. 2008;49(3):390-398.

327. Nestor PJ, Fryer TD, Smielewski P, Hodges JR. Limbic hypometabolism in Alzheimer's disease and mild cognitive impairment. *Ann Neurol*. 2003;54(3):343-351.

328. Ouchi Y, Nobezawa S, Okada H, Yoshikawa E, Futatsubashi M, Kaneko M. Altered glucose metabolism in the hippocampal head in memory impairment. *Neurology*. 1998;51(1):136-142.

329. Sakamoto S, Ishii K, Sasaki M, et al. Differences in cerebral metabolic impairment between early and late onset types of Alzheimer's disease. *J Neurol Sci*. 2002;200(1-2): 27-32.

330. Silverman DH, Small GW, Chang CY, et al. Positron emission tomography in evaluation of dementia: regional brain metabolism and long-term outcome. *JAMA*. 2001;286(17):2120-2127.

331. Herholz K, Nordberg A, Salmon E, et al. Impairment of neocortical metabolism predicts progression in Alzheimer's disease. *Dement Geriatr Cogn Disord*. 1999;10(6):494-504.

332. Jagust WJ, Haan MN, Eberling JL, Wolfe N, Reed BR. Functional imaging predicts cognitive decline in Alzheimer's disease. *J Neuroimaging*. 1996;6(3):156-160.

333. Lee DY, Seo EH, Choo IH, et al. Neural correlates of the Clock Drawing Test performance in Alzheimer's disease: a FDG-PET study. *Dement Geriatr Cogn Disord*. 2008;26(4):306-313.

334. Fellgiebel A, Siessmeier T, Scheurich A, et al. Association of elevated phospho-tau levels with Alzheimer-typical 18F-fluoro-2-deoxy-D-glucose positron emission tomography findings in patients with mild cognitive impairment. *Biol Psychiatry*. 2004;56(4):279-283.

335. Yamaguchi S, Meguro K, Itoh M, et al. Decreased cortical glucose metabolism correlates with hippocampal atrophy in Alzheimer's disease as shown by MRI and PET. *J Neurol Neurosurg Psychiatry*. 1997;62(6):596-600.

336. Azari NP, Pettigrew KD, Schapiro MB, et al. Early detection of Alzheimer's disease: a statistical approach using positron emission tomographic data. *J Cereb Blood Flow Metab*. 1993;13(3):438-447.

337. Dobert N, Pantel J, Frolich L, Hamscho N, Menzel C, Grunwald F. Diagnostic value of FDG-PET and HMPAO-SPET in patients with mild dementia and mild cognitive impairment: metabolic index and perfusion index. *Dement Geriatr Cogn Disord*. 2005;20(2-3):63-70.

338. Herholz K, Perani D, Salmon E, et al. Comparability of FDG PET studies in probable Alzheimer's disease. *J Nucl Med*. 1993;34(9):1460-1466.

339. Herholz K, Salmon E, Perani D, et al. Discrimination between Alzheimer dementia and controls by automated analysis of multicenter FDG PET. *Neuroimage*. 2002;17(1):302-316.

340. Kippenhan JS, Barker WW, Nagel J, Grady C, Duara R. Neural-network classification of normal and Alzheimer's disease subjects using high-resolution and low-resolution PET cameras. *J Nucl Med*. 1994;35(1):7-15.

341. Minoshima S, Frey KA, Koeppe RA, Foster NL, Kuhl DE. A diagnostic approach in Alzheimer's disease using three-dimensional stereotactic surface projections of fluorine-18-FDG PET. *J Nucl Med*. 1995;36(7):1238-1248.

342. Herholz K. PET studies in dementia. *Ann Nucl Med*. 2003;17(2):79-89.

343. Magistretti PJ, Pellerin L. The contribution of astrocytes to the 18F-2-deoxyglucose signal in PET activation studies. *Mol Psychiatry*. 1996;1(6):445-452.

344. Rocher AB, Chapon F, Blaizot X, Baron JC, Chavoix C. Resting-state brain glucose utilization as measured by PET is directly related to regional synaptophysin levels: a study in baboons. *Neuroimage*. 2003;20(3):1894-1898.

345. Alexander GE, Chen K, Pietrini P, Rapoport SI, Reiman EM. Longitudinal PET evaluation of cerebral metabolic decline in dementia: a potential outcome measure in Alzheimer's disease treatment studies. *Am J Psychiatry*. 2002;159(5):738-745.

346. Hirono N, Hashimoto M, Ishii K, Kazui H, Mori E. One-year change in cerebral glucose metabolism in patients with Alzheimer's disease. *J Neuropsychiatry Clin Neurosci*. 2004;16(4):488-492.

347. Reiman EM, Caselli RJ, Chen K, Alexander GE, Bandy D, Frost J. Declining brain activity in cognitively normal apolipoprotein E epsilon 4 heterozygotes: a foundation for using positron emission tomography to efficiently test treatments to prevent Alzheimer's disease. *Proc Natl Acad Sci U S A*. 2001;98(6):3334-3339.

348. Small GW, Ercoli LM, Silverman DH, et al. Cerebral metabolic and cognitive decline in persons at genetic risk for Alzheimer's disease. *Proc Natl Acad Sci U S A*. 2000;97(11):6037-6042.

349. Smith GS, de Leon MJ, George AE, et al. Topography of cross-sectional and longitudinal glucose metabolic deficits in Alzheimer's disease. Pathophysiologic implications. *Arch Neurol*. 1992;49(11):1142-1150.

350. de Leon MJ, Convit A, Wolf OT, et al. Prediction of cognitive decline in normal elderly subjects with 2-[(18)F]fluoro-2-deoxy-D-glucose/poitron-emission tomography (FDG/PET). *Proc Natl Acad Sci U S A*. 2001;98(19):10966-10971.

351. Kennedy AM, Frackowiak RS, Newman SK, et al. Deficits in cerebral glucose metabolism demonstrated by positron emission tomography in individuals at risk of familial Alzheimer's disease. *Neurosci Lett*. 1995;186(1):17-20.

352. Mosconi L, Tsui WH, Pupi A, et al. (18)F-FDG PET database of longitudinally confirmed healthy elderly individuals improves detection of mild cognitive impairment and Alzheimer's disease. *J Nucl Med*. 2007;48(7):1129-1134.

353. Reiman EM, Caselli RJ, Yun LS, et al. Preclinical evidence of Alzheimer's disease in persons homozygous for the epsilon 4 allele for apolipoprotein E. *N Engl J Med*. 1996;334(12):752-758.

354. Reiman EM, Chen K, Alexander GE, et al. Functional brain abnormalities in young adults at genetic risk for late-onset Alzheimer's dementia. *Proc Natl Acad Sci U S A*. 2004;101(1):284-289.

355. Reiman EM, Chen K, Alexander GE, et al. Correlations between apolipoprotein E epsilon4 gene dose and brain-imaging measurements of regional hypometabolism. *Proc Natl Acad Sci U S A*. 2005;102(23):8299-8302.

356. Rimajova M, Lenzo NP, Wu JS, et al. Fluoro-2-deoxy-D-glucose (FDG)-PET in APOEepsilon4 carriers in the Australian population. *J Alzheimers Dis*. 2008;13(2):137-146.

357. Small GW, Mazziotta JC, Collins MT, et al. Apolipoprotein E type 4 allele and cerebral glucose metabolism in relatives at risk for familial Alzheimer disease. *JAMA*. 1995;273(12):942-947.

358. Anchisi D, Borroni B, Franceschi M, et al. Heterogeneity of brain glucose metabolism in mild cognitive impairment and clinical progression to Alzheimer disease. *Arch Neurol*. 2005;62(11):1728-1733.

359. Arnaiz E, Jelic V, Almkvist O, et al. Impaired cerebral glucose metabolism and cognitive functioning predict deterioration in mild cognitive impairment. *Neuroreport*. 2001;12(4):851-855.

360. Berent S, Giordani B, Foster N, et al. Neuropsychological function and cerebral glucose utilization in isolated memory

360. impairment and Alzheimer's disease. *J Psychiatr Res.* 1999;33(1):7-16.

361. Caselli RJ, Chen K, Lee W, Alexander GE, Reiman EM. Correlating cerebral hypometabolism with future memory decline in subsequent converters to amnestic pre-mild cognitive impairment. *Arch Neurol.* 2008;65(9):1231-1236.

362. Chetelat G, Desgranges B, de la Sayette V, Viader F, Eustache F, Baron JC. Mild cognitive impairment: can FDG-PET predict who is to rapidly convert to Alzheimer's disease? *Neurology.* 2003;60(8):1374-1377.

363. Chetelat G, Eustache F, Viader F, et al. FDG-PET measurement is more accurate than neuropsychological assessments to predict global cognitive deterioration in patients with mild cognitive impairment. *Neurocase.* 2005;11(1): 14-25.

364. Drzezga A, Grimmer T, Riemenschneider M, et al. Prediction of individual clinical outcome in MCI by means of genetic assessment and (18)F-FDG PET. *J Nucl Med.* 2005;46(10):1625-1632.

365. Drzezga A, Lautenschlager N, Siebner H, et al. Cerebral metabolic changes accompanying conversion of mild cognitive impairment into Alzheimer's disease: a PET follow-up study. *Eur J Nucl Med Mol Imaging.* 2003;30(8):1104-1113.

366. Mosconi L, De Santi S, Li J, et al. Hippocampal hypometabolism predicts cognitive decline from normal aging. *Neurobiol Aging.* 2008;29(5):676-692.

367. Mosconi L, Perani D, Sorbi S, et al. MCI conversion to dementia and the APOE genotype: a prediction study with FDG-PET. *Neurology.* 2004;63(12):2332-2340.

368. Heiss WD, Kessler J, Mielke R, Szelies B, Herholz K. Long-term effects of phosphatidylserine, pyritinol, and cognitive training in Alzheimer's disease. A neuropsychological, EEG, and PET investigation. *Dementia.* 1994;5(2):88-98.

369. Kadir A, Darreh-Shori T, Almkvist O, et al. PET imaging of the in vivo brain acetylcholinesterase activity and nicotine binding in galantamine-treated patients with AD. *Neurobiol Aging.* 2008;29(8):1204-1217.

370. Mega MS, Cummings JL, O'Connor SM, et al. Cognitive and metabolic responses to metrifonate therapy in Alzheimer disease. *Neuropsychiatry Neuropsychol Behav Neurol.* 2001;14(1):63-68.

371. Potkin SG, Anand R, Fleming K, et al. Brain metabolic and clinical effects of rivastigmine in Alzheimer's disease. *Int J Neuropsychopharmacol.* 2001;4(3):223-230.

372. Teipel SJ, Drzezga A, Bartenstein P, Moller HJ, Schwaiger M, Hampel H. Effects of donepezil on cortical metabolic response to activation during (18)FDG-PET in Alzheimer's disease:adouble-blindcross-overtrial.*Psychopharmacology (Berl).* 2006;187(1):86-94.

373. Tune L, Tiseo PJ, Ieni J, et al. Donepezil HCl (E2020) maintains functional brain activity in patients with Alzheimer disease: results of a 24-week, double-blind, placebo-controlled study. *Am J Geriatr Psychiatry.* 2003;11(2):169-177.

374. Backman L, Andersson JL, Nyberg L, Winblad B, Nordberg A, Almkvist O. Brain regions associated with episodic retrieval in normal aging and Alzheimer's disease. *Neurology.* 1999;52(9):1861-1870.

375. Kessler J, Herholz K, Grond M, Heiss WD. Impaired metabolic activation in Alzheimer's disease: a PET study during continuous visual recognition. *Neuropsychologia.* 1991;29(3):229-243.

376. Moulin CJ, Laine M, Rinne JO, et al. Brain function during multi-trial learning in mild cognitive impairment: a PET activation study. *Brain Res.* 2007;1136(1):132-141.

377. Schroder J, Buchsbaum MS, Shihabuddin L, et al. Patterns of cortical activity and memory performance in Alzheimer's disease. *Biol Psychiatry.* 2001;49(5):426-436.

378. Woodard JL, Grafton ST, Votaw JR, Green RC, Dobraski ME, Hoffman JM. Compensatory recruitment of neural resources during overt rehearsal of word lists in Alzheimer's disease. *Neuropsychology.* 1998;12(4):491-504.

379. Klunk WE, Lopresti BJ, Ikonomovic MD, et al. Binding of the positron emission tomography tracer Pittsburgh compound-B reflects the amount of amyloid-beta in Alzheimer's disease brain but not in transgenic mouse brain. *J Neurosci.* 2005;25(46):10598-10606.

380. Lockhart A, Lamb JR, Osredkar T, et al. PIB is a non-specific imaging marker of amyloid-beta (Abeta) peptide-related cerebral amyloidosis. *Brain.* 2007;130(Pt 10):2607-2615.

381. Johnson KA, Gregas M, Becker JA, et al. Imaging of amyloid burden and distribution in cerebral amyloid angiopathy. *Ann Neurol.* 2007;62(3):229-234.

382. Bacskai BJ, Frosch MP, Freeman SH, et al. Molecular imaging with Pittsburgh Compound B confirmed at autopsy: a case report. *Arch Neurol.* 2007;64(3): 431-434.

383. Ikonomovic MD, Klunk WE, Abrahamson EE, et al. Postmortem correlates of in vivo PiB-PET amyloid imaging in a typical case of Alzheimer's disease. *Brain.* 2008;131(Pt 6):1630-1645.

384. Leinonen V, Alafuzoff I, Aalto S, et al. Assessment of beta-amyloid in a frontal cortical brain biopsy specimen and by positron emission tomography with carbon 11-labeled Pittsburgh Compound B. *Arch Neurol.* 2008;65(10): 1304-1309.

385. Kemppainen NM, Aalto S, Wilson IA, et al. Voxel-based analysis of PET amyloid ligand [11C]PIB uptake in Alzheimer disease. *Neurology.* 2006;67(9):1575-1580.

386. Kemppainen NM, Aalto S, Wilson IA, et al. PET amyloid ligand [11C]PIB uptake is increased in mild cognitive impairment. *Neurology.* 2007;68(19):1603-1606.

387. Li Y, Rinne JO, Mosconi L, et al. Regional analysis of FDG and PIB-PET images in normal aging, mild cognitive impairment, and Alzheimer's disease. *Eur J Nucl Med Mol Imaging.* 2008;35(12):2169-2181.

388. Lowe VJ, Kemp BJ, Jack CR Jr, et al. Comparison of 18F-FDG and PiB PET in cognitive impairment. *J Nucl Med.* 2009;50(6):878-886.

389. Mintun MA, Larossa GN, Sheline YI, et al. [11C]PIB in a nondemented population: potential antecedent marker of Alzheimer disease. *Neurology.* 2006;67(3):446-452.

390. Ng S, Villemagne VL, Berlangieri S, et al. Visual assessment versus quantitative assessment of 11C-PIB PET and 18F-FDG PET for detection of Alzheimer's disease. *J Nucl Med.* 2007;48(4):547-552.

391. Pike KE, Savage G, Villemagne VL, et al. Beta-amyloid imaging and memory in non-demented individuals: evidence for preclinical Alzheimer's disease. *Brain.* 2007;130(Pt 11):2837-2844.

392. Rabinovici GD, Furst AJ, O'Neil JP, et al. 11C-PIB PET imaging in Alzheimer disease and frontotemporal lobar degeneration. *Neurology*. 2007;68(15):1205-1212.

393. Rowe CC, Ng S, Ackermann U, et al. Imaging beta-amyloid burden in aging and dementia. *Neurology*. 2007;68(20):1718-1725.

394. Wiley CA, Lopresti BJ, Venneti S, et al. Carbon 11-labeled Pittsburgh Compound B and carbon 11-labeled (R)-PK11195 positron emission tomographic imaging in Alzheimer disease. *Arch Neurol*. 2009;66(1):60-67.

395. Ziolko SK, Weissfeld LA, Klunk WE, et al. Evaluation of voxel-based methods for the statistical analysis of PIB PET amyloid imaging studies in Alzheimer's disease. *Neuroimage*. 2006;33(1):94-102.

396. Edison P, Archer HA, Hinz R, et al. Amyloid, hypometabolism, and cognition in Alzheimer disease: an [11C]PIB and [18F]FDG PET study. *Neurology*. 2007;68(7):501-508.

397. Engler H, Forsberg A, Almkvist O, et al. Two-year follow-up of amyloid deposition in patients with Alzheimer's disease. *Brain*. 2006;129(Pt 11):2856-2866.

398. Forsberg A, Engler H, Almkvist O, et al. PET imaging of amyloid deposition in patients with mild cognitive impairment. *Neurobiol Aging*. 2008;29(10):1456-1465.

399. Grimmer T, Henriksen G, Wester HJ, et al. Clinical severity of Alzheimer's disease is associated with PIB uptake in PET. *Neurobiol Aging*. 2009;30(12):1902-1909.

400. Villemagne VL, Pike KE, Darby D, et al. Abeta deposits in older non-demented individuals with cognitive decline are indicative of preclinical Alzheimer's disease. *Neuropsychologia*. 2008;46(6):1688-1697.

401. Dickerson BC, Bakkour A, Salat DH, et al. The cortical signature of Alzheimer's disease: regionally specific cortical thinning relates to symptom severity in very mild to mild AD dementia and is detectable in asymptomatic amyloid-positive individuals. *Cereb Cortex*. 2009;19(3): 497-510.

402. Kemppainen NM, Aalto S, Karrasch M, et al. Cognitive reserve hypothesis: Pittsburgh Compound B and fluorodeoxyglucose positron emission tomography in relation to education in mild Alzheimer's disease. *Ann Neurol*. 2008;63(1):112-118.

403. Fagan AM, Mintun MA, Mach RH, et al. Inverse relation between in vivo amyloid imaging load and cerebrospinal fluid Abeta42 in humans. *Ann Neurol*. 2006;59(3): 512-519.

404. Grimmer T, Riemenschneider M, Forstl H, et al. Beta amyloid in Alzheimer's disease: increased deposition in brain is reflected in reduced concentration in cerebrospinal fluid. *Biol Psychiatry*. 2009;65(11):927-934.

405. Koivunen J, Pirttila T, Kemppainen N, et al. PET amyloid ligand [11C]PIB uptake and cerebrospinal fluid beta-amyloid in mild cognitive impairment. *Dement Geriatr Cogn Disord*. 2008;26(4):378-383.

406. Klunk WE, Mathis CA, Price JC, Lopresti BJ, DeKosky ST. Two-year follow-up of amyloid deposition in patients with Alzheimer's disease. *Brain*. 2006;129(Pt 11): 2805-2807.

407. Price JC, Klunk WE, Lopresti BJ, et al. Kinetic modeling of amyloid binding in humans using PET imaging and Pittsburgh Compound-B. *J Cereb Blood Flow Metab*. 2005;25(11):1528-1547.

408. Wolk DA, Price JC, Saxton JA, et al. Amyloid imaging in mild cognitive impairment subtypes. *Ann Neurol*. 2009;65(5):557-568.

409. Okello A, Koivunen J, Edison P, et al. Conversion of amyloid positive and negative MCI to AD over 3 years: an 11C-PIB PET study. *Neurology*. 2009;73(10):754-760.

410. Aizenstein HJ, Nebes RD, Saxton JA, et al. Frequent amyloid deposition without significant cognitive impairment among the elderly. *Arch Neurol*. 2008;65(11):1509-1517.

411. Reiman EM, Chen K, Liu X, et al. Fibrillar amyloid-beta burden in cognitively normal people at 3 levels of genetic risk for Alzheimer's disease. *Proc Natl Acad Sci U S A*. 2009;106(16):6820-6825.

412. Davies P, Maloney AJ. Selective loss of central cholinergic neurons in Alzheimer's disease. *Lancet*. 1976;2(8000): 1403.

413. Bohnen NI, Kaufer DI, Ivanco LS, et al. Cortical cholinergic function is more severely affected in parkinsonian dementia than in Alzheimer disease: an in vivo positron emission tomographic study. *Arch Neurol*. 2003;60(12): 1745-1748.

414. Davis KL, Mohs RC, Marin D, et al. Cholinergic markers in elderly patients with early signs of Alzheimer disease. *JAMA*. 1999;281(15):1401-1406.

415. Eggers C, Herholz K, Kalbe E, Heiss WD. Cortical acetylcholine esterase activity and ApoE4-genotype in Alzheimer disease. *Neurosci Lett*. 2006;408(1):46-50.

416. Herholz K, Weisenbach S, Zundorf G, et al. In vivo study of acetylcholine esterase in basal forebrain, amygdala, and cortex in mild to moderate Alzheimer disease. *Neuroimage*. 2004;21(1):136-143.

417. Iyo M, Namba H, Fukushi K, et al. Measurement of acetylcholinesterase by positron emission tomography in the brains of healthy controls and patients with Alzheimer's disease. *Lancet*. 1997;349(9068):1805-1809.

418. Kuhl DE, Koeppe RA, Minoshima S, et al. In vivo mapping of cerebral acetylcholinesterase activity in aging and Alzheimer's disease. *Neurology*. 1999;52(4):691-699.

419. Poirier J, Delisle MC, Quirion R, et al. Apolipoprotein E4 allele as a predictor of cholinergic deficits and treatment outcome in Alzheimer disease. *Proc Natl Acad Sci U S A*. 1995;92(26):12260-12264.

420. Rinne JO, Kaasinen V, Jarvenpaa T, et al. Brain acetylcholinesterase activity in mild cognitive impairment and early Alzheimer's disease. *J Neurol Neurosurg Psychiatry*. 2003;74(1):113-115.

421. Shinotoh H, Namba H, Fukushi K, et al. Progressive loss of cortical acetylcholinesterase activity in association with cognitive decline in Alzheimer's disease: a positron emission tomography study. *Ann Neurol*. 2000;48(2):194-200.

422. Herholz K, Weisenbach S, Kalbe E, Diederich NJ, Heiss WD. Cerebral acetylcholine esterase activity in mild cognitive impairment. *Neuroreport*. 2005;16(13):1431-1434.

423. Bohnen NI, Kaufer DI, Hendrickson R, et al. Degree of inhibition of cortical acetylcholinesterase activity and cognitive effects by donepezil treatment in Alzheimer's disease. *J Neurol Neurosurg Psychiatry*. 2005;76(3): 315-319.

424. Shinotoh H, Aotsuka A, Fukushi K, et al. Effect of donepezil on brain acetylcholinesterase activity in patients with AD measured by PET. *Neurology*. 2001;56(3):408-410.

425. O'Brien JT, Colloby SJ, Pakrasi S, et al. Alpha4beta2 nicotinic receptor status in Alzheimer's disease using 123I-5IA-85380 single-photon-emission computed tomography. *J Neurol Neurosurg Psychiatry.* 2007;78(4):356-362.

426. Sabri O, Kendziorra K, Wolf H, Gertz HJ, Brust P. Acetylcholine receptors in dementia and mild cognitive impairment. *Eur J Nucl Med Mol Imaging.* 2008;35(Suppl 1):S30-S45.

427. Fukuchi K, Hashikawa K, Seike Y, et al. Comparison of iodine-123-iomazenil SPECT and technetium-99m-HMPAO-SPECT in Alzheimer's disease. *J Nucl Med.* 1997;38(3):467-470.

428. Soricelli A, Postiglione A, Grivet-Fojaja MR, et al. Reduced cortical distribution volume of iodine-123 iomazenil in Alzheimer's disease as a measure of loss of synapses. *Eur J Nucl Med.* 1996;23(10):1323-1328.

429. Blin J, Baron JC, Dubois B, et al. Loss of brain 5-HT2 receptors in Alzheimer's disease. In vivo assessment with positron emission tomography and [18F]setoperone. *Brain.* 1993;116(Pt 3):497-510.

430. Hasselbalch SG, Madsen K, Svarer C, et al. Reduced 5-HT2A receptor binding in patients with mild cognitive impairment. *Neurobiol Aging.* 2008;29(12):1830-1838.

431. Kepe V, Barrio JR, Huang SC, et al. Serotonin 1A receptors in the living brain of Alzheimer's disease patients. *Proc Natl Acad Sci U S A.* 2006;103(3):702-707.

432. Meltzer CC, Price JC, Mathis CA, et al. PET imaging of serotonin type 2A receptors in late-life neuropsychiatric disorders. *Am J Psychiatry.* 1999;156(12):1871-1878.

433. Versijpt J, Van Laere KJ, Dumont F, et al. Imaging of the 5-HT2A system: age-, gender-, and Alzheimer's disease-related findings. *Neurobiol Aging.* 2003;24(4):553-561.

434. Kemppainen N, Laine M, Laakso MP, et al. Hippocampal dopamine D2 receptors correlate with memory functions in Alzheimer's disease. *Eur J Neurosci.* 2003;18(1):149-154.

435. Kemppainen N, Ruottinen H, Nagren K, Rinne JO. PET shows that striatal dopamine D1 and D2 receptors are differentially affected in AD. *Neurology.* 2000;55(2):205-209.

436. Meguro K, Yamaguchi S, Itoh M, Fujiwara T, Yamadori A. Striatal dopamine metabolism correlated with frontotemporal glucose utilization in Alzheimer's disease: a double-tracer PET study. *Neurology.* 1997;49(4):941-945.

437. Pizzolato G, Chierichetti F, Fabbri M, et al. Reduced striatal dopamine receptors in Alzheimer's disease: single photon emission tomography study with the D2 tracer [123I]-IBZM. *Neurology.* 1996;47(4):1065-1068.

438. Haga S, Akai K, Ishii T. Demonstration of microglial cells in and around senile (neuritic) plaques in the Alzheimer brain. An immunohistochemical study using a novel monoclonal antibody. *Acta Neuropathol.* 1989;77(6):569-575.

439. Venneti S, Wiley CA, Kofler J. Imaging microglial activation during neuroinflammation and Alzheimer's disease. *J Neuroimmune Pharmacol.* 2009;4(2):227-243.

440. Cagnin A, Brooks DJ, Kennedy AM, et al. In-vivo measurement of activated microglia in dementia. *Lancet.* 2001;358(9280):461-467.

441. Edison P, Archer HA, Gerhard A, et al. Microglia, amyloid, and cognition in Alzheimer's disease: an [11C](R) PK11195-PET and [11C]PIB-PET study. *Neurobiol Dis.* 2008;32(3):412-419.

442. Okello A, Edison P, Archer HA, et al. Microglial activation and amyloid deposition in mild cognitive impairment: a PET study. *Neurology.* 2009;72(1):56-62.

443. Tomasi G, Edison P, Bertoldo A, et al. Novel reference region model reveals increased microglial and reduced vascular binding of 11C-(R)-PK11195 in patients with Alzheimer's disease. *J Nucl Med.* 2008;49(8):1249-1256.

444. Versijpt JJ, Dumont F, Van Laere KJ, et al. Assessment of neuroinflammation and microglial activation in Alzheimer's disease with radiolabelled PK11195 and single photon emission computed tomography. A pilot study. *Eur Neurol.* 2003;50(1):39-47.

445. Yasuno F, Ota M, Kosaka J, et al. Increased binding of peripheral benzodiazepine receptor in Alzheimer's disease measured by positron emission tomography with [11C] DAA1106. *Biol Psychiatry.* 2008;64(10):835-841.

446. Groom GN, Junck L, Foster NL, Frey KA, Kuhl DE. PET of peripheral benzodiazepine binding sites in the microgliosis of Alzheimer's disease. *J Nucl Med.* 1995;36(12):2207-2210.

447. O'Brien JT. Role of imaging techniques in the diagnosis of dementia. *Br J Radiol.* 2007;80(Spec No 2):S71-S77.

448. Roman GC, Tatemichi TK, Erkinjuntti T, et al. Vascular dementia: diagnostic criteria for research studies. Report of the NINDS-AIREN International Workshop. *Neurology.* 1993;43(2):250-260.

449. Kalaria RN. Small vessel disease and Alzheimer's dementia: pathological considerations. *Cerebrovasc Dis.* 2002;13(Suppl 2):48-52.

450. Kalaria RN. Vascular factors in Alzheimer's disease. *Int Psychogeriatr.* 2003;15(Suppl 1):47-52.

451. Mills S, Cain J, Purandare N, Jackson A. Biomarkers of cerebrovascular disease in dementia. *Br J Radiol.* 2007;80(Spec No 2):S128-S145.

452. De Groot JC, De Leeuw FE, Oudkerk M, et al. Periventricular cerebral white matter lesions predict rate of cognitive decline. *Ann Neurol.* 2002;52(3):335-341.

453. Meyer JS, Rauch GM, Crawford K, et al. Risk factors accelerating cerebral degenerative changes, cognitive decline and dementia. *Int J Geriatr Psychiatry.* 1999;14(12):1050-1061.

454. McKeith IG, Dickson DW, Lowe J, et al. Diagnosis and management of dementia with Lewy bodies: third report of the DLB Consortium. *Neurology.* 2005;65(12):1863-1872.

455. Burton EJ, Karas G, Paling SM, et al. Patterns of cerebral atrophy in dementia with Lewy bodies using voxel-based morphometry. *Neuroimage.* 2002;17(2):618-630.

456. Whitwell JL, Weigand SD, Shiung MM, et al. Focal atrophy in dementia with Lewy bodies on MRI: a distinct pattern from Alzheimer's disease. *Brain.* 2007;130(Pt 3):708-719.

457. Ishii K, Hosaka K, Mori T, Mori E. Comparison of FDG-PET and IMP-SPECT in patients with dementia with Lewy bodies. *Ann Nucl Med.* 2004;18(5):447-451.

458. Lobotesis K, Fenwick JD, Phipps A, et al. Occipital hypoperfusion on SPECT in dementia with Lewy bodies but not AD. *Neurology.* 2001;56(5):643-649.

459. O'Brien JT, Colloby S, Fenwick J, et al. Dopamine transporter loss visualized with FP-CIT SPECT in the differential diagnosis of dementia with Lewy bodies. *Arch Neurol.* 2004;61(6):919-925.

460. Colloby SJ, Williams ED, Burn DJ, Lloyd JJ, McKeith IG, O'Brien JT. Progression of dopaminergic degeneration in dementia with Lewy bodies and Parkinson's disease with and without dementia assessed using 123I-FP-CIT SPECT. *Eur J Nucl Med Mol Imaging*. 2005;32(10):1176-1185.

461. McKeith I, O'Brien J, Walker Z, et al. Sensitivity and specificity of dopamine transporter imaging with 123I-FP-CIT SPECT in dementia with Lewy bodies: a phase III, multicentre study. *Lancet Neurol*. 2007;6(4):305-313.

462. Boxer AL, Miller BL. Clinical features of frontotemporal dementia. *Alzheimer Dis Assoc Disord*. 2005;19(Suppl 1):S3-S6.

463. Du AT, Schuff N, Kramer JH, et al. Different regional patterns of cortical thinning in Alzheimer's disease and frontotemporal dementia. *Brain*. 2007;130(Pt 4):1159-1166.

464. Good CD, Scahill RI, Fox NC, et al. Automatic differentiation of anatomical patterns in the human brain: validation with studies of degenerative dementias. *Neuroimage*. 2002;17(1):29-46.

465. Laakso MP, Frisoni GB, Kononen M, et al. Hippocampus and entorhinal cortex in frontotemporal dementia and Alzheimer's disease: a morphometric MRI study. *Biol Psychiatry*. 2000;47(12):1056-1063.

466. Whitwell JL, Jack CR Jr, Baker M, et al. Voxel-based morphometry in frontotemporal lobar degeneration with ubiquitin-positive inclusions with and without progranulin mutations. *Arch Neurol*. 2007;64(3):371-376.

467. Whitwell JL, Jack CR Jr, Parisi JE, et al. Rates of cerebral atrophy differ in different degenerative pathologies. *Brain*. 2007;130(Pt 4):1148-1158.

468. Whitwell JL, Jack CR Jr, Senjem ML, Josephs KA. Patterns of atrophy in pathologically confirmed FTLD with and without motor neuron degeneration. *Neurology*. 2006;66(1): 102-104.

469. Galton CJ, Patterson K, Graham K, et al. Differing patterns of temporal atrophy in Alzheimer's disease and semantic dementia. *Neurology*. 2001;57(2):216-225.

470. Foster NL, Heidebrink JL, Clark CM, et al. FDG-PET improves accuracy in distinguishing frontotemporal dementia and Alzheimer's disease. *Brain*. 2007;130 (Pt 10):2616-2635.

471. McNeill R, Sare GM, Manoharan M, et al. Accuracy of single-photon emission computed tomography in differentiating frontotemporal dementia from Alzheimer's disease. *J Neurol Neurosurg Psychiatry*. 2007;78(4):350-355.

472. Gatz M, Reynolds CA, Fratiglioni L, et al. Role of genes and environments for explaining Alzheimer disease. *Arch Gen Psychiatry*. 2006;63(2):168-174.

473. Potkin SG, Turner JA, Guffanti G, et al. Genome-wide strategies for discovering genetic influences on cognition and cognitive disorders: methodological considerations. *Cogn Neuropsychiatry*. 2009;14(4-5):391-418.

474. Shen L, Kim S, Risacher SL, et al. Whole genome association study of brain-wide imaging phenotypes for identifying quantitative trait loci in MCI and AD: A study of the ADNI cohort. *Neuroimage*. 2010 Jan 25; in press, doi:10.1016/j.neuroimage.2010.01.042.

475. Storandt M, Grant EA, Miller JP, Morris JC. Longitudinal course and neuropathologic outcomes in original vs revised MCI and in pre-MCI. *Neurology*. 2006;67(3):467-473.

476. Caselli RJ, Reiman EM, Locke DE, et al. Cognitive domain decline in healthy apolipoprotein E epsilon4 homozygotes before the diagnosis of mild cognitive impairment. *Arch Neurol*. 2007;64(9):1306-1311.

477. Jack CR Jr, Petersen RC, Grundman M, et al. Longitudinal MRI findings from the vitamin E and donepezil treatment study for MCI. *Neurobiol Aging*. 2008;29(9):1285-1295.

478. Fox NC, Black RS, Gilman S, et al. Effects of Abeta immunization (AN1792) on MRI measures of cerebral volume in Alzheimer disease. *Neurology*. 2005;64(9):1563-1572.

479. Fox NC, Cousens S, Scahill R, Harvey RJ, Rossor MN. Using serial registered brain magnetic resonance imaging to measure disease progression in Alzheimer disease: power calculations and estimates of sample size to detect treatment effects. *Arch Neurol*. 2000;57(3):339-344.

480. Mechelli A, Price CJ, Friston KJ, Ashburner J. Voxel-based morphometry of the human brain: methods and applications. *Curr Med Imaging Rev*. 2005;1(1):1-9.

Chapter 20
Application of Neuroimaging Methods to Define Cognitive and Brain Abnormalities Associated with HIV

Jodi Heaps, Jennifer Niehoff, Elizabeth Lane, Kuryn Kroutil, Joseph Boggiano, and Robert Paul

Introduction

Human immunodeficiency virus (HIV) is a retrovirus that invades and inactivates T-lymphocyte cells of the immune system leading to Acquired Immune Deficiency Syndrome (AIDS). In 2007, there were 33 million people living with HIV. That year alone, 2.7 million people became infected with the virus, and 2 million people died of HIV-related causes.[1] These numbers are not evenly distributed globally and tend to be disproportionately concentrated in countries least able to financially shoulder the burden of providing medical care to patients. In 2007, an estimated 1.9 million people were newly infected with HIV in sub-Saharan Africa, bringing the total number of people living with HIV to 22 million in that area. The number of people infected in sub-Saharan Africa represents a full 67% of the global total of people with HIV, and 75% of all AIDS deaths in 2007.[1]

In 1996, combinations of antiretroviral medications known as highly active antiretroviral therapy (HAART) were introduced to treat HIV-positive individuals. The use of antiretroviral drugs effectively suppresses viral replication and reconstitutes immune function to levels that prevent the development of opportunistic infections that were so often fatal prior to the advent of combination therapy. Without HAART, the life expectancy of a patient from time of infection was 11 years, but with medications patients are living in excess of 20 years.[1] Longer life expectancy in patients and continued incidence of new

infections is resulting in an ever increasing number of people living with chronic HIV.

Even though HAART has been very effective at restoring immune function, it tends to have poor penetration into the central nervous system (CNS).[2] This is a primary concern as HIV enters the CNS and exerts a variety of deleterious effects soon after systemic infection. The virus crosses the blood–brain barrier (BBB) via infected macrophages, infected cell transmission across the choroid plexus,[3] and the passage of free virons across areas of damaged BBB.[4] Neuronal damage is not caused by direct infection of the virus, but indirectly through the inflammatory response to infection of macrophages and microglia with the virus and the build-up of inflammatory cytokines. Ensuing cognitive dysfunction manifests as a frontal–subcortical pattern of impairment with prominent involvement of fine motor movements, learning new information, attention and concentration, and executive functions.

The most recent terminology to classify varying degrees of cognitive impairment takes into account not only decreases in cognitive performance (as demonstrated through neuropsychological testing) but also the impact these cognitive declines have on everyday functioning or activities of daily living.[5] Additional criteria consider the presence of other comorbid diseases, disorders, or substance abuse related to cognitive dysfunction, and whether or not the observable impairment meets criteria for delirium or dementia.[5] A patient who shows impairment in at least two domains of cognitive function without any observed or self-reported difficulties with everyday functions may be classified as having asymptomatic cognitive impairment (ANI). To qualify for a diagnosis of mild neurocognitive disorder (MND) patients must demonstrate impairment in at least two cognitive domains, however, the impairments must also interfere mildly with

R. Paul (✉)
Department of Psychology, Division of Behavioral Neuroscience, University of Missouri, One University Blvd., Stadler, 412, St. Louis, MO 63121, USA
e-mail: paulro@umsl.edu

R.A. Cohen and L.H. Sweet (eds.), *Brain Imaging in Behavioral Medicine and Clinical Neuroscience*, DOI 10.1007/978-1-4419-6373-4_20, © Springer Science+Business Media, LLC 2011 everyday functioning validated by self-report or the observation of others. A diagnosis of HIV-associated dementia (HAD) is characterized by more severe impairments in at least two domains of cognitive function, resulting in marked interference with everyday activities, and the impairment does meet criteria for dementia (but cannot meet criteria for delirium). To reiterate an earlier set of diagnostic criteria, ANI, MND, or HAD cannot be diagnosed in the presence of comorbidities that may confound the diagnosis, such as the presence of depression, history of other CNS disorders, opportunistic infections, or active substance abuse.

Comorbid conditions can affect the progression and severity of cognitive disturbances associated with HIV. Individuals coinfected with hepatitis C and HIV, which is fairly common especially in injecting drug users, tend to demonstrate greater cognitive dysfunction than either HIV or hepatitis C.[2] In addition, when compared with HIV patients who do not use illicit drugs, those patients who abuse drugs have more rapid progression to severe forms of neurocognitive dysfunction, and, in fact, some HIV-infected drug abusers may have an accelerated form of HAD.[6] Depression, also commonly observed among HIV patients, can be difficult to distinguish from the initial stages of HAD, with symptoms of fatigue, pain, anorexia, and insomnia common in both conditions.[7] Additionally, depression has been linked to immune suppression and lack of adherence to medication,[8] which can affect progression of neurological symptoms. Another major comorbid condition is age. As the population of HIV patients' ages, the comorbidity of age-related vascular disease, metabolic disturbances, and neurodegenerative diseases with chronic HIV infection complicates diagnosis and treatment of HAD.[9] Finally, emerging data suggest that inflammation and toxicity due to HIV predisposes the brain to pathological effects similar to those seen in Alzheimer's disease (AD) patients.[10]

Longer periods of infection, even with better immune function and lower viral loads due to HAART, have led to a decrease in the incidence of HAD, but an increased prevalence of more mild forms of cognitive dysfunction.[11] The distribution of antiretrovirals across the BBB and into the CNS tends to be poor, but even with effective medication the inflammatory response may continue.[10] Because these inflammatory factors continue in the presence of low viral load and high CD4+ counts, traditional plasma indicators of disease progression have not shown a strong correlation with CNS involvement and cognitive functioning.[11] New indicators of CNS status would prove useful tools in the diagnosis and treatment of HIV-associated cognitive dysfunction.

Common MRI Findings in HIV

Numerous neuroimaging studies have now been completed that describe the neural signatures of HIV-related brain impairment. In this section, we briefly review the literature that provides neuropathological support for the validity of neuroimaging abnormalities in HIV. Studies involving postmortem examinations have verified MRI findings in patients with progressive HIV by demonstrating that cortical atrophy and white matter alterations (WMA) are both present in the brain and relate to the amount of HIV present in the brain, with more pronounced atrophy evident in severe states of infection.[12–17] Jernigan et al.[18] found that nondemented patients with AIDS showed increases in cerebrospinal fluid (CSF) and reduced gray matter volumes compared to asymptomatic HIV-positive individuals and HIV-negative control groups. Although atrophy is related to the severity of HIV infection and neurological complication, a study completed by Post et al.[19] – prior to the introduction of HAART – reported cortical atrophy in both neurologically asymptomatic and symptomatic groups. Among the asymptomatic subjects, seven of 13 individuals with abnormal MRI scans showed mild-to-moderate sulcal enlargement. Of the symptomatic group, five subjects of ten displayed abnormalities, with four of those participants exhibiting sulcal enlargements. Post et al.[20] also found mild to marked cortical atrophy in patients with HIV encephalitis. An additional pre-HAART study using MRI to detect cortical atrophy reported significantly more atrophy, most notably in the temporal lobes, in AIDS patients compared to patients at earlier disease stages.[12] The preceding studies demonstrate that MRI is an effective technique in detecting cortical atrophy in the early manifestation of HIV infection in the brain.

Another common finding in HIV studies is subcortical atrophy, which is more pronounced on MRI as HIV infection progresses.[12–14,17,21–27] Later stages of

HIV infection including AIDS and HAD all show pronounced atrophy in the ventricle and the area around the region of the caudate nucleus.[14,22–26,28] In two additional studies, reduction of gray matter volume, especially in the area of the caudate, was significantly related to HIV dementia, suggesting that atrophy of the basal ganglia and the area of the caudate nucleus are important MRI markers of HIV dementia.[22,29] Aylward et al.,[28] in an MRI study focusing on the basal ganglia, confirmed reports that general atrophy is related to severity of HIV infections and that basal ganglia volumes are significantly related to HIV dementia.

Structural MRI and Cognitive Performance

Volumetric MRI has provided an important method to identify relationships between atrophy, both cortical and subcortical, in HIV and deficits on specific cognitive abilities. Poutiainen et al.[14] found a statistically significant inverse relationship between peripheral atrophy and memory scores in individuals with AIDS. In a study by Harrison et al.,[17] poor results on aspects of verbal memory, psychomotor speed, and cognitive flexibility were specifically related to wide sulci in HIV patients. Levin et al.[13] identified slowing of response speed that was significantly related to severity of cerebral atrophy as measured by the enlargement of ventricular area and CSF space. Patel et al.[15] found a significant negative correlation between atrophy assessed by using whole brain parenchymal volume (PBV) and performance of motor sequencing assessed using the grooved pegboard task.

The severity of atrophy around the caudate nucleus is most often linked to specific cognitive performance deficits in domains of gross motor functioning, mental flexibility, tactile perception, and fine motor skills.[13,15,23–25] A number of studies[23–25] reported statistically significant relationships between caudate volume and neuropsychological performance. Specifically, these studies reported significant relationships between caudate atrophy and fine/complex motor functioning as assessed by using the grooved pegboard test. The relationship between atrophy of the caudate and fine/complex motor skills was the most robust finding, but all three studies also showed a significant relationship between caudate atrophy and mental processing speed.[24,25] MRI in relation to performance on the grooved pegboard test may be a good indicator of change and severity of HIV infection, especially in later stages of HIV (AIDS, HAD). Hestad et al.[23] reported a significant relationship between caudate atrophy and performance on Trails B, a measure of mental flexibility. Recently, in a study by Paul et al.,[30] apathy ratings in HIV patients significantly correlated with nucleus accumbens volume. The degree of apathy was directly related to magnitude of the decrease in volume of the nucleus accumbens. This corroborates earlier findings that the decrement of neurological function relates to the severity of HIV infection (Fig. 20.1).[12–16,23–26,28,29,31,32]

Contrary to the number of studies indicating atrophy in the subcortical region, some recent work has found enlargement of the putamen in HIV-positive patients demonstrating mild cognitive symptoms.[33] The enlarged

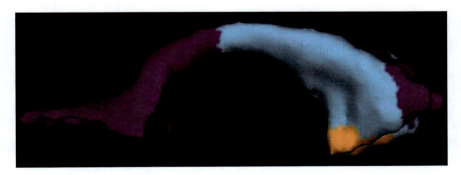

Fig. 20.1 3D reconstruction of the nucleus accumbens (*yellow*) and caudate (*blue*) and lateral ventricles (*purple*). Lower volumes of the nucleus accumbens correlate with increased ratings of apathy and lower volumes of the caudate correlate with poorer performances on tests of executive function among HIV patients

putamen was related to slow motor speed and immune status (left and right putamen, respectively), and the authors suggested that inflammation or dysfunction of the dopamine system in the putamen might explain the findings of hypertrophy in this nucleus. Additional work is needed to determine the evolution of MRI volumetric changes in HIV, and the relationship between these changes and both immune markers and cognitive performance. Once these studies are complete, a more comprehensive understanding of nonlinear changes in brain volume and cognitive status will be obtained.

White Matter Abnormalities in HIV

A second common structural MRI finding in HIV studies includes WMA. As with atrophy, WMA increase in severity with the progression of HIV infection, with the most severe abnormalities in patients with AIDS-related dementia.[16–18,21,26,27,29,31,32,34–37] Studies have also revealed relationships between white matter changes and cognitive performance, but it is important to note that there is no consensus regarding these findings. Harrison et al.[17] identified a[17] significant relationship between patients with changes in white matter and performance on Trails B, symbol digit, and tests in the nonverbal memory domain. Similar results have been reported in other studies[29]; however, there have also been studies finding a relationship between WMA and age, but no relationship was noted between WMA and disease factors.[38]

MRI studies have also been employed to examine the effects of treatment – in the form of HAART, protease inhibitors, and monotherapeutic treatments – on structural changes.[35,39–41] In all instances where treatment was reported, MRI follow-ups showed the regression or halting of WMA and/or atrophy; however, structural observations sometimes took up to 20 months to appear on MRI.[40] These findings show that MRI can be used to track the effectiveness of various treatment regimens through imaging of WMAs and atrophied regions of the brain.

Magnetic Resonance Spectroscopy and HIV

Magnetic resonance spectroscopy (H[1]-MRS) has also been used as a tool to examine the manifestation of HIV damage in the CNS.[4,42,43] Studies have found that H[1]-MRS reliably detects damage, such as AIDS encephalopathy, more effectively than MRI or neuropsychological testing.[42] Proton, or H[1]-MRS, is the most frequently used method of MRS; however, it is also possible to use carbon 13 and phosphorous 31 to measure different compounds associated with cellular processes. Using H[1]-MRS, a number of common metabolite concentrations and ratios have been identified as important markers of inflammation and neuronal decline. In HIV, the most common compounds measured using H[1]-MRS are choline (Cho), creatine (Cr), myo-inositol (mI), and N-acetyl aspartate (NAA) either in absolute concentrations or ratios.[4]

H[1]-MRS is able to detect certain metabolites in the brain and therefore the markers used and the brain regions under review in most studies are relatively standard. Choline is a protein that is often found in membrane structures and is active in phospholipid metabolism in the CNS.[42] Increases in Cho are thought to reflect damage to myelinated tissues.[4,42] Creatine (Cr) is found in similar concentrations throughout gray and white matter and is used by the mitochondria of cells as a component of cellular metabolism. It is often used in ratio with other compounds due to its consistent concentration in the different tissue types. Decreases in Cr indicate a reduction in the normal cellular metabolism. Myo-inositol (mI) is commonly referred to as a glial marker and increases in mI reflect a propagation of astrocytes in damaged tissue, although the increase in mI may reflect other factors as well.[4] Finally, NAA is produced by the mitochondria of neurons and decreases are thought to reflect neuronal damage among other factors.

There is some debate over the use of absolute concentrations or ratios of the metabolites and which is more accurate in identifying CNS damage in HIV. Studies have found significant results using both methods; however, since the metabolites have shown to be affected with relation to the disease,[44] the use of ratios may dilute results compared to absolute concentrations. Furthermore, the use of ratios adds to the complexity of explaining the relationship between the variables and how the disease affects the metabolic processes in the CNS.

Early studies using H[1]-MRS examined differences between HIV-positive patients who demonstrated varying degrees of cognitive changes, from ANI to HAD. Chang et al.[45] measured elevated concentrations of mI and Cho in patients with varying levels of cognitive dysfunction compared to healthy controls, but did not find any differences in NAA between the HIV groups. Low CD4 count and higher CNS viral loads were found to be related to elevated mI and Cho. The researchers postulated that the lack of changes in NAA indicates that neuronal damage is not yet present in early stages of cognitive decline; however, with increasing severity of cognitive impairment reductions in NAA is evident. Meyerhoff et al.[46] observed similar results in subcortical regions, with NAA reduced only in patients who demonstrated severe cognitive impairments. A later study by Chang et al.[44] examined the relationship between metabolite concentrations, CD4, viral loads (plasma and CSF), and performance on an executive function task in HAART naïve patients. They again reported increased mI, Cho, and Cr in frontal areas, but basal ganglia (BG) Cr was reduced. All metabolite changes were related to increasing disease severity. Low CD4 and higher plasma viral load correlated with increased mI. The difference in the levels of Cr between the BG and the frontal region led the researchers to recommend the use of absolute metabolite concentrations rather than ratios to provide more meaningful results. Also, these results are important in understanding how metabolite concentrations may vary among brain regions over the course of the disease.

Additional studies, using multiple imaging techniques, have reported metabolite alterations that correlate with other imaging indices. Functional MRI and MRS have been used in combination to investigate the relationship between metabolites, blood oxygen level-dependent (BOLD) signal and working memory.[47] Paul et al.[48] observed that HIV patients, who scored in the MCI range for ADC, had higher levels of Cho/Cr and lower levels of NAA/Cho in the putamen of the basal ganglia compared to controls. Using quantitative MRI, putamen size correlated significantly with the NAA/Cr ratio in the basal ganglia, while all other MRI and MRS correlations were not significant. Sacktor et al.,[49] as part of a multicenter study, investigated both single voxel-MRS (SV-MRS) and MRS together to determine the possibility of using both to detect metabolite abnormalities. The different techniques use different echo times and voxel sizes in MRS are slightly smaller than in SV-MRS, but both produced results indicating alterations in the metabolites. Specifically, impaired HIV patients had reduced NAA/Cr in frontal white matter using SV-MRS. Using MRS, impaired HIV patients had increased Cho/Cr and reduced NAA/Cr in the caudate compared with HIV patients who demonstrated no impairments.

There are a number of factors beyond HIV alone that investigators consider when studying MRS indices in this population. The use of antiretroviral medication, current and prior drug use, and age all could impact the metabolite concentrations found using H^1-MRS. Age has been used as a covariate in a number of the studies and has been shown to attenuate the relationships between disease and NAA values.[50,51] Additionally, Chang et al.[45] reported normalization of some MRS metabolites after HAART though it remains unclear if these alterations hold over time.

A few studies have reported the effects of methamphetamine use, marijuana use, and alcoholism on MRS indices in HIV.[52-54] Chang et al.[52] determined that HIV subjects with a history of chronic methamphetamine use demonstrated additive effects of HIV and drug use resulting in significantly lower NAA in the three regions measured (BG, FWM, FGM) and increased mI in FWM compared to HIV-negative patients with no drug use. NAA and Cr reductions were observed in the cortexes of HIV-positive (without HAD diagnosis) patients with alcoholism.[54] The investigators noted that when the metabolites were expressed as a ratio, the results were nonsignificant, again indicating the benefits of using absolute measures of metabolites over the use of ratios. Also, neither groups of individuals with HIV nor alcoholism alone showed significant metabolite abnormalities.

The use of marijuana is common in HIV patients, but there are very few studies reporting the possible effects of the drug on cognitive function in HIV. In 2006, a study by Chang et al.[53] identified a combined effect of chronic marijuana use and HIV on increased Cr in the thalamus. Additionally, the team examined glutamate levels and reported a reduction in glutamate in frontal white matter in the HIV and marijuana groups individually. Reductions in glutamate could be due to a disruption of neuronal or glial processes. Interestingly, the HIV-positive group who used marijuana chronically demonstrated near-normal glutamate levels in the frontal region. Additional research needs to be done in this area in order to determine the combined effects of HIV and drug use on metabolite concentrations and CNS functional integrity.

Sample sizes used in most HIV neuroimaging studies are often small and consist of samples selected on criteria that differ across studies. These differences as well as the use of various methods of image acquisition can affect the results of the studies. The HIV-MRS Consortium was formed to help diminish the effects of these differences and find regional effects of HIV using MRS.[55] Lee and colleagues conducted a preliminary study to determine the reliability of multiple centers using H[1]-MRS to examine metabolite differences in the CNS of HIV patients. Importantly, the consortium identified elevated Cho/Cr and mI/Cr ratios in the BG of HAD participants compared to controls. Also, mI/Cr ratios were elevated in FWM and NAA/Cr were reduced in the HAD group in the FWM. A follow-up study examined metabolite patterns in HIV patients with ADC, HIV neuroasymptomatic (NAS) patients, and a control group to compare metabolite ratios and their relationships with clinical markers such as CD4, viral loads, and effects of aging.[56] The ratios of mI/Cr and Cho/Cr were elevated for the NAS patients compared with controls and further elevated for the ADC group in the BG and FWM. Additionally, NA/Cr in the FWM was reduced in the ADC group compared with NAS. CSF viral load correlated with the metabolites in the white matter, and HIV and aging showed additive effects on the Cho/Cr and mI/Cr ratios in the BG independent of dementia severity. These results are similar to the early findings, with a pattern of subcortical alteration in glial metabolites even in NAS patients, and reductions in NA compounds (marking neuronal loss) only found with more severe cognitive impairment.

HIV and fMRI

Functional MRI (fMRI) is used to determine changes in the blood oxygenation level-dependent (BOLD) signal during MRI. The BOLD signal provides a measure of changes in the regional blood flow during specific cognitive tasks. While the BOLD signal arises from changes in blood flow and not from changes in neuronal activity, these changes correlate with activity at the neuronal level. Studies using fMRI have often used a clinical and control sample to compare activation changes in the brain during specific cognitive tasks. The use of fMRI in HIV populations is still a relatively novel approach as few studies have employed this type of imaging to date.

The fronto-striatal circuit has been heavily studied with regard to HIV, since most of the damage seen in HIV patients occurs in this network and is associated with the executive function deficits identified in this population. An fMRI study by Melrose et al.[57] investigated the difference in the prefrontal cortex and basal ganglia between an HIV-positive group and healthy controls by using a semantic event sequencing task, previously found to activate the prefrontal cortex and basal ganglia, to determine if this system was affected by the disease. Functional connectivity analysis revealed that the HIV group had greater connectivity between the basal ganglia and the anterior parietal regions, as opposed to the control group that had greater connectivity between the basal ganglia and the prefrontal cortex. Additionally, these changes appeared to have taken place prior to any significant volumetric changes within these structures in the HIV group, suggesting that the metabolite alterations may precede anatomical changes.

Attention and memory are both heavily studied within the area of HIV and fMRI. Both of these abilities, along with other executive functions, are dependent upon an intact fronto-striatal system in the brain. Studies have consistently found deficits in these areas and evidence for these deficits on fMRI. One such study by Chang et al.[58] observed that on tasks of working memory and attention subjects with HIV activated the same areas as controls and displayed greater activation in several other areas. As task difficulty increased, individuals with HIV showed greater BOLD activation in the left prefrontal cortex and supplementary motor areas, both of which are areas adjacent to or in the periphery of the normal activation regions.

In an fMRI study on attention, Chang et al.[59] observed the recruitment of additional areas of the brain in the HIV group compared to the control group, though no differences in performance on the task was noted. The additionally recruited areas in the HIV group were peripheral, adjacent, or contralateral to the regions activated in the healthy controls. Additionally, HIV individuals exhibited less activation in the traditional attention networks, including the prefrontal, dorsal, parietal, and cerebellar regions.

In a study of working memory, asymptomatic HIV subjects were found to have greater BOLD activation and activation volume in the lateral prefrontal cortex compared with healthy controls, even when their performances were the same on neuropsychological tests.[60] Another study by Ernst et al.[47] used both fMRI and MRS to investigate whether glial markers showing abnormal brain metabolism correlated with BOLD acquisition on fMRI. Positive correlations between BOLD signal strength and glial metabolites such as Cho, mI, and Cr were noted, but no relationship with NAA were observed, leading the researchers to determine that glial changes may reduce processing efficiency without marked neuronal changes taking place. Results also indicated that glial markers in the basal ganglia and frontal white matter correlate with BOLD signal, suggesting that working memory deficits may be driven by glial abnormalities and inflammation in these areas.

Although the majority of the literature has focused on the damage that takes place involving the fronto-striatal system, some evidence suggests that HIV also causes damage to the hippocampal region of the brain. To investigate this relationship, Castelo et al.[61] employed an episodic memory task to determine whether the BOLD signal was different in HIV individuals. The results indicated a decreased signal in the medial temporal regions and areas of the prefrontal cortex with increased activation in the frontal and parietal regions surrounding the prefrontal area normally associated with this task. This study suggests the possible role of hippocampal damage in HIV. A recent study[62] employed fMRI to investigate hippocampal function during episodic memory tasks in HIV-positive and HIV-negative women.[62] The results indicated a decrease in bilateral hippocampal activation during the encoding phase of the task and increased activation during the delayed recognition task in the HIV-positive group compared with the HIV-negative group. The differences in activation also correlated with worse performance on the episodic verbal memory task.

A limitation to fMRI studies specific to HIV is that not many studies have looked at whether there are alterations in the hemodynamic blood flow of HIV positive individuals. This is important to investigate, since fMRI is dependent upon normal blood flow in the brain. If HIV results in altered blood flow in the brain, then comparisons to healthy controls will not necessarily indicate differences in blood flow due to neuronal activation. One such study[63] noted significant differences in HIV/AIDS patients when stratified on their neurological symptoms.[63] The patients who exhibited neurological symptoms displayed significantly longer hemodynamic response compared with asymptomatic HIV/AIDS patients. More studies of the same nature should be done in order to investigate this issue and determine the utility of using fMRI in an HIV population.

Diffusion Tensor Imaging and HIV

Diffusion tensor imaging (DTI) is a magnetic resonance imaging technique utilizing diffusion gradients to measure directional diffusion of water molecules. In white matter tracts, diffusion occurs most easily along the length of the axon. Damage to myelin, inflammation, or damage to the axon is reflected in increased diffusion perpendicular to axons. This indicator of integrity of white matter tracts makes DTI especially useful in studying diseases associated with demyelination and altered neuronal integrity.[64]

DTI is a powerful imaging method to understand neuropathogenesis in this population due to the impact of HIV on the brain white matter. Thurnher et al.[65] examined frontal white matter using measures of both fractional anisotropy (FA) and apparent diffusion coefficient (ADC). FA is a scalar measure of the degree of anisotropy or directional movement of water, in a given voxel. Low FA values indicate low directionality of diffusion and therefore loss of axonal organization. ADC measures the magnitude of random diffusion, with low values indicating little random diffusivity, and therefore intact organization of white matter tracts, and high values indicating a loss of this organization. Thurnher et al.[65] reported both reduced FA and increased ADC in frontal white matter of HIV patients when compared with healthy controls. These results would seem to support the use of DTI for determining white matter changes in HIV, but as the results were not statistically significant, the authors concluded that the imaging, as conducted, was not a useful tool for detecting frontal white matter damage in HIV.

DTI has been used to examine the status of the entire brain in HIV patients. In two studies, one research identified reduced whole brain FA among HIV patients compared with healthy controls, and these reduced values were significantly associated with severity of dementia on multiple standardized measures.[66] ADC values generally tend to increase with the severity of dementia. Evaluation of the whole brain using DTI could prove useful in determining general extent of CNS involvement in HIV infection.

Memory difficulties have been observed in HIV patients, leading researchers to examine damage to the hippocampus. Thurnher et al.[65] identified both reduced FA values and higher ADC values in the hippocampi of HIV patients when compared with healthy controls, though the differences did not reach statistical significance. DTI has also been utilized to identify neuropathological abnormalities in the basal ganglia. Ragin et al.[67] compared FA and mean diffusivity (MD) values with test results for various cognitive domains. MD is similar to ADC and is referred to as a scalar measure of the total diffusion within a determined volume of tissue, with low values indicating low diffusion of water within tissue. This study also examined the caudate and putamen of HIV patients and reported significant relationships between increased MD in the putamen and verbal memory deficits. Significant correlations were also observed with FA measurements of both caudate and putamen related to measures of visual memory, and reduced FA values in the putamen were significantly correlated with working memory deficits. FA values in the putamen were also significantly correlated with overall degree of impairment in HIV patients, as ascertained by the average of all measured cognitive functions. Other studies have reported relationships between reduced FA in the white matter of HIV patients and performance on tests of visuoconstruction.[67]

A few DTI studies have examined the corpus callosum in HIV patients. Thurnher et al.[65] reported that the FA values in the genu were significantly reduced in HIV patients when compared with healthy controls. FA values for the splenium were also reduced, but not significantly, and ADC values were higher in the genu in HIV-positive patients than in controls. Further, ADC values were higher in the splenium, but not to the level of statistical significance observed in additional studies. Wu et al.[3] reported that the reduced FA in the splenium of HIV patients was significantly correlated with multiple standardized measures of dementia. The MD values for the splenium of HIV patients were significantly increased over that of control subjects. Both the FA and MD alterations observed in HIV patients were also significantly correlated with measures of motor speed. The results from the Wu et al. study indicate that DTI might be a useful tool in predicting cognitive decline. Most recently, researchers have looked at the axial and radial diffusivity values and found that HIV had a larger effect on radial diffusivity compared with axial diffusivity, which could indicate that disease progresses primarily due to demyelinating processes.[68]

New Imaging Possibilities in HIV

Several new methods of imaging have significant promise in assessing the structural brain changes and cognitive dysfunction in HIV infection. Few of these methods have been cited in the literature in brain imaging of HIV infection to date though it is expected subsequent studies will incorporate these methods with greater frequency. In this section, we review a few methods that have significant potential to enhance our understanding of HIV neuropathogenesis, including arterial spin labeling (ASL), quantified tractography in DTI, diffusion spectrum imaging (DSI), and near-infrared light imaging.

ASL is a method of perfusion imaging, which utilizes magnetically inverted water movement to measure blood flow to tissue. The inverted water molecules are labeled and used as endogenous tracers within vessels.[69] Water movement can be measured in both gray and white matter, but is measured primarily in small vessels and the tissue around them.[70] ASL is generally separated into two techniques, pulsed and continuous. A recent study used continuous ASL to assess caudate blood flow and volume in an HIV-infected population.[71] Results indicate reduced blood flow and volume in the caudate among individuals with cognitive impairment compared with (healthy) controls. This finding is important, because blood flow changes may precede changes in structural integrity and may also be related to the degree of cognitive impairment in this population. Additionally, ASL can be employed in functional studies to assess brain activation during tasks.[72] This method may be useful in individuals with HIV because impairment is seen in multiple areas of cognition. It may be possible to quantify activity in differing areas of the brain while monitoring pathway disconnections associated with impaired functioning by assessing the amount of water movement using ASL during cognitive tasks. Another new method of ASL, velocity selective ASL, may prove useful in assessing inflow to structures and measuring tissue damage.[73]

Velocity selective ASL (VSASL) is another method of perfusion tensor imaging. Again, VSASL has the potential to measure local inflow to structures to determine tissue damage.[73] A unique characteristic of VSASL is that it is not dependent upon a spatiotemporal delay, unlike pulsed and continuous ASL, making it a superior method of measuring inflow to areas of low perfusion. Continuous and pulsed ASL are dependent upon the spatiotemporal delay related to the time needed for the inverted hydrogen molecules to reach the region of interest, potentially causing measurement errors. VSASL, on the other hand, measures hydrogen moving at a specified velocity[74] resulting in fewer measurement errors.[74] Thus, VSASL may be superior over pulsed or continuous ASL in measuring blood flow in damaged or occluded brain structures.

Quantified tractography is used as a metric for measuring specific orientation and curvature[75] of white matter pathways to determine structural integrity in DTI.[76] Changes in the white matter due to damage or pathology, as measured by a decrease in linear anisotropy possibly due to axonal loss[77] reflect changes in tractography generated streamtube algorithms. The streamtubes may increase or decrease in number and length, depending on the type of white matter damage. Thus, by measuring the change in streamtube algorithms, changes in white matter integrity can be quantified. Using this method, it may be possible to observe subtle pathway differences between diseased and healthy populations[76] including HIV.[76] A study by Paul et al.[78] used quantified DTI and FLAIR imaging in addition to a neuropsychological evaluation to determine the integrity of brain systems in an HIV-infected individual with progressive multifocal leukoencephalopathy. Results indicated the patient performed significantly worse than HIV monoinfected comparisons on neuropsychological testing. The patient had multiple white matter abnormalities, and quantified DTI was able to identify abnormalities, which were not apparent on FLAIR images. Our group is currently utilizing quantified DTI to examine fiber length and number among individuals infected with clade C HIV (Fig. 20.2).

DSI is a second novel diffusion imaging technique with potential applications in the imaging of HIV. The capabilities of DSI improve upon DTI techniques such that DSI is capable of identifying cross fibers, or intersecting tracts, within a single voxel in the brain. DSI can also identify long fiber tracts and the route and termination sites of white matter pathways.[79] In a 2008 study, DSI was employed in adult formalin-fixed brains of macaques as well as in healthy human brains. DSI revealed fiber crossings in multiple brain structures, including the caudate nucleus, which DTI was unable to capture.[80] This finding is particularly important considering HIV infection targets the head of the caudate nucleus.

Techniques such as near-infrared imaging (NIRI) and near-infrared spectroscopy (NIRS) utilize visible as well as near-infrared light, passing through tissue to gain a better understanding of the structure of that tissue.[81] Functional near-infrared spectroscopy has been

Left panel: Seropositive HIV patient   **Right panel: Seronegative individual**

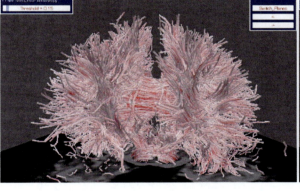 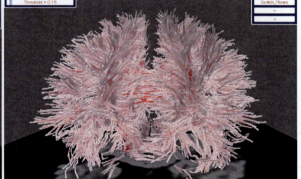

Fig. 20.2 Quantified tractrography results. Streamtubes represent individual white matter pathways

Quantified results of the images above

Measure	Clade C Seropositive (n=3)	Seronegative (n=1)
Total length (mm)*	189,840 (46,368)	258,141
Number of tubes*	6,819 (791)	10,161
Average FA.	42 (.02)	.50

used in functional imaging for neurological conditions such as Parkinson's disease,[82,83] but not yet in HIV. Parkinson's disease is a subcortical, neurodegenerative disease like HIV. Both conditions produce frontal lobe abnormalities due to integrated frontal-subcortical circuitry, suggesting that functional near-infrared spectroscopy may have a role in the functional imaging of HIV.

Finally, a method of positron emission tomography (PET) utilizing Pittsburgh compound B (PiB) as a tracer to identify amyloid-beta plaque formation in the brain is currently being explored as a method of imaging HIV. PiB has frequently been used in Alzheimer's disease research as amyloid-beta plaque formation is thought to be a major factor in developing AD. Research utilizing PiB is still relatively new, with the work of Klunk et al. in 2004[84] at the University of Pittsburgh, being the first publication using PiB to study AD. PiB has also been used in research associated with the aging process[85] and in Lewy body dementia.[86,87] Increased amyloid-beta plaque formation is one of the two major histological markers associated with AD, although plaque formation has been observed in cognitively healthy elderly individuals using PiB,[85] thus the exact cause of AD is still unknown. Studies are currently ongoing at several major research centers but results of PiB imaging have not been published. However, we expect that PiB imaging will facilitate our understanding of the HIV neuropathogenesis, with particular focus on the interaction between HIV and neuronal degeneration associated with the disease.

Summary and Conclusions

It is clear from the literature described above that neuroimaging methods have played a major role in facilitating our understanding of the impact of HIV on the brain. Collectively, neuroimaging has provided a window into the brain that is not possible with behavioral observations and examinations. Evidence of macrostructural and microstructural changes to neuronal integrity is found in studies using volumetrics, diffusion imaging, and MRS, while functional properties of the brain have been defined via BOLD MRI. Several neuroimaging methods (e.g., MRS) appear sensitive to the earliest changes in CNS integrity, and in fact these changes may

precede any other expression of disease burden in the brain, as well as effective response to treatment.

Some surprising findings have emerged from the neuroimaging literature, including potential for biphasic or nonlinear trends such as putamen hypertrophy among nondemented patients,[33] and perhaps subsequently, basal ganglia atrophy in the context of dementia.[28] Similar findings have been reported in the white matter of HIV patients, with evidence of increased FA which may represent inflammatory processes[88] early in the disease process, whereas later stages might be more typically characterized by decreased FA (more consistent with neuronal compromise).

Another very interesting finding is in regard to hippocampal involvement in HIV. Neuropathological studies have previously demonstrated a relationship between hippocampal abnormalities in the brain and cognitive impairment,[89] but only recently have these abnormalities been visualized using fMRI.[62] These findings are of particular interest because HIV has classically been defined as a "subcortical" disease with both the anatomy and behavioral expression of dysfunction more consistent with deep brain region involvement compared to damage to the structures of the medial temporal lobe and cortical mantle. At present the impact of HIV on the hippocampus is unclear, particularly since most patients do not exhibit the amnestic memory dysfunction consistent with AD. Perhaps studies incorporating PiB, fMRI, and volumetrics will shed light on these novel findings.

Despite all of the advances that have occurred in the field of neuroimaging of HIV in the past decade, many questions remain. Perhaps most intriguing is the neuropathogenesis of HIV, and both host and viral factors that moderate expression of the disease. It remains unclear why some individuals exhibit significant (perhaps profound) cognitive impairment, whereas other individuals exhibit little if any cognitive compromise. We also continue to have a limited understanding of the evolution of brain dysfunction associated with HIV when dysfunction does occur. Do all patients with specific risk factors progress from mild impairment to dementia, is the course of the evolution linear or nonlinear, or does it fluctuate significantly with continuous changes in immune status? We believe the answers to these questions, and many other questions, will be obtained in the near future and neuroimaging will play a critical role in unraveling these mysteries.

References

1. Joint United Nations Programme on HIV/AIDS. *Second guidance paper: joint UN programmes and teams on AIDS: practical guidelines on implementing effective and sustainable joint teams and programmes of support.* Geneva, Switzerland: Joint United Nations Programme on HIV/AIDS; 2008.
2. Letendre SL, Cherner M, Ellis RJ, et al. The effects of hepatitis C, HIV, and methamphetamine dependence on neuropsychological performance: biological correlates of disease. *AIDS.* 2005;19(Suppl 3):S72–S78.
3. Wu Y, Storey P, Cohen BA, Epstein LG, Edelman RR, Ragin AB. Diffusion alterations in corpus callosum of patients with HIV. *AJNR Am J Neuroradiol.* 2006;27(3):656–660.
4. Avison MJ, Nath A, Berger JR. Understanding pathogenesis and treatment of HIV dementia: a role for magnetic resonance? *Trends Neurosci.* 2002;25(9):468–473.
5. Antinori A, Arendt G, Becker JT, et al. Updated research nosology for HIV-associated neurocognitive disorders. *Neurology.* 2007;69(18):1789–1799.
6. Nath A, Maragos WF, Avison MJ, Schmitt FA, Berger JR. Acceleration of HIV dementia with methamphetamine and cocaine. *J Neurovirol.* 2001;7(1):66–71.
7. Dube B, Benton T, Cruess DG, Evans DL. Neuropsychiatric manifestations of HIV infection and AIDS. *J Psychiatry Neurosci.* 2005;30(4):237–246.
8. Hartzell JD, Janke IE, Weintrob AC. Impact of depression on HIV outcomes in the HAART era. *J Antimicrob Chemother.* 2008;62(2):246–255.
9. Valcour V, Paul R. HIV infection and dementia in older adults. *Clin Infect Dis.* 2006;42(10):1449–1454.
10. Hult B, Chana G, Masliah E, Everall I. Neurobiology of HIV. *Int Rev Psychiatry.* 2008;20(1):3–13.
11. Nath A, Schiess N, Venkatesan A, Rumbaugh J, Sacktor N, McArthur J. Evolution of HIV dementia with HIV infection. *Int Rev Psychiatry.* 2008;20(1):25–31.
12. Elovaara I, Poutiainen E, Raininko R, et al. Mild brain atrophy in early HIV infection: the lack of association with cognitive deficits and HIV-specific intrathecal immune response. *J Neurol Sci.* 1990;99(2–3):121–136.
13. Levin HS, Williams DH, Borucki MJ, et al. Magnetic resonance imaging and neuropsychological findings in human immunodeficiency virus infection. *J Acquir Immune Defic Syndr.* 1990;3(8):757–762.
14. Poutiainen E, Elovaara I, Raininko R, et al. Cognitive performance in HIV-1 infection: relationship to severity of disease and brain atrophy. *Acta Neurol Scand.* 1993;87(2):88–94.
15. Patel SH, Kolson DL, Glosser G, et al. Correlation between percentage of brain parenchymal volume and neurocognitive performance in HIV-infected patients. *AJNR Am J Neuroradiol.* 2002;23(4):543–549.
16. Broderick DF, Wippold FJ 2nd, Clifford DB, Kido D, Wilson BS. White matter lesions and cerebral atrophy on MR images in patients with and without AIDS dementia complex. *AJR Am J Roentgenol.* 1993;161(1):177–181.
17. Harrison MJ, Newman SP, Hall-Craggs MA, et al. Evidence of CNS impairment in HIV infection: clinical, neuropsychological, EEG, and MRI/MRS study. *J Neurol Neurosurg Psychiatry.* 1998;65(3):301–307.
18. Jernigan TL, Archibald S, Hesselink JR, et al. Magnetic resonance imaging morphometric analysis of cerebral volume loss in human immunodeficiency virus infection. The HNRC Group. *Arch Neurol.* 1993;50(3):250–255.
19. Post MJ, Berger JR, Duncan R, Quencer RM, Pall L, Winfield D. Asymptomatic and neurologically symptomatic HIV-seropositive subjects: results of long-term MR imaging and clinical follow-up. *Radiology.* 1993;188(3):727–733.
20. Post MJ, Tate LG, Quencer RM, et al. CT, MR, and pathology in HIV encephalitis and meningitis. *AJR Am J Roentgenol.* 1988;151(2):373–380.
21. Grant I, Atkinson JH, Hesselink JR, et al. Evidence for early central nervous system involvement in the acquired immunodeficiency syndrome (AIDS) and other human immunodeficiency virus (HIV) infections. Studies with neuropsychologic testing and magnetic resonance imaging. *Ann Intern Med.* 1987;107(6):828–836.
22. Dal Pan GJ, McArthur JH, Aylward E, et al. Patterns of cerebral atrophy in HIV-1-infected individuals: results of a quantitative MRI analysis. *Neurology.* 1992;42(11):2125–2130.
23. Hestad K, McArthur JH, Dal Pan GJ, et al. Regional brain atrophy in HIV-1 infection: association with specific neuropsychological test performance. *Acta Neurol Scand.* 1993;88(2):112–118.
24. Hall M, Whaley R, Robertson K, Hamby S, Wilkins J, Hall C. The correlation between neuropsychological and neuroanatomic changes over time in asymptomatic and symptomatic HIV-1-infected individuals. *Neurology.* 1996;46(6):1697–1702.
25. Kieburtz K, Ketonen L, Cox C, et al. Cognitive performance and regional brain volume in human immunodeficiency virus type 1 infection. *Arch Neurol.* 1996;53(2):155–158.
26. Stout JC, Ellis RJ, Jernigan TL, et al. Progressive cerebral volume loss in human immunodeficiency virus infection: a longitudinal volumetric magnetic resonance imaging study. HIV Neurobehavioral Research Center Group. *Arch Neurol.* 1998;55(2):161–168.
27. Sonnerborg A, Saaf J, Alexius B, Strannegard O, Wahlund LO, Wetterberg L. Quantitative detection of brain aberrations in human immunodeficiency virus type 1-infected individuals by magnetic resonance imaging. *J Infect Dis.* 1990;162(6):1245–1251.
28. Aylward EH, Henderer JD, McArthur JC, et al. Reduced basal ganglia volume in HIV-1-associated dementia: results from quantitative neuroimaging. *Neurology.* 1993;43(10):2099–2104.
29. Aylward EH, Brettschneider PD, McArthur JC, et al. Magnetic resonance imaging measurement of gray matter volume reductions in HIV dementia. *Am J Psychiatry.* 1995;152(7):987–994.
30. Paul RH, Brickman AM, Navia B, et al. Apathy is associated with volume of the nucleus accumbens in patients infected with HIV. *J Neuropsychiatry Clin Neurosci.* 2005;17(2):167–171.
31. Post MJ, Berger JR, Quencer RM. Asymptomatic and neurologically symptomatic HIV-seropositive individuals: prospective evaluation with cranial MR imaging. *Radiology.* 1991;178(1):131–139.
32. Raininko R, Elovaara I, Virta A, Valanne L, Haltia M, Valle SL. Radiological study of the brain at various stages of human immunodeficiency virus infection: early development of brain atrophy. *Neuroradiology.* 1992;34(3):190–196.

33. Castelo JM, Courtney MG, Melrose RJ, Stern CE. Putamen hypertrophy in nondemented patients with human immunodeficiency virus infection and cognitive compromise. *Arch Neurol.* 2007;64(9):1275–1280.

34. Kieburtz KD, Ketonen L, Zettelmaier AE, Kido D, Caine ED, Simon JH. Magnetic resonance imaging findings in HIV cognitive impairment. *Arch Neurol.* 1990;47(6):643–645.

35. Olsen WL, Longo FM, Mills CM, Norman D. White matter disease in AIDS: findings at MR imaging. *Radiology.* 1988;169(2): 445–448.

36. Chrysikopoulos HS, Press GA, Grafe MR, Hesselink JR, Wiley CA. Encephalitis caused by human immunodeficiency virus: CT and MR imaging manifestations with clinical and pathologic correlation. *Radiology.* 1990;175(1):185–191.

37. Jarvik JG, Hesselink JR, Kennedy C, et al. Acquired immunodeficiency syndrome. Magnetic resonance patterns of brain involvement with pathologic correlation. *Arch Neurol.* 1988;45(7):731–736.

38. McMurtray A, Nakamoto B, Shikuma C, Valcour V. Cortical Atrophy and White Matter Hyperintensities in HIV: the Hawaii Aging with HIV Cohort Study. *J Stroke Cerebrovasc Dis.* 2008;17(4):212–217.

39. Post MJ, Levin BE, Berger JR, Duncan R, Quencer RM, Calabro G. Sequential cranial MR findings of asymptomatic and neurologically symptomatic HIV+ subjects. *AJNR Am J Neuroradiol.* 1992;13(1):359–370.

40. Thurnher MM, Schindler EG, Thurnher SA, Pernerstorfer-Schon H, Kleibl-Popov C, Rieger A. Highly active antiretroviral therapy for patients with AIDS dementia complex: effect on MR imaging findings and clinical course. *AJNR Am J Neuroradiol.* 2000;21(4):670–678.

41. Filippi CG, Sze G, Farber SJ, Shahmanesh M, Selwyn PA. Regression of HIV encephalopathy and basal ganglia signal intensity abnormality at MR imaging in patients with AIDS after the initiation of protease inhibitor therapy. *Radiology.* 1998;206(2):491–498.

42. Boska MD, Mosley RL, Nawab M, et al. Advances in neuroimaging for HIV-1 associated neurological dysfunction: clues to the diagnosis, pathogenesis and therapeutic monitoring. *Curr HIV Res.* 2004;2(1):61–78.

43. Foerster BR, Thurnher MM, Malani PN, Petrou M, Carets-Zumelzu F, Sundgren PC. Intracranial infections: clinical and imaging characteristics. *Acta Radiol.* 2007;48(8):875–893.

44. Chang L, Ernst T, Witt MD, Ames N, Gaiefsky M, Miller E. Relationships among brain metabolites, cognitive function, and viral loads in antiretroviral-naive HIV patients. *Neuroimage.* 2002;17(3):1638–1648.

45. Chang L, Ernst T, Leonido-Yee M, Walot I, Singer E. Cerebral metabolite abnormalities correlate with clinical severity of HIV-1 cognitive motor complex. *Neurology.* 1999;52(1):100–108.

46. Meyerhoff DJ, Bloomer C, Cardenas V, Norman D, Weiner MW, Fein G. Elevated subcortical choline metabolites in cognitively and clinically asymptomatic HIV+ patients. *Neurology.* 1999;52(5):995–1003.

47. Ernst T, Chang L, Arnold S. Increased glial metabolites predict increased working memory network activation in HIV brain injury. *Neuroimage.* 2003;19(4):1686–1693.

48. Paul RH, Ernst T, Brickman AM, et al. Relative sensitivity of magnetic resonance spectroscopy and quantitative magnetic resonance imaging to cognitive function among nondemented individuals infected with HIV. *J Int Neuropsychol Soc.* 2008;14(5):725–733.

49. Sacktor N, Skolasky RL, Ernst T, et al. A multicenter study of two magnetic resonance spectroscopy techniques in individuals with HIV dementia. *J Magn Reson Imaging.* 2005;21(4):325–333.

50. Ernst T, Chang L. Effect of aging on brain metabolism in antiretroviral-naive HIV patients. *AIDS.* 2004;18(Suppl 1): S61–S67.

51. Paul RH, Yiannoutsos CT, Miller EN, et al. Proton MRS and neuropsychological correlates in AIDS dementia complex: evidence of subcortical specificity. *J Neuropsychiatry Clin Neurosci.* 2007;19(3):283–292.

52. Chang L, Ernst T, Speck O, Grob CS. Additive effects of HIV and chronic methamphetamine use on brain metabolite abnormalities. *Am J Psychiatry.* 2005;162(2):361–369.

53. Chang L, Cloak C, Yakupov R, Ernst T. Combined and independent effects of chronic marijuana use and HIV on brain metabolites. *J Neuroimmune Pharmacol.* 2006;1(1):65–76.

54. Pfefferbaum A, Adalsteinsson E, Sullivan EV. Cortical NAA deficits in HIV infection without dementia: influence of alcoholism comorbidity. *Neuropsychopharmacology.* 2005;30(7):1392–1399.

55. Lee PL, Yiannoutsos CT, Ernst T, et al. A multi-center 1H MRS study of the AIDS dementia complex: validation and preliminary analysis. *J Magn Reson Imaging.* 2003;17(6):625–633.

56. Chang L, Lee PL, Yiannoutsos CT, et al. A multicenter in vivo proton-MRS study of HIV-associated dementia and its relationship to age. *Neuroimage.* 2004;23(4):1336–1347.

57. Melrose RJ, Tinaz S, Castelo JM, Courtney MG, Stern CE. Compromised fronto-striatal functioning in HIV: an fMRI investigation of semantic event sequencing. *Behav Brain Res.* 2008;188(2):337–347.

58. Chang L, Speck O, Miller EN, et al. Neural correlates of attention and working memory deficits in HIV patients. *Neurology.* 2001;57(6):1001–1007.

59. Chang L, Tomasi D, Yakupov R, et al. Adaptation of the attention network in human immunodeficiency virus brain injury. *Ann Neurol.* 2004;56(2):259–272.

60. Ernst T, Chang L, Jovicich J, Ames N, Arnold S. Abnormal brain activation on functional MRI in cognitively asymptomatic HIV patients. *Neurology.* 2002;59(9):1343–1349.

61. Castelo JM, Sherman SJ, Courtney MG, Melrose RJ, Stern CE. Altered hippocampal-prefrontal activation in HIV patients during episodic memory encoding. *Neurology.* 2006;66(11):1688–1695.

62. Maki PM, Cohen MH, Weber K, et al. Impairments in memory and hippocampal function in HIV-positive vs HIV-negative women: a preliminary study. *Neurology.* 2009;72(19): 1661–1668.

63. Juengst SB, Aizenstein HJ, Figurski J, Lopez OL, Becker JT. Alterations in the hemodynamic response function in cognitively impaired HIV/AIDS subjects. *J Neurosci Methods.* 2007;163(2):208–212.

64. Tucker KA, Robertson KR, Lin W, et al. Neuroimaging in human immunodeficiency virus infection. *J Neuroimmunol.* 2004;157(1–2):153–162.

65. Thurnher MM, Castillo M, Stadler A, Rieger A, Schmid B, Sundgren PC. Diffusion-tensor MR imaging of the brain in human immunodeficiency virus-positive patients. *AJNR Am J Neuroradiol.* 2005;26(9):2275–2281.

66. Ragin AB, Storey P, Cohen BA, Epstein LG, Edelman RR. Whole brain diffusion tensor imaging in HIV-associated cognitive impairment. *AJNR Am J Neuroradiol.* 2004; 25(2):195–200.

67. Ragin AB, Wu Y, Storey P, Cohen BA, Edelman RR, Epstein LG. Diffusion tensor imaging of subcortical brain injury in patients infected with human immunodeficiency virus. *J Neurovirol.* 2005;11(3):292–298.

68. Chen Y, An H, Zhu H, et al. White matter abnormalities revealed by diffusion tensor imaging in non-demented and demented HIV+ patients. *Neuroimage.* 2009;47(4):1154–1162.

69. Wong EC, Buxton RB, Frank LR. Implementation of quantitative perfusion imaging techniques for functional brain mapping using pulsed arterial spin labeling. *NMR Biomed.* 1997;10(4–5):237–249.

70. Ye FQ, Mattay VS, Jezzard P, Frank JA, Weinberger DR, McLaughlin AC. Correction for vascular artifacts in cerebral blood flow values measured by using arterial spin tagging techniques. *Magn Reson Med.* 1997;37(2):226–235.

71. Ances BM, Roc AC, Wang J, et al. Caudate blood flow and volume are reduced in HIV+ neurocognitively impaired patients. *Neurology.* 2006;66(6):862–866.

72. Silva AC. Perfusion-based fMRI: insights from animal models. *J Magn Reson Imaging.* 2005;22(6):745–750.

73. Frank LR, Lu K, Wong EC. Perfusion tensor imaging. *Magn Reson Med.* 2008;60(6):1284–1291.

74. Wong EC, Cronin M, Wu WC, Inglis B, Frank LR, Liu TT. Velocity-selective arterial spin labeling. *Magn Reson Med.* 2006;55(6):1334–1341.

75. Xue R, van Zijl PC, Crain BJ, Solaiyappan M, Mori S. In vivo three-dimensional reconstruction of rat brain axonal projections by diffusion tensor imaging. *Magn Reson Med.* 1999;42(6):1123–1127.

76. Correia S, Lee SY, Voorn T, et al. Quantitative tractography metrics of white matter integrity in diffusion-tensor MRI. *Neuroimage.* 2008;42(2):568–581.

77. Beaulieu C. The basis of anisotropic water diffusion in the nervous system - a technical review. *NMR Biomed.* 2002; 15(7–8):435–455.

78. Paul RH, Laidlaw DH, Tate DF, et al. Neuropsychological and neuroimaging outcome of HIV-associated progressive multifocal leukoencephalopathy in the era of antiretroviral therapy. *J Integr Neurosci.* 2007;6(1):191–203.

79. Schmahmann JD, Pandya DN, Wang R, et al. Association fibre pathways of the brain: parallel observations from diffusion spectrum imaging and autoradiography. *Brain.* 2007;130(Pt 3):630–653.

80. Wedeen VJ, Wang RP, Schmahmann JD, et al. Diffusion spectrum magnetic resonance imaging (DSI) tractography of crossing fibers. *Neuroimage.* 2008;41(4):1267–1277.

81. Benaron DA, Contag PR, Contag CH. Imaging brain structure and function, infection and gene expression in the body using light. *Philos Trans R Soc Lond B Biol Sci.* 1997;352(1354):755–761.

82. Murata Y, Katayama Y, Oshima H, et al. Changes in cerebral blood oxygenation induced by deep brain stimulation: study by near-infrared spectroscopy (NIRS). *Keio J Med.* 2000;49(Suppl 1):A61–A63.

83. Sakatani K, Katayama Y, Yamamoto T, Suzuki S. Changes in cerebral blood oxygenation of the frontal lobe induced by direct electrical stimulation of thalamus and globus pallidus: a near infrared spectroscopy study. *J Neurol Neurosurg Psychiatry.* 1999;67(6):769–773.

84. Klunk WE, Engler H, Nordberg A, et al. Imaging brain amyloid in Alzheimer's disease with Pittsburgh Compound-B. *Ann Neurol.* 2004;55(3):306–319.

85. Aizenstein HJ, Nebes RD, Saxton JA, et al. Frequent amyloid deposition without significant cognitive impairment among the elderly. *Arch Neurol.* 2008;65(11):1509–1517.

86. Gomperts SN, Rentz DM, Moran E, et al. Imaging amyloid deposition in Lewy body diseases. *Neurology.* 2008;71(12): 903–910.

87. Maetzler W, Liepelt I, Reimold M, et al. Cortical PIB binding in Lewy body disease is associated with Alzheimer-like characteristics. *Neurobiol Dis.* 2009;34(1):107–112.

88. Stebbins GT, Smith CA, Bartt RE, et al. HIV-associated alterations in normal-appearing white matter: a voxel-wise diffusion tensor imaging study. *J Acquir Immune Defic Syndr.* 2007;46(5):564–573.

89. Moore DJ, Masliah E, Rippeth JD, et al. Cortical and subcortical neurodegeneration is associated with HIV neurocognitive impairment. *AIDS.* 2006;20(6):879–887.

Chapter 21
Neuroimaging and Cognitive Function in Multiple Sclerosis

Lawrence H. Sweet and Susan D. Vandermorris

Multiple Sclerosis (MS) is a degenerative disease of uncertain etiology that affects the central nervous system. It is the most common nontraumatic disabling neurological disorder among adults under 60 years of age,[79] with approximately 12,000 individuals receiving a diagnosis of MS in the United States each year.[1] MS affects women more frequently than men (1.7:1),[11] and the risk for MS increases the farther one lives from the equator.[35]

The precise etiological and neuropathological mechanisms of MS are unclear; however, it appears to result from autoimmune dysfunction that targets the neuronal myelin sheath, causing white matter inflammation, demyelination, and consequently disrupted axonal transmission. Traditionally, MS has been characterized as a subcortical disease, with diffuse lesions primarily located in the periventricular white matter and spinal cord. Recent research has shown that gray matter lesions and cortical thinning are also present.[2,10,76,90,91,103] It is not known if the same etiological factors underlie white matter and gray matter damage in MS and how these interact to result in symptoms.

Clinical course of MS is variable and is categorized into four subtypes based on the pattern and rate of progression of the disease. Relapsing-remitting MS is characterized by periods of symptom exacerbation and recovery. Secondary progressive MS is characterized by an initial relapsing-remitting course that later develops into a course of gradual worsening, with or without occasional relapses or minor remissions. Progressive-relapsing MS is characterized by a pattern of acute relapses overlaid on an underlying course of steady progressive decline. Primary progressive MS is characterized by a gradual and continuous worsening of symptoms, with no notable relapsing and remitting pattern.[58] Course varies greatly between patients. Approximately 10% of patients exhibit a benign course, while approximately 10% meet the criteria for dementia.[78] Relapsing–remitting is the most common early course (approximately 90%), and the majority exhibit a secondary progressive course later in the disease process.[79]

MS is associated with a variety of autonomic, sensory, motor, cognitive, and psychiatric symptoms which also vary substantially across individuals. These presenting symptoms have pronounced implications for quality of life and functional status for afflicted individuals. Motor weakness, fatigue, tremor, parasthesia, ataxia, optic neuritis, pain, and urinary, bowel, and sexual dysfunction are common.[79] Approximately 50% of MS patients experience depression during their life[31,59,85] which represents a more than a threefold increase in lifetime prevalence compared to the general population.[4,51] Prevalence of Bipolar Affective Disorder is estimated to be at least twice the normal rate, and may be much higher.[59]

Although sensorimotor symptoms, fatigue, and mood disorders complicate assessment, it has been well documented that cognitive deficits are present in 43–70% of MS cases.[3,29,80] Notable individual differences in presence, pattern, and severity of cognitive deficits are common in MS; however, as a group, individuals with MS have generally been found to show consistent impairment on neuropsychological tests of processing speed, working memory, and episodic memory. Deficits in other cognitive domains have also been described, including spatial processing, verbal fluency, and executive function (for reviews see refs. [20,23,29]).

L.H. Sweet (✉)
Department of Psychiatry and Human Behavior,
Warren Alpert Medical School of Brown University,
Providence, RI 02912, USA
e-mail: lawrence_sweet@brown.edu

R.A. Cohen and L.H. Sweet (eds.), *Brain Imaging in Behavioral Medicine and Clinical Neuroscience*,
DOI 10.1007/978-1-4419-6373-4_21, © Springer Science+Business Media, LLC 2011

As magnetic resonance imaging (MRI) has become a critical feature of the MS diagnostic workup, it is not surprising that a great deal of research has been directed towards optimizing imaging techniques for detecting MS-related neuropathology, and consensus diagnostic criteria for MS have evolved over time to reflect these advances.[58,74] Fluid attenuated inversion recovery (FLAIR) T1-weighted and T2-weighted MRI sequences are routinely used in clinical settings to reveal the extent of neuropathology in MS. While inflammation and demyelination have long been known to be key features of neuronal changes in MS, there is a growing recognition of neuronal loss in both white and gray matter in MS.[2,10,76,91,103] This neuronal loss may have a differential regional impact; with some evidence that this loss may preferentially affect temporal and frontal cortical gray matter regions.[10,76,90]

The growing focus on structural imaging of gray matter pathology and interest in regional brain effects on cognitive function in MS has converged with functional neuroimaging research, which inherently examines gray matter. Functional neuroimaging techniques not only examine regional gray matter function but also allow targeted functional challenges, and in the case of functional MRI (FMRI), the possibility to assess gray matter structural and functional integrity during the same scanning session. The remainder of this chapter focuses on the investigation of higher order cognitive function in MS using structural and functional neuroimaging. We begin with a brief overview of structural imaging findings, review functional imaging research, and discuss future directions in neuroimaging in MS.

Structural Imaging

The demyelination characteristic of MS produces multifocal lesions primarily located in the central nervous system white matter. Historically, the cognitive impairment observed in MS has been hypothesized to be a result of disrupted neural transmission caused by these lesions. Although lesions are usually more numerous in periventricular regions, corpus callosum, and the white matter regions of the frontal lobes, they may occur anywhere, including cortical and subcortical gray matter.[2,25,79,90,91,103]

Neuroimaging studies have examined relationships between lesions and cognitive function for more than two decades using structural MRI. These studies have consistently reported moderate correlations between whole-brain white matter lesion load and cognitive performance, such that greater lesion burden is associated with greater cognitive dysfunction.[5,32,40,46,60,72,82,87,93,100] For example, Franklin and colleagues[40] found that number and size of total lesions was significantly positively correlated with a neuropsychological battery summary score. Rao and colleagues[82] found a significant relationship between total lesion area and recent memory, conceptual reasoning, and visuospatial problem solving. Comi and colleagues[32] reported that total lesion area was associated with lower scores on most neuropsychological measures in a comprehensive test battery. Investigators have also demonstrated that white matter lesion load predicts cognitive decline.[86,93]

Despite consistent support for the relationship between total lesion load and a variety of cognitive functions, evidence for a link between regional lesions and associated cognitive functions has been mixed, with early studies failing to demonstrate sensitivity and specificity of regional pathology in predicting cognitive dysfunction. For example, Huber and colleagues reported that greater total lesion area was associated with worse performance on neuropsychological tests of memory, executive function, interhemispheric transfer, and psychomotor speed; however, regional lesion area was not related to any of the neuropsychological measures.[47] Foong and colleagues reported significant correlations between scores on measures of executive function and extent of frontal lesions; however, executive function scores were also significantly correlated with whole-brain lesion area.[37]

More recently, a growing number of studies have shown support for the specificity of regional white matter lesions in predicting performance on associated cognitive domains.[5,12,52,89,93,100,102] For example, Arnett and colleagues[5] found that patients categorized with a high level of frontal lesions made more errors and achieved fewer categories on the Wisconsin Card Sorting Test (WCST) than a low frontal lesion group with equivalent total lesion area. Swirsky-Sacchetti and colleagues[100] found that verbal fluency, confrontation naming, and conceptual reasoning were associated with bilateral frontal lobe lesion load, while visuospatial problem-solving ability, auditory attention, and verbal learning were associated with parietooccipital lesion load. Tsolaki and colleagues[102] found that memory impairments were correlated significantly with increased number of lesions in the corona radiata, insula, and hippocampus. Sperling and colleagues[93] reported frontal and parietal lesion areas each inversely related to Selective Reminding Test Continuous Long-Term Recall and Paced Auditory Serial Addition Task performance.

While structural imaging studies of white matter pathology in MS have produced support for hypothesized mechanisms of symptom expression, a developing body of structural imaging research in MS involves the assessment of brain atrophy. Studies of whole-brain atrophy, ventricular enlargement, and regional atrophy have demonstrated associations between these measures and cognitive impairment in MS.[2,14,15,17,30,45,105,106] Huber and colleagues found corpus callosum atrophy to be related to slower cognitive processing speed and interhemispheric transfer,[47] as well as dementia,[48] in MS patients. Rao and colleagues[82] reported a correlation between corpus callosum atrophy and slowed cognitive processing. Tsolaki and colleagues[102] found that memory impairments were correlated significantly with increased size of the third ventricle. Comi and colleagues[32] reported that corpus callosum atrophy, ventricular dilation, cerebral atrophy, and total lesion area were associated with lower scores on most neuropsychological measures in their comprehensive test battery.

Regional specificity of atrophy has been shown in a number of studies, with evidence for an association between thalamic atrophy and cognitive status,[14,45] as well as evidence of higher correlations between subcortical atrophy and cognition as compared to that of whole-brain atrophy or lesion load.[15,18] There is some evidence for a longitudinal association between cognitive decline and increasing brain atrophy.[44,70,106] For example, early progression of brain atrophy has been shown to predict cognitive impairment at a 5-year follow-up interval.[96]

With the focus of neuroimaging research on MS traditionally on white matter, and some limitations to the parcelation and quantification of cortical regions, the implications of gray matter cortical atrophy have not been studied extensively, and relationships between cortical atrophy and subcortical pathology have not been defined. There is a growing recognition of neuronal loss in both white and gray matter in MS.[2,90,91,103] This neuronal loss may have a differential regional impact; with some evidence that this loss may preferentially affect

temporal and frontal cortical gray matter regions.[90] There is some evidence that the extent of regional cortical atrophy may correspond to the degree of cognitive impairment observed in patients with MS.[15,61,73] For example, one recent study of the clinical relevance of specific regional cortical atrophy has documented associations between left frontal atrophy with verbal memory and right frontal atrophy with visual memory and working memory.[101]

Functional Neuroimaging

Functional neuroimaging studies involving challenges of higher order cognitive functions in MS have been published only in the past decade. These studies have used functional magnetic resonance imaging (FMRI) techniques and focus on the domains frequently impaired in neuropsychological studies, including working memory, executive function, and episodic memory. Of these cognitive domains, verbal working memory has received the most attention, employing cognitive testing paradigms including the Paced Auditory Serial Addition Task and its variants, the n-Back task and the Sternberg task.

The Paced Auditory Serial Addition Task (PASAT) was designed as a measure of complex processing speed for the assessment of traumatic brain injury.[41] However, it is also considered to be a verbal working memory challenge highly sensitive to cognitive dysfunction in MS.[33] As a standardized measure with normative data, the PASAT has been frequently employed in both clinical assessments and behavioral research studies of MS.[13,16,81] It has also been incorporated as a primary component of the MS Functional Composite, a scale used to quantify MS-related disability.[33] Development of this scale stemmed from recognition in the late 1980s that cognitive impairments substantially contributed to disability in MS and that traditional disability scales did not assess higher order cognitive functions.

During the standard version of the PASAT, the examinee is asked to attend to a series of single-digit numbers spoken aloud at a consistent interval. Beginning with the second number, the examinee is asked to report the sum of the two consecutive numbers and retain the latter of the two digits presented for addition to the next number presented. Numbers are presented in an initial series with an interval rate of 3 s, followed by a more challenging series with an interval rate of 2 s.

Despite differences in task parameters, FMRI studies employing PASAT-type paradigms reveal similar patterns of task-related brain response in healthy participants. These include bilateral (left more frequently reported than right) dorsolateral prefrontal regions, posterior parietal cortices, and the supplementary motor area.[8,28] Patients with MS and clinically isolated syndrome (CIS, a term used to describe those patients who show some MS symptoms, but do not meet full criteria for MS and can be considered to be at high risk for developing the disorder), exhibit similar patterns, with evidence for increased activity in expected regions, unexpected regions, or both, when compared to controls. Although activation in frontal regions is commonly observed in both patients with MS and controls,[8,9,28,56] there is some evidence that the pattern of frontal activity may differ between groups, with greater right-sided frontal activation in patients with MS compared to controls in some studies[28,94] and greater left-sided prefrontal activation in at least one other study.[38] For example, Audoin and colleagues found greater right-sided frontal activation in patients diagnosed with CIS compared to controls.[9]

Some studies have provided evidence for greater magnitude of activation in patients with MS compared to healthy controls in specific regions, including the bilateral parietal lobes,[28,56] bilateral temporal lobes,[56] and right cerebellum.[9] Such overactivation in terms of magnitude or extent has often been called *compensatory activity*, particularly when it can be demonstrated that performance levels do not significantly differ. Greater dispersion of task-related activation in patients with MS compared with controls has been demonstrated in prefrontal regions, parietal lobes, and the anterior cingulate.[28,56,94] Alterations within working memory network connectivity have also been demonstrated in patients with MS compared to controls.[6,7] It is important to note that correlations with behavioral performance levels have shown that worse performance on PASAT tasks is associated with increased activation in right frontal and parietal regions.[28] This important finding suggests that the frequent finding of overactivation in regions typically associated with verbal working memory challenges in MS patients is actually related to the verbal working memory challenge and not solely a function of potential differences in baseline states or physiological responses.

Studies of MS patients with and without working memory impairment have also shown differences in patterns of task-related activation on FMRI,[8,28,56] although methodological differences between these studies complicate interpretation of differing results. Data from Forn and colleagues[38] showed greater left-sided prefrontal activation in an MS group in the context of an absence of performance differences between MS and control groups. The authors point to these results in interpreting their findings as evidence of cortical reorganization in the MS group. Other evidence of cortical reorganization in MS across the disease course comes from a comparison of patients with CIS, MS, and controls on PVSAT (a visual PASAT variant) which revealed no significant performance level differences across groups, but greater hippocampal and parahippocampal activation in the MS group compared with the CIS group and greater activation of anterior cingulate in the CIS group compared to controls.[77]

The *n*-Back task is another frequently administered measure of verbal working memory that is highly amenable to functional neuroimaging research. During the *n*-Back task, a series of sequential stimuli are presented individually. For each stimulus, the examinee's task is to decide if it is the same as the stimulus presented "*n*" items before. For example, during a 2-Back task (i.e., $n = 2$), the response would be "yes" if the stimulus currently presented matches the stimulus presented two earlier. Examinees usually respond with a button. The most common levels of "*n*" are 1-Back, 2-Back, and 3-Back, with a 0-Back control task frequently used for baseline performance in functional neuroimaging experiments. During the 0-Back, the examinee is asked to respond with "yes" each time a predetermined target appears and usually with "no" to other stimuli. Collectively, these levels comprise the *n*-Back paradigm, enabling systematic escalation of working memory demands. There are numerous versions of the *n*-Back paradigm, and several different versions have been designed to assess visual, spatial, and verbal working memory. Stimuli are usually presented visually using a computer screen or projector; however, auditory stimulus presentation is also common. Typical stimuli include letters, words, figures, spatial locations, and photographs. In functional neuroimaging research, stimuli are presented in blocks, usually including the 0-Back baseline control task, which is alternated with blocks of one or more *n*-Back levels. Consistent activation patterns have been associated with the *n*-Back among healthy controls regardless of stimulus type. These include bilateral activity centered on the inferior parietal lobule, rostral middle frontal gyrus, caudal middle frontal gyrus, superior frontal gyrus, anterior superior frontal gyrus, and the inferior frontal gyrus, often including Broca's area and the anterior insula.[65]

A number of FMRI studies comparing patients with MS and controls using n-Back paradigms have shown similar patterns of frontal and parietal cortical activity in both groups.[27,99,104] Some authors have found evidence for greater activity in these regions in patients with MS compared to controls,[39,99] although other others have shown decreased activation in frontal regions in a less disabled group of patients with MS compared to controls.[104]

Three studies have employed n-Back paradigms in a context of graded task difficulty. Penner and colleagues employed a graded task difficulty strategy using a simple reaction time task, a spatial stroop task, and a 2-Back task.[71] MS patients with mild cognitive impairment showed increased frontal and posterior parietal activation relative to controls, an effect which decreased with increasing task complexity. MS patients with severe impairment showed increased parietal activation only. Interestingly, the observed magnitude of overactivation relative to controls in mildly impaired subjects was notably greater than that of the more severely impaired patients, suggesting a failure of adaptive over-recruitment of neural regions in the more severely impaired patients. Sweet and colleagues, employing a gradient of working memory task difficulty (1, 2, and 3-Back), replicated prior findings of greater activation in working memory regions in MS compared with control across all tasks but found that task-related activation in the MS group diminished in the 3-Back condition, suggesting a demand threshold whereby those with MS are able to employ compensatory activation only up to a certain level of task difficulty.[98]

The Sternberg task is a third measure of working memory amenable to functional neuroimaging studies. During this task, a set of stimuli (e.g., numbers) are presented, followed by a delay and presentation of a single number. The task is to determine if the single number presented was included in the initial set. Two studies have employed the Sternberg paradigm in patients with MS. One study found increased activation in right prefrontal and temporal areas in patients with MS compared to controls, with poorer performance in the patient group associated with greater

right frontal and temporal activation.[43] A second study found decreased bilateral cerebellar activation in patients with MS compared to controls.[54]

Complementing the extensive body of literature on functional imaging of working memory, a small number of studies have examined executive functions. Executive functions are multifaceted and include skills such as planning, problem solving, mental flexibility, and resistance to cognitive interference. Although executive function is key to successful performance of verbal working memory tasks described above, a handful of studies have examined specific executive functions such as planning and resistance to interference using the Tower of London task,[92] modifications of the n-Back task, and a counting Stroop task.[26]

Lazeron and colleagues assessed neuroimaging correlates of planning and problem solving using a modification of the Tower of London task in a sample of patients with MS and healthy controls. This widely used neuropsychological test of executive function consists of three pegs and beads of three different colors. The task involves several problem-solving items during which beads must be moved from one peg to the other to create a pattern following a set of basic rules (e.g., only one bead may be moved at a time). Results showed similar levels of activation in bilateral frontal and parietal lobes, as well as the cerebellum, in patients to controls, in the context of poorer behavioral performance on the task in the MS group.[53] The authors interpreted this pattern of findings as consistent with the depletion of adaptive overrecruitment of neural regions in the patient group.

Using a n-back task modified to increase executive function demands by employing both single- and dual-task conditions, Nebel and colleagues found that patients with MS with cognitive deficits showed worse performance on both behavioral tasks, reduced activation in superior and inferior frontal gyrus during the single task n-Back, and decreased activity within the middle and inferior frontal gyrus, inferior parietal structures, and occipital areas during the dual-task n-Back.[64] MS Patients without cognitive impairment did not differ in terms of behavioral performance or FMRI activity from controls. The authors suggest that this study did not provide evidence of compensatory neural mechanisms in patients with MS with or without specific cognitive deficits; rather these findings support reduced cortical activity in patients with specific deficits.

Using a counting Stroop task, Parry and colleagues examined group differences in performance and activation in a group of patients with MS compared with healthy controls. During this task sets of up to four identical neutral words (e.g., cat or dog) or up to four identical number words (i.e., one, two, three, or four) were presented. The participant's task was to report the number of items presented in the set via a button press. During the interference trial, the number words did not match the number of items in the set. Results showed comparable behavioral performance levels and overall patterns of activation, with greater left prefrontal activation in patients compared with controls and greater right frontal activation in controls than patients.[68]

Episodic memory is another cognitive domain frequently impacted in MS and is amenable to study in functional imaging paradigms. To date, just two studies have examined functional imaging correlates of episodic memory performance. One study investigated FMRI activation patterns during performance of a delayed recognition task. Despite similar performance levels, MS patients exhibited greater activity in left posterior parietal cortex and attenuated deactivation in the rostral anterior cingulate compared to controls. The authors concluded that these patterns were likely due to compensatory overactivation as a result of neural inefficiency.[62] In another study, Bobholz and colleagues examined the association of T2-weighted lesions and FMRI activation during a verbal episodic memory recognition task.[21] They demonstrated significant correlations between increasing regional brain activation with increasing lesion volume, particularly in frontal and parietal association areas. These correlations were stronger during the retrieval phase, compared with the encoding phase of the memory task, a finding that the authors interpreted as consistent with prior behavioral finding that memory retrieval processes are preferentially affected by MS pathology.

Other Functional Imaging Modalities

Other functional neuroimaging techniques such as positron emission tomography (PET),[19,24,69,84,97] single photon emission computed tomography (SPECT),[55,75] and perfusion MRI[49] have been used to examine MS. Overall, these studies have reported lower resting regional and global cerebral blood flow and glucose metabolism in patients with MS. These reductions generally relate to deficits in higher order cognitive impairment. For instance, Paulesu and colleagues[69] examined glucose metabolism in 15 MS patients with long-term memory impairment, 13 MS patients without cognitive impairment, and 10 healthy control participants. Impaired MS participants exhibited less bilateral activation in the hippocampus, cingulate, thalamus, cerebellum, and occipital cortex compared to the normal control group, and less bilateral hippocampus and left thalamus activation than the unimpaired MS group. Additional PET studies have reported that global oxygen utilization significantly predicts Mini Mental State Exam scores ($n = 20$),[97] estimated IQ decline, and cerebral atrophy ($n = 15$).[24] A SPECT study of seventeen patients with mild cognitive impairment[75] reported a significant association between abnormal left temporal metabolism and deficits in verbal fluency and verbal memory tasks. Regional specificity of cerebral blood flow perfusion and volume observed using perfusion MRI has been documented in MS,[49] with significant correlations observed between deep gray matter blood perfusion and visuoconstruction and executive function.

These studies suggest that greater cognitive impairment is associated with less activation in cortical and subcortical regions in MS patients. Impairments of long-term memory and verbal fluency may be related to lower than expected temporal lobe activation; however, other regions may also be involved. While these findings on cerebrovascular function suggest possible mechanisms of cognitive impairment in MS, they also raise questions about baselines used in FMRI paradigms.

Conclusions and Future Directions

This is an exciting time for MS researchers. With numerous established neuroimaging techniques, rapidly developing new techniques, and the potential of innovative combinations of these methods, previously unanswerable research questions are rapidly coming within reach. MS is already an excellent example of a disease process for which neuroimaging techniques rapidly advanced from research to clinical applications. Structural MRI, such as T1-weighted, T2-weighted, and FLAIR sequences have become well established as key indicators in the diagnosis of MS. It is likely that more research techniques will transition to clinical applications in the near future. Meanwhile, innovative research methods, including new analyses of traditional structural MRI output, continue to have a major impact on our understanding of cognitive dysfunction in MS. Although neuroimaging techniques used to assess higher order cognitive function of individual patients are not used in clinical settings, several promising neuroimaging techniques designed to quantify structural integrity will likely complement the more traditional MRI sequences in the near future. In the longer term, it is also possible that functional neuroimaging methods will inform treatment decisions and be used to monitor intervention efficacy in clinical trials.

Other Neuroimaging Techniques

Several neuroimaging methods show outstanding promise for accelerating impact in clinical research over the next few years. Although these have been applied to the study of MS, they are methodologically more complex than the more common neuroimaging techniques already described, with less conventional acquisition, analysis, and interpretations pipelines. Each has unique strengths and limitations that make them worth considering for addition to existing MS neuroimaging protocols.

One particularly interesting neuroimaging technique for MS research is diffusion tensor imaging (DTI), which is a noninvasive structural MRI application that enables quantification of white matter tracts by measuring the directionality (or fractional anisotropy) of water molecules. DTI has clear utility in quantifying white matter pathology associated with demyelination, yet early studies of DTI have yielded mixed results, with one study documenting an association between whole-brain fractional anisotropy and cognitive performance[83] and another showing no such association.[88] However, changes in brain structure in normal appearing tissue on conventional imaging has revealed associations between brain structure and cognition using measures using DTI-derived

measures of specific cortical and subcortical regions.[88] DTI and other advanced white matter imaging methods have the advantage that more specific information may be gathered about particular white matter tracks and presumably the functions associated with the associated gray matter regions they connect.

Another rapidly developing neuroimaging technique is magnetic resonance spectroscopy (MRS), which is an MR application that quantifies regional metabolite levels. Certain findings, such as greater N-acetyl aspartate (NAA) levels suggest neuronal loss. MRS has shown utility by demonstrating significant correlations between neuropathology and cognitive function, particularly in otherwise normal-appearing white matter.[36,95] Pan and colleagues have demonstrated significant associations between high periventricular NAA levels and cognitive impairment.[66] Mathiesen and colleagues found significant group differences in patients with MS with and without cognitive impairment in terms of a whole-brain MRS indicator of neuronal integrity (i.e., NAA/creatine ratio[57]). Evidence for regional specificity of structural brain changes with cognitive status has been seen using MRS, where correlations were observed between left periventricular area measures of neural integrity with verbal memory, as well as between right periventricular area integrity and an executive functioning measure.[66]

Susceptibility weighted imaging (SWI) offers a novel approach to assess lesion characteristics, such as iron deposition and venous connectivity. It has been useful in detecting lesions in otherwise normal appearing tissue.[42] Therefore, it is a complementary and potentially more sensitive method for quantification and classification of lesions.

Perfusion MRI has several possible uses in clinical research, including MS. It is a reasonable alternative to radiological techniques such as PET and SPECT for assessment of baseline perfusion levels, which has been associated with cognitive dysfunction. Perfusion MRI may also be used to determine if baseline differences in perfusion levels might confound BOLD FMRI experiments. Moreover, perfusion FMRI may eventually become a feasible alternative to BOLD FMRI. Currently, technical limitations such as relatively low signal to noise ratio and partial brain acquisition must be overcome before perfusion FMRI can compete with other functional neuroimaging approaches.

Improvements in Analyses of Traditional Neuroimaging Data

Another key methodological development has been the creation of new methods of analysis of the images routinely acquired for clinical assessments (e.g., T1, FLAIR). More accurate, automated, and objective methods for the quantification of white and gray matter have been refined over the past decade. Important examples include voxel-based morphometry and cortical thickness measurements using T1 images. As discussed above, the importance of gray matter pathology in the development of cognitive deficits has received greater appreciation in recent years. Improving analytic methods available to reliably quantify gray matter volume, thickness, and lesion areas enables better examination of how gray matter integrity relates to other disease factors. A major advantage of this new direction is the ability to link gray matter pathology with a large body of existing literature on underlying white matter pathology.

Assessment of gray matter pathology has become a hot topic in MS research, with encouraging initial findings in relation to cognitive function. In the research setting, measurements of regional cortical thinning are easily tested for relationships to expected cognitive functions, and initial findings are promising. In the clinic, such measures are likely to eventually inform diagnosis, prognosis, and treatment efficacy in the near future. However, several steps must be taken which will likely parallel the rise of white matter lesion load as a clinical indicator, before this method may be used clinically. Specifically, standardized assessment and evaluation procedures must be developed which will need to be validated through clinical research. Eventually, functional imaging techniques may be used for the same purpose suggested for quantification of regional cortical thinning, with the added advantage that the expected cognitive domains may be directly challenged and brain response observed. With several investigators reporting compensatory activity during equal cognitive performance in MS patients, it is possible that functional neuroimaging may be used to detect cognitive problems before they manifest behaviorally.

Multisequence MRI

It is interesting to note that the majority of neuroimaging in MS has been done using MRI. While PET and SPECT has been used in early neuroimaging studies of MS, these studies were aimed at detecting correlations between resting cerebral blood flow and cognitive impairments. More recently even this type of research has been done using arterial spin labeling (ASL) MRI sequences.[49] The numerous scanning modalities available on the MRI make it an ideal venue for efficient multisequence imaging. While multisequence MRI is already conducted in routine clinical assessments using T1, T2, and FLAIR sequences, these sequences are prescribed to assess only lesion load. Therefore, a new direction in clinical neuroimaging research, including MS, is the use of multisequence MRI for evaluation of lesion load, and other features such as tract integrity, cortical atrophy, neural response function, cerebrovascular perfusion, and metabolism in the same scanning session. In the future, multisequence neuroimaging is likely to provide the clinician with a variety of complementary information relevant to diagnosis, severity, prognosis, and treatment efficacy. With several sequences available in one scanning session, and more under development, MRI holds great potential for efficient and comprehensive neuroimaging assessment.

In research, multisequence imaging allows identification and control of key confounding variables, such as differences in lesion types in lesion quantification studies or potentially differing baseline perfusion levels in FMRI experiments. It is now feasible to determine, for example, relative contributions of regional gray matter pathology, white matter pathology in specific tracts, hemodynamic abnormalities, and neural dysfunction in a single study employing a single MRI assessment session.

One excellent example of multisequence MRI research was conducted by Bonzano and colleagues. They combined FMRI using the PVSAT and DTI to examine the potential effects of white matter pathology on cortical reorganization. They identified the superior longitudinal fasciculus as the primary white matter tract connecting areas active during the PVSAT FMRI challenge. Using DTI functional anisotropy assessments of this tract, they identified two subgroups. Patients with greater tract integrity appeared similar to controls; however, patients with lower tract integrity exhibited additional significant bilateral activity, suggesting bilateralization of function when tracts are damaged.[22]

Several examples of multimodal imaging exist in other clinical populations. One in particular will be critical in the evaluation of FMRI research in MS. That is the combination of perfusion imaging and FMRI.

Several investigators have reported the phenomenon of compensatory activity in MS. The common interpretation of this finding is that greater activity in the patient group represents increased brain activity relative to baseline to perform normally on the cognitive challenge. However, this assumes that the MS patients and control group do not differ on the baseline tasks necessary in FMRI, including resting baseline. Since it is known from early PET and SPECT work in MS that baselines may differ in MS patients, this is a critical confound that may be controlled using perfusion MRI at baseline.

A related research direction is assessment of the default network. The default network is another hot topic in functional neuroimaging relevant to MS and any other group where perfusion appears to differ at baseline. There are two general possibilities for this effect. First, there may be cerebrovascular abnormalities patients with MS. Second, there may be abnormalities in the function of neurons in the default network.

Paradigms

Several factors have made FMRI the method of choice when examining brain function in MS patients. Advantages include cost, availability, noninvasiveness, and temporal and spatial resolution (see Chap. 3). However, there are disadvantages to this method. Since verbal responses are difficult to collect during loud FMRI sequences and result in head movement during the scan acquisition, investigators often use versions modified for use in FMRI studies. For example, the PASAT task requires verbal responses to auditory-presented stimuli. Adaptations for use in the FMRI scanner include the use of covert verbal responses or further modification such as the use of visually presented stimuli and a multiple choice response format in the PVSAT.[77] However, as the PVSAT also differs in format and cognitive demands from the original PASAT, the inability to use existing test norms after modification is perhaps an opportunity missed. Nonetheless, the existence of test norms for the similar original version offers some more support for construct validity compared to other verbal working memory challenges such as the n-Back, which does not have a history of clinical use. On the other hand, when covert responding is used, additional procedures such as retesting outside of the scanner are needed to determine

performance levels, and above chance performance in the scanner cannot be directly verified. These issues of validity and generalizability are not specific to the PASAT, but faced by investigators who wish to adopt any existing cognitive test for FMRI experiments, and the similarity of FMRI findings across studies suggests convergent construct validity.

The types and sophistication of cognitive challenges has also been limited. For instance, although processing speed and cognitive fatigue are core cognitive deficits in patients with MS, few functional neuroimaging studies have investigated processing speed in the absence of simultaneous higher order complex attention, working memory, or executive demands. Similarly, efforts to isolate the functional effects of fatigue and processing speed in these more complicated designs have also been limited.

Beyond Cognitive Function

Although considerable efforts are underway to examine relationships between neuroimaging variables and higher order cognitive functions, a handful have addressed the impact of neural pathology on everyday function. Although it is assumed that cognitive impairments ultimately generalize to impairments in daily function, a more direct approach has been taken by neuroimaging researchers. These efforts may provide more ecologically relevant information about prognosis for activities of daily living and other functional outcomes. One important recent study of 111 MS patients and 46 control participants found that worse performance on neuropsychological measures of conceptual reasoning was associated with greater brain pathology (atrophy and lesion volume), unemployment, and disability.[67] In other research, inverse relationships have been reported between brain pathology and quality of life. In one study of 60 patients, lesion load and atrophy in the parietal cortices were specifically associated with the MS Quality of Life – 54 (MSQOL-54) assessed role limitations, sexual dysfunction, and mental health.[50] Greater supratentorial lesion load has been associated with lower social role performance as assessed by the Short Form 36 Health Survey (SF-36) among 156 MS patient early in their disease course.[34] A recent large volumetric study of 507 MS patients has found that lower global white and particularly gray matter volumes and global lesion load were associated with poorer emotional well-being and worse reported thinking/fatigue levels assessed with the Health-Related Quality-of-Life questionnaire (HRQOL).[63] Together, these studies suggest a direct link between brain pathology, functional outcomes, and quality of life and support potential mediation via cognitive function.

Summary

While the precise etiological and neuropathological mechanisms of MS remain to be determined, neuroimaging has provided many critical discoveries and is leading the way toward an ever-growing understanding of the nature of this disease. Therefore, MS is likely to remain on the forefront of the transition of research neuroimaging techniques to clinical applications. Promising new methods are being developed to help address unresolved questions in MS research. These include new imaging techniques and new analysis methods applied in the analysis of routinely acquired imaging data. Basic questions remain to be clarified about mechanisms of lesions and atrophy and how white and gray matter pathology interact to affect brain function and cognitive performance. Multisequence MRI is needed to address these types of questions. For instance, functional neuroimaging provides objective assessment of subjective states, such as fatigue and depressed mood that can be examined for relationships with structural indices and cognitive performance. Overall, the recent focus on gray matter structure and function in MS is promising. The convergence of research on gray matter function using FMRI and gray matter pathology using newer quantification methods allows for more direct inferences about disease mechanisms and about how brain dysfunction affects cognitive dysfunction.

References

1. Alonso A, Hernan MA. Temporal trends in the incidence of multiple sclerosis: a systematic review. *Neurology.* 2008;71(2):129–135.
2. Amato MP, Bartolozzi ML, Zipoli V, et al. Neocortical volume decrease in relapsing-remitting MS patients with mild cognitive impairment. *Neurology.* 2004;63(1):89–93.

3. Amato MP, Zipoli V, Portaccio E. Cognitive changes in multiple sclerosis. *Expert Rev Neurother.* 2008;8(10):1585–1596.
4. APA. *Diagnostic and Statistical Manual – IV.* Washington, DC: American Psychiatric Association; 1994.
5. Arnett P, Rao SM, Bernardin L, Grafman J, Yetkin F, Lobeck L. Relationship between frontal lobe lesion and Wisconsin card sorting test performance in patients with MS. *Neurology.* 1994;44:420–425.
6. Au Duong MV, Audoin B, Boulanouar K, et al. Altered functional connectivity related to white matter changes inside the working memory network at the very early stage of MS. *J Cereb Blood Flow Metab.* 2005;25(10):1245–1253.
7. Au Duong MV, Boulanouar K, Audoin B, et al. Modulation of effective connectivity inside the working memory network in patients at the earliest stage of multiple sclerosis. *Neuroimage.* 2005;24(2):533–538.
8. Audoin B, Ibarrola D, Au Duong MV, et al. Functional MRI study of PASAT in normal subjects. *Magma.* 2005;18(2):96–102.
9. Audoin B, Ibarrola D, Ranjeva JP, et al. Compensatory cortical activation observed by fMRI during a cognitive task at the earliest stage of MS. *Hum Brain Mapp.* 2003;20(2):51–58.
10. Bakshi R, Benedict RH, Bermel RA, Jacobs L. Regional brain atrophy is associated with physical disability in multiple sclerosis: semiquantitative magnetic resonance imaging and relationship to clinical findings. *J Neuroimaging.* 2001;11(2):129–136.
11. Baum HM, Rothschild BB. The incidence and prevalence of reported multiple sclerosis. *Ann Neurol.* 1981;10(5):420–428.
12. Baumhefner RW, Tourtellotte WW, Syndulko K, et al. Quantitative multiple sclerosis plaque assessment with magnetic resonance imaging. Its correlation with clinical parameters, evoked potentials, and intra-blood–brain barrier IgG synthesis. *Arch Neurol.* 1990;47(1):19–26.
13. Beatty WW, Goodkin DE, Monson N, Beatty PA. Cognitive disturbances in patients with relapsing remitting multiple sclerosis. *Arch Neurol.* 1989;46:1113.
14. Benedict RH, Bruce JM, Dwyer MG, et al. Neocortical atrophy, third ventricular width, and cognitive dysfunction in multiple sclerosis. *Arch Neurol.* 2006;63(9):1301–1306.
15. Benedict RH, Carone DA, Bakshi R. Correlating brain atrophy with cognitive dysfunction, mood disturbances, and personality disorder in multiple sclerosis. *J Neuroimaging.* 2004;14(3 suppl):36S–45S.
16. Benedict RH, Fischer JS, Archibald CJ, et al. Minimal neuropsychological assessment of MS patients: a consensus approach. *Clin Neuropsychol.* 2002;16(3):381–397.
17. Berg D, Maurer M, Warmuth-Metz M, Rieckmann P, Becker G. The correlation between ventricular diameter measured by transcranial sonography and clinical disability and cognitive dysfunction in patients with multiple sclerosis. *Arch Neurol.* 2000;57(9):1289–1292.
18. Bermel RA, Bakshi R, Tjoa C, Puli SR, Jacobs L. Bicaudate ratio as a magnetic resonance imaging marker of brain atrophy in multiple sclerosis. *Arch Neurol.* 2002;59:275.
19. Blinkenberg M, Rune K, Jensen CV, et al. Cortical cerebral metabolism correlates with MRI lesion load and cognitive dysfunction in MS. *Neurology.* 2000;54(3):558–564.

20. Bobholz JA, Rao SM. Cognitive dysfunction in multiple sclerosis: a review of recent developments. *Curr Opin Neurol.* 2003;16(3):283–288.

21. Bobholz JA, Rao SM, Lobeck L, et al. fMRI study of episodic memory in relapsing-remitting MS: correlation with T2 lesion volume. *Neurology.* 2006;67(9):1640–1645.

22. Bonzano L, Pardini M, Mancardi GL, Pizzorno M, Roccatagliata L. Structural connectivity influences brain activation during PVSAT in multiple sclerosis. *Neuroimage.* 2009;44(1):9–15.

23. Brassington JC, Marsh NV. Neuropsychological aspects of multiple sclerosis. *Neuropsychol Rev.* 1998;8(2):43–77.

24. Brooks DJ, Leenders KL, Head G, Marshall J, Legg NJ, Jones T. Studies on regional cerebral oxygen utilisation and cognitive function in multiple sclerosis. *J Neurol Neurosurg Psychiatry.* 1984;47(11):1182–1191.

25. Brownell B, Hughes JT. The distribution of plaques in the cerebrum in multiple sclerosis. *J Neurol Neurosurg Psychiatry.* 1962;25:315.

26. Bush G, Whalen PJ, Rosen BR, Jenike MA, McInerney SC, Rauch SL. The counting Stroop: an interference task specialized for functional neuroimaging–validation study with functional MRI. *Hum Brain Mapp.* 1998;6(4):270–282.

27. Cader S, Cifelli A, Abu-Omar Y, Palace J, Matthews PM. Reduced brain functional reserve and altered functional connectivity in patients with multiple sclerosis. *Brain.* 2006;129(pt 2):527–537.

28. Chiaravalloti N, Hillary F, Ricker J, et al. Cerebral activation patterns during working memory performance in multiple sclerosis using FMRI. *J Clin Exp Neuropsychol.* 2005; 27(1):33–54.

29. Chiaravalloti ND, DeLuca J. Cognitive impairment in multiple sclerosis. *Lancet Neurol.* 2008;7(12):1139–1151.

30. Christodoulou C, Krupp LB, Liang Z, et al. Cognitive performance and MR markers of cerebral injury in cognitively impaired MS patients. *Neurology.* 2003;60(11):1793–1798.

31. Chwastiak L, Ehde DM, Gibbons LE, Sullivan M, Bowen JD, Kraft GH. Depressive symptoms and severity of illness in multiple sclerosis: epidemiologic study of a large community sample. *Am J Psychiatry.* 2002;159(11):1862–1868.

32. Comi G, Filippi M, Martinelli V, et al. Brain magnetic resonance imaging correlates of cognitive impairment in multiple sclerosis. *J Neurol Sci.* 1993;115(suppl):S66–73.

33. Cutter GR, Baier ML, Rudick RA, et al. Development of a multiple sclerosis functional composite as a clinical trial outcome measure. *Brain.* 1999;122(pt 5):871–882.

34. de Groot V, Beckerman H, Twisk JW, et al. Vitality, perceived social support and disease activity determine the performance of social roles in recently diagnosed multiple sclerosis: a longitudinal analysis. *J Rehabil Med.* 2008; 40(2):151–157.

35. Ebers GC, Sadovnick AD. Epidemiology. In: Paty DW, Ebers GC, eds. *Multiple Sclerosis.* Philadelphia, PA: FA Davis Co; 1998:5–28.

36. Filippi M, Tortorella C, Rovaris M, et al. Changes in the normal appearing brain tissue and cognitive impairment in multiple sclerosis. *J Neurol Neurosurg Psychiatry.* 2000;68(2): 157–161.

37. Foong J, Rozewicz L, Quaghebeur G, et al. Executive function in multiple sclerosis. The role of frontal lobe pathology. *Brain.* 1997;120(1):15–26.

38. Forn C, Barros-Loscertales A, Escudero J, et al. Cortical reorganization during PASAT task in MS patients with preserved working memory functions. *Neuroimage.* 2006;31(2): 686–691.

39. Forn C, Barros-Loscertales A, Escudero JN, et al. Compensatory activations in patients with multiple sclerosis during preserved performance on the auditory N-back task. *Hum Brain Mapp.* 2007;28(5):424–430.

40. Franklin GM, Heaton RK, Nelson LM, Filley CM, Seibert C. Correlation of neuropsychological and MRI findings in chronic/progressive multiple sclerosis. *Neurology.* 1988;38(12): 1826–1829.

41. Gronwall DM. Paced auditory serial-addition task: a measure of recovery from concussion. *Percept Mot Skills.* 1977; 44(2):367–373.

42. Haacke EM, Makki M, Ge Y, et al. Characterizing iron deposition in multiple sclerosis lesions using susceptibility weighted imaging. *J Magn Reson Imaging.* 2009;29(3): 537–544.

43. Hillary FG, Chiaravalloti ND, Ricker JH, et al. An investigation of working memory rehearsal in multiple sclerosis using fMRI. *J Clin Exp Neuropsychol.* 2003;25(7):965–978.

44. Hohol MJ, Guttmann CRG, Orav J, et al. Serial neuropsychological assessment and magnetic resonance imaging analysis in multiple sclerosis. *Arch Neurol.* 1997;54(8):1018–1025.

45. Houtchens MK, Benedict RH, Killiany R, et al. Thalamic atrophy and cognition in multiple sclerosis. *Neurology.* 2007;69(12):1213–1223.

46. Huber SJ, Bornstein RA, Rammohan KW, Christy JA. Magnetic resonance imaging correlates of executive function impairments in multiple sclerosis. *Neuropsychiatry Neuropsychol Behav Neurol.* 1992;5(1):33–36.

47. Huber SJ, Bornstein RA, Rammohan KW, Christy JA. Magnetic resonance imaging correlates of neuropsychological impairment in multiple sclerosis. *J Neuropsychiatry Clin Neurosci.* 1992;4(2):152–158.

48. Huber SJ, Paulson GW, Shuttleworth EC, et al. Magnetic resonance imaging correlates of dementia in multiple sclerosis. *Arch Neurol.* 1987;44(7):732–736.

49. Inglese M, Adhya S, Johnson G, et al. Perfusion magnetic resonance imaging correlates of neuropsychological impairment in multiple sclerosis. *J Cereb Blood Flow Metab.* 2008;28(1):164–171.

50. Janardhan V, Bakshi R. Quality of life and its relationship to brain lesions and atrophy on magnetic resonance images in 60 patients with multiple sclerosis. *Arch Neurol.* 2000;57(10):1485–1491.

51. Kessler RC, Berglund P, Demler O, et al. The epidemiology of major depressive disorder: results from the National Comorbidity Survey Replication (NCS-R). *JAMA.* 2003; 289(23):3095–3105.

52. Lazeron RH, Boringa JB, Schouten M, et al. Brain atrophy and lesion load as explaining parameters for cognitive impairment in multiple sclerosis. *Mult Scler.* 2005;11(5): 524–531.

53. Lazeron RH, Rombouts SA, Scheltens P, Polman CH, Barkhof F. An fMRI study of planning-related brain activity in patients with moderately advanced multiple sclerosis. *Mult Scler.* 2004;10(5):549–555.

54. Li Y, Chiaravalloti ND, Hillary FG, et al. Differential cerebellar activation on functional magnetic resonance

imaging during working memory performance in persons with multiple sclerosis. *Arch Phys Med Rehabil.* 2004; 85(4):635–639.

55. Lycke J, Wikkelso C, Bergh AC, Jacobsson L, Andersen O. Regional cerebral blood flow in multiple sclerosis measured by single photon emission tomography with technetium-99m hexamethylpropyleneamine oxime. *Eur Neurol.* 1993;33(2):163–167.

56. Mainero C, Caramia F, Pozzilli C, et al. fMRI evidence of brain reorganization during attention and memory tasks in multiple sclerosis. *Neuroimage.* 2004;21(3):858–867.

57. Mathiesen HK, Jonsson A, Tscherning T, et al. Correlation of global N-acetyl aspartate with cognitive impairment in multiple sclerosis. *Arch Neurol.* 2006;63(4):533–536.

58. McDonald WI, Compston A, Edan G, et al. Recommended diagnostic criteria for multiple sclerosis: guidelines from the International Panel on the diagnosis of multiple sclerosis. *Ann Neurol.* 2001;50(1):121–127.

59. Minden SL, Schiffer RB. Affective disorders in multiple sclerosis. Review and recommendations for clinical research. *Arch Neurol.* 1990;47(1):98–104.

60. Moller A, Wiedemann G, Rohde U, Backmund H, Sonntag A. Correlates of cognitive impairment and depressive mood disorder in multiple sclerosis. *Acta Psychiatr Scand.* 1994;89(2):117–121.

61. Morgen K, Sammer G, Courtney SM, et al. Evidence for a direct association between cortical atrophy and cognitive impairment in relapsing-remitting MS. *Neuroimage.* 2006;30(3):891–898.

62. Morgen K, Sammer G, Courtney SM, et al. Distinct mechanisms of altered brain activation in patients with multiple sclerosis. *Neuroimage.* 2007;37(3):937–946.

63. Mowry EM, Beheshtian A, Waubant E, et al. Quality of life in multiple sclerosis is associated with lesion burden and brain volume measures. *Neurology.* 2009;72(20):1760–1765.

64. Nebel K, Wiese H, Seyfarth J, et al. Activity of attention related structures in multiple sclerosis patients. *Brain Res.* 2007;1151:150–160.

65. Owen AM, McMillan KM, Laird AR, Bullmore E. N-back working memory paradigm: a meta-analysis of normative functional neuroimaging studies. *Hum Brain Mapp.* 2005; 25(1):46–59.

66. Pan JW, Krupp LB, Elkins LE, Coyle PK. Cognitive dysfunction lateralizes with NAA in multiple sclerosis. *Appl Neuropsychol.* 2001;8(3):155–160.

67. Parmenter BA, Zivadinov R, Kerenyi L, et al. Validity of the Wisconsin Card Sorting and Delis–Kaplan Executive Function System (DKEFS) Sorting Tests in multiple sclerosis. *J Clin Exp Neuropsychol.* 2007;29(2):215–223.

68. Parry AM, Scott RB, Palace J, Smith S, Matthews PM. Potentially adaptive functional changes in cognitive processing for patients with multiple sclerosis and their acute modulation by rivastigmine. *Brain.* 2003;126(12):2750–2760.

69. Paulesu E, Perani D, Fazio F, et al. Functional basis of memory impairment in multiple sclerosis: a [18F]FDG PET study. *Neuroimage.* 1996;4(2):87–96.

70. Pelletier J, Suchet L, Witjas T, et al. A longitudinal study of callosal atrophy and interhemispheric dysfunction in relapsing-remitting multiple sclerosis. *Arch Neurol.* 2001; 58(1):105–111.

71. Penner IK, Rausch M, Kappos L, Opwis K, Radu EW. Analysis of impairment related functional architecture in MS patients during performance of different attention tasks. *J Neurol.* 2003;250(4):461–472.

72. Piras MR, Magnano I, Canu ED, et al. Longitudinal study of cognitive dysfunction in multiple sclerosis: neuropsychological, neuroradiological, and neurophysiological findings. *J Neurol Neurosurg Psychiatry.* 2003;74(7):878–885.

73. Portaccio E, Amato MP, Bartolozzi ML, et al. Neocortical volume decrease in relapsing-remitting multiple sclerosis with mild cognitive impairment. *J Neurol Sci.* 2006;245(1–2): 195–199.

74. Poser CM, Brinar VV. Diagnostic criteria for multiple sclerosis: an historical review. *Clin Neurol Neurosurg.* 2004;106(3):147–158.

75. Pozzilli C, Passafiume D, Bernardi S, et al. SPECT, MRI and cognitive functions in multiple sclerosis. *J Neurol Neurosurg Psychiatry.* 1991;54(2):110–115.

76. Prinster A, Quarantelli M, Orefice G, et al. Grey matter loss in relapsing-remitting multiple sclerosis: a voxel-based morphometry study. *Neuroimage.* 2006;29(3):859–867.

77. Rachbauer D, Kronbichler M, Ropele S, Enzinger C, Fazekas F. Differences in cerebral activation patterns in idiopathic inflammatory demyelination using the paced visual serial addition task: an fMRI study. *J Neurol Sci.* 2006;244(1–2):11–16.

78. Rao SM. Neuropsychological studies in chronic progressive multiple sclerosis. *Ann N Y Acad Sci.* 1984;436:495–497.

79. Rao SM. *Neurobehavioral Aspects of Multiple Sclerosis.* New York: Oxford University Press; 1990.

80. Rao SM, Leo GJ, Bernardin L, Unverzagt F. Cognitive dysfunction in multiple sclerosis. I. Frequency, patterns, and prediction. *Neurology.* 1991;41(5):685–691.

81. Rao SM, Leo GJ, Ellington L, Nauertz T, Bernardin L, Unverzagt F. Cognitive dysfunction in multiple sclerosis. II. Impact on employment and social functioning. *Neurology.* 1991;41(5):692–696.

82. Rao SM, Leo GJ, Haughton VM, St Aubin-Faubert P, Bernardin L. Correlation of magnetic resonance imaging with neuropsychological testing in multiple sclerosis. *Neurology.* 1989;39(1):161–166.

83. Roca M, Torralva T, Meli F, et al. Cognitive deficits in multiple sclerosis correlate with changes in fronto-subcortical tracts. *Mult Scler.* 2008;14(3):364–369.

84. Roelcke U, Kappos L, Lechner-Scott J, et al. Reduced glucose metabolism in the frontal cortex and basal ganglia of multiple sclerosis patients with fatigue: a 18F-fluorodeoxyglucose positron emission tomography study. *Neurology.* 1997;48(6):1566–1571.

85. Ron MA. Multiple sclerosis: psychiatric and psychometric abnormalities. *J Psychosom Res.* 1986;30(1):3–11.

86. Rovaris M, Filippi M, Falautano M, et al. Relation between MR abnormalities and patterns of cognitive impairment in multiple sclerosis. *Neurology.* 1998;50(6):1601–1608.

87. Rovaris M, Filippi M, Minicucci L, et al. Cortical/subcortical disease burden and cognitive impairment in patients with multiple sclerosis. *AJNR Am J Neuroradiol.* 2000; 21(2):402–408.

88. Rovaris M, Iannucci G, Falautano M, et al. Cognitive dysfunction in patients with mildly disabling relapsing-remitting

multiple sclerosis: an exploratory study with diffusion tensor MR imaging. *J Neurol Sci.* 2002;195(2):103–109.

89. Ryan L, Clark C, Klonoff H, Li D, Paty D. Patterns of cognitive impairment in relapsing-remitting multiple sclerosis and their relationship to neuropathy on MRI. *Neuropsychology.* 1996;10:176–193.

90. Sailer M, Fischl B, Salat D, et al. Focal thinning of the cerebral cortex in multiple sclerosis. *Brain.* 2003;126(8): 1734–1744.

91. Sanfilipo MP, Benedict RH, Weinstock-Guttman B, Bakshi R. Gray and white matter brain atrophy and neuropsychological impairment in multiple sclerosis. *Neurology.* 2006; 66(5):685–692.

92. Shallice T. Specific impairments of planning. *Philos Trans R Soc Lond B Biol Sci.* 1982;298(1089):199–209.

93. Sperling RA, Guttmann CR, Hohol MJ, et al. Regional magnetic resonance imaging lesion burden and cognitive function in multiple sclerosis: a longitudinal study. *Arch Neurol.* 2001;58(1):115–121.

94. Staffen W, Mair A, Zauner H, et al. Cognitive function and fMRI in patients with multiple sclerosis: evidence for compensatory cortical activation during an attention task. *Brain.* 2002;125(6):1275–1282.

95. Staffen W, Zauner H, Mair A, et al. Magnetic resonance spectroscopy of memory and frontal brain region in early multiple sclerosis. *J Neuropsychiatry Clin Neurosci.* 2005; 17(3):357–363.

96. Summers M, Swanton J, Fernando K, et al. Cognitive impairment in multiple sclerosis can be predicted by imaging early in the disease. *J Neurol Neurosurg Psychiatry.* 2008;79(8):955–958.

97. Sun X, Tanaka M, Kondo S, Okamoto K, Hirai S. Clinical significance of reduced cerebral metabolism in multiple sclerosis: a combined PET and MRI study. *Ann Nucl Med.* 1998;12(2):89–94.

98. Sweet LH, Rao SM, Primeau M, Durgerian S, Cohen RA. Functional magnetic resonance imaging response to increased verbal working memory demands among patients with multiple sclerosis. *Hum Brain Mapp.* 2006;27(1): 28–36.

99. Sweet LH, Rao SM, Primeau M, Mayer AR, Cohen RA. Functional magnetic resonance imaging of working memory among multiple sclerosis patients. *J Neuroimaging.* 2004;14(2):150–157.

100. Swirsky-Sacchetti T, Mitchell DR, Seward J, et al. Neuropsychological and structural brain lesions in multiple sclerosis: a regional analysis. *Neurology.* 1992;42(7): 1291–1295.

101. Tekok-Kilic A, Benedict RH, Zivadinov R. Update on the relationships between neuropsychological dysfunction and structural MRI in multiple sclerosis. *Expert Rev Neurother.* 2006;6(3):323–331.

102. Tsolaki M, Drevelegas A, Karachristianou S, Kapinas K. Correlation of dementia, neuropsychological and MRI findings in multiple sclerosis. *Dementia.* 1994;5(1): 48–52.

103. Valsasina P, Benedetti B, Rovaris M, Sormani MP, Comi G, Filippi M. Evidence for progressive gray matter loss in patients with relapsing-remitting MS. *Neurology.* 2005;65(7): 1126–1128.

104. Wishart HA, Saykin AJ, McDonald BC, et al. Brain activation patterns associated with working memory in relapsing-remitting MS. *Neurology.* 2004;62(2):234–238.

105. Zivadinov R, De Masi R, Nasuelli D, et al. MRI techniques and cognitive impairment in the early phase of relapsing-remitting multiple sclerosis. *Neuroradiology.* 2001;43(4):272–278.

106. Zivadinov R, Sepcic J, Nasuelli D, et al. A longitudinal study of brain atrophy and cognitive disturbances in the early phase of relapsing-remitting multiple sclerosis. *J Neurol Neurosurg Psychiatry.* 2001;70(6):773–780.

Chapter 22
Neuroimaging of Fatigue

Helen M. Genova, Glenn R. Wylie, and John DeLuca

Fatigue is a common problem afflicting up to 40% of the population based on community samples.[1] It is often one of the primary complaints in visits to primary care and the hospital, as well as to family physicians[2] and can have a significant negative effect on quality of life.[3] Fatigue is also a nonspecific symptom observed in numerous neurological, psychiatric and other medical disorders. Although elusive, definitions of fatigue have been based primarily on its subjective nature. For instance, the Multiple Sclerosis Council for Clinical Practice Guidelines[4] defines fatigue as "a subjective lack of physical and/or mental energy that is perceived by the individual or caregiver to interfere with usual and desired activities." One of the challenges of studying fatigue is that it is clearly not a unitary concept. For instance, fatigue can be operationalized as behavioral performance decrements (objective fatigue) or as a person's perception of fatigue (subjective fatigue) (for review see ref. [5]). Fatigue can also be divided into other components such as central and peripheral fatigue, or as cognitive and physical fatigue. Fatigue has also been conceptualized as both a symptom and an illness. Adding to the confusion is the construct contamination often observed in studies of fatigue. For instance, inventories meant to assess fatigue often include items on sleepiness and cognition, both of which may not be directly associated with fatigue (c.f. ref. [5]).

Fatigue has been reported to be one of the most common symptoms in medical disorders such as Multiple Sclerosis (MS), Chronic Fatigue Syndrome (CFS), Traumatic Brain Injury (TBI), Cancer, and Parkinson's Disease, to name a few. It may manifest as a primary symptom of the disorder (e.g., from neurological damage) or as a secondary symptom, such as a side effect of medications. Due to the multifaceted nature of fatigue and its presence in many clinical disorders with varying physiologies, the causes of fatigue are, for the most part, unknown. The purpose of the present chapter is to review the contribution of neuroimaging studies to our understanding of fatigue.

Figure 22.1 illustrates the number of studies that have been performed using neuroimaging techniques to study fatigue in various clinical conditions. Despite its frequency as a symptom in many medical disorders, fatigue research using neuroimaging has been limited primarily two disorders: MS and CFS. Therefore, the present chapter will focus primarily in reviewing the existing neuroimaging research on fatigue in MS and CFS, although we will provide a very brief discussion on other populations as well.

Fatigue in MS

Fatigue is one of the most common symptoms reported in persons with MS.[6] It is the most common symptom reported in over 90% of persons with MS (Schapiro 2006)[73] and was reported as the worst symptom in over two-thirds of MS patients.[6] Fatigue is associated with a high degree of disability such as reduced activities of daily living,[7] altered mood and ability to cope,[8] reduced energy and endurance,[9] and decreased quality of life.[10] There is also evidence that fatigue negatively affects employment and social relationships in MS.[6,11]

Although the pathophysiology of fatigue in MS remains elusive, several hypotheses have been offered

J. DeLuca (✉)
Kessler Foundation Research Center, 1199 Pleasant Valley Way, West Orange, NJ 07052, USA
and
Department of Physical Medicine and Rehabilitation, University of Medicine and Dentistry of New Jersey – New Jersey Medical School, Newark, NJ, USA
e-mail: jdeluca@kesslerfoundation.org

R.A. Cohen and L.H. Sweet (eds.), *Brain Imaging in Behavioral Medicine and Clinical Neuroscience*,
DOI 10.1007/978-1-4419-6373-4_22, © Springer Science+Business Media, LLC 2011

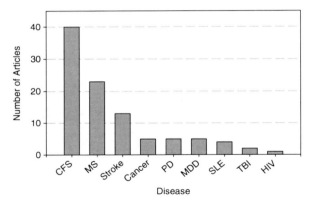

Fig. 22.1 Number of neuroimaging articles published on fatigue by clinical group. *CFS* chronic fatigue syndrome, *MS* multiple sclerosis, *PD* Parkinson's disease, *MDD* major depressive disorder, *SLE* systemic lupus erythematosus, *TBI* traumatic brain injury, *HIV* human immunodeficiency virus. For each clinical group, we initially searched the PubMed data base with the terms [magnetic resonance imaging (MRI)] or [diffusion tensor imaging (DTI)] or [magnetic resonance spectroscopy (MRS)] or [positron emission tomography (PET)] or [single photon emission computerized tomography (SPECT)] or [magnetoencephalography (MEG)] or [magnetic resonance (MR)] or [functional magnetic resonance imaging (fMRI)] or "neuroimaging," then within those results, we searched for "fatigue," and then within those results, we searched for each of the disease types. Reviews and case studies were excluded

based on recent research. These include immune system dysregulation, neuroendocrine alterations,[12] presence of circulating cytokines,[13] impaired nerve conduction, neurotransmitter dysregulation, autonomic nervous system involvement, demyelination, and energy depletion (for review see ref. [6]). Secondary effects of MS might also be contributing to fatigue, such as medications, increased pain, sleep disturbances, and comorbidity of mood disorders.

A great deal of research has focused on damage to the central nervous system (CNS) as the major contributing factor to MS-related fatigue. In particular, research using neuroimaging has begun to provide evidence that several distinct areas of the CNS may be specifically involved in fatigue.

Structural MRI Studies of Fatigue in MS

Several studies have been conducted examining the relationship between self-reported measures of fatigue and structural damage in MS using MRI. Early studies focused primarily on lesion burden analysis using MRI, and showed little to no relationship between these indices of pathology and self-reported fatigue, although more recent research using more modern techniques have been somewhat more successful.

Of the early studies, van der Werf et al[14] examined the relationship between subjective fatigue severity (i.e., Checklist Individual Strength subscale of fatigue CIS-FATIGUE) and cerebral abnormalities (i.e., T2- and T1-weighted total lesion load in discrete cerebral areas, total lesion load, and cerebral atrophy). No relationship was found between cerebral abnormalities and fatigue. Similarly, Bakshi et al[15] found no relationship between fatigue severity and lesion load or atrophy in a sample of 71 patients with MS. Additionally when the sample was divided into fatigued and nonfatigued subjects, no differences in terms of MRI measures were detected between groups.

Mainero et al[16] suggested that increased fatigue in MS may be related to blood–brain barrier disruption, which would allow cytokines to infiltrate the CNS. It was hypothesized that the presence of gadolinium enhancing (Gd+) lesions on MRI scans would be indicative of blood–brain barrier disruption. Eleven patients with relapsing–remitting MS underwent enhanced MRI after standard-dose and triple-dose injection of gadolinium–diethylene triaminopentaacetic acid (Gd–DTPA). No relationship was found between the number and volume of Gd-enhancing lesions and fatigue severity at any time point studied. Several other studies utilizing MRI have attempted to detect a relationship between pathology and self-reported fatigue have also failed to find a relationship.[17-19]

While most studies using MRI in MS have failed to find a significant relationship between structural indices and subjective fatigue, a few studies have reported positive results. Colombo et al[20] divided their MS subjects into two groups: (1) patients with fatigue (fatigue severity scale; FSS) ≥ 25 and complaints of fatigue and (2) patients without fatigue (FSS<25 and no complaints of fatigue). Results showed that the fatigued MS group had significantly more lesions in the parietal lobe, internal capsule, and periventricular trigone compared to the nonfatigued group. These authors suggested that controlling for neurological disability by only including persons with mild disability increased the likelihood of detecting a relationship between fatigue and structural MRI variables and fatigue.

Marrie et al[21] examined the relationship between pathological changes on MRI and subjective fatigue longitudinally over 8 years. While no relationship between pathology and fatigue was observed after 2 years, a significant fatigue effect was observed over the 8-year period. This relationship remained significant even after adjusting for disability, mood, and the subjects' baseline MRI. These data may suggest that self-perception of fatigue may predate the observation of pathological changes that can be detected by MRI. As such, longitudinal design might be more sensitive in observing the relationship between fatigue and structural MRI variables.

Tedeschi et al[22] studied a large sample of MS subjects ($n=222$) and controlled for disability by only including subjects with EDSS scores ≤ 2. Whereas some earlier studies used methods to quantify pathology that were operator dependent and semiautomated, the Tedeschi et al study utilized a "fully automated, operator independent, multiparametric segmentation method" to measure various indices of pathology including white matter fraction (lower white matter fraction would indicate white matter atrophy), abnormal white matter fraction (i.e., lesion loads), and gray matter fraction (lower gray matter fraction would indicate gray matter atrophy). Results showed that MS subjects with high fatigue (higher FSS scores) had a significantly greater white matter atrophy, greater T1- and T2-lesion loads, and greater gray matter atrophy. A significant relationship was also found between higher scores on the FSS and lower white matter and gray matter fractions.

Fatigue in MS Using Advanced MRI Imaging

Although traditional MRI has provided inconsistent findings regarding the fatigue–pathology relationship in MS, more advanced MRI neuroimaging methods may be more sensitive to the changes in the brain which correlate with self-reported fatigue.

One technique that has been used to study neurometabolism is magnetic resonance spectroscopy (^{1}H-MRS). ^{1}H-MRS allows for the detection of differing metabolite levels, such as choline (Cho), lactate (Lac), creatine (Cr), and N-acetyl-l-aspartate (NAA). Each of these metabolites provides valuable information regarding neuronal and axonal damage in MS, as they each correlate with particular aspects of neural function. Most research in MS using this technique has examined levels of NAA, the second most abundant amino acid in the brain. As it is found almost exclusively in normal mature neurons, NAA is considered a marker for neuronal integrity and density.[23] Generally, in MS, NAA levels have been shown to be decreased compared to controls, reflecting pathological changes in neuronal tissue. These decreases in NAA have also been shown to correlate with disability (for review see ref. [24]). ^{1}H-MRS has also allowed researchers to detect pathology in normal appearing white matter (NAWM). Damage to NAWM has also been shown to contribute to neurologic impairment.[24] In order to study NAA levels in the brain and their differences between groups, it is common practice to measure a metabolite ratio difference rather than absolute concentration differences (see ref. [25] for review). Such ratios are thought to correct for certain experimental conditions, such as field inhomogeneities and localization method differences.[25] Frequently, when examining NAA in the brain, the ratio of NAA to Creatine (Cr) is the ratio of interest, because creatine is thought to be stable in normal adults as well as clinical samples.[26,27]

Tartaglia et al[17] examined the relationship between axonal damage and subjective fatigue in MS using ^{1}H-MRS. They examined neurometabolite levels specifically in an area covering the corpus callosum and adjacent periventricular white matter in MS subjects which they divided into a high-fatigue group and low-fatigue group. After controlling for EDSS score and age, they found that the high-fatigue group had lower NAA/Cr ratio (i.e., reduced neuronal integrity) than the low-fatigue group. These findings remained significant after controlling for depression. Thus, MS subjects with greater complaints of fatigue had significantly greater levels of neuronal pathology. As mentioned above, these authors also examined the relationship between lesion load and fatigue and found no significant relationship. Taken together, these findings suggest that ^{1}H-MRS is more sensitive to pathological changes in the brain which may be correlated to subjective fatigue compared to traditional structural MRI indices.

Téllez et al[18] examined NAA/Cr levels in frontal white matter and the basal ganglia to determine whether the neurometabolite levels correlated with scores on both the FSS and the modified fatigue impact scale (mFIS). They divided their MS sample into a fatigued group and a nonfatigued group to examine whether differences in axonal damage could be identified between groups. A significant decrease in NAA/Cr in the lentiform nucleus of the basal ganglia was observed in patients with fatigue, a finding that remained after controlling for EDSS scores and depression. Additionally, a correlation was found between NAA/Cr levels of the basal ganglia and a subscale of the mFIS, such that NAA/Cr levels diminished as mFIS scores increased. Interestingly, no relationship between NAA/Cr and fatigue was found in white matter nor did the NAA/Cr levels in white matter differ between fatigued and nonfatigued MS subjects. These data suggest that localized damage (e.g., basal ganglia) may be related to subjective fatigue, suggesting that studies that have examined lesion load across brain regions may have been "washing out" the effect of interest. No relationship was found between fatigue and T2-lesion load, again suggesting that MRS may be more sensitive in detecting damage than MRI, at least when examining fatigue effects.

Not all of the studies using more advanced MRI techniques have found a relationship between subjective fatigue and neuropathology. For example, two relatively new techniques for studying pathology are diffusion tensor imaging (DTI) and magnetization transfer imaging (MTI). DTI is a technique that measures the integrity of white matter in vivo, by measuring the diffusivity of water.[28,29] MTI is a technique for improving image contrast in MR imaging. This technique may allow for the subcategorization of MS lesions into those due to demylination vs. those due to inflammation and swelling. Codella et al[30] found no difference in gray matter pathology (assessed by MTI and DTI) between fatigued and nonfatigued MS patients. Furthermore, no correlation was detected between the FSS and any MT/DTI measures. The same group published a similar study[31] examining overall pathology using DTI/MT and reported similarly that no relationship existed between pathology and subjective fatigue. While more work is needed, the initial research suggests that damage detected by MT and DTI may be unrelated to fatigue and that other neuroimaging measures may be more sensitive in persons with MS.

Functional Neuroimaging Techniques to Examine Fatigue in MS

Functional neuroimaging techniques to study fatigue in MS consist primarily of and Positron Emission Tomagraphy (PET) and functional magnetic resonance imaging (fMRI).

Roelcke et al[32] used 18F-fluorodeoxyglucose PET to measure cerebral glucose metabolism in a sample of 47 persons with MS. The MS sample was divided into those with vs. without fatigue based on self-report using the FSS. They found significantly reduced glucose metabolism in prefrontal regions and premotor cortex, putamen, and in the right supplementary motor area in the fatigued MS group compared to the nonfatigue MS group. The fatigued MS group also showed hypometabolism in white matter extending from the rostral putamen toward the lateral head of the caudate nucleus, and a negative correlation between FSS scores and glucose metabolism in the right prefrontal cortex. In contrast, elevated glucose metabolism was observed in the nonfatigued MS group in the cerebellar vermis and anterior cingulate. Roelcke et al[32] concluded that both the basal ganglia and the prefrontal regions are critical for the expression of fatigue in MS.

Most of the functional imaging studies of fatigue in MS have utilized fMRI. Based on the FSS, Filippi et al[19] examined 15 MS subjects with subjective fatigue and 14 MS subjects without fatigue and measured BOLD activation during performance of a simple motor task. The fatigued MS group had significantly less cerebral activation than the nonfatigued MS group in several regions involved in motor planning and execution. These included the ipsilateral cerebellar hemisphere, ipsilateral precuneus, contralateral thalamus, and contralateral middle frontal gyrus. A negative correlation was observed between FSS scores and cerebral activation in the thalamus. Given the role of the thalamus as a relay station between prefrontal regions and basal ganglia, the authors suggested that the observed findings were due to a disruption of cortical–subcortical circuits in the MS subjects with fatigue. While the fatigued MS group showed under-recruitment of motor regions, they also displayed increased activation in the anterior cingulate compared to the nonfatigued group. Filippi et al[19] suggested that the recruitment of the anterior cingulate in the fatigued group may represent a "compensatory mechanism" due to the increased effort required for the fatigued MS subjects to perform the task. Interestingly, in their analysis of the structural MRI data, no significant differences in lesion load quantity was observed between the fatigued and nonfatigued MS groups, suggesting that functional cerebral changes may be more sensitive than structural imaging indices in identifying brain regions associated with fatigue.

The functional imaging studies reviewed thus far have utilized subjective report as the measure of fatigue. More recently, several investigators have attempted to obtain objective measures of cognitive fatigue rather than focusing on subjective measure which have little specificity. Objective measurements of cognitive fatigue have focused on behavioral performance during cognitive challenges. To accomplish this, cognitive fatigue has been conceptualized in at least two different ways: (1) performance during a *prolonged period of time* (e.g., beginning to end of workday) and (2) performance during *sustained mental effort*. Of these two, successful attempts at objective measurement of cognitive fatigue have been observed almost exclusively on decreased behavioral performance on tasks requiring *sustained mental effort* (c.f. ref. [5] for a review). This approach is conceptually similar to that of motor fatigue where fatigue has been defined as a failure to maintain a required force or output of power during sustained or repeated muscle contraction. This idea of objectively measuring cognitive fatigue during fMRI acquisition has been utilized recently in persons with MS to examine brain regions associated with fatigue.

DeLuca et al[33] administered four trials of a sustained attention task (i.e., modified symbol digit modalities task or mSDMT) during fMRI acquisition, attempting to induce cognitive fatigue in persons with MS and in healthy controls. The fMRI literature has shown that with repeated administration of a task, cerebral activation in healthy subjects decreases over time.[34-36] Thus, DeLuca et al[33] hypothesized that healthy individuals would show a *decrease* in cerebral activation to repeated administration of the mSDMT tasks over time. In contrast, they hypothesized that participants with MS would show a greater *increase* in cerebral activity, while performing the mSDMT across time compared to healthy controls. That is, DeLuca et al[33] operationally defined "cognitive fatigue" as an increase in cerebral activation across the four trials of a processing speed task in individuals with MS, relative to the control group (who would exhibit a decrease in brain activity across time). No group differences in performance accuracy across the four trials of the cognitive task were observed, although the MS performed the task more slowly. As hypothesized, the MS group showed increased cerebral activation in key areas of the brain, whereas the healthy group showed decreased activation (see Figs. 22.2 and 22.3). These regions

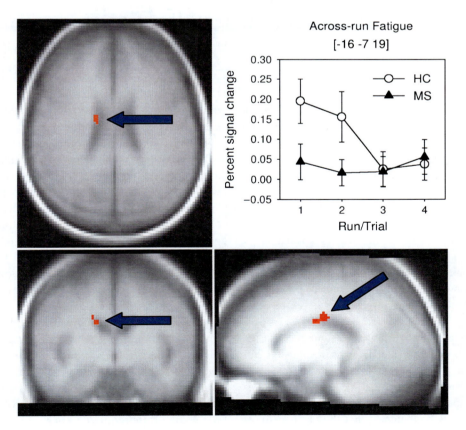

Fig. 22.2 Activity in Caudate in the interaction (*inset graph*) between MS and HC groups. From DeLuca et al[33].

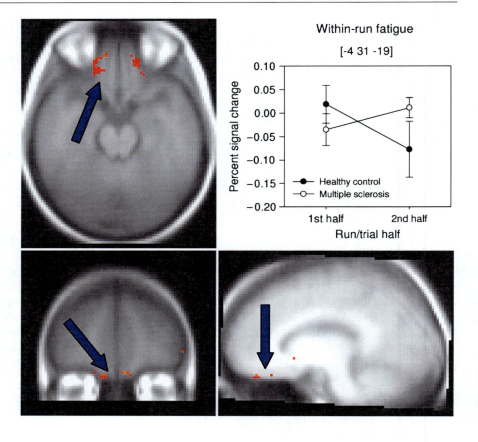

Fig. 22.3 Activity in orbital frontal gyrus. The axial, coronal, and sagital views are shown for the interaction (*inset graph*) between group (MS and HC) and within-run fatigue. From DeLuca et al[33].

included the precuneus, superior parietal lobe (BA 7), medial/orbital frontal gyrus, inferior parietal lobe, and the caudate in the basal ganglia. The authors suggested that the increased activation in the MS group (i.e., cognitive fatigue) may represent the increased "cerebral effort" to maintain adequate performance. While other authors have hypothesized that the extra "cerebral effort" may represent compensation,[37,38] DeLuca et al's[33] construct of cognitive fatigue provides an alternative explanation for the effort hypothesis. Unfortunately, DeLuca et al[33] did not assess subjective fatigue in their study. As such, it was unclear how the objective performance-based measure of cognitive fatigue correlates with self-reported fatigue in MS.

The DeLuca et al[33] study was designed to test the current model of brain mechanisms responsible for central fatigue proposed by Chaudhuri and Behan.[39,40] This model hypothesizes that "central fatigue" is derived from the nonmotor function of the basal ganglia. Chaudhuri and Behan suggest that the mechanism of fatigue was due to altered communication within the basal ganglia system affecting feedback between striato-thalamo-cortical fibers. The results of the DeLuca et al[33] study show altered cerebral activation within the basal ganglia and frontal lobes during a cognitively fatiguing task, and thus lend direct support to the Chaudhuri and Behan model.

Tartaglia et al[41] also conducted a behavioral study designed to objectively assess cognitive fatigue in persons with MS. They hypothesized that induced cognitive fatigue could alter cerebral activation patterns associated with subsequent motor performance. This was based on the idea that fatigue in MS may be related to "greater demands being placed on diminishing functional neural circuits, resulting in reduced capacity to respond to new demands.[41]" examined fMRI activation in three stages. First, subjects performed a motor task (stage 1), followed by a challenging cognitive task (the PASAT; stage 2), finally, they were required to perform the motor task again (stage 3). The healthy control (HC) group showed no significant difference in cerebral activation during the motor task in stage 1 compared with the same task in stage 3 (i.e., pre- vs. post-PASAT). The MS group displayed increased activity in multiple brain regions after performance of the PASAT relative to controls. These included bilateral cingulate gyrus, the postcentral gyrus, and the right prefrontal cortex. As hypothesized, while the HCs showed decreased activation on the motor task after PASAT performance (i.e., stage 3 vs. stage 1), in the MS group the activation in all recruited areas was increased. The authors concluded that induced cognitive fatigue could alter brain activation in an unrelated motor task in persons with MS.

In summary, structural MRI studies have yielded mixed results in identifying the underlying cerebral structures associated with fatigue in MS. Much more success has been observed in studies employing functional imaging, particularly fMRI. While most studies have utilized subjective report as the primary index of fatigue, a few have measured cognitive fatigue using objective performance during the imaging session.

Chronic Fatigue Syndrome

CFS is a heterogeneous illness characterized by severe and debilitating fatigue as well as infectious, rheumatological, and neuropsychiatric symptoms.[42] As illustrated in Fig. 22.1, many structural and functional imaging studies have been conducted in persons with CFS. One could expect that because fatigue is the defining characteristic of CFS, neuroimaging studies would reveal much about fatigue itself. However, this may not be the case. Most neuroimaging studies with CFS subjects were not conducted to specifically address fatigue per se, but rather to examine CFS as an illness. As such, some of the differences in brain structure and function between individuals with CFS and healthy controls might be related to differences in subject characteristics (e.g., psychopathology) rather than fatigue. Thus, only studies, which measure fatigue and use this measurement in the imaging data can be used to make inferences about brain mechanisms involved in fatigue in CFS. Unfortunately, only a handful of more recent studies have employed this approach in CFS.

Structural Neuroimaging in CFS and Fatigue

Most of the early studies in CFS have focused on identifying structural changes in the brain between CFS and controls. These studies have led to mixed results. When structural problems have been observed in CFS, they have been primarily associated with white matter hyperintensities. While several studies have found an increased number of white matter hyperintensities on MRI in CFS vs. healthy controls,[43,44] several other studies have not.[45,46] One possible reason for this was suggested by a study by[47] who found significantly more subcortical white matter hyperintensities in CFS subjects without psychiatric illness (concurrent or historic) compared to the CFS group with concurrent psychiatric illness. Similar findings were reported by.[48]

After dividing their CFS sample into those with and without cerebral abnormalities,[49] found significantly more impairments in physical functioning on the SF-36 in the CFS group with cerebral abnormalities relative to those without cerebral abnormalities. Lange et al[50] measured cerebral volume using MRI and found larger lateral ventrical volumes in the CFS group compared to healthy controls. Significantly reduced gray matter volume in prefrontal areas bilaterally has been observed in CFS as well.[51] In the Okada et al study, gray matter volume in the right prefrontal cortex was correlated with the severity of self-reported fatigue. The authors suggested that the prefrontal cortex may play a prominent role in the phenomenology of fatigue. de Lange et al[52] have reported that reduced gray matter volume in CFS can be partially reversed with cognitive behavioral therapy.

Functional Neuroimaging of Fatigue in CFS

Schwartz et al[53] used single proton emission computerized tomography (SPECT) and reported increased perfusion in lateral frontal cortex as well as lateral and medial temporal cortex in their CFS group. Machale et al[54] also reported increased perfusion in CFS using SPECT in the right thalamus and basal ganglia (pallidum and putamen).

In contrast, Costa et al[55] reported hypoperfusion using SPECT in the brainstem of their CFS sample. Taken together, while these SPECT studies show significant differences in cerebral blood flow (CBF) in persons with CFS, the relationship between CBF and fatigue is unclear. Fischler et al,[56] on the other hand, examined whether there was a relationship between physical and mental fatigue and cerebral perfusion using SPECT in persons with CFS. No relationship between cerebral perfusion and fatigue was found.

Using 18-flourodeoxyglucose PET (FDG-PET), Tirelli et al[57] reported significant decreases in cerebral metabolism in the frontal lobes of persons with CFS. Siessmeier et al[58] reported abnormalities in the anterior cingulate gyrus/mesial frontal cortex and orbital frontal cortex in about half of their CFS sample. Yet, no significant relationships were observed between reductions in glucose metabolism and subjective fatigue in CFS.

While the above studies using SPECT and PET utilized self-reported measures of fatigue, more recent studies have employed paradigms designed to induce fatigue during scanning. In such studies, subjects are required to perform a challenging task that one might expect would induce fatigue, and the pattern of cerebral activity is investigated in CFS relative to HCs. Using this approach, Schmaling et al[59] found that the CFS group displayed more widespread and diffuse rCBF in frontal, temporal, and thalamic regions relative to controls during SPECT scanning. Lange et al[60] required subjects to perform a challenging cognitive task during fMRI and found that persons with CFS showed more diffuse and bilateral activity than healthy controls. Specifically, healthy control subjects showed left-sided activity in frontal and parietal regions, while persons with CFS showed bilateral activity in frontal and parietal regions. Caseras et al[61] reported that as the difficulty of a working memory task increased, cerebral activation in the right prefrontal cortex also increased in the CFS group. While all of these studies that utilized challenging tasks as the experimental paradigm have shown group differences between individuals with CFS and controls, it remains unclear if these differences have anything to do with fatigue itself as no specific relationship with measures of fatigue were made.

More recent studies in CFS have included measures of fatigue in the analysis of the functional imaging data. One recent study using fMRI showed a relationship between subjective fatigue and functional brain activity during performance of a cognitive task (modified PASAT) in CFS.[62] These authors reported that subjective reports of fatigue were associated with task performance and were associated with significant activation in several brain regions including the cerebellum (vermis), the cingulate region (middle and posterior), inferior frontal gyrus, superior temporal gyrus, parietal regions, and the hippocampus. Using a similar approach, Tanaka et al[63] used fMRI to examine functional brain activity associated with both a difficult, fatiguing visual search task, and brain activity associated with a completely extraneous, task-irrelevant change in auditory stimulation. The CFS group showed significantly less cerebral activity than the healthy control group during the task-irrelevant change in auditory stimulation, and the activity was correlated with subjective ratings of fatigue. In contrast, the functional activity associated with the search task did not differ between the CFS and control groups, nor did it correlate with subjective ratings of fatigue. The authors suggested that CFS subjects may have less processing "capacity" and therefore have less ability to process task-irrelevant stimuli than healthy controls.

Caseras et al[64] utilized a novel approach to the study of fatigue in persons with CFS. These authors analyzed the BOLD response while persons with CFS were watching either a fatigue-inducing scenario (video clip) or an anxiety-inducing scenario. Following each scenario, subjects rated their feelings of fatigue and anxiety. Results showed that for both the CFS and healthy control groups, the fatiguing clips induced significantly greater feelings of fatigue than the anxiety-clips, and that the induced fatigue was significantly greater in the CFS group relative to controls. While watching the fatiguing clips, the CFS group showed significantly increased activity in cerebellum and occipito-parietal regions bilaterally extending toward the cingulate gyrus, the left hippocampal gyrus, and the left caudate nucleus. In the healthy group, significantly increased activity was observed while watching the fatigue clip relative to the anxiety clip in the right dorsolateral and bilateral medial prefrontal cortex (extending toward the anterior cingulate), right insula and right caudate nucleus. Fatigue was associated with activity in the basal ganglia (caudate) for both the CFS and healthy control groups. Interestingly, more activations were observed in the CFS group in posterior brain regions and those associated with emotion (cingulate), whereas the healthy control group showed more activity in frontal regions associated with executive control. Importantly, although the two studies used very different paradigms and analyses, the brain regions activated in the CFS group in the Caseras et al[64] study largely overlap with those reported by Cook et al[62]

In summary, despite evidence of structural changes in white matter and gray matter volume in persons with CFS, how these changes are associated with fatigue per se is unclear. Functional neuroimaging studies offer greater promise in understanding the cerebral mechanisms of fatigue in CFS. However, most of the existing functional imaging studies in CFS did not specifically examine fatigue, and thus must be interpreted with caution. When fatigue was specifically studied and related to functional brain activity, areas that appear to be significantly associated with fatigue in CFS included the basal ganglia, the cingulate, the cerebellum, and the parietal cortex. Many of these structures, particularly the basal ganglia, support the Chaudhuri and Behan[39,40] model of fatigue.

Functional Neuroimaging in Other Clinical Populations

Relative to the work completed in persons with CFS and MS, very few functional imaging studies examining fatigue have been completed in other populations (see Fig. 22.1). In persons with systemic lupus erythematosus, it has been reported that no relationship exists between subjective fatigue and regional cerebral blood flow.[65] In HIV-positive individuals, one study found no relationship between subjective fatigue and FDG-PET brain abnormalities.[66] However, in Major Depressive Disorder (MDD), fatigue was found to covary with measures of functional brain activity in one study.[67] Brody et al[67]

examined the association between changes in depressive symptoms and changes in regional brain metabolism using PET from before to after treatment in patients with MDD. It was observed that improvement in fatigue from pre- to posttreatment correlated with decreases in ventral PFC activity (metabolism) bilaterally.

Parkinson's disease (PD) is another disease where fatigue is a common debilitating symptom. Two studies examined the availability of dopamine in the basal ganglia and its relationship with fatigue in PD using SPECT. Schifitto et al[68] compared patients with PD who were fatigued to nonfatigued patients, and found no difference in their measure of striatal dopamine transporter density, $[^{123}I]$-β-CIT SPECT in the striatum, caudate, or putamen. Weintraub et al[69] also did not find a significant relationship between fatigue and striatal dopamine availability in PD. In contrast, Abe et al[70] found that higher fatigue scores were associated with less frontal perfusion in PD using SPECT.

One study has investigated fatigue in persons with TBI, using a paradigm similar to that employed by DeLuca et al[33] in an attempt to objectively measure cognitive fatigue using fMRI.[71] A cognitive task requiring sustained attention (i.e., SDMT) was administered three times consecutively during fMRI acquisition for both TBI and HC subjects. Like the DeLuca et al[33] study in MS, (see also above) Kohl et al hypothesized that TBI participants would show an *increase* in cerebral activity on the mSDMT in areas of the brain hypothesized to be associated with fatigue, while healthy controls would show *decreased* activation across time. This relative increase in cerebral activation with the cognitive challenge in persons with TBI was operationally defined "cognitive fatigue." Behaviorally, no significant difference in performance accuracy was observed between the TBI and HC group, although the TBI group was significantly slower in performing the task. However, in the fMRI data, relative increases in cerebral activation in the TBI groups was observed in the middle frontal gyrus (BA 10), the superior parietal lobe (BA 7), the basal ganglia (the putamen), and the anterior cingulate (BA 32) (see Fig. 22.4). These data were interpreted as supporting the Chaudhuri and Behan[39,40] model of central fatigue.

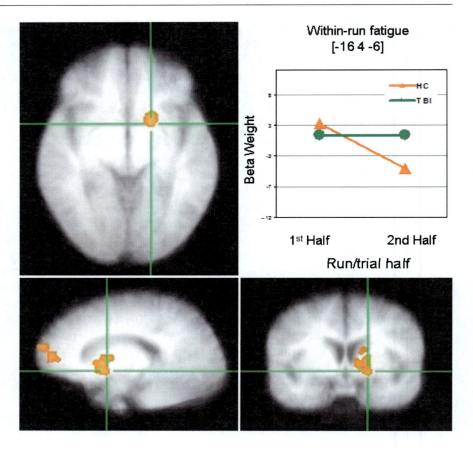

Fig. 22.4 Activity in the left basal ganglia (caudate/putamen). Axial, coronal, and sagital views of the interaction between group (TBI and HC) and fatigue. From Kohl et al.[71]

Conclusions

It is clear from the present review that there are relatively few neuroimaging studies geared toward understanding the neural architecture of fatigue, and that this research is in its infancy. Most of the studies of fatigue using neuroimaging have been conducted in persons with CFS or MS, with relatively few studies in other clinical populations. While the structural imaging studies have yielded largely mixed results, the newer functional imaging studies hold significant promise concerning the functional organization of fatigue in the brain. Unfortunately, most of these studies are again focused mainly on CFS or MS. One of the major challenges of fatigue research in general is that despite over 100 years of inquiry (see ref. [72]), the definition and conceptualization of fatigue as a construct remains elusive. Despite the fact that we have known for decades that fatigue is multidimensional in nature, clinicians and researchers continue to utilize self-report as the "gold standard." However, numerous authors have questioned the validity and utility of this single-minded approach (see ref. [5,12]). The vast majority of neuroimaging research has utilized self-reported fatigue as the preferred mode of assessing fatigue. Assessment of subjective fatigue benefits from ease of administration, but suffers from significant difficulties in interpretation. For example, we know that self-reported fatigue is most often correlated with degree of psychopathology.[12] In addition, with over a century of inquiry, one thing we know for sure is that self-reported fatigue does not correlate with objective measures of fatigue.[5,72] As a result, when functional imaging studies show a relationship between self-reported fatigue and functional activation in regions of the brain, one must remain cautious about the interpretation of these results. More recent functional imaging studies have attempted a novel approach of assessing fatigue behaviorally during scanning and relating such objective measures of fatigue with cerebral activation. However, it remains unclear if this novel approach of operationally defining fatigue behaviorally will provide a more valid paradigm in understanding the elusive construct of fatigue.

While fatigue is extraordinarily common as a symptom in many neurological and psychiatric diseases, we know very little about its precise mechanism. Current models of fatigue hypothesize that the nonmotor functions of the basal ganglia play a key role in central fatigue.[39,40] These authors posit that fatigue is due to "alterations in the normal flow of sequential activation within the basal ganglia system affecting the neural integrator and the cortical feedback by the associated loop of the striato-thalamo-cortical fibers is a possible mechanism of central fatigue ..." (p40). Thus, major functional interaction between the basal ganglia, the frontal cortex, the thalamus, and the amygdala are hypothesized to play a critical role in central fatigue. Overall, the functional imaging studies reviewed in this chapter tend to provide preliminary support for this model of fatigue. If indeed fatigue is associated with functional impairment in a cortical–subcortical circuit, studies which have examined structural damage (e.g., total lesion load throughout the brain) may simply not provide the sensitivity required to detect a relationship between fatigue and pathology. As such, functional neuroimaging techniques promise to provide an exciting potential for significant advances in our elusive understanding of the brain mechanisms associated with fatigue in clinical populations.

References

1. Lewis G, Wessely S. The epidemiology of fatigue: more questions than answers. *J Epidemiol Commun Health*. 1992;46: 92–97.
2. Manu P, Lane T, Matthews D. Chronic fatigue syndromes in clinical practice. *Psychother Psychosom*. 1992;58(2):60–68.
3. Nelson E, Kirk J, McHugo G, et al. Chief complaint fatigue: a longitudinal study from the patient's perspective. *Fam Pract Res J*. 1987;6(4):175–188.
4. Paralyzed Veterans of America. *Fatigue and Multiple Sclerosis: Evidenced-Based Management Strategies for Fatigue in Multiple Sclerosis*. Washington, DC: Multiple Sclerosis Council for Clinical Practice Guidelines; 1998.

5. DeLuca J. Fatigue: its definition, its study and its future. In: DeLuca J, ed. *Fatigue as a Window to the Brain*. Cambridge, MA: MIT; 2005:319–325.
6. Krupp L, Christodoulou C, Schombert H. Multiple sclerosis and fatigue. In: DeLuca J, ed. *Fatigue as a Window to the Brain*. Cambridge, MA: MIT; 2005:61–71.
7. Barak Y, Achiron A. Cognitive fatigue in multiple sclerosis: findings from a two-wave screening project. *J Neurol Sci*. 2006;245(1–2):73–76.
8. Ritvo PG, Fisk JD, Archibald CJ, Murray TJ, Field C. Psychosocial and neurological predictors of mental health in multiple sclerosis. *J Clin Epidemiol*. 1996;49:467–472.
9. Ng AV, Kent-Baun JA. Quantitation of lower physical activity in persons with multiple sclerosis. *Med Sci Sprots Exerc*. 1997;29:517–523.
10. Schwartz CE, Coulthard-Morris L, Zeng Q. Psychosocial correlates of fatigue in multiple sclerosis. *Arch Phys Med Rehabil*. 1996;7:165–170.
11. Skerrett T, Moss-Morris R. Fatigue and social impairment in multiple sclerosis: the role of patients' cognitive and behavioral responses to their symptoms. *J Psychosom Res*. 2006;61(5):587–593.
12. Wessely S, Hotopf M, Sharpe D. *Chronic Fatigue and Its Syndromes*. New York: Oxford University Press; 1998.
13. Iriarte J, Subira ML, Castro P. Modalities of fatigue in multiple sclerosis: correlation with clinical and biological factors. *Mult Scler*. 2000;6:124–130.
14. van der Werf S, Jongen P, Lycklama à Nijeholt G, Barkhof F, Hommes O, Bleijenberg G. Fatigue in multiple sclerosis: interrelations between fatigue complaints, cerebral MRI abnormalities and neurological disability. *J Neurol Sci*. 1998;160(2):164–170.
15. Bakshi R, Miletich R, Henschel K, et al. Fatigue in multiple sclerosis: cross-sectional correlation with brain MRI findings in 71 patients. *Neurology*. 1999;53(5):1151–1153.
16. Mainero C, Faroni J, Gasperini C, et al. Fatigue and magnetic resonance imaging activity in multiple sclerosis. *J Neurol*. 1999;246(6):454–458.
17. Tartaglia M, Narayanan S, Francis S, et al. The relationship between diffuse axonal damage and fatigue in multiple sclerosis. *Arch Neurol*. 2004;61(2):201–207.
18. Téllez N, Alonso J, Río J, et al. The basal ganglia: a substrate for fatigue in multiple sclerosis. *Neuroradiology*. 2008;50(1):17–23.
19. Filippi M, Rocca M, Colombo B, et al. Functional magnetic resonance imaging correlates of fatigue in multiple sclerosis. *Neuroimage*. 2002;15(3):559–567.
20. Colombo B, Boneschi F, Rossi P, et al. MRI and motor evoked potential findings in nondisabled multiple sclerosis patients with and without symptoms of fatigue. *J Neurol*. 2000;247(7):506–509.
21. Marrie R, Fisher E, Miller D, Lee J, Rudick R. Association of fatigue and brain atrophy in multiple sclerosis. *J Neurol Sci*. 2005;228(2):161–166.
22. Tedeschi G, Dinacci D, Lavorgna L, et al. Correlation between fatigue and brain atrophy and lesion load in multiple sclerosis patients independent of disability. *J Neurol Sci*. 2007;263(1–2):15–19.
23. Simmons ML, Frondoza CG, Coyle JT. Immunocytochemical localization of N-acetyl-aspartate with monoclonal antibodies. *Neuroscience*. 1991;45(1):37–45.

24. Miller DH, Thompson AJ, Filippi M. Magnetic resonance studies of abnormalities in the normal appearing white matter and grey matter in multiple sclerosis. *J Neurol.* 2003;250(12):1407–1419.

25. Li BS, Wang H, Gonen O. Metabolite ratios to assumed stable creatine level may confound the quantification of proton brain MR spectroscopy. *Magn Reson Imaging.* 2003;21(8): 923–928.

26. Tartaglia MC, Narayanan S, De Stefano N, et al. Choline is increased in pre-lesional normal appearing white matter in multiple sclerosis. *J Neurol.* 2002;249(10):1382–1390.

27. De Stefano N, Narayanan S, Francis SJ, et al. Diffuse axonal and tissue injury in patients with multiple sclerosis with low cerebral lesion load and no disability. *Arch Neurol.* 2002;59(10):1565–1571.

28. Hoptman MJ, Volavka J, Johnson G, Weiss E, Bilder RM, Lim KO. Frontal white matter microstructure, aggression, and impulsivity in men with schizophrenia: a preliminary study. *Biol Psychiatry.* 2002;52(1):9–14.

29. Lim KO, Hedehus M, Moseley M, de Crespigny A, Sullivan EV, Pfefferbaum A. Compromised white matter tract integrity in schizophrenia inferred from diffusion tensor imaging. *Arch Gen Psychiatry.* 1999;56(4):367–374.

30. Codella M, Rocca M, Colombo B, Martinelli-Boneschi F, Comi G, Filippi M. Cerebral grey matter pathology and fatigue in patients with multiple sclerosis: a preliminary study. *J Neurol Sci.* 2002;194(1):71–74.

31. Codella M, Rocca M, Colombo B, Rossi P, Comi G, Filippi M. A preliminary study of magnetization transfer and diffusion tensor MRI of multiple sclerosis patients with fatigue. *J Neurol.* 2002;249(5):535–537.

32. Roelcke U, Kappos L, Lechner-Scott J, et al. Reduced glucose metabolism in the frontal cortex and basal ganglia of multiple sclerosis patients with fatigue: a 18F-fluorodeoxyglucose positron emission tomography study. *Neurology.* 1997;48(6): 1566–1571.

33. DeLuca J, Genova H, Hillary F, Wylie G. Neural correlates of cognitive fatigue in multiple sclerosis using functional MRI. *J Neurol Sci.* 2008;270(1–2):28–39.

34. Petersen S, van Mier H, Fiez J, Raichle M. The effects of practice on the functional anatomy of task performance. *Proc Natl Acad Sci USA.* 1998;95(3):853–860.

35. Raichle M, Fiez J, Videen T, et al. Practice-related changes in human brain functional anatomy during nonmotor learning. *Cereb Cortex.* 1994;4(1):8–26.

36. Koch K, Wagner G, von Consbruch K, et al. Temporal changes in neural activation during practice of information retrieval from short-term memory: an fMRI study. *Brain Res.* 2006;1107:140–150.

37. Lange G, Steffener J, Cook D, et al. Objective evidence of cognitive complaints in Chronic Fatigue Syndrome: a BOLD fMRI study of verbal working memory. *Neuroimage.* 2005;26(2):513–524.

38. Christodoulou C, DeLuca J, Ricker J, et al. Functional magnetic resonance imaging of working memory impairment following traumatic brain injury. *J Neurol Neurosurg Psychiatry.* 2001;71:161–168.

39. Chaudhuri A, Behan P. Fatigue and basal ganglia. *J Neurol Sci.* 2000;179(suppl 1–2):34–42.

40. Chaudhuri A, Behan P. Fatigue in neurological populations. *Lancet.* 2004;363:978–988.

41. Tartaglia M, Narayanan S, Arnold D. Mental fatigue alters the pattern and increases the volume of cerebral activation required for a motor task in multiple sclerosis patients with fatigue. *Eur J Neurol.* 2008;15(4):413–419.

42. Fukuda K, Straus SE, Hickie I, Sharpe MC, Dobbins JG, Komaroff A. The chronic fatigue syndrome: a comprehensive approach to its definition and study. *Ann Intern Med.* 1994;121:953–959.

43. Buchwald D, Cheney P, Peterson D, et al. A chronic illness characterized by fatigue, neurologic and immunologic disorders, and active human herpes virus type 6 infection. *Ann Intern Med.* 1992;116(2):103–113.

44. Natelson B, Cohen J, Brassloff I, Lee H. A controlled study of brain magnetic resonance imaging in patients with the chronic fatigue syndrome. *J Neurol Sci.* 1993;120(2):213–217.

45. Schwartz R, Garada B, Komaroff A, et al. Detection of intracranial abnormalities in patients with chronic fatigue syndrome: comparison of MR imaging and SPECT. *AJR Am J Roentgenol.* 1994;162(4):935–941.

46. Cope H, Pernet A, Kendall B, David A. Cognitive functioning and magnetic resonance imaging in chronic fatigue. *Br J Psychiatry.* 1995;167(1):86–94.

47. Lange G, DeLuca J, Maldjian J, Lee H, Tiersky L, Natelson B. Brain MRI abnormalities exist in a subset of patients with chronic fatigue syndrome. *J Neurol Sci.* 1999;171(1):3–7.

48. Greco A, Tannock C, Brostoff J, Costa D. Brain MR in chronic fatigue syndrome. *AJNR Am J Neuroradiol.* 1997;18(7): 1265–1269.

49. Cook D, Lange G, DeLuca J, Natelson B. Relationship of brain MRI abnormalities and physical functional status in chronic fatigue syndrome. *Int J Neurosci.* 2001;107(1–2):1–6.

50. Lange G, Holodny A, DeLuca J, et al. Quantitative assessment of cerebral ventricular volumes in chronic fatigue syndrome. *Appl Neuropsychol.* 2001;8(1):23–30.

51. Okada T, Tanaka M, Kuratsune H, Watanabe Y, Sadato N. Mechanisms underlying fatigue: a voxel-based morphometric study of chronic fatigue syndrome. *BMC Neurol.* 2004;4(1):14.

52. de Lange F, Koers A, Kalkman J, et al. Increase in prefrontal cortical volume following cognitive behavioural therapy in patients with chronic fatigue syndrome. *Brain.* 2008;131(pt 8): 2172–2180.

53. Schwartz R, Garada B, Komaroff A, et al. Detection of intracranial abnormalities in patients with chronic fatigue syndrome: comparison of MR imaging and SPECT. *AJR Am J Roentgenol.* 1994;162(4):935–941.

54. MacHale S, Lawrie S, Cavanagh J, et al. Cerebral perfusion in chronic fatigue syndrome and depression. *Br J Psychiatry.* 2000;176:550–556.

55. Costa D, Tannock C, Brostoff J. Brainstem perfusion is impaired in chronic fatigue syndrome. *QJM.* 1995;88(11):767–773.

56. Fischler B, D'Haenen H, Cluydts R, et al. Comparison of 99m Tc HMPAO SPECT scan between chronic fatigue syndrome, major depression and healthy controls: an exploratory study of clinical correlates of regional cerebral blood flow. *Neuropsychobiology.* 1996;34(4):175–183.

57. Tirelli U, Chierichetti F, Tavio M, et al. Brain positron emission tomography (PET) in chronic fatigue syndrome: preliminary data. *Am J Med.* 1998;105(3A):54S–58S.

58. Siessmeier T, Nix W, Hardt J, Schreckenberger M, Egle U, Bartenstein P. Observer independent analysis of cerebral glucose metabolism in patients with chronic fatigue syndrome. *J Neurol Neurosurg Psychiatry.* 2003;74(7):922–928.

59. Schmaling K, Lewis D, Fiedelak J, Mahurin R, Buchwald D. Single-photon emission computerized tomography and neurocognitive function in patients with chronic fatigue syndrome. *Psychosom Med*. 2003;65(1):129–136.

60. Lange G, Steffener J, Christodoulou C, et al. FMRI of auditory verbal working memory in severe fatiguing illness. *Neuroimage*. 2000;11(5 suppl 1):S95–S95.

61. Caseras X, Mataix-Cols D, Giampietro V, et al. Probing the working memory system in chronic fatigue syndrome: a functional magnetic resonance imaging study using the *n*-back task. *Psychosom Med*. 2006;68(6):947–955.

62. Cook D, O'Connor P, Lange G, Steffener J. Functional neuroimaging correlates of mental fatigue induced by cognition among chronic fatigue syndrome patients and controls. *Neuroimage*. 2007;36(1):108–122.

63. Tanaka M, Sadato N, Okada T, et al. Reduced responsiveness is an essential feature of chronic fatigue syndrome: a fMRI study. *BMC Neurol*. 2006;6:9.

64. Caseras X, Mataix-Cols D, Rimes K, et al. The neural correlates of fatigue: an exploratory imaginal fatigue provocation study in chronic fatigue syndrome. *Psychol Med*. 2008;38(7):941–951.

65. Omdal R, Sjöholm H, Koldingsnes W, et al. Fatigue in patients with lupus is not associated with disturbances in cerebral blood flow as detected by SPECT. *J Neurol*. 2005;252:78–83.

66. Andersen AB, Law I, Ostrowski S, et al. Self-reported fatigue common among optimally treated HIV patients: no correlation with cerebral FDG-PET scanning abnormalities. *Neuroimmunomodulation*. 2006;13:69–75.

67. Brody AL, Saxena S, Makdelkern MA, et al. Brain metabolic changes associated with symptom factor improvement in major depressive disorder. *Biol Psychiatry*. 2001;50:171–178.

68. Schifitto G, Friedman JH, Oakes D, et al. Fatigue in levodopa-naive subjects with Parkinson disease. *Neurology*. 2008;71:481–485.

69. Weintraub D, Newberg AB, Cary MS, et al. Striatal dopamine transporter imaging correlates with anxiety and depression symptoms in Parkinson's disease. *J Nucl Med*. 2005;46(2):227–232.

70. Abe K, Takanashi M, Yanagihara T. Fatigue in patients with Parkinson's disease. *Behav Neurol*. 2000;12:103–106.

71. Kohl AD, Wylie GR, Genova HM, Hillary FG, DeLuca J. The neural correlates of cognitive fatigue in traumatic brain injury using functional MRI. *Brain Inj*. 2009;23(5):420–432.

72. Mosso A. *Fatigue*. London: Swan Sonnenschein and Co.; 1904.

73. Schapiro, R. The pathophysiology of MS-related fatigue: What is role of wake promotion. Intl J MS Care, Supplement, November, 2002:6–8.

Chapter 23
Brain Imaging in Behavioral Medicine and Clinical Neuroscience: Synthesis

Ronald A. Cohen and Lawrence H. Sweet

It has been less than two decades since Ogawa, Kwong, and other neuroimaging pioneers published the first studies demonstrating that blood oxygen level-dependent (BOLD) changes could be detected using magnetic resonance (MR)-based methods.[1-4] These results rapidly spurred functional magnetic resonance imaging (FMRI) investigations of the effects of sensory stimulation, motor function, and basic cognitive processes[5-11] that complemented parallel work that had been emerging a few years before using radiological methods like positron emission tomography (PET).[12] Since then, there has been an explosion of interest and research in the field of functional brain imaging, along with major methodological advancements. Functional brain imaging has evolved to the point that many universities now have research-dedicated MR scanners independent of the clinical facilities that are often available within affiliated medical center settings. Furthermore, a number of psychology departments have installed MR systems in their on-campus buildings which, given the costs associated with having a dedicated scanners, reflects a growing perception that this technology is likely to have a major impact on cognitive and behavioral science in the years to come.

The development of FMRI has been of particular interest to psychologists and behavioral scientists because it has become the best and most versatile technique for examination of brain activity associated with cognitive, emotional, and behavioral processes. Given that the correlation of brain and behavior has been a primary goal of psychologists and other behavioral scientists over the past century, it is not surprising that FMRI has received such attention in recent years. For this reason, many of the chapters in this book emphasized the application of FMRI and other functional imaging methods in behavioral medicine and clinical neuroscience. However, it is important to recognize that for some disciplines, FMRI is not the primary imaging modality of interest. For example, neurologists who evaluate and treat acute stroke are much more focused on structural and perfusion/diffusion imaging, which can provide information about alterations in cerebral blood flow and early ischemic damage to brain tissue (see Chap. 18). Similarly, structural imaging sequences such as T1, T2, and FLAIR have become routine in the diagnosis and clinical management of Multiple Sclerosis (MS). Despite a remarkable and rapidly growing body of research on MS using FMRI, clinical applications have not yet been developed (see Chap. 21). In fact, given the proliferation of significant FMRI research findings, it is surprising that this type of neuroimaging has not been well integrated into clinical medicine to date. Historically, it is noteworthy that the initial development of most MR-based imaging methods occurred at roughly the same time as FMRI, about two decades ago. Therefore, more rapid integration into clinical practice reflects the fact that some MR sequences had more immediate utility in the assessment and diagnosis of particular neurological conditions.

The oldest and most routine type of neuroimaging is structural brain imaging. It remains the primary method for identifying neuroanatomic abnormalities in the brain and also for detecting chronic lesions from infarction, trauma, or other causes. We have not focused extensively on routine structural imaging in

R.A. Cohen (✉)
Department of Psychiatry and Human Behavior,
and the Institute for Brain Science Warren Alpert Medical School of Brown University, Providence, RI 02912, USA
e-mail: RCohen@lifespan.org

R.A. Cohen and L.H. Sweet (eds.), *Brain Imaging in Behavioral Medicine and Clinical Neuroscience*,
DOI 10.1007/978-1-4419-6373-4_23, © Springer Science+Business Media, LLC 2011

this book. Clinical MR and radiological methods for structural brain imaging are well developed and now quite routine. There are many books and atlases available that provide reference for interpreting anatomic data from structural imaging. For clinicians and researchers working with other neuroimaging modalities, including FMRI, magnetic resonance spectroscopy (MRS), and diffusion-weighted and perfusion-weighted imaging, the anatomic data obtained from traditional structural MRI remains the gold standard for the measurement of neuroanatomy, with T1-weighted images routinely acquired in the same imaging session for coregistration and anatomical localization. Only a few years ago, the identification and measurement of particular brain areas required manual tracing. Structural analysis methods and programs such as voxel-based morphometry (VBM)[13] and Freesurfer[14-17] now exist, enabling the quantitative measurement of cortical and subcortical volumes, cortical thickness, and lesion load. These programs continue to be refined, and while some degree of manual verification is still necessary for quality control, such morphometric analyses can now be conducted in large batches with good reliability. It seems probable that in the next few years, the quality of these programs will be such that most analyses can be conducted with automatic segmentation and parcellation-based tissue types and brain regions. These structural neuroanatomic analysis methods will probably continue to have their greatest direct impact on the clinical neurosciences, where there is typically a compelling need. For example, to determine whether the volumes of cortical and subcortical structures are reduced or ventricles enlarged in neurodegenerative diseases, where atrophy is expected, and when identification of lesions is critical. For behavioral medicine clinicians and investigators focusing on other types of neuroimaging, these structural imaging methods are still essential, as they provide the foundation upon which interpretation of other types of imaging can occur.

In the remainder of this chapter, we highlight some of the key concepts, technological advances, and future directions of neuroimaging in behavioral medicine and neuroscience which have relevance across the topics introduced by the contributors of this volume. We begin with methodological considerations, followed by highlights of current issues in clinical research and practice, and an overview of future directions.

Methodological Considerations

Physiological and Metabolic Neuroimaging

While structural and functional neuroimaging generally receive the most attention from behavioral researchers, a recurring theme throughout this book relates to the fact that these methods are ultimately driven by the physiology of the brain. The fact that water-containing fluids (e.g., blood) have biomagnetic and metabolic properties enables them to be detected by MR and radiological methods. Therefore, cerebral circulation and the perfusion of brain tissues sets up the conditions necessary for the various types of imaging that we have discussed. Blood perfusion and diffusion varies as a function of the characteristics of particular brain tissue and whether it is physiologically healthy or not. The link between physiology and neuroimaging is most obvious in the case of functional imaging, where the neuronal response that is the object of the measurement is highly integrated with physiological responses of cerebral perfusion and oxygen metabolism. However, it is important to note that even structural imaging of neuroanatomy ultimately depends on the physiological characteristics of tissue being measured. For example, a lesion resulting from cerebral infraction no longer has normal physiological function, resulting in altered MR characteristics.

The power of neuroimaging as a clinical and research tool in behavioral medicine and clinical neuroscience becomes fully apparent when one examines other MR methods that are aimed directly at specific physiological processes, such as cerebral perfusion and tissue diffusion, as well as cerebral metabolite abnormalities via MRS. These imaging modalities have been discussed to varying degrees in the chapters of this book. The fact that it is possible to measure physiological, metabolic imaging, in addition to FMRI and structural neuroanatomic imaging, creates the necessary conditions for being able to study brain structure–function together with the neuropathological processes that may mediate disturbances or individual differences in these relationships. We will visit some of these methods again later in this chapter as we review neuroimaging of the specific disorders and behaviors discussed in this book.

Multimodal Imaging

An emerging trend in neuroimaging is the use of multimodal imaging methods within a single assessment session with a given patient or research participant. This trend towards multimodal imaging is implicit in the material presented most of the clinical chapters of the book, and is explicitly discussed in many chapters. For example, in the context of acute stroke, procedures are described for the routine assessment of patients presenting with suspected cerebral infarction. These now involve a combination of structural CT or MRI, in addition to other methods, to assess the degree of regional hypoperfusion and evidence of recoverable versus unrecoverable tissue function in the penumbra. Researchers and clinicians studying other brain disorders, such as Alzheimer's disease (AD), multiple sclerosis (MS), and HIV-and cardiovascular disease-associated brain dysfunction increasingly are incorporating multimodal imaging as well.

Besides providing a means for integrating pathophysiology with brain structure and function, multimodal imaging also may be used to improve interpretation of data from a particular type of imaging. For example, in our current studies of patients with heart failure, a central problem stems from the fact that assumptions about normal hemodynamic function cannot be assumed among patients with severe vascular disturbances. By measuring both FMRI and cerebral blood flow through a method such as ASL, it is possible to examine the influence of altered cerebral perfusion on the BOLD response. Given that the BOLD FMRI signal occurs as a function of both cerebral blood flow (CBF) and neuronal response, there is value in being able to dissociate these components. Such strategy has also been applied to recent studies of AD and mild cognitive impairment (MCI).[18,19]

A number of other related developments are occurring in the area of multimodal imaging. For example, measuring oxygen consumption rate is possible using calibrated FMRI, providing a way of examining the brain's metabolic response in relationship to cerebral blood flow on FMRI. Some of these efforts are described in Chap. 15, including studies by Hoge and his colleagues examining how CBF and the BOLD response covary over time.[20-22] It is now possible quantify oxygen consumption and the BOLD response during FMRI paradigms,[23,24] although considerable research is needed to work out the logistics of this process to make it more available in clinical and routine research contexts.

Advantages and Limitations of Neuroimaging Techniques

To a great extent these issues have been covered earlier in the book. For example, the relative advantages of FMRI and other neuroimaging methods are discussed in Chaps. 1 and 2, and in many other specific chapters that followed. Chapter 8 (Chiou and Hillary) discusses important conceptual and methodological considerations for neuroimaging in clinical populations and should be reviewed by individuals contemplating research or clinical neuroimaging applications. We briefly outline some of the major advantages and limitations of MR and radiological methods below.

MR-Based Methods Advantages

- Noninvasive for the most part and consequently lower physical risk
- Less expensive than some radiological techniques
- Now widely available in both medical and university settings in the United States
- Excellent spatial resolution, especially for neuroanatomy
- Very good temporal resolution
- Experiments can be designed with multiple tasks and sequences within a single session
- Functional and physiological imaging data can be integrated quite well, and coregistration with neuroanatomy is relatively straightforward.
- Flexibility in experimental research designs

MR-Based Methods Limitations

- MR methods cannot provide the millisecond temporal resolution available from electrophysiology. Hemodynamic-based functional imaging methods have inherent time lags that limited temporal resolution compared to EEG. Therefore, visualization of the temporal evolution of short-duration cognitive events in real time is unlikely in near horizon.
- MR-based methods cannot yet provide the type of neurotransmitter and metabolic information that is available through the analysis of response to ligands

and specific tracers available with PET. This makes FMRI somewhat less useful for studying neurotransmitter disturbances.

- MR methods exclude certain segments of the population, in particular people with some types of metal implants, including electrical devices (e.g., pacemakers).
- Some people find lying in the scanner for long periods uncomfortable, particularly if they have anxiety disorders.

Radiological Imaging

Many of the advantages and disadvantages of radiological imaging mirror the issues discussed above.

- PET and SPECT imaging are invasive and involve the introduction of a radioactive ligand into the body. This raises potential risks and limits the number of imaging sessions that can be conducted with a single participant. This issue makes short-term longitudinal less feasible.
- The cost of PET, particularly the radioisotopes that have to be generated by cyclotron, is prohibitive.
- The temporal and spatial resolution of these methods are not as high as those available with FMRI.
- A major advantage is that analysis of cerebral neurotransmitter systems and peptides is more readily available than with MR methods.
- Direct measures of absolute cerebral metabolic activity in the resting state can be derived from methods like PET more readily than MR methods, which require comparison of brain response during two different conditions (e.g., cognitive activity vs. rest). As we discuss below, this limitation may be less of an issue than in the past with the development of resting FMRI methods.

Clinical Neuroimaging: Current Landscape

Neuroimaging in Neurology

It seems intuitive that neuroimaging methods would have their greatest initial impact in clinical neuroscience with respect to the assessment of brain disorders. This is, in fact, largely the case. Structural imaging

with either CT or MRI is now routinely conducted whenever a brain disorder is suspected in a patient. This is particularly true when there has been a sudden change in mental status or behavioral capacity. For example, patients presenting with severe unilateral headache, sensory changes, and other neurological signs now often are referred for a brain scan to insure that a neoplasm or some other insidious process is not occurring. Not too many years ago, this was also accompanied by routine EEG, though currently electrophysiological assessment is not conducted unless there is evidence of altered consciousness, possible seizure disorder, or some other findings that warrant the characterization of the brain's electrical activity. Structural brain imaging has become the standard and is often where neuroimaging stops for most patients, unless there is evidence of a brain disorder.

Although neuroimaging methods are now beginning to be broadly applied in many different areas of clinical neuroscience and behavioral medicine research, it is in the field of neurology, specifically stroke, where their clinical use is most routine. Protocols now exist for the type of imaging that should be conducted for patients at different stages of stroke (see Chap. 18). Imaging is initially conducted to confirm that a suspected stroke is embolic or hemorrhagic. If the stroke is determined to be embolic based on certain imaging findings on standard CT or MRI, perfusion- and diffusion-weighted imaging are conducted to determine the extent of the penumbra and the cerebral infarct and to provide a baseline for therapeutic intervention. Standardized decision processes have been established that depend, in part, on the type of neuroimaging equipment available in a particular medical center. An essential element of stroke neuroimaging is that it now routinely employs multimodal imaging to help sort out the pathophysiology of the evolving infarction. While there continue to be many new developments occurring on a regular basis, the field of stroke neuroimaging has evolved to the point that it can now be considered a relative mature clinical assessment, with certain procedures being widely accepted as the standard of practice. It is noteworthy that while functional imaging is of interest to many stroke researchers, it has not been integrated in clinical practice, in large part, because it currently does not provide as much information about acute pathophysiology associated with the evolving stroke as other methods.

Of course, brain imaging plays an important part in the neurodiagnostic process and treatment planning for other disorders besides stroke. If stroke neuroimaging is considered as a model for how multimodal neuroimaging can be used to aid in assessing brain disturbances and guiding treatment, most of the other disorders and behavioral processes discussed in this book remain as clinical frontiers, though their stage of clinical development varies along a relatively broad spectrum. For instance, neurosurgeons rely not only on standard structural imaging but also increasingly on other types of neuroimaging to inform the strategy that they will undertake during surgery. In this regard, new neuroimaging methods are finding their way into routine practice. Examples include ablation of neoplasms, surgical treatments for epilepsy, and hydrocephalus. Neurosurgeons planning removal of brain tumors are increasingly obtaining DTI tractography data to enable them to navigate around important white matter tracts.[25-33] While this application is somewhat less well established than the protocols for stroke, it is another example of the clinical application of multimodal imaging.

Epilepsy surgery provides another example of the application of multimodal imaging over the past several years. FMRI has been shown to be sensitive to brain areas that are the locus of seizure.[34-38] Furthermore, FMRI has been used to identify brain areas involved in language and memory, as an adjunct or potentially in lieu of the intracarotid sodium amobarbital procedure (Wada Test) or other similar procedures in which the brain is selectively anesthetized by hemisphere to test for language and memory localization,[34] with sequential assessments conducted pre- and postsurgery.[35] These efforts are still in their early stage, although in some states, it is now possible to bill for presurgical FMRI.

The assessment of Alzheimer's disease (AD) and other neurodegenerative brain disorders represents the other major area where the clinical application of neuroimaging is becoming routine. As Dr. Saykin and his colleagues described in Chap. 19, compelling information can be obtained through FMRI in conjunction with other types of neuroimaging. The value of neuroimaging for the assessment of dementia is that it provides a biomarker of brain degeneration that is independent of the neurocognitive measures obtained by the neuropsychologists, and converging evidence from these different types of data can help to validate diagnosis. Structural imaging, including the use of fluid attenuated inversion recovery (FLAIR) imaging to characterize white matter lesions, is now routinely conducted in the initial assessment of AD, and increasingly, functional neuroimaging is also performed.[39-48]

PET or SPECT imaging is now the most common form of functional imaging for AD,[41-48] and this is generally limited to interpretation of findings from resting activity. As discussed in Chap. 19, there are many areas open for clinical development and research inquiry in the neuroimaging of neurodegenerative diseases, such as AD, and at this point in time, neuroimaging in AD research is still in its developmental stage. In the future, standard procedures for assessing the effects of cognitive enhancers and other drugs to slow the progression of AD will likely employ FMRI and other functional methods to assess for therapeutic outcome.

Multiple sclerosis (Chap. 21) provides an illustration in which considerable functional neuroimaging work has been conducted, which when considered together with data on white matter integrity and other biomarkers provides insights into the direction that clinical neuroimaging may be taking in the future. MS also shows how the focus of neuroimaging is evolving with respect to brain disorders. When neuropsychologists and clinical neurologists first studied the brain effects of MS, they largely focused on white matter lesions and alterations in neurotransmission along these myelinated pathways. This work is an excellent example of how rapidly neuroimaging may transition from a research technique to a key routine diagnostic tool. MS has been shown to also affect the cortex and associated cognitive processing increasingly, possibly due to inflammatory processes associated with disease. This puts added emphasis on the need to employ methods that will inform about the functional integrity of cortical response (e.g., FMRI). However, FMRI is not a routine part of the neurodiagnostic assessment for MS. FMRI investigations using challenges of common disease-related impairments, including fatigue (Chap. 22), are likely to inform clinical decisions in the near future. While fatigue is a cardinal symptom of MS, it is also present is several disorders covered in this book. Therefore, advances in our understanding of structural and functional correlates of fatigue will likely provide an objective index for diagnosis, prognosis, and treatment efficacy for a number of disorders in the future.

Neuroimaging in Medical Conditions that Affect the Brain

HIV and cardiovascular disease (CVD) are examples of conditions/disorders that typically are not viewed as primarily brain disorders, but where there is compelling evidence of brain dysfunction among many patients. In many respects, diseases such as CVD and HIV represent the boundary between behavioral medicine and clinical neuroscience. In the case of HIV, behavioral factors, most notably substance abuse and sexual activity, play major roles in the transmission of the infection and also in adherence to treatment. In the case of CVD, the various behavioral risk factors discussed in Part 2 of the book, including exercise, obesity, alcohol, and nicotine use, greatly influence functional outcome, as well as the likelihood that patients will experience associated brain dysfunction. At this point in time, clinical neuroimaging is primarily used for purposes of detecting gross abnormalities by standard structural imaging with either CT or MRI. For example, patients with HIV routinely undergo MRI to determine whether there is evidence of opportunistic brain infection, such as toxoplasmosis or PML. Yet, there is now a wealth of evidence showing that both cerebral metabolite abnormalities on MRS and subtle morphometric brain changes occur in the course of chronic infection that may not be apparent on standard imaging (Chap. 20).

Similarly, patients with CVD often receive structural neuroimaging to rule out large vessel infarction, particularly in the context of cardiothoracic surgery. Yet, there is evidence that many people with chronic CVD have significant quantities of white matter lesion that may reflect microvascular disease and that over time changes occur that are best characterized by examining cerebral perfusion, structural brain changes, functional brain response, and neurocognitive function simultaneously over time (Chap. 23). It is now relatively common for patients undergoing cardiac surgery to have ultrasound assessment during the course of surgery, as a way of monitoring microemboli released into the blood. However, for the most part, neuroimaging remains a research topic, and not a primary consideration of clinicians working with HIV and CVD patients.

Neuroimaging in Behavioral Medicine

While some inroads have occurred in the application of functional and physiological imaging methods for assessment and diagnosis in the clinical neuroscience,

the application of neuroimaging for the broader field of behavioral medicine is still in its infancy. Brain imaging is not routinely performed for any of the behavioral conditions discussed in Part 2 of the book, with exception of chronic pain syndromes, when the goal is to rule out brain tumor or aneurysm in the case of head ache, or when some type of brain disturbance is thought to be contributing to a peripheral pain disorder. Nonetheless, neuroimaging has been the subject of increasing research inquiry over the past decade, and these efforts will likely increase in the coming years. Several factors are driving this interest, including: (1) Desire to better delineate the neurobehavioral mechanisms underlying conditions, such as obesity, reduced activity levels, smoking, and other behaviors that contribute to chronic disease, (2) Realization that not all people respond in a uniform manner to behavioral interventions, pointing to the need for ways of characterizing different phenotypes of nicotine dependence, smoking, etc., (3) The need to identify objective physiological measures of certain problem behaviors, like pain, and (4) The hope that functional neuroimaging may provide potentially powerful biomarkers that can be used for testing whether behavioral interventions are affecting the brain responses relevant to the problem behaviors of people being treated in behavioral medicine. Active neuroimaging research is now occurring on all of the topics discussed in Part 2. Some of these areas of investigation have the potential for translation into clinical practice in the not too distant future. These include functional imaging for the management of nicotine and other type of substance abuse, mood, and pain.

In many cases of chronic pain (Chap. 17), it is now relatively well established that sensory processes may not be the primary factor driving the pain experience, but rather brain processes that cause an application of the pain response. There would be considerable value in having functional brain imaging methods that could help to characterize increases in certain brain response associated with chronic pain that could then be targeted for intervention. Functional imaging can also be coupled with behavioral and pharmacologic interventions, as a way of determining whether an interpretation is actually causing a change in the response of particular brain responses associated with the experience of pain.[49-51]

Neuroimaging also provides a potentially powerful clinical tool for examining both the effects of using and withdrawing nicotine and other drugs of abuse. A number of research groups are now employing functional imaging in conjunction with behavioral and pharmacological interventions (see Chaps. 9, 11, and 12). In the next few years, these methods are likely to become more fully integrated into the clinical protocols for the treatment of these conditions. The neuroimaging of these disorders also illustrates the relative value offered by MR versus radiological methods. FMRI has been helpful in characterizing task-associated differences in brain response to smoking cues, cognitive and affective processes associated with drug use, and the functional systems underlying these conditions. However, radiological methods such as PET provide considerable value because of their greater ability at this time to image the activity of particular neurotransmitters and peptides in the brain. This is also certainly true when studying mood disorders (Chap. 10).

The behavioral medicine topics of eating disorders, obesity, physical activity, metabolic syndrome, and fatigue (Chaps. 12–15) are all in early stages of neuroimaging research development. It seems less likely that neuroimaging will be implemented in routine clinical assessment or treatment of these conditions in the near term. Accordingly, current neuroimaging research on these topics is motivated, in large part, by the goal of better understanding the neural mechanisms underlying why some people are obese and others are not, or why some people are more sedentary than others. For each of these topics, two different types of neuroimaging research questions tend to exist: (1) How to better understand the brain processes contributing to the behavioral condition of interest, and (2) Efforts to understand the effects of the particular behavior or behavioral outcome on brain function. This second goal is probably most amenable to clinical application in the nearer term. For example, many clinical researchers now believe that increasing physical activity in the elderly may have neuroprotective brain effects. This possibility can be tested through FMRI. Similarly, there is preliminary evidence that obesity may have negative cognitive consequences and that weight loss may improve cognitive function. We are currently conducting FMRI studies of patients of pre- and postbehavioral weight loss and also bariatric surgery, to examine how weight loss as well as changes in other risk factors affects brain response.

The application of neuroimaging for the assessment of fatigue is a particularly valuable line of research.

Like pain, fatigue is a subjective experience, but one that has objective manifestations. Fatigue can be extremely debilitating. Fatigue is common in neurological conditions like MS. Patients with chronic HIV also describe fatigue as a major problem. Fatigue is one of the most difficult to diagnosis and treat problems in medicine, and conditions such as chronic fatigue syndrome tend to befuddle most physicians. FMRI provides a method for studying how the brain's response to task demands change with sustained performance or under conditions of sleep deprivation and fatigue induced by other factors. Fatigue is also another problem that bridges the fields of clinical neuroscience and behavioral medicine. FMRI is now being employed to examine the effects of sustained performance, cognitive load, and the subjective experience of fatigue (Chap. 22).

Future Directions

Functional Brain Imaging: Future Clinical Directions

The unprecedented potential of FMRI to examine brain–behavior relationships has been employed in the development of numerous innovative applications. Some promising clinical applications are briefly reviewed below.

- *Presurgical mapping*: Currently, the only functional imaging method that has been adopted for clinical use and is reimbursable by some insurance companies is FMRI for presurgical localization of language and other cognitive functions in the context of epilepsy surgery. It is likely that in the future, brain mapping using FMRI will be available prior to brain surgery for other conditions.
- *Recovery of function*: Currently, methods such as diffusion weighted- and perfusion-weighted imaging are used primarily in the context of acute stroke. In the future, it is likely that standard protocols will be developed for measuring recovery of longer-term brain function following stroke, traumatic brain injury, and other conditions. In this regard, greater understanding of the nature of compensatory brain response is needed, and this literature will likely expand.

- *Treatment efficacy*: Clinical treatment outcome studies are likely to increasingly incorporate FMRI and potentially other neuroimaging metrics (e.g., MRS) as functional outcome measures to provide indices that are independent of behavioral performance.
- *Measurement of subjective states*: Studies of subjective experience of pain and fatigue are currently being conducted. There is beginning to be greater interest in examining functional brain response during other subjective states, such as meditation and hypnosis. Studies of the nature of consciousness are only now beginning to emerge.
- *Functional imaging of sleep disorders*: Currently, EEG is the primary method for studying sleep disorders. Other functional neuroimaging methods are likely to be integrated into this clinical field.
- *Malingering and lie-detection*: Studies are already emerging on the use of FMRI for assessment of malingering and lie detection. Given that memory encoding causes activation of particular brain regions, FMRI provides a means of determining whether the brain of patients being evaluated for possible malingering is activated in anticipation during cognitive processing, independent of objective performance.[52,53]

The Frontier: New and Emerging Imaging Methods

There are many technological developments occurring in the field of neuroimaging which are revolutionizing the neuroscience at a remarkable rate. While it is difficult to predict which methods will have the greatest impact in the future several developments appear to be particularly important.

- *Multimodal neuroimaging*: This has been a recurring theme in many of these chapters. Increasingly, multimodal imaging is being conducted in the research setting. However, integrating all of the data available from these methods is very challenging and typically requires that different analysis systems be programmed to communicate with each other. Methodological developments over the next few years are likely to make this task much easier.
- *Functional ASL*: The more general theme is that the neuroimaging methods that we have discussed in this book are ultimately highly related to each other.

Some are now generally thought of as structural imaging methods, while others are thought of as functional methods. Yet, for most methods, there is nothing inherent that limits it to one use or another. For example, diffusion weighted-imaging is currently used to provide information about ischemic data in cortical tissue, while diffusion tensor imaging, which is based on DWI, is used primarily to characterize white matter tracts. In the future, hybrid methods will likely exist that acquire multiple types of information simultaneously. Functional ASL is an example of this. ASL methods were developed as a way of measuring regional cerebral blood flow, without the need of a contrast agent. However, this method can also be used for functional imaging, as an alternative to BOLD.

- *Standardized paradigms*: One of the major challenges limiting the use of certain neuroimaging methods in clinical settings is the lack of normative data and standardization of tasks for use in the scanner. This is particularly true for FMRI, where each lab often has their own task versions, resulting in differences in results across settings. Eventually, agreements on standard tasks to be used across sites will likely occur, enabling greater reliability of these methods.
- *High field strength MRI*: There is a continual upgrading of magnet strength across imaging centers. Currently, 3-Telsa MRI systems are common in university medical centers in this country. However, even with this field strength, there are limits to what can be imaged. Increasingly high-field strength and high-resolution systems will become mainstream at imaging centers, greatly increasing the power of the methods that are available.
- *Whole-brain and nonhydrogen based MRS methods*: Magnetic resonance spectroscopy is one of the oldest MR-based imaging methods. Single voxel MRS is relatively simple to implement, but only provides information on a few metabolites from a single location. Each voxel takes about 5–10 min to acquire. Whole-brain MRS methods have been developed which enable acquisition across all of the brain's voxels. The total time for this method is only somewhat more than the time to do three voxels currently. While these methods are currently available, the analytic approaches for interpreting this quantity of data are far from ideal, and further development is needed before this method is readily available for research or clinical applications. Furthermore, other types of MRS imaging are also available including

scanning that is responsive to phosphorus and carbon in tissue. These methods provide the possibility of imaging other metabolites and peptides, besides what is obtainable through standard single-voxel MRS. However, the cost and logistics of these methods are currently very prohibitive.

- *Pittsburgh Compound B (PIB)*: This compound is a benzothiazole derivative that binds to β-amyloid in brain and is currently used as a PET imaging agent in studies of AD and also HIV.[54-56] Discoveries of ligands of this type are likely to revolutionize the study of neurodegerative brain disorders.
- *Nanotech contrast agents*: Nanotechnology, the emerging branch of science dedicated to the development of methods for controlling matter at an atomic or molecular scale, and devices of this scale with application in medicine and other technologies. There are already efforts underway to develop nanoparticles and devices that can be used in conjunction with MR imaging. Nanotech contrast agents have the potential to enhancement of MR imaging, including making these methods for sensitive to metabolic events, including neurotransmitter and peptide function.[57-59]

Conclusions

We are at the cusp of a revolutionary era in the field of neuroimaging that undoubtedly will have major implications for clinical neuroscience and behavioral medicine. Most of the methodological constraints that currently exist and limit the application of neuroimaging methods for clinical use will likely be overcome in the coming decades. Behavioral and neuroscientists will increasingly be called upon to integrate methods from neuroimaging with behavioral and cognitive approaches that have been developed over the past century. These are truly exciting times to be involved in this frontier of behavioral and brain science.

First demonstration of endogenous BOLD effects:

Ogawa S, Lee TM, Kay AR, Tank DW. Brain magnetic resonance imaging with contrast dependent on blood oxygenation. *Proc Natl Acad Sci USA*. 1990;87:9868-9872.
Ogawa S, Lee TM, Nayak AS, Glynn P. Oxygenation-sensitive contrast in magnetic resonance image of rodent brain at high magnetic fields. *Magn Reson Med*. 1990;14(1):68-78.

First demonstration of BOLD in humans (published simultaneously to give both authors credit):

Ogawa S, Tank DW, Menon R, Ellermann JM, Kim S-G, Merkle H, Ugurbil K. Intrinsic signal changes accompanying sensory stimulation: functional brain mapping with magnetic resonance imaging. *Proc Natl Acad Sci USA*. 1992;89:5951-5955.
Kwong KK, Belliveau JW, Chesler DA, Goldberg IE, Weisskoff RM, Poncelet BP, Kennedy DN, Hoppel BE, Cohen MS, Turner R, Cheng H-M, Brady TJ, Rosen BR. Dynamic magnetic resonance imaging of human brain activity during primary sensory stimulation. *Proc Natl Acad Sci USA*. 1992;89:5675-5679.

References

1. Kwong KK, Belliveau JW, Chesler DA, et al. Dynamic magnetic resonance imaging of human brain activity during primary sensory stimulation. *Proc Natl Acad Sci USA*. 1992;89:5675–5679.
2. Ogawa S, Tank DW, Menon R, et al. Intrinsic signal changes accompanying sensory stimulation: functional brain mapping with magnetic resonance imaging. *Proc Natl Acad Sci USA*. 1992;89:5951–5955.
3. Ogawa S, Lee TM, Kay AR, Tank DW. Brain magnetic resonance imaging with contrast dependent on blood oxygenation. *Proc Natl Acad Sci USA*. 1990;87(24):9868–9872.
4. Ogawa S, Lee TM, Nayak AS, Glynn P. Oxygenation-sensitive contrast in magnetic resonance image of rodent brain at high magnetic fields. *Magn Reson Med*. 1990;14(1):68–78.
5. Bandettini PA, Kwong KK, Davis TL, et al. Characterization of cerebral blood oxygenation and flow changes during prolonged brain activation. *Hum Brain Mapp*. 1997;5(2):93–109.
6. Belliveau JW, Kennedy DN Jr, McKinstry RC, et al. Functional mapping of the human visual cortex by magnetic resonance imaging. *Science*. 1991;254(5032):716–719.
7. Buckner RL, Goodman J, Burock M, et al. Functional-anatomic correlates of object priming in humans revealed by rapid presentation event-related fMRI. *Neuron*. 1998;20(2):285–296.
8. Malach R, Reppas JB, Benson RR, et al. Object-related activity revealed by functional magnetic resonance imaging in human occipital cortex. *Proc Natl Acad Sci USA*. 1995;92(18):8135–8139.
9. Cohen MS, Kosslyn SM, Breiter HC, et al. Changes in cortical activity during mental rotation. A mapping study using functional MRI. *Brain*. 1996;119(Pt 1):89–100.
10. Cramer SC, Weisskoff RM, Schaechter JD, et al. Motor cortex activation is related to force of squeezing. *Hum Brain Mapp*. 2002;16(4):197–205.
11. Rao SM, Bobholz JA, Hammeke TA, et al. Functional MRI evidence for subcortical participation in conceptual reasoning skills. *Neuroreport*. 1997;8(8):1987–1993.
12. Petersen SE, Fox PT, Posner MI, Mintun M, Raichle ME. Positron emission tomographic studies of the cortical anatomy of single-word processing. *Nature*. 1988;331(6157):585–589.
13. Ashburner J, Friston KJ. Voxel-based morphometry – the methods. *Neuroimage*. 2000;11(6 Pt 1):805–821.

14. Dale AM, Fischl B, Sereno MI. Cortical surface-based analysis I: segmentation and surface reconstruction. *Neuroimage.* 1999;9(2):179–194.

15. Fischl B, Sereno MI, Dale AM. Cortical surface-based analysis II: inflation, flattening, and a surface-based coordinate system. *Neuroimage.* 1999;9(2):195–207.

16. Fischl B, van der Kouwe A, Destrieux C, et al. Automatically parcellating the human cerebral cortex. *Cereb Cortex.* 2004;14:11–22.

17. Fischl B, Salat DH, Busa E, et al. Whole brain segmentation: automated labeling of neuroanatomical structures in the human brain. *Neuron.* 2002;33:341–355.

18. Bangen KJ, Restom K, Liu TT, et al. Differential age effects on cerebral blood flow and BOLD response to encoding: associations with cognition and stroke risk. *Neurobiol Aging.* 2009;30(8):1276–1287.

19. Restom K, Bangen KJ, Bondi MW, Perthen JE, Liu TT. Cerebral blood flow and BOLD responses to a memory encoding task: a comparison between healthy young and elderly adults. *Neuroimage.* 2007;37(2):430–439.

20. Hoge RD, Atkinson J, Gill B, Crelier GR, Marrett S, Pike GB. Investigation of BOLD signal dependence on cerebral blood flow and oxygen consumption: the deoxyhemoglobin dilution model. *Magn Reson Med.* 1999;42(5):849–863.

21. Hoge RD, Atkinson J, Gill B, Crelier GR, Marrett S, Pike GB. Linear coupling between cerebral blood flow and oxygen consumption in activated human cortex. *Proc Natl Acad Sci USA.* 1999;96(16):9403–9408.

22. Hoge RD, Atkinson J, Gill B, Crelier GR, Marrett S, Pike GB. Stimulus-dependent BOLD and perfusion dynamics in human V1. *Neuroimage.* 1999;9(6 Pt 1):573–585.

23. Brown GG, Eyler Zorrilla LT, Georgy B, Kindermann SS, Wong EC, Buxton RB. BOLD and perfusion response to finger-thumb apposition after acetazolamide administration: differential relationship to global perfusion. *J Cereb Blood Flow Metab.* 2003;23(7):829–837.

24. Brown GG, Perthen JE, Liu TT, Buxton RB. A primer on functional magnetic resonance imaging. *Neuropsychol Rev.* 2007;17(2):107–125.

25. Guye M, Parker GJ, Symms M, et al. Combined functional MRI and tractography to demonstrate the connectivity of the human primary motor cortex in vivo. *Neuroimage.* 2003;19(4):1349–1360.

26. Mori S, Frederiksen K, van Zijl PC, et al. Brain white matter anatomy of tumor patients evaluated with diffusion tensor imaging. *Ann Neurol.* 2002;51(3):377–380.

27. Inoue T, Ogasawara K, Beppu T, Ogawa A, Kabasawa H. Diffusion tensor imaging for preoperative evaluation of tumor grade in gliomas. *Clin Neurol Neurosurg.* 2005;107(3): 174–180.

28. Laundre BJ, Jellison BJ, Badie B, Alexander AL, Field AS. Diffusion tensor imaging of the corticospinal tract before and after mass resection as correlated with clinical motor findings: preliminary data. *AJNR Am J Neuroradiol.* 2005;26(4):791–796.

29. Kamada K, Sawamura Y, Takeuchi F, et al. Functional identification of the primary motor area by corticospinal tractography. *Neurosurgery.* 2005;56(1 suppl):98–109. discussion 198–109.

30. Nimsky C, Ganslandt O, Hastreiter P, et al. Intraoperative diffusion-tensor MR imaging: shifting of white matter tracts during neurosurgical procedures – initial experience. *Radiology.* 2005;234(1):218–225.

31. Gossl C, Fahrmeir L, Putz B, Auer LM, Auer DP. Fiber tracking from DTI using linear state space models: detectability of the pyramidal tract. *Neuroimage.* 2002;16(2):378–388.

32. Misaki T, Beppu T, Inoue T, Ogasawara K, Ogawa A, Kabasawa H. Use of fractional anisotropy value by diffusion tensor MRI for preoperative diagnosis of astrocytic tumors: case report. *J Neurooncol.* 2004;70(3):343–348.

33. Tropine A, Vucurevic G, Delani P, et al. Contribution of diffusion tensor imaging to delineation of gliomas and glioblastomas. *J Magn Reson Imaging.* 2004;20(6):905–912.

34. Moeller F, Tyvaert L, Nguyen DK, et al. EEG-fMRI: adding to standard evaluations of patients with nonlesional frontal lobe epilepsy. *Neurology.* 2009;73(23):2023–2030.

35. Donaire A, Falcon C, Carreno M, et al. Sequential analysis of fMRI images: A new approach to study human epileptic networks. *Epilepsia.* 2009;50(12):2526–2537.

36. Donaire A, Bargallo N, Falcon C, et al. Identifying the structures involved in seizure generation using sequential analysis of ictal-fMRI data. *Neuroimage.* 2009;47(1):173–183.

37. Auer T, Veto K, Doczi T, et al. Identifying seizure-onset zone and visualizing seizure spread by fMRI: a case report. *Epileptic Disord.* 2008;10(2):93–100.

38. Jacobs J, Rohr A, Moeller F, et al. Evaluation of epileptogenic networks in children with tuberous sclerosis complex using EEG-fMRI. *Epilepsia.* 2008;49(5):816–825.

39. Ott BR, Heindel WC, Whelihan WM, Caron MD, Piatt AL, Noto RB. A single-photon emission computed tomography imaging study of driving impairment in patients with Alzheimer's disease. *Dement Geriatr Cogn Disord.* 2000;11(3): 153–160.

40. Bauer M, Langer O, Dal-Bianco P, et al. A positron emission tomography microdosing study with a potential antiamyloid drug in healthy volunteers and patients with Alzheimer's disease. *Clin Pharmacol Ther.* 2006;80(3):216–227.

41. Small GW, Bookheimer SY, Thompson PM, et al. Current and future uses of neuroimaging for cognitively impaired patients. *Lancet Neurol.* 2008;7(2):161–172.

42. Rowe CC, Ackerman U, Browne W, et al. Imaging of amyloid beta in Alzheimer's disease with 18F-BAY94-9172, a novel PET tracer: proof of mechanism. *Lancet Neurol.* 2008;7(2):129–135.

43. Jagust W, Reed B, Mungas D, Ellis W, Decarli C. What does fluorodeoxyglucose PET imaging add to a clinical diagnosis of dementia? *Neurology.* 2007;69(9):871–877.

44. McKeith I, O'Brien J, Walker Z, et al. Sensitivity and specificity of dopamine transporter imaging with 123I-FP-CIT SPECT in dementia with Lewy bodies: a phase III, multicentre study. *Lancet Neurol.* 2007;6(4):305–313.

45. Nordberg A. PET imaging of amyloid in Alzheimer's disease. *Lancet Neurol.* 2004;3(9):519–527.

46. Kemppainen N, Ruottinen H, Nagren K, Rinne JO. PET shows that striatal dopamine D1 and D2 receptors are differentially affected in AD. *Neurology.* 2000;55(2):205–209.

47. Ishii K, Imamura T, Sasaki M, et al. Regional cerebral glucose metabolism in dementia with Lewy bodies and Alzheimer's disease. *Neurology.* 1998;51(1):125–130.

48. Duara R, Grady C, Haxby J, et al. Positron emission tomography in Alzheimer's disease. *Neurology.* 1986;36(7): 879–887.

49. Dube AA, Duquette M, Roy M, Lepore F, Duncan G, Rainville P. Brain activity associated with the electrodermal reactivity to acute heat pain. *Neuroimage.* 2009;45(1): 169–180.
50. Burgmer M, Pogatzki-Zahn E, Gaubitz M, Wessoleck E, Heuft G, Pfleiderer B. Altered brain activity during pain processing in fibromyalgia. *Neuroimage.* 2009;44(2): 502–508.
51. Kufahl P, Li Z, Risinger R, et al. Expectation modulates human brain responses to acute cocaine: a functional magnetic resonance imaging study. *Biol Psychiatry.* 2008;63(2):222–230.
52. Browndyke JN, Paskavitz J, Sweet LH, et al. Neuroanatomical correlates of malingered memory impairment: event-related fMRI of deception on a recognition memory task. *Brain Inj.* 2008;22(6):481–489.
53. Lee TM, Liu HL, Chan CC, Ng YB, Fox PT, Gao JH. Neural correlates of feigned memory impairment. *Neuroimage.* 2005;28(2):305–313.
54. Reiman EM, Chen K, Liu X, et al. Fibrillar amyloid-beta burden in cognitively normal people at 3 levels of genetic

risk for Alzheimer's disease. *Proc Natl Acad Sci USA.* 2009;106(16):6820–6825.
55. Klunk WE, Lopresti BJ, Ikonomovic MD, et al. Binding of the positron emission tomography tracer Pittsburgh compound-B reflects the amount of amyloid-beta in Alzheimer's disease brain but not in transgenic mouse brain. *J Neurosci.* 2005;25(46):10598–10606.
56. Klunk WE, Engler H, Nordberg A, et al. Imaging brain amyloid in Alzheimer's disease with Pittsburgh Compound-B. *Ann Neurol.* 2004;55(3):306–319.
57. Cormode DP, Skajaa T, Fayad ZA, Mulder WJ. Nanotechnology in medical imaging: probe design and applications. *Arterioscler Thromb Vasc Biol.* 2009;29(7): 992–1000.
58. Namdeo M, Saxena S, Tankhiwale R, Bajpai M, Mohan YM, Bajpai SK. Magnetic nanoparticles for drug delivery applications. *J Nanosci Nanotechnol.* 2008;8(7): 3247–3271.
59. Sun C, Lee JS, Zhang M. Magnetic nanoparticles in MR imaging and drug delivery. *Adv Drug Deliv Rev.* 2008;60(11): 1252–1265.

Index

A

Acute drug effects, 164–165
Acute ischemic stroke
  acute period, 307
  approaches, 293
  cerebral infarction evolution
    CBF, 294–295
    MRI images, 301
    stages, 294
  CT
    angiography, 298–299
    noncontrast CT, 295, 296
    perfusion imaging, 295, 297, 298
    stable Xenon, 303
  Diamox, 304
  hyperacute period, 306–307
  MRI
    angiography, 302, 304, 305
    continuous arterial spin labeling perfusion, 303
    DWI (*see* Diffusion weighted imaging)
    perfusion-weighted imaging (PWI), 302, 307
  penumbra, 294, 305, 306
  PET, 303
  rationale, 295
  shadow, 294
  treatment, 293
AD. *See* Alzheimer's disease
ADC. *See* Apparent diffusion coefficient
ADHD. *See* Attention-deficit/hyperactivity disorder
Advanced glycation end products (AGEs), 204
Affective-emotional system, 276
Alzheimer's disease (AD)
  APOE, 309, 310
  assessment, 387
  biomarkers, 311
  blood brain barrier dysfunction, 217–218
  capillaries and cerebral arterioles disruption, 219
  clinical symptoms, 310
  clinical trials, 324
  CT, 311
  early detection, 309
  early diagonsis, 323–324

  genomics, 322–323
  insulin resistance, 204–205
  LOAD, 309–310
  microvascular disease, 217
  neurobiology and neuropathology, 310
  pathophysiology, 217
  PET
    AD *vs.* MCI, 318–319
    amyloid imaging, 319–321
    cerebral metabolism, 319
    FDG, 319
    neuroinflammation, microglia, 321
    neurotransmitter, 321
  SPECT, 318
  structural MRI
    brain atrophy, 313–314
    DWI/DTI techniques, 314
    episodic memory, 315–317
    functional and resting-state connectivity, 317–318
    functional MRI, 315
    vs. global GM density, 312, 313
    hippocampal volume and EC thickness, 311, 312
    MCI-converters, 313–314
    MRS, 314–315
    perfusion MRI, 315
  treatment, 310–311
  VaD, 216–217, 322
Alzheimer's Disease Neuroimaging Initiative (ADNI), 311
Amphetamine, 164–165
Amyloid plaques, 310
ANI. *See* Asymptomatic cognitive impairment
Anorexia nervosa (AN)
  abnormal body image perception, 186–187
  brain structural changes, 187
  clinical diagnosis, 184
  disturbed food relationship, 186
  global and regional brain function, 185
  serotonin and dopamine transmission, 185–186
  structural abnormalities, 184, 185

395

Anxiety and depression
  fibromyalgia, 281
  neural substrate, 280
  noxious thermal stimulus, 280
  PTSD, 281
  visual signal, 280
Apolipoprotein E (APOE), 309, 310
Apparent diffusion coefficient (ADC)
  diffusion measurement, brain, 51
  DWI/DTI, 314
  HIV, 347
Arterial input function (AIF), 68
Arterial spin-labeling (ASL)
  absolute perfusion quantification, 77–78
  continuous technique, 75–76
  HIV, 348–349
  image readout module
    background suppression, 79
    fast imaging technique, 78
    macrovascular signal suppression, 79
    magnetic field strength implication, 79–80
    spin-echo *vs.* gradient echo, 78
    volumetric acquisition, 79
  nuclear magnetization, 70
  perfusion MRI, 315
  pulsed technique
    bolus passage curve, 68–69
    EPISTAR, 73–74
    FAIR, 74–75
    hypercapnia induction, 72
    limitations, 72
    magnetization transfer effects, 73
    PICORE, 75
    quantitative tracer kinetic model, 72
    180° RF pulse, blood supply, 71
  tagging method, 77
  track changes, blood flow, 41
  velocity sensitive, 76–77
ASL. *See* Arterial spin-labeling
Asymptomatic cognitive impairment (ANI), 341
Attention and distraction, 282–283
Attention-deficit/hyperactivity disorder (ADHD), 209–210

B
Balloon analogue risk task (BART), 172
BDNF. *See* Brain-derived neurotrophic factor
BED. *See* Binge eating disorder
Beer–Lambert law, 94
Behavioral medicine and clinical neuroscience
  fMRI, 383
  functional ASL and high field strength MRI, 390
  malingering and lie-detection, 390
  MR-based methods
    advantages, 385
    limitations, 385–386

MRS, 390–391
  multimodal imaging, 385, 390
  nanotech contrast agents, 391
  neuroanatomic abnormalities identification, 383
  neuroimaging
    application, 389
    chronic pain, 388
    HIV and CVD, 387–388
    neurology, 386–387
    nicotine, 388–389
  physiological and metabolic neuroimaging, 384
  PIB, 391
  pre-surgical mapping, 389
  radiological imaging, 386
  sleep disorders and standardized paradigms, 390
  stroke, 389
  structural analysis methods and programs, 384
  subjective states measurement, 390
  treatment efficacy, 390
Binge eating disorder (BED), 179, 182
Blood oxygen level dependent (BOLD) signal, 6
  cerebral perfusion, 234–235
  fNIRS, 96
  functional brain response, 229
Body mass index (BMI), 193, 194
Brain activation, 287
Brain-derived neurotrophic factor (BDNF), 260–261
Brain parenchymal volume (PBV), 343
Bulimia nervosa (BN)
  brain response, 184
  definition, 182
  food cues, 183–184
  serotonin, 183
  structural and global functional abnormalities,
    182–183

C
Cardiovascular disease (CVD)
  AD
    blood brain barrier dysfunction, 217–218
    capillaries and cerebral arterioles disruption, 219
    microvascular disease, 217
    pathophysiology, 217
    VaD, 216–217
  brain dysfunction, 215
  effects, 215
  mechanisms, 225
  neurocognition and brain dysfunction (*see*
    Neurocognition and brain dysfunction)
  neuroimaging, 387–388 (*see also* Neuroimaging)
Cerebral blood flow, 297
Cerebrospinal fluid (CSF), 14
Cerebrovascular hypoperfusion, 44
CFS. *See* Chronic fatigue syndrome
Chronic drug effects, 165–166

Index

Chronic fatigue syndrome (CFS)
  functional neuroimaging, 375–377
  number of neuroimaging articles, 369, 370
  structural neuroimaging, 375
Cocaine, 165, 166
Cognitive fatigue, 373
Cognitive process, 2
Computed tomography (CT)
  acute ischemic stroke
    angiography, 298–299
    noncontrast CT, 295, 296
    perfusion imaging, 295, 297, 298
    stable Xenon, 303
  AD, 311
  neurocognition and brain dysfunction, 226
  obesity, 193
  radiological imaging, 4
Craving, 166
CSF. *See* Cerebrospinal fluid
Cue reactivity, 138, 139
CVD. *See* Cardiovascular disease

D

Data acquisition
  head motion and noise source, 104–105
  MRI environment, 103–104
Data interpretation
  activation, 110–112
  cognitive subtraction, 112–113
  mood/affect influence, 113
Data processing and BOLD signal analysis
  activation detection and statistical consideration,
    105–106
  data preparation, 105
  exogenous substances/medication effects, 109–110
  injury and pathological effects, 108–109
  natural heterogeneity, 107
  normal developmental effects, 107–108
  test-retest reliability and reproducibility, 106–107
Deep white matter lesions (DWML), 322
Default mode network (DMN), 318
Default network, 43
Dementia with Lewy bodies (DLB), 322
Deoxygenated hemoglobin (deoxy-Hb), 93
Diffusion-encoding gradient pulse, 50
Diffusion tensor imaging (DTI), 231–232, 372
  AD, 314
  ADC, 51
  clinical application
    alcohol abuse, 61
    diabetes and metabolic syndrome, 60–61
    HIV Infection, 62–63
    hypertension, 60
    nicotine and substance use, 61–62
  data acquisition, 52–53

degree of signal attenuation, 51
  DWI, 51, 52
  ellipsoids, different magnitudes, 54–55
  HIV, 347–348
  imaging artifacts, 58–59
  in vivo brain structural connectivity, 63
  limitation, 51–52
  MS, functional neuroimaging, 361
  obesity, 197–198
  quantitative analysis, data
    quantitative tractography, 57–58
    ROI approach, 56–57
    VBM, 57
  random motion, pollen particles, 49
  squared displacement, water molecules, 49
  Stejskal–Tanner pulsed gradient spin echo acquisition, 52
  TBSS, 58
  utilization, data
    scalar metrics, 53–55
    tractography, 55–56
  water diffusion, 50
  white matter fiber, 50
Diffusion weighted imaging (DWI), 51, 52
  acute ischemic stroke
    ADC, 301
    advantages, 301
    anterior cerebral artery (ACA) territory, 299, 302
    chronic infarct, anterior cerebral artery, 302
    embolic infarction, 299, 303
    fluid attenuated inversion recovery (FLAIR), 299
    infarction evolution, 299, 301
    middle cerebral artery, 299, 306
    pontine infarction, 302, 305
    posterior cerebral artery, 299, 300
    subacute infarction, 299, 300
  AD, 314
  obesity, 194
Distinct nociceptive processing systems, 276
DLB. *See* Dementia with Lewy bodies
Dopamine D4 receptor (DRD4), 264
Dopamine D2 receptors (DRD2), 180
Dopamine signaling, 186
Dorsal prefrontal cortex (DPFC), 181
DRD4. *See* Dopamine D4 receptor
DTI. *See* Diffusion tensor imaging
Dynamic susceptibility contrast (DSC) method, 70
Dysynchiria, 279

E

Eating disorders
  AN (*see* Anorexia nervosa)
  BED, 179, 182
  BN (*see* Bulimia nervosa)
  clinical manifestation, 179
  definition, 179

Eating disorders (*Cont.*)
  overeating
    definition, 179
    food consumption, 181–182
    functional neuroimaging, 179–180
    sensory cues, 180–181
Echo-planar imaging (EPI), 24
Echo-planar imaging and signal targeting with alternating
    radio frequency (EPISTAR), 73–74
Echo time, 85–86
Electroencephalography (EEG), 2, 119, 277
Electrophysiological method, 3
Endophenotypes, 119–120
EPI. *See* Echo-planar imaging
Episodic memory, 315–317
ERPs. *See* Event-related potentials
Event-related optical signal (EROS), 94
Event-related potentials (ERPs), 3, 119
Exercise and brain
  adherence
    DRD4 allele, 265–266
    Hedonic Theory, 264–265
    Learning Theory, 265
  cognition effects, neural mechanism
    AD, 261–262
    angiogenesis and neurogenesis, 259
    BDNF, 261
    blood volume changes, 259
    children and young adults, 258–259
    fMRI, cardiovascular fitness, 260–261
    meta-analysis, 258, 259
    older adults, 258
    P3 component, 260
    physical fitness, 257–258
    stroke exercise, 262
  health benefits and effects, 257
  MDD
    neural structures, 264
    neurobiological disturbance, 263
    symptoms, 263
    treatment, 263–264
  normal affective function, 262–263

F
Fatigue Severity Scale (FSS), 370, 371
[18]F-fluorodeoxyglucose (FDG), 182
FID. *See* Free induction decay
Flow alternating inversion recovery (FAIR), 74–75
fMRI. *See* Functional magnetic resonance imaging
Focal lesion, 1
Fractional anisotropy (FA), 314, 347
Free induction decay (FID), 14, 83
Frontotemporal dementia (FTD), 322
Functional brain imaging evolution
  brain disorder, 7

cognition, 6–7
physiological condition, 6
systemic diseases, 7
Functional magnetic resonance imaging (fMRI)
  abnormal brain function, 37
  annual totals, Medline Indexed Publications, 38
  BOLD
    signal, 6
    signal quantification and experimental design, 39–40
    strength and limitation, 40–42
    subtraction and cross-correlation analyses, 37
  brain function localization, 38
  cardiovascular disease, 43
  cerebrovascular hypoperfusion, 44
  data acquisition
    head motion and noise source, 104–105
    MRI environment, 103–104
  data interpretation
    activation, 110–112
    cognitive subtraction, 112–113
    mood/affect influence, 113
  data processing and BOLD signal analysis
    activation detection and statistical consideration,
      105–106
    data preparation, 105
    exogenous substances/medication effects, 109–110
    injury and pathological effects, 108–109
    natural heterogeneity, 107
    normal developmental effects, 107–108
    test-retest reliability and reproducibility, 106–107
  default network, 43
  HIV, 346–347
  metabolic activity, 6
  multiple regression analyses, 38
  multi-sequence imaging, 44
  nicotine dependence, 118
  nociception and pain identification, 277–278
  non-echoplanar sequences, 43
  psychiatric disorder, 38
  T_1 and T_2 relaxation, 5
Functional near-infrared spectroscopy (fNIRS)
  apparatus, 94–95
  application, 98–99
  BOLD-based signal, 96
  fMRI, 95–96
  hemodynamic response, 93
  limitation, 97
  neural function direct methods, 95
  neural function indirect methods, 95–96
  principles, 93–94
  strength, 96–97
  validation effort, 97–98
Functional neuroimaging
  CFS
    BOLD response analysis, 376
    data analysis, 376

Index

left basal ganglia activity, 377, 378
pattern of cerebral activity, 376
SPECT, perfusion, 375–376
structural changes, white and gray matter, 377
task performance, 376
multiple sclerosis
n-Back task, 358–359
compensatory activity, 358
counting Stroop task, 360
DTI, 361
episodic memory, 360
executive functions, 359
fatigue, 372–374, 377
left-sided prefrontal activation, 358
MRS, 361
PASAT, 357, 358
PET and SPECT, 360
Sternberg task, 359
SWI, 361
nicotine dependence
abstinence effects, 128–135, 140–141
activation pattern, smoking cue presentation, 138–139
activation reward pathway, 138
advantages and disadvantages, 120
cognition and working memory tasks, 139
EEG and ERP, 119
fMRI, 118
germinal cue reactivity, 138
imaging genomics, 119–120, 142
implications, 142–143
International Affective Picture Series (IAPS), 120, 138
MEG, 119
mesocorticolimbic dopamine system, 117
MRS, 119
neurobiology, 117–118
neurological pathways, 119, 120
nicotine and tobacco effects, 124–128, 140
PET, 118, 119
regions of interest (ROI), 138
SPECT, 118
studies, 121–124
task-free approaches, 135–137, 141–142
overeating, 179–180
techniques
caudate activity, 373
cerebral activation, 374
compensatory mechanism, 372
effort, cerebral, 374
fMRI, 373
glucose metabolism, 372
objective measurements, cognitive fatigue, 372–373
orbital frontal gyrus activity, 373, 374
PD (*see* Parkinson's disease)
TBI, 377
thalamus, 372

G
Gray matter pathology, 362

H
HAART. *See* Highly active antiretroviral therapy
HAD. *See* HIV-associated dementia
Hedonic Theory, 264–265
Hemodynamic response, 93
Highly active antiretroviral therapy (HAART), 341
HIV-associated dementia (HAD), 342
5-HT1A receptor, 186
5-HT2A receptor, 185–186
Human immunodeficiency virus (HIV)
acquired immune deficiency syndrome (AIDS), 341
ANI, 341
ASL, 348–349
comorbid condition, 342
DTI, 347–348
fMRI, 346–347
HAART, 341
imaging possibility, 348–350
magnetic resonance spectroscopy, 344–346
MND, 341
MRI finding, 342–343
PET, 350
quantified tractography, 349
structural MRI and cognitive performance, 343–344
VSASL, 348–349
white matter abnormality, 344
Hypertension
cognition, 206–207
neuroimaging, 207–208

I
Image standardization, 105
Imaging genomics, 10, 119–120
Impaired response inhibition and salience attribution model (I-RISA), 171
Incentive sensitization model, 171
Insulin resistance
cognitive functioning, 202–203
diabetes, neuroimaging, 205, 206
glucose regulation, 202
neuropathology and neuroimaging
AD, 204–205
AGEs, 204
cerebral vascular reactivity, 204
dysfunction, capillary recruitment, 203
hippocampus, 203
hyperglycemia, 203, 204
insulin signaling pathway, 204
Intravenous nicotine infusion, 140
Irritable bowel syndrome (IBS), 286
Ischemic penumbra, 294, 305, 306

L

Laminae I and V, 276
Larmor frequency, 83
Late-onset AD (LOAD), 309–310
Learning Theory, 265
Lesion analysis approach, 1
Light-emitting diode (LED), 94

M

Magnetic encephalography (MEG), 3
Magnetic resonance angiography (MRA), 302, 304, 305
Magnetic resonance imaging (MRI)
    acute ischemic stroke
        angiography, 302, 304, 305
        continuous arterial spin labeling perfusion, 303
        DWI, 299–302
        multiple embolic infarctions, 299, 303
        perfusion-weighted imaging (PWI), 302, 307
    environment, data acquisition, 103–104
    findings, HIV, 194
    multiple sclerosis, 356
Magnetic resonance (MR) signal
    contrast
        brain fMRI scanning, 30
        partial saturation, 25
        saturation recovery, 26
        signal intensity $vs.$ TR, 25–26
        tissue type, 25
        T_2 weighting, 26–27
    image acquisition pulse sequences
        echo-planar imaging (EPI) method, 24
        frequency encoding, 23
        gradient echo sequence, 21
        multiple-shot acquisition, 24–25
        phase encode gradient, 22
        primer-crusher gradient, 24
        pulse sequence diagram, 24
    MRI hardware
        gradient system, 31–32
        magnet, 30–31
        RF coil, 32–35
    nuclear induction signal
        flip angle, 13
        Larmor frequency, 12
        magnetization vector, 12, 13
        polarization, 12
        quantum mechanical approach, 11
        radiofrequency resonator/coil, 13
        spin angular momentum, 11
    relaxation
        cerebrospinal fluid (CSF), 14
        free induction decays (FID), 14
        longitudinal Bloch equation, 13
        longitudinal magnetization, 16

        magnetization $vs.$ postsaturation, 15
        shimming, 14
        spin echo pulse and signal diagram, 15–16
        transverse magnetization decay, 14
    safety, 35–36
    signal-to-noise ratio, 28–30
    spatial encoding
        clinical scanner, 16
        field of view (FOV), 21
        Fourier transform of signal, 18
        frequency encoding, 18
        gradient waveform shape function, 20
        isocenter, 17
        linear gradient application effect, 17
        phase encoding process, 20
        signal energy distribution in k-space, 21–22
        three-lobed waveform, 19
        zero-crossings and bandwidth interval, 19
Magnetic resonance spectroscopy (MRS)
    behavioral medicine and clinical neuroscience, 390–391
    multiple sclerosis, 361
    neuroimaging, 235–236
    nicotine dependence, 119
    radiological imaging, 5
    structural MRI, 314–315
Magnetization transfer imaging (MTI), 372
Magnetoencephalography (MEG), 119, 277
Major depressive disorder (MDD)
    acetylcholine concentration reduction, 152
    anticholinesterase inhibitor, 151
    $vs.$ bipolar disorder (BP), 150
    cholinergic hyperactivity, 150–151
    forced swim test (FST), 151
    mood stabilizers, 152
    nAChR antagonists, antidepressants, 151–152
    neural structures, 264
    neurobiological disturbance, 263
    nicotine administration, 150
    symptoms, 149, 150, 263
    treatment, 263–264
MCI. See Mild cognitive impairment
Mean diffusivity (MD). See Apparent diffusion coefficient
MEG. See Magnetoencephalography
Mesocorticolimbic dopamine system, 117
Metabolic dysfunction
    health effects, 201
    hypertension
        cognition, 206–207
        neuroimaging, 207–208
    insulin resistance
        cognition, 202–203
        diabetes, neuroimaging, 205, 206
        glucose regulation, 202
        neuropathology and neuroimaging, 203–205
    metabolic syndrome, 201

Index

obesity
  brain function, 210–211
  neuropsychology, 208–210
Metabolic syndrome, 201
Methamphetamine (METH), 62
  acute drug effects, 165
  chronic drug effects, 165–166
Midzolam, 282
Mild cognitive impairment (MCI), 310
Mild neurocognitive disorder (MND), 341
Monoamine oxidase (MAO) inhibitors, 149
Mood, stress and tobacco smoking relationship
  MAO inhibitors, 149
  nAChR
    anatomical localization, 148
    neuronal α and β subunits, 147–148
    serotonin, 150
    in vivo imaging, $\beta2$, 148, 149
  nicotine dependence
    MDD (see Major depressive disorder)
    PSTD (see Post-traumatic stress disorder)
  nicotine effects, 147
MRS. See Magnetic resonance spectroscopy
Multiple sclerosis (MS), 106, 387
  autoimmune dysfunction, 355
  beyond cognitive function, 363–364
  functional neuroimaging
    n-Back task, 358–359
    compensatory activity, 358
    counting Stroop task, 360
    DTI, 361
    episodic memory, 360
    executive functions, 359
    left-sided prefrontal activation, 358
    MRS, 361
    PASAT, 357, 358
    PET and SPECT, 360
    Sternberg task, 359
    SWI, 361
  MRI, 356
  multi-sequence MRI, 362–363
  paradigms, 363
  relapsing-remitting course, 355
  structural imaging, 356–357
  traditional neuroimaging data analysis, 362
Multiple sclerosis fatigue
  advanced MRI imaging, 371–372
  CFS (see Chronic fatigue syndrome)
  CNS, 370
  definition, fatigue, 369
  degree of disability, 369
  functional neuroimaging techniques
    caudate activity, 373
    cerebral activation, 374
    compensatory mechanism, 372

effort, cerebral, 374
fMRI, 373
glucose metabolism, 372
objective measurements, cognitive fatigue, 372–373
orbital frontal gyrus activity, 373, 374
PD (see Parkinson's disease)
TBI, 377
thalamus, 372
non-specific symptom, 369
number of neuroimaging articles, 369–370
pathophysiology, 369–370
structural MRI, 370–371

N

nAChR. See Nicotinic acetylcholine receptors
Neurocognition and brain dysfunction
  cardiac rehabilitation, 219
  cerebral hypoperfusion, 221
  cerebral perfusion, 221
  CVD, 219, 220, 225
  heart failure function, 220
  neuroimaging
    advantages, 225–226
    cerebral perfusion, 232–235
    CT, 226
    diffusion imaging, 231
    DTI, 231–232
    functional brain response, 228–231
    MRS, 235–236
    structural brain abnormalities, 226–227
    white matter damage, 227, 228
  systemic vascular contribution
    cardiac output, 222
    cerebral hemodynamic autoregulatory failure, 222
    cytokines and inflammatory process, 224–225
    endothelial disturbance, 223
    measurement, 223, 224
    neurocognitive function, 224
    vascular burden, 222–223
  vascular and metabolic risk factors, 220–221
Neurofibrillary tangles, 310
Neuroimaging
  advantages, 225–226
  application, 389
  cerebral perfusion
    AD patients, 232, 233
    hemodynamic, BOLD response, 234–235
    PET/SPECT, 233
    transcranial Doppler imaging, 234
  chronic pain, 388
  CT, 226
  diffusion imaging, 231
  DTI, 231–232

Neuroimaging (*Cont.*)
functional brain response
aging, 228–229
BOLD response alterations, 229
cortical recruitment, working memory, 230–231
hypertension (HTN), 230
networks and ROI, 228
HIV and CVD, 387–388
MRS, 235–236
neurodegenerative brain disease, 216
neurology, 386–387
nicotine, 388–389
structural brain abnormalities, 226–227
VCI (*see* Vascular cognitive impairment)
white matter damage, 227–228
Neuropsychology, 1
Nicotinic acetylcholine receptors (nAChR)
anatomical localization, 148
in vivo imaging, β2, 148, 149
serotonin, 150
α and β subunits, 147–148
Nociceptors, 276
Noninvasive neuroimaging technique. *See* Functional
magnetic resonance imaging
Non-invasive nicotine/tobacco administration, 140
Normalization. *See* Image standardization

O
Obesity
AD, 197, 198
brain function, 210–211
DTI, 197–198
functional brain alterations
consumption, food, 196
dopamine availability, 197
eating behavior, functional imaging, 195, 196
neural response *vs.* lean control, 196
impacts, older adults, 198
morphological brain alterations
CT, 193
DWI and MRI, 194
PET and MRS, 194–195
neuropsychology
ADHD, 209–210
BMI, 209
cognition, 208–209
hypertension, 209
risk factors, 193
mμ-Opioid system activation, 284
Optical window, 94
Overeating
definition, 179
food consumption, 181–182
functional neuroimaging, 179–180
sensory cues, 180–181
Oxygenated hemoglobin (oxy-Hb), 93

P
Paced Auditory Serial Addition Task (PASAT),
358, 375
Pain coping skills training, 285–286
Pain neuroimaging
CBT, 285–286
experimentally induced pain, 278–279
functional anatomy, nociception and pain, 277–278
gate control theory, 275
hypnosis, 286–287
meditation, 287
neural correlation, 276
neuromatrix theory, 275
pain reconceptualization, 286
pain stimulus, 288
placebo analgesia
bowel distention, 284
fMRI, 284
manipulation, 284–285
pain anticipation, 284
pain neurosignature, 285
rACC and PAG activation, 284
psychological factors
anxiety and depression, 280–281
attention and distraction, 282–283
empathy, 283
pain anticipation, 281–282
pain catastrophizing, 279–280
psychological interventions effects, 283
structural anatomy, nociception and pain, 276–277
Parkinson's disease (PD), 377
PBV. *See* Brain parenchymal volume
Perfusion MRI
ASL
absolute perfusion quantification, 77–78
evolution, 71–76
image readout module, 78–80
nuclear magnetization, 70
pulse sequences, 71
tagging method, 77
velocity sensitive, 76–77
definition, 67
DSC method
AIF, 68
bolus passage curve, 68–69
cerebral blood volume (CBV), 69
Gadolinium-DTPA contrast agent, 68–69
pulse sequences, 68
reliability, 70
steady-state technique, 70
Perfusion-weighted imaging (PWI), 302, 307
Periaqueductal gray (PAG), 284
PET. *See* Positron emission tomography
Pittsburgh compound B (PIB), 319, 320, 391
Positron emission tomography (PET), 5, 277–278
acute ischemic stroke, 303
AD *vs.* MCI, 318–319

amyloid imaging, 319–321
cerebral metabolism, 319
FDG, 319
HIV, 350
morphological brain alterations, 194–195
multiple sclerosis, 360
neuroinflammation, microglia, 321
neurotransmitter, 321
nicotine dependence, 118, 119
Post-traumatic stress disorder (PTSD), 281
brain and cognition, 153–154
hippocampus, 155
β_2-nAChR availability, 154
vs. never-smoking healthy controls, 154
nicotinic acetylcholinergic system, 153
symptomatology, 153
Prader–Willi syndrome, 196
Prefrontal cortex, 279
Probabilistic tractography, 56
Proton magnetic resonance spectroscopy (^{1}H MRS)
echo time, 85–86
hardware, 85
localization and volume-of-interest, 85
principles, 83–84
quantification, 87
shimming, 86–87
spin-lattice and spin-spin relaxation time, 86
visible metabolites, neurobiological significance
choline, phosphocholine and glycerophosphocholine, 88
creatine and phosphocreatine, 88
glucose (Glc), 89
glutamate (Glu), 89
myo-inositol (mI), 88–89
N-acetyl-aspartate (NAA), 88
water suppression, 86–87
Proximal inversion with control for off-resonance effects (PICORE), 75
Pseudoatrophy, 184
Psychostimulants
acute drug effects, 164–165
between-person factors
age, 169, 170
alcohol consumption, 170
dopamine release, 169
dopamine response, 170–171
drug dependence, 168
family history, 168–170
gender drug abusers, 168, 169
populations and study drugs, 169
temperament/personality, 169–171
vulnerability, 171–173
chronic drug effects, 165–166
craving, 166

methodology
ethics, research, 164
neuroimaging studies, 163–164
sample heterogeneity and size, 164
overarching models, 171
public health impact, 163
real-time fMRI technology, 173
relapse, 167–168
treatment options, 173
withdrawal, 166–167

Q
Quantified tractography, 349
Quantitative imaging of perfusion using a single subtraction (QUIPSS), 77
Quantitative tractography, 57–58

R
Radioactive ligands, 119
Radiological imaging
autoradiographic method, 5
CT imaging, 4
MRS, 5
Receptor for advanced glycation endproducts (RAGE), 218
Region of interest (ROI) approach, 56–57
Resting-state connectivity, 318
Retrospective image correction (RETROICOR), 105
Rostral ACC (rACC), 284

S
Scopolamine, 151
Shimming process, 86–87
Single photon emission computed tomography (SPECT)
acute ischemic stroke, 304
AD, 318
cerebral perfusion, 233
CFS fatigue, 375–376
multiple sclerosis, 360
nAChR, in vivo imaging, 148
neurotransmitter PET, 321
nicotine dependence research, 118, 120
Parkinson's disease, 377
radiological imaging, 5
SPECT. *See* Single photon emission computed tomography
Susceptibility weighted imaging (SWI), 361

T
Tract-based spatial statistics (TBSS), 58
Transcranial Doppler imaging, 234
Two factor dopamine model, 171

V

Variable number of tandem repeats (VNTR)
  polymorphism, 142
Vascular cognitive impairment (VCI)
  AD, 216
  blood-brain barrier dysfunction, 217–218
  capillaries and cerebral arterioles disruption, 219
  microvascular disease, 217
  pathophysiology, 217
  VaD, 216, 217
Vascular dementia (VaD), 216–217, 322
Vascular psychophysiology, 4
Velocity selective arterial spin labeling (VSASL), 348–349
Velocity sensitive ASL (VSASL), 76–77
Voxel-based morphometry (VBM), 57, 194
VSASL. *See* Velocity selective arterial spin labeling

W

White matter hyperintensity (WMHI) volumes, 208
White matter lesions (WMLs), 205, 208
White matter pathology, 357